Essential
Primary Care

BMA

This book is dedicated to

Mina, Robbie and Laura Blythe
Walter, Sam, Isobel and Rufus Buchan

With our love

Andrew Blythe and Jessica Buchan

Essential Primary Care

Edited by

Andrew Blythe
General Practitioner at Gaywood House Surgery, Bristol;
Director of Assessments and Feedback for the MB ChB Programme,
Faculty of Health Sciences, University of Bristol

Jessica Buchan
General Practitioner;
Teaching Fellow, University of Bristol

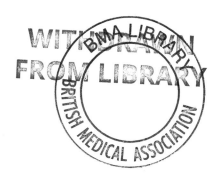

WILEY Blackwell

This edition first published 2017 © 2017 by John Wiley & Sons, Ltd

Registered Office
John Wiley & Sons, Ltd, The Atrium, Southern Gate, Chichester, West Sussex,
PO19 8SQ, UK

Editorial Offices
9600 Garsington Road, Oxford, OX4 2DQ, UK
The Atrium, Southern Gate, Chichester, West Sussex, PO19 8SQ, UK
111 River Street, Hoboken, NJ 07030-5774, USA

For details of our global editorial offices, for customer services and for information about how to
apply for permission to reuse the copyright material in this book please see our website at
www.wiley.com/wiley-blackwell

The right of Andrew Blythe and Jessica Buchan to be identified as the authors of this work has been
asserted in accordance with the UK Copyright, Designs and Patents Act 1988.

Library of Congress Cataloging-in-Publication Data

Essential primary care / edited by Andrew Blythe, Jessica Buchan.
     p. ; cm.
     Includes bibliographical references and index.
     ISBN 978-1-118-86761-7 (pbk.)
I. Blythe, Andrew, 1965–, editor.   II. Buchan, Jessica, editor.
     [DNLM: 1. Primary Health Care–Great Britain. W 84.6 FA1]
     RA440
     362.1071422′6–dc23

                                                    2015033626

A catalogue record for this book is available from the British Library.

Wiley also publishes its books in a variety of electronic formats. Some content that appears in print
may not be available in electronic books.

Cover image: http://www.gettyimages.co.uk/detail/photo/senior-health-care-house-call-royalty-free-
image/157649298

Set in 10/12pt Adobe Garamond by SPi Global, Pondicherry, India
Printed and bound in Singapore by Markono Print Media Pte Ltd

1   2017

Contents

Middle and old age

Contributors

All of the contributors are practising GPs and are members of the Centre for Academic Primary Care at the University of Bristol.

Andrew Blythe
Senior Teaching Fellow

Jessica Buchan
Teaching Fellow in Primary Care

Polly Duncan
Academic Clinical Fellow

Gene Feder
Professor of Primary Care

Alastair Hay
Professor of Primary Care

Sarah Jahfar
Teaching Fellow in Primary Care

Lucy Jenkins
Teaching Fellow in Primary Care

David Kessler
Reader in Primary Care Mental Health

Barbara Laue
Senior Teaching Fellow in Primary Care

Matthew Ridd
Consultant Senior Lecturer in Primary Care

Trevor Thompson
Reader in Healthcare Education

Simon Thornton
Academic Clinical Fellow

Foreword

For many medical students, the first place they will encounter patients will be in general practice. Later in their course, they will have extended attachments to practices and will have the chance to consult with patients themselves. The experience can be exciting and interesting, but also a bit overwhelming. Patients come to the GP to talk about anything and everything. They present with physical, psychological or social problems, and sometimes all three types of problem at once. They do not turn up and describe a neatly packaged problem, but often have a jumble of symptoms which don't obviously correspond to any of the anatomical or physiological systems. How can a medical student know where to start when faced with such a wide range of potential problems?

This book is designed to help medical students and doctors in training for a career in general practice by providing an essential guide. If you know what the patient is likely to be coming to discuss, reading about the topic beforehand can help you feel prepared. But one of challenges of general practice is that you rarely know in advance what problem you are going to be faced with. If you read the relevant section of this book after seeing a patient, it will help you to make sense of what you have just encountered. Many students find that it's much easier to remember about a medical condition if they read about it soon after experiencing a real case.

All of the chapters in this book have been written by colleagues from the Centre for Academic Primary Care involved in teaching medical students at the University of Bristol. The content and the approach reflect their many years of teaching medical students at all stages of the curriculum. The content is practical and pitched at an appropriate level, but is also evidence-based.

General practice is the first point of contact with the health service for most people when they become ill. It accounts for the vast majority of patient–doctor contacts, with about a million consultations in general practice every working day in England. GPs are trusted more than any other group of professionals. General practice is also the most common career destination for medical students, so it's important that they have every opportunity to make the most of their attachments in primary care.

My hope is that this book will inspire students and doctors in training to gain a better understanding of the variety, challenge, responsibility and enjoyment of working in general practice.

Chris Salisbury
Professor of Primary Health Care
Head, Centre for Academic Primary Care
University of Bristol

Preface

This book is written primarily for medical students. It grew from the teaching of primary care that we give to our students at the University of Bristol, from their first year through to their final year of study. All the authors are GPs who work within the Centre of Academic Primary Care at the University of Bristol. We hope this is a book which students will want to refer to throughout their time at medical school and in their foundation years. For those who choose to enter general practice as a career, it should be helpful during their time as a GP registrar.

Studying primary care can seem daunting because it encompasses the entire breadth of medicine: from birth to death, from minor to life-threatening illness. It considers the social, physical and psychological aspects of health and disease. So, where should you start? The purpose of this book is to provide a basic grounding, giving a realistic perspective of what is common, without focussing on detail at the expense of missing the big picture. It is designed to provide practical advice on how to consult with patients, make sense of their symptoms, explain things to them and manage their problems.

We have tried to make the chapters enjoyable and easy to read. They contain case studies which reflect the variety of primary care and top tips for consulting with patients. In the case studies, we present the reader with questions about what to do next and then offer advice. The online version of this book also contains an extensive range of self-test questions (best-of-five questions, extended-matching questions, true/false questions and scenarios for objective structured clinical examinations) which should help to consolidate the reader's learning and prepare them for their undergraduate exams, including finals.

The book has five parts. Part 1 covers the building blocks of primary care: its structure and its connection with secondary care, the consultation, the process of making a diagnosis, prescribing and ethical issues. Part 2 deals with some key topics in health promotion. Part 3 deals with patients' problems in roughly chronological life order. Part 4 is on cancer and Part 5 discusses death and palliative care.

You don't have to read all the chapters in order. You should be able to dip into sections at any stage of your learning. For example, if you are going on a GP attachment and have not yet studied child health, the chapters in this book should be enough to get you started and help you to get the most out of your attachment. Rereading these chapters should provide you with a solid foundation for your revision. Each chapter has a list of references which, if you want to pursue a topic in greater depth, should be a good place to start.

Writing any book is a major undertaking, and this one was no exception. In addition to all our co-authors, we are particularly grateful to Barbara Laue for helping with the final reading. Most of all, we are very grateful to our families for all the support and time they have given throughout the long gestation. This book is dedicated to them.

Andrew Blythe and Jessica Buchan
Bristol

How to use your textbook

Features contained within your textbook

Every chapter begins with a list of **Key topics** and of the chapter's **Learning objectives**.

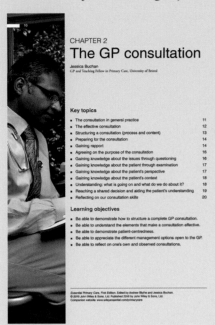

CHAPTER 2
The GP consultation

Jessica Buchan
GP and Teaching Fellow in Primary Care, University of Bristol

Key topics

- The consultation in general practice — 11
- The effective consultation — 12
- Structuring a consultation (process and content) — 13
- Preparing for the consultation — 14
- Gaining rapport — 14
- Agreeing on the purpose of the consultation — 16
- Gaining knowledge about the issues through questioning — 16
- Gaining knowledge about the patient through examination — 17
- Gaining knowledge about the patient's perspective — 17
- Gaining knowledge about the patient's context — 18
- Understanding: what is going on and what do we do about it? — 18
- Reaching a shared decision and aiding the patient's understanding — 19
- Reflecting on our consultation skills — 20

Learning objectives

- Be able to demonstrate how to structure a complete GP consultation.
- Be able to understand the elements that make a consultation effective.
- Be able to demonstrate patient-centredness.
- Be able to appreciate the different management options open to the GP.
- Be able to reflect on one's own and observed consultations.

Essential Primary Care, First Edition. Edited by Andrew Blythe and Jessica Buchan.
© 2016 John Wiley & Sons, Ltd. Published 2016 by John Wiley & Sons, Ltd.
Companion website: www.wileyessential.com/primarycare

CHAPTER 1
The structure and organisation of primary care

Andrew Blythe
General Practitioner at Gaywood House Surgery, Bristol; Director of Assessments and Feedback for the MB ChB Programme, Faculty of Health Sciences, University of Bristol

Key topics

- What is primary care? — 4
- Organisation of primary care in the UK — 5
- What can be done in primary care? — 8

Learning objectives

- Understand the benefits of a health service that is based on primary care.
- Understand the scope and limitations of primary care in the UK.
- Appreciate how primary care is evolving in the UK.

Essential Primary Care, First Edition. Edited by Andrew Blythe and Jessica Buchan.
© 2016 John Wiley & Sons, Ltd. Published 2016 by John Wiley & Sons, Ltd.
Companion website: www.wileyessential.com/primarycare

Key topics give a summary of the topics covered in the chapter.

Learning objectives describe the main learning points in the chapter.

Top tips: prescribing antidepressants

- SSRIs are the first choice among the antidepressants.
- Patients should always be advised that it is likely to be a few weeks before they feel any benefit from the drugs.
- Patients should be advised that they may experience adverse effects: gastrointestinal upset, temporary increase in anxiety and sexual dysfunction are all common.
- The patient should be reviewed after 2 weeks. If there is improvement, this interval can be increased, although ongoing support is an important part of GP care.
- It is recommended that drug treatment is continued for at least 6 months, if effective.
- These drugs should not be stopped suddenly, but over a period of about 4 weeks; otherwise, a discontinuation syndrome (commonly, dizziness, headache, nausea and lethargy) can occur.

Top tips highlight key information to be aware of.

Case study 4.1

Josephine Jenkins is a 79-year-old widow who was discharged from hospital 10 days ago. Her daughter phones the GP to request a home visit because she is becoming breathless and seems to be having difficulty getting around the house. Mrs Jenkins lives by herself in a house with one toilet at the top of the stairs. She has suffered from COPD for the last 10 years. She is on treatment for hypertension, had a myocardial infarction 5 years ago and has osteoarthritis of her hips. She uses a stick to walk and is able to get up and down the stairs because there is a hand rail on both sides.

Mrs Jenkins' discharge letter states that while she was in hospital, she was treated for an infective exacerbation of her COPD with a course of antibiotics and steroids. She had an echocardiogram, which showed mild to moderate left ventricular failure. During her admission, her amlodipine was stopped and she was started on furosemide. She was discharged with a month's supply of the following medication:

- Aspirin dispersible tablets 75 mg daily.
- Ramipril capsules 5 mg daily.
- Simvastatin tablets 40 mg at night.
- Seretide Accuhaler 500 (fluticasone proprionate 500 μg/ salmeterol 50 μg) one puff twice a day.
- Tiotropium bromide inhaler 18 μg daily.
- Salbutamol inhaler 100 μg per inhalation, two puffs when needed.
- Paracetamol 500 mg tablets, two tablets four times a day.
- Codeine phosphate tablets 30 mg, two tablets a day if needed.
- Furosemide tablets 40 mg daily (at 8 am).

What aspects of Mrs Jenkins' medication should the GP review during the home visit?

The GP should find out what medicines she is actually taking. On returning home, she may have reverted to taking her usual list of tablets, which doesn't include furosemide. It appears that she has been diagnosed with left ventricular failure; this accounts for some of her breathlessness. The furosemide has been prescribed to treat this and to help her breathlessness. Another possibility is that she has stopped the furosemide intentionally because it makes her go to the toilet often, which she finds difficult because it means going up and down the stairs frequently. She may not understand what the furosemide is for.

The GP should check her inhaler technique. Her breathlessness may be partly due to an inability to use the salbutamol inhaler. She might find it easier to use a spacer device with the inhaler.

Her worsening mobility may be because of the pain in her hips. The GP needs to check how often she is taking the paracetamol. Is she taking it four times a day? She has been prescribed codeine to take as top-up pain relief. This may be making her constipated. If so, she will need some sort of laxative. Fear of becoming constipated may be preventing her from taking the codeine.

Excluding the codeine, she is meant to take a total of 12 tablets/capsules a day. She might find it easier to remember to take all of these if they were put in a cassette with compartments for each day of the week.

Case studies give further insight into real-life patient scenarios.

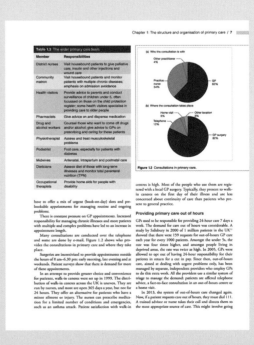

Chapter 1: The structure and organisation of primary care / 7

Table 1.3 The wider primary care team

Member	Responsibilities
District nurses	Visit housebound patients to give palliative care, insulin and other injections and wound care
Community matron	Visit housebound patients and monitor patients with multiple chronic diseases; emphasis on admission avoidance
Health visitors	Provide advice to parents and conduct surveillance of children under 5, often focussed on those on the child protection register; some health visitors specialise in providing care to older people
Pharmacists	Give advice on and dispense medication
Drug and alcohol workers	Counsel those who want to come off drugs and/or alcohol; give advice to GPs on prescribing and caring for these patients
Physiotherapist	Assess and treat musculoskeletal problems
Podiatrist	Foot care, especially for patients with diabetes
Midwives	Antenatal, intrapartum and postnatal care
Dieticians	Assess diet of those with long-term illnesses and monitor total parenteral nutrition (TPN)
Occupational therapists	Provide home aids for people with disability

Figure 1.2 Consultations in primary care.

Your textbook is full of **illustrations and tables**.

The **website icon** indicates that you can find accompanying self-assessment resources on the book's companion website.

About the companion website

Don't forget to visit the companion website for this book:

 www.wileyessential.com/primarycare

There you will find valuable material designed to enhance your learning, including:

- Cases
- EMQs
- MCQs
- OSCE checklists
- PowerPoint slides of all the figures from the book, for you to download.

Scan this QR code to visit the companion website:

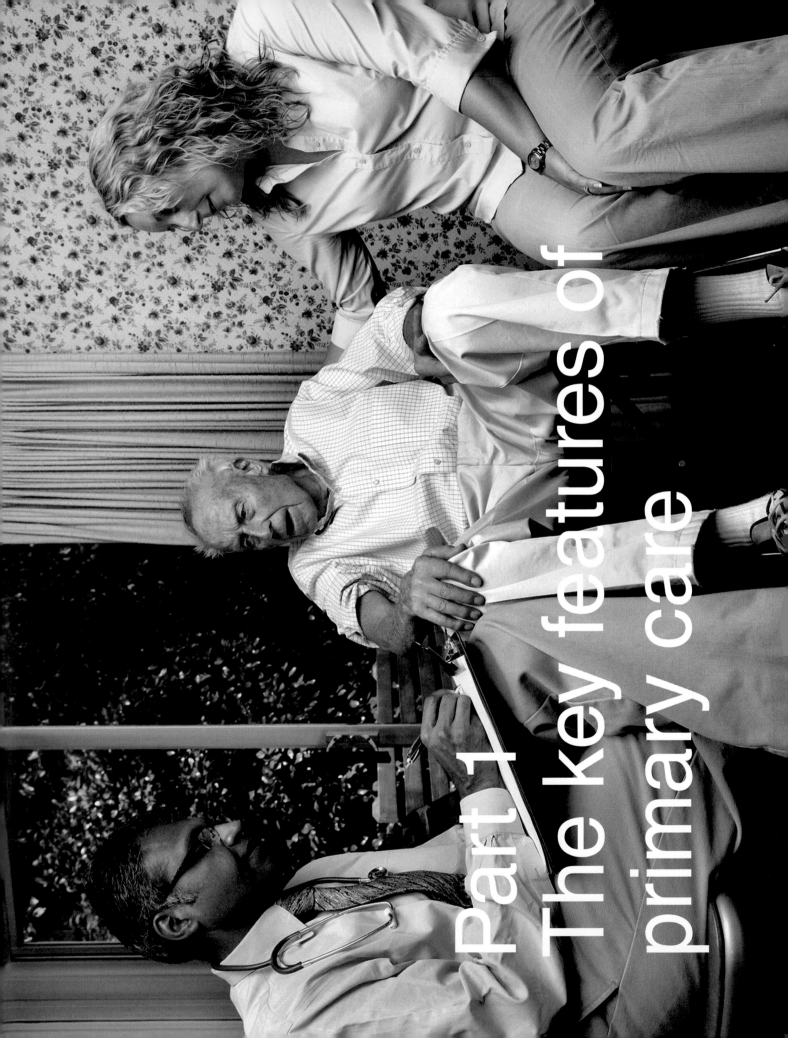

Part 1
The key features of primary care

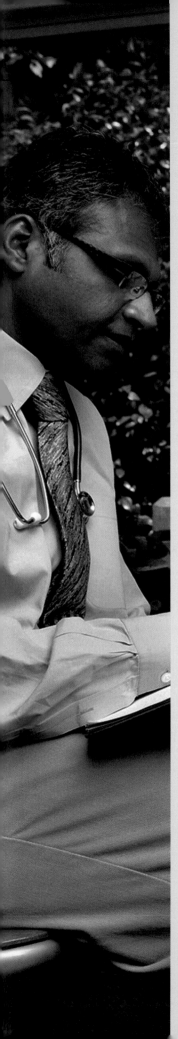

CHAPTER 1
The structure and organisation of primary care

Andrew Blythe
GP and Senior Teaching Fellow, University of Bristol

Key topics

Learning objectives

- Understand the benefits of a health service that is based on primary care.
- Understand the scope and limitations of primary care in the UK.
- Appreciate how primary care is evolving in the UK.

Essential Primary Care, First Edition. Edited by Andrew Blythe and Jessica Buchan.
© 2017 John Wiley & Sons, Ltd. Published 2017 by John Wiley & Sons, Ltd.
Companion website: www.wileyessential.com/primarycare

What is primary care?

Primary care is first-contact care provided by health care professionals to local populations. Primary care attempts to manage the health needs of individuals within these defined populations in a coordinated, comprehensive and continuous fashion from birth until death. Because patients present with unsorted problems, primary care health care professionals must be generalists who have an expert understanding of the causes of health and illness throughout a person's life.

In many countries primary care provides the foundation upon which the rest of the country's health system is built. This is certainly true in the UK. Everyone in the UK is entitled to register with a local general medical practitioner (GP). Once registered, the person is entitled to consult with a GP or nurse in the practice to which that GP belongs as often as they like. Most of the time, the GP is able to manage the patient's problem within the primary care team. Sometimes, the GP needs to refer the patient to the next tier of the health service – secondary care – for further investigation and treatment. In so doing, the GP acts as a 'gatekeeper' to the rest of the National Health Service (NHS), ensuring appropriate use of more expensive secondary care services, which are normally based in hospital.

The importance of primary care

The importance of having a strong primary care sector in every country was highlighted by the World Health Organization (WHO) in 1978 at an international conference at Alma-Ata, in what is now known as Uzbekistan.[1] The Alma-Ata declaration set out the aspiration of providing health for all by a primary care-led service. Here is its definition of primary care:

> Primary health care is essential health care based on practical, scientifically sound and socially acceptable methods and technology made universally accessible to individuals and families in the community through their full participation and at a cost that the community and country can afford to maintain at every stage of their development in the spirit of selfreliance and self-determination. It forms an integral part both of the country's health system, of which it is the central function and main focus, and of the overall social and economic development of the community. It is the first level of contact of individuals, the family and community with the national health system bringing health care as close as possible to where people live and work, and constitutes the first element of a continuing health care process.
>
> *Article VI, Alma-Ata Declaration, WHO, 1978*[1]

The aspirations of the Alma-Ata declaration have not yet been fully realised, but many countries are attempting to improve the health care that they offer their citizens by building a stronger base in primary care. China, for example, aims to train a further 300 000 GPs over the next 10 years, so that there will be 1 GP for every 3000–5000 people.[2]

The last 2 decades have seen the publication of a lot of evidence suggesting that countries which have a strong primary care sector have better health care outcomes. Professor Barbara Starfield, from the Johns Hopkins School of Public Health in the USA, published a seminal paper on this topic in 1994,[3] in which she ranked developed countries according to their health care outcomes and the strength of their primary care services. Countries which had the most developed primary care services had the best health care outcomes. The USA, which had the least developed primary care system at the time, had the worst health care outcomes. In the same paper, Professor Starfield showed that the countries which spent the least per capita on health care were the countries which had the most developed systems of primary care.

A more recent analysis of data from 31 European countries[4] has confirmed that health care outcomes are better in those countries which have a strong primary care base, as measured by the density of primary care providers and the quality of their environment. However, this analysis has not confirmed that these better outcomes are provided more cheaply. Today, countries in Europe which have well-developed primary care services tend to spend a larger proportion of their gross domestic product (GDP) on health than countries with less robust primary care services. According to the World Bank, in 1995 the UK spent 6.8% of its GDP on health; by 2012, it was spending 9.4%.[5]

Knowing the patient

> In hospitals the diseases stay and the people come and go; in general practice, the people stay and the diseases come and go.
>
> *Iona Heath, Past President of the Royal College of General Practitioners*[6]

One of the central features of primary care in the UK has been the relationship between the patient and 'their GP'. Patients are registered with a GP for years (the mean is 11 years), and in this time GPs often get to know their patients well. GPs' knowledge of their patients helps them with diagnosing and addressing the patients' worries. When a new diagnosis is made, patients want to know why and how it has happened to them. Knowledge of the patient makes it easier for the GP to provide this explanation and help the patient chose the best plan of action.

> In many instances knowing the person who has the disease is as important as knowing the disease that person had.
>
> *James McCormick*[7]

Case study 1.1 may help to explain why knowledge of the patient is so important in primary care.

Case study 1.1

Stephen Stockman is a 60-year-old widower who works on the railways. He is on treatment for high blood pressure. Recently, he saw the practice nurse for a blood pressure check; it was high, so the nurse told him to consult his GP. Last week he also went to see his optician for a routine eye check and was told that he might need referral to the Eye Hospital because the appearance of the back of his right eye indicated that he might have glaucoma. He hasn't noticed any change in his vision.

What finally prompts him to make an appointment with the doctor is neither of these things: it's the fact that he has a cough that has gone on for 3 weeks. He could have made an appointment to see one of the other doctors in the practice a bit sooner, but he decides to wait for the next available appointment with his usual GP, Dr Jones. When he comes to the GP, he starts out by mentioning the cough.

How does the GP's prior knowledge of this patient help to sort out these problems?
Dr Jones got to know Mr Stockman well when his wife was dying of lung cancer. Dr Jones made regular home visits to provide palliative care and issued the death certificate.

Afterwards, she had a few consultations with Mr Stockman to support him through his bereavement. The GP established a strong, trusting relationship with Mr Stockman.

Knowing that his wife died of lung cancer, Dr Jones suspects Mr Stockman is worried that his cough is the first sign of cancer, so she takes particular care to check out this possibility.

Dr Jones holds the entire set of medical records for Mr Stockman, dating back to childhood. Dr Jones knows when Mr Stockman was diagnosed with hypertension and has records of the medication he has tried so far and the tablets he had to stop because of side effects. Thus, Dr Jones is in the best position to decide what new or additional tablet Mr Stockman could try to control his blood pressure better.

Amongst the medical records are all the consultant letters from visits to hospital. One of the letters is from a consultant whom Mr Stockman saw at the Eye Hospital 6 years ago. In this letter, the consultant describes the same appearance of the right fundus that the optician is describing now. The consultant had ruled out glaucoma. Mr Stockman had forgotten this.

Organisation of primary care in the UK

The UK has a national network of GP practices. All GP practices operate as independent small businesses that are subcontracted by the NHS to provide primary care services to specified geographical areas. There are restrictions on the number of practices in a given area. In many parts of the country, particularly in urban areas, there are several practices with overlapping boundaries. Therefore, many patients have a choice about which practice they register with. Members of a given household tend to be registered with the same practice, but this is not always the case. About 98% of the UK population is registered with a GP.

The GP workforce

The number of full time-equivalent GPs in the UK has grown very slowly in recent years, but the way in which they have been organised has changed quite rapidly. The number of single-handed practices continues to fall, as practices merge and grow. All GPs used to work as partners, but a change to the GP contract in 2004 made it financially advantageous for partnerships to employ salaried doctors. Now, over a quarter of the GP workforce is salaried. The average number of patients registered per full time-equivalent GP is about 1500, but this is considerably smaller in rural areas, where the population is much more sparsely scattered. Other key statistics on general practice in England are presented in Table 1.1.

Table 1.1 Facts and figures on primary care workforce in NHS, England, 2014.

Number of full time-equivalent, fully-trained GPs	32 628 (23 763 GP partners + 8 865 salaried/locum GPs)
Number of full time-equivalent nurses in general practice	15 062
Number of full time-equivalent other staff working in general practice	73 334
Number of practices	7 875
Average number of patients registered at each practice	7 171
Number of GPs per 100 000 patients	66.5

Source: NHS Workforce: *Summary of staff in NHS: results from September 2014 census*. 25 March 2015. www.hscic.gov.uk.

Before they can start work as independent GPs in the UK, doctors must complete 3 years of further training following the 2 year foundation programme. They must also pass the membership exam of the Royal College of General Practitioners (MRCGP). The Royal College of General Practitioners would like training for GPs to be extended to 4 years, and the

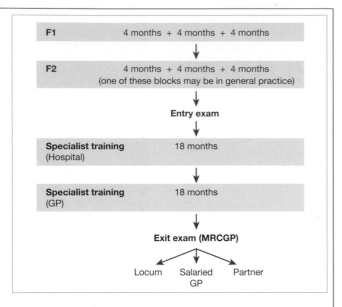

Figure 1.1 Training pathway for GPs in UK.

Table 1.2 The practice team.

Member	Responsibilities
Practice nurse	Wound management, vaccinations, minor illness clinics, chronic disease clinics, cervical smears, contraceptive services
Health care assistant	Phlebotomy, weight-loss clinics, smoking-cessation clinics, health checks
Receptionist	Booking appointments, processing requests for repeat prescriptions
Secretary	Typing referral letters and reports, booking hospital appointments, chasing results, reports and appointments at hospital
Data clerk	Summarising notes, coding information in letters and discharge summaries
Prescribing advisor	Conducting audits, reviewing quality and cost-effectiveness of prescribing
Practice manager	Managing the team (human resources), managing practice accounts and contracts

Department of Health says it shares this aim. At present, the funds that would be needed to make this happen have not been identified. Figure 1.1 shows the current training pathway for GPs in the UK.

The practice primary care team

GPs employ many people in order to provide comprehensive care, including practice nurses, health care assistants, receptionists, secretaries, data clerks and practice managers. Their roles are summarised in Table 1.2.

Practice nurses

The role of the practice nurse expanded significantly when practices took on responsibility for a large part of chronic disease management. In most practices, it is the practice nurses who run the asthma, chronic obstructive pulmonary disease (COPD), hypertension and diabetes clinics, with support and advice from a GP.

Increased workload, resource constraints and changes to legislation have led to a blurring of boundaries between roles. Much work previously done by GPs has been taken up by nurses, and nurse tasks are being carried out by health care assistants (HCAs) and phlebotomists

Some practice nurses have had extended training and are able to write prescriptions and work as nurse practitioners; these nurses can run minor illness clinics and assist with running urgent surgeries.

An increasing volume of work in primary care is being undertaken by practice nurses; in 2008–09, practice nurses were doing 34% of all consultations. There is evidence to support this expansion of the nurse role: practice nurses are effective in giving lifestyle advice;[8] they have been shown to be instrumental in improving outcomes in chronic diseases such as diabetes;[9] and patient satisfaction with nurse consultations is high.[10]

Consultations with practice nurses are longer, which increases patient satisfaction but counterbalances the lower salary costs. As yet, there is no evidence that substituting GPs with nurses is cost-effective. GPs run shorter appointments, deal with several problems in a single consultation and have expertise in managing undifferentiated symptoms.

Attached to each practice or group of practices is a team of district nurses. Sometimes these nurses have a base in the same building as the GPs; sometimes they are located elsewhere. Patients can be referred to a district nurse by a GP or can refer themselves directly. District nurses provide medical care to patients who are housebound. Patients may be housebound temporarily, such as after a major operation, or they may be permanently confined to their houses, as the result of a disability or terminal illness. The district nursing service is under considerable pressure and is constantly exploring new ways of working. Most district nursing teams have a skill mix from the most highly trained and experienced community matrons to workers with less training, such as HCAs and phlebotomists.

A number of other professionals work in the community with the primary care team, but are usually based and employed outside the GP practice; these are listed in Table 1.3.

The demand for consultations

In England, about 340 million consultations take place in primary care every year; that's about five to six consultations per patient per year. Consultation rates are much higher for young children and the elderly. Women consult more often than men.

All practices have to provide appointments between 8 am and 6.30 pm Monday to Friday. During these hours, practices

Table 1.3 The wider primary care team.

Member	Responsibilities
District nurses	Visit housebound patients to give palliative care, insulin and other injections and wound care
Community matron	Visit housebound patients and monitor patients with multiple chronic diseases; emphasis on admission avoidance
Health visitors	Provide advice to parents and conduct surveillance of children under 5, often focussed on those on the child protection register; some health visitors specialise in providing care to older people
Pharmacists	Give advice on and dispense medication
Drug and alcohol workers	Counsel those who want to come off drugs and/or alcohol; give advice to GPs on prescribing and caring for these patients
Physiotherapist	Assess and treat musculoskeletal problems
Podiatrist	Foot care, especially for patients with diabetes
Midwives	Antenatal, intrapartum and postnatal care
Dieticians	Assess diet of those with long-term illnesses and monitor total parenteral nutrition (TPN)
Occupational therapists	Provide home aids for people with disability

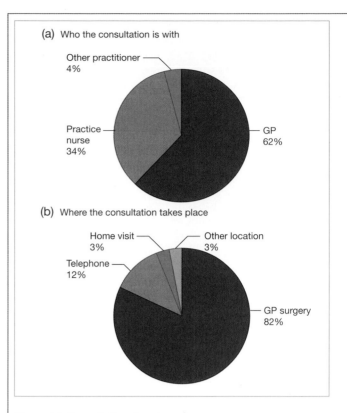

Figure 1.2 Consultations in primary care.

have to offer a mix of urgent (book-on-day) slots and pre-bookable appointments for managing routine and ongoing problems.

There is constant pressure on GP appointments. Increased responsibility for managing chronic illnesses and more patients with multiple and complex problems have led to an increase in appointment length.

Many consultations are conducted over the telephone and some are done by e-mail. Figure 1.2 shows who provides the consultations in primary care and where they take place.

Surgeries are incentivised to provide appointments outside the hours of 8 am–6.30 pm: early morning, late evening and at weekends. Patient surveys show that there is demand for more of these appointments.

In an attempt to provide greater choice and convenience for patients, walk-in centres were set up in 1999. The distribution of walk-in centres across the UK is uneven. They are run by nurses, and most are open 365 days a year, but not for 24 hours. They offer an alternative for patients who have a minor ailment or injury. The nurses can prescribe medication for a limited number of conditions and emergencies, such as an asthma attack. Patient satisfaction with walk-in

centres is high. Most of the people who use them are registered with a local GP surgery. Typically, they present to walk-in centres on the first day of their illness and are less concerned about continuity of care than patients who present to general practice.

Providing primary care out of hours

GPs used to be responsible for providing 24-hour care 7 days a week. The demand for care out of hours was considerable. A study by Salisbury in 2000 of 1 million patients in the UK[11] showed that there were 159 requests for out-of-hours GP care each year for every 1000 patients. Amongst the under 5s, the rate was four times higher, and amongst people living in deprived areas, the rate was twice as high. In 2005, GPs were allowed to opt out of having 24-hour responsibility for their patients in return for a cut in pay. Since then, out-of-hours care, aimed at dealing with urgent problems only, has been managed by separate, independent providers who employ GPs to do this extra work. All the providers use a similar system of triage to manage the demand: patients are offered telephone advice, a face-to-face consultation in an out-of-hours centre or a home visit.

In 2013, the system of out-of-hours care changed again. Now, if a patient requests care out of hours, they must dial 111. A trained advisor or nurse takes their call and directs them to the most appropriate source of care. This might involve going to a pharmacist, going to accident and emergency or consulting with the out-of-hours GP provider.

The repeated changes to the provision of out-of-hours services and the introduction of walk-in centres has created confusion for patients. Out-of-hours care used to be reserved for urgent problems that could not wait until the GP surgery opened again. It is unclear if this is still the case. Should the NHS provide routine primary care round the clock? A similar question is being asked of secondary care.

What can be done in primary care?

Primary care in the UK has many resources at its disposal.

GPs can prescribe almost anything that is listed in the British National Formulary (BNF); 90% of all prescriptions are issued in primary care. GPs have a notional budget for their prescribing and are under pressure to stick to this. Trained pharmacists work within the practice as prescribing advisors to ensure cost-effective prescribing.

GPs can refer patients to almost any hospital in the UK through a national booking system called Choose and Book.

GPs have the right to admit patients to their local district hospital, where their care is transferred to a consultant. Some GPs also have access to beds in community hospitals, where they can continue to look after their own patients.

Record-keeping

GPs are the guardians of the entire set of their patients' medical records. They are the only people who hold this record. When the NHS was created, it was decided that whenever someone is seen within the service, a report of that encounter should be sent to their GP. GPs used to keep all these reports in cardboard wallets together with their own paper records. Medical records are often fascinating historical documents, and tell a story of a patient's life. Now all the letters are scanned and stored electronically. All GP practices have computer systems to hold their patient records. Initially, these computer systems were set up to cope with the volume of repeat prescriptions, but soon they were used to hold disease registers and the notes written by GPs at each consultation. Every component of the patient record can be coded, which means the records can be searched easily. For instance, with a few clicks, any practice can tell you how many patients they have who are taking a particular medicine and how many have had their blood pressure checked in the last 6 months. This is a powerful tool for research. This information is also sought by insurance companies, who want to know what risk they are taking on when offering life insurance. Patients, of course, have to give their permission for this information to be disclosed and have the right to withhold it.

Legal powers

GPs have considerable legal powers. They have the right to issue death certificates (see Chapter 40) and can decide whether or not someone is fit to work. In the UK, someone who is ill or injured can sign themselves off work for the first 7 days by completing a self-certificate, obtained from their employer. If, after this time, they have not recovered sufficiently to return to work, they need to obtain a Statement of Fitness to Return to Work (Fit Note) from a doctor. GPs can use this note to make recommendations about the conditions that would enable their patient to return to work. Alternatively, they can indicate on the note that their patient is completely unfit to work. Overall, being in work is good for an individual's health. It is better for someone to work in a modified or reduced capacity than not to work at all. This is why, in 2010, the doctor's 'Sick Note' was redesigned and rebadged as a 'Fit Note'. GPs feel that the format of the Fit Note has helped them talk to patients about returning to work and has encouraged more of their patients to make a phased return to work.[12]

Once a patient has been unfit for work for more than 3 months, the GP's responsibility for certification ends and an agent of the Department of Work and Pensions assesses the patient to decide if they are entitled to long-term benefits.

Perhaps the greatest strength of GPs is their knowledge of health and illness. This enables them to anticipate future problems, to reassure patients who will get better, to prepare those who may get worse and to identify those who may have a serious disease. GPs might not be able to offer a cure or treatment, but they can always help patients make sense of their problems and offer comfort.

SUMMARY

Primary care describes the health care which patients can obtain directly without having to be referred by someone else. Primary care health workers have to deal with undifferentiated problems in patients of any age. The health care system in the UK has a strong primary care base and a large workforce of primary care physicians (general practitioners). One in four doctors in the UK are GPs.

GPs work in group practices alongside many other types of health care worker. They provide a local service and offer continuity of care. The majority of their consultations are done in GP premises, but they also visit patients who are housebound. In the UK, GPs have substantial resources and powers at their disposal. This means they are able to investigate and diagnose problems, manage patients with chronic disease and refer patients to specialists when necessary. Primary care services outside of normal working hours have been reorganised several times, and this has created considerable confusion for patients.

Now visit **www.wileyessential.com/primarycare** to test yourself on this chapter.

REFERENCES

1. Anonymous. Declaration of Alma-Ata. International Conference on Primary Health Care, Alma-Ata, USSR, 6–12 September 1978. Available from: http://www.who.int/publications/almaata_declaration_en.pdf (last accessed 6 October 2015).

2. Wang Y, Wilkinson M, Ng E, Cheng KK. Primary care reform in China. *Br J Gen Pract* 2012;**62**:546.

3. Starfield B. Is primary care essential? *Lancet* 1994;**334**:1129–33.

4. Kringos DS, Boerma W, van der Zee J, Groenewegen P. Europe's strong primary care systems are linked to better population health but also to higher health spending. *Health Affairs* 2013;**32**:686–94.

5. World Bank. Health expenditure, total (% of GDP). Available from: http://data.worldbank.org/indicator/SH.XPD.TOTL.ZS (last accessed 6 October 2015).

6. Heath I. Keeping the particular alive in general practice 2006. Available from: https://www.icgp.ie/assets/26/D2AF6FE9-DEFF-4524-9ABEADC5FB3B7AC4_document/Iona.pdf (last accessed 6 October 2015).

7. McCormick J. Death of the personal doctor. *Lancet* 1996;**348**:667–8.

8. Sargent GM, Forrest LE, Parker RM. Nurse delivered lifestyle interventions in primary health care to treat chronic disease risk factors associated with obesity: a systematic review. *Obes Rev* 2012;**13**(12):1148–71.

9. Clark CE, Smith LFP, Taylor RS, Campbell JL. Nurse-led interventions used to improve control of high blood pressure in people with diabetes: a systematic review and meta-analysis. *Diabet Med* 2011;**28**(3):250–61.

10. Laurant M, Reeves D, Hermens R, et al. Substitution of doctors by nurses in primary care. *Cochrane Database Syst Rev* 2005 Apr 18;(2):CD001271.

11. Salisbury C, Trivella M, Bruster S. Demand for and supply of out of hours care from general practitioners in England and Scotland: observational study based on routinely collected data. *BMJ* 2000;**320**:618–21.

12. Hann M, Sibbald B. General practitioners' attitudes towards patients' health and work, 2010–12. DWP Research Report 835. Available from: http://www.gov.uk/government/uploads/system/uploads/attachment_data/file/207514/rrep835.pdf (last accessed 6 October 2015).

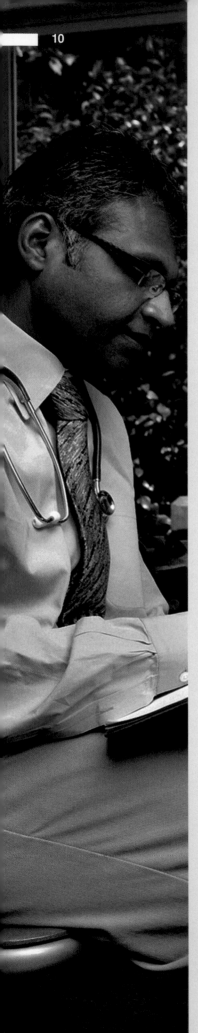

CHAPTER 2
The GP consultation

Jessica Buchan
GP and Teaching Fellow in Primary Care, University of Bristol

Key topics

Learning objectives

- Be able to demonstrate how to structure a complete GP consultation.
- Be able to understand the elements that make a consultation effective.
- Be able to demonstrate patient-centredness.
- Be able to appreciate the different management options open to the GP.
- Be able to reflect on one's own and observed consultations.

Essential Primary Care, First Edition. Edited by Andrew Blythe and Jessica Buchan.
© 2017 John Wiley & Sons, Ltd. Published 2017 by John Wiley & Sons, Ltd.
Companion website: www.wileyessential.com/primarycare

The consultation in general practice

Traditionally, doctors are taught how to take a comprehensive clinical history (see Box 2.1) in a structured way. This model is good for making a deductive diagnosis, but in general practice, patients don't always come for a diagnosis. They may come for a review of their medication, for support in managing a chronic illness or sick relative or for advice about preventing ill health. Sometimes, they might come in unprepared for bad news the GP needs to give them. The traditional clinical history-taking model doesn't really tell doctors how to approach these types of consultation.

Although making a diagnosis is a large and important part of any doctor's role, many consultations don't end with the diagnosis. Before patients leave the consultation room, they need an explanation of what is going on, what is going to happen next, and what they must do (e.g. how to take the medication they have been prescribed). Patients also need to know what to do if things don't go according to plan (e.g. there could be unexpected worsening of their symptoms or serious side effects from medication they have been prescribed). GPs need to answer patients' questions and decide on a timescale and a method for follow-up.

GPs generally have 10 minutes for each patient, and by the time the patient has got into the room, they may have only 8 or 9 minutes to consult in. GPs also have to fit a number of other tasks into the consultation:

- **Chronic disease management** (e.g. ongoing review of a patient with diabetes or heart failure).
- **Reviewing medication** (e.g. checking blood pressure control in a patient taking antihypertensive medication and reviewing adherence and side effects).
- **Health promotion** (e.g. organising screening tests, such as a cervical smear).
- **Prevention of ill health** (e.g. motivating a patient to stop smoking).

Consultations have to be focused; the GP has to learn to collect relevant information, rather than as much information as possible. In general practice, it helps that doctors may already know their patients and be able to put their symptoms in the context of their personality, habits and background. GPs usually have access to the patient's medical record: a comprehensive record of the patient's recent consultations, past medical history, correspondence (including results and hospital letters), current medication, past drug history and allergies.

Why are consultation skills important?

With all these tasks to achieve in 10 minutes, do we have time for communication skills? And how much do they matter? Communication skills in medical practice involve far more than just 'being nice' to the patient. The General Medical Council (GMC),[1] British Medical Association (BMA)[2] and Royal Colleges of General Practitioners (RCGP), Physicians (RCP) and Surgeons (RCS) all recognise that communication skills are essential to being a good and effective doctor. For revalidation, doctors have to produce evidence of patient satisfaction with their performance. All the Royal Colleges assess communication skills within their membership examinations. In the UK, communication skills are embedded in medical training through the GMC document, Tomorrow's Doctors.[1]

Good communication skills are important for the following reasons.

Listening can save time

The physician Sir William Osler (1849–1919) is credited with the aphorism, 'Listen to your patient, he is telling you the diagnosis'. We can learn all the 'right' questions to ask our patients, but are we really listening? We should also listen to what the patient is trying to say, not just the words that they use. To be effective, we need to use all our senses to consult, as often body language and facial expression speak volumes.

Box 2.1 Traditional clinical history-taking model

Imagine a patient comes to you saying, 'I've got a cough'.
The traditional way of taking a clinical history might follow this sequence:

- **Presenting complaint (PC):** Cough.
- **History of the presenting complaint (HPC):** Ask about the character of the cough, its duration and any associated symptoms (e.g. fever, sputum or weight loss).
- **Review of systems (ROS):** Systematically go through other systems and check no symptoms have been missed (e.g. asking about gastrointestinal symptoms may prompt the patient to tell you about his heartburn; this might be relevant to the presenting complaint, as acid reflux can cause a chronic cough).

- **Drug history (DH):** Is the cough a side effect of medication (e.g. from ACE inhibitors)? Is the patient on inhalers, indicating known asthma or chronic obstructive pulmonary disease (COPD)?
- **Past medical history (PMH):** Is there a known respiratory condition such as COPD or asthma, or a risk of lung disease such as prematurity with ventilation.
- **Family history (FH):** Consider alpha-1-antitrypsin deficiency with a family history of COPD in young relatives or nonsmokers.
- **Social history (SH):** Does the patient smoke? Is there a potential occupational or environmental cause for their cough (e.g. risk of occupational asthma or asbestosis)?

Poor consultation skills lead to misdiagnosis and errors in treatment

As much as 28% of medical error is diagnostic, of which half is potentially serious.[3] Closed questioning and running through a huge list of questions without really hearing the patient's story can lead to a narrow and inaccurate differential diagnosis. Hurrying patients by putting words in their mouths leads to the doctor making assumptions. If patients do not understand their doctor's medical jargon, they may unintentionally mislead and say what they think the doctor wants to hear.

Teamwork relies on good communication

For patient safety, we also have to communicate well with our colleagues. Being a good doctor means being able to work in teams, whatever area of medicine we practice in.

Good communication about treatment improves concordance

Patients whose doctors fail to elicit their ideas and expectations of their illness and treatment are less likely to understand their illness, adhere to medication or feel satisfied with the consultation.[2,3] A patient may not adhere to their blood pressure medication because they didn't realise they were supposed to keep taking the tablets. Perhaps they were 'told', but they didn't 'hear' the doctor, who mumbled and was facing their computer screen.

Good communication reduces patient dissatisfaction and complaints

Patients react badly when talked down to, intimidated, bullied or not listened to – just as we would in their position.

The effective consultation

It is more important to know what sort of person has a disease than to know what sort of disease a person has.
Hippocrates (c. 400 BC)

There is no 'right way' to consult. But good, effective consultations share some attributes:

- **Preparation**: The doctor sees the right person, ideally at the right time, and has the necessary information to hand. The doctor should also be mentally prepared to focus on the patient.
- **Rapport**: The doctor gets on with their patients; this results in more satisfied patients and a doctor who is less frustrated and more satisfied by their work.[4] To enable communication, the patient needs to feel that the doctor is listening, and to feel comfortable telling the doctor what may be difficult and sensitive information. For patients in need of counselling, feeling understood and supported by their doctor can also be an end in itself. In the 1950s and 60s, the psychoanalyst Michael Balint, who worked with GPs, described the therapeutic role of the doctor and introduced the concept of the 'doctor as the drug'.[5]

Case study 2.1a

Betty Bright is 62. She sees a new GP at the practice, Dr Ben Meecham. Dr Meecham introduces himself and asks Betty to take a seat. He asks why she has come to see him today.

Betty replies: 'Well, I think I'm probably just upset, I had the cat put down last week. She was old, but, you know, it still gets you. So I've not been sleeping and this cough isn't helping, I'm worn out and wondered if I needed something? My neighbour said I ought to come because it could be an infection. Oh, and I keep meaning to tell you about my knee.'

Why do you think Betty has come to the doctor today?
A few reasons for Betty's attendance may be going through Dr Meecham's mind: Is she experiencing grief from the death of her pet? Is she depressed? Lonely? Has she got a chest infection? Is this a presentation of insomnia? Tiredness? And what about her knee? Is the knee painful? Is it affecting her mobility?

Dr Meecham may be tempted to choose a problem to focus on. However, this could result in Betty saying,

'But what about my knee? That's what I *really* came about,' after 8 minutes spent dealing with her cough. This could turn into an ineffective consultation, with a frustrated doctor, unsure whether to run over time, who may blame the patient for having unrealistic expectations, and a patient who leaves feeling rushed, not listened to, and let down because her problems weren't properly addressed.

Outcome
Dr Meecham is aware that he needs to spend more time with Betty agreeing on an agenda for the consultation (see Case study 2.1b). Patients don't have presenting complaints: they have stories, and often experience a number of different symptoms. Their symptoms impact on their life, and the meaning they give their symptoms, and how they act upon them, depends on factors such as their experience, knowledge and belief and the opinions of those around them. Understanding this helps us consult effectively and reduces frustration for ourselves and our patients.

Box 2.2 How to elicit ideas, concerns and expectations

- You may find out the patient's perspective on their problem simply through allowing their story to unfold, asking open questions and clarifying points you don't fully understand. Attentive listening and curiosity help the patient open up and help you hear the clues the patient is giving you about their beliefs, worries and wishes.
- You can also explicitly probe for the patient's perspective by asking questions like: 'How did that make you feel?', 'What did that mean to you?', 'What did that make you think?', 'What went through your mind?', or even 'What ideas have you had about what's going on?' and 'What's been worrying you about the headaches?'
- Be careful about asking what the patient is expecting from you, as it can sound rude. It can be better to say: 'When you thought about coming here today, what did you hope for?' or 'What would you like to do about blood pressure pills?'
- You can reflect back either on something the patient has said or something you notice: 'Upset…?', 'You look worried when you talk about your daughter', 'I get the sense that you're worried?', 'Sounds like you were concerned about feeling your heart beating?'
- You can use empathic statements to put yourself in the patient's shoes: 'I can understand the hospital visit would have made you upset', 'I imagine you're wondering if you need an X-ray?' Patients are usually quick to correct you if you guess wrong, and in doing so often tell you what they did feel, or do expect.
- When it's hard for patients to admit they are worried, you can take the pressure off them by relating to hypothetical patients, or your experience of common concerns: 'I'd like to reassure you that this sort of rash isn't serious. In my experience, parents often worry when their child has a rash that it might mean something serious like meningitis. Is that something that had gone through your mind?' or 'Most people worry when they get chest pain that it's a problem with the heart. Is that what you were thinking?'
- Eliciting expectations can be tricky ahead of offering the patient options – they may not want to second-guess you. It can help to ask after you've offered some choices: 'We could meet again after you've spoken to your boss. I could refer you for counselling or give you something to read about stress. Is there anything else you were hoping for that I've not mentioned?'

- **Agree on the purpose of the consultation**: It is useful to spend time at the beginning of the consultation finding out the patient's reason for attendance. When the doctor and patient agree on the purpose of the consultation and the tasks that need to be achieved, there is less frustration and more satisfaction for both parties. We often talk about the patient's 'ideas, concerns and expectations' about their symptoms. These can also be used at any time during the consultation to check with the patient that the consultation is going to plan (see Box 2.2).
- **Knowledge**: Consultations go wrong when the doctor doesn't gain enough information about the patient. This includes gaining enough of the right medical information to make an accurate diagnosis, but also gaining knowledge about the patient's medical, social and psychological context. The knowledge required depends on the type of consultation and the situation. For example, it is never easy to give bad news to a patient, but understanding what that patient already knows, what they are expecting and what they have experienced so far can help. For a consultation to be effective, the doctor also needs up-to-date medical knowledge and the ability to apply it.
- **Understanding**: It is one thing for patients to tell us what they are experiencing, but quite another to really understand what they mean. When a patient tells us they have 'heartburn', do they mean a retro-sternal burning sensation after eating, with an acidic taste in the mouth, or are they actually describing the symptoms of angina? Patients may

not understand their doctors. Sometimes patients are full of praise for a doctor's manner or thoroughness but do not understand what is wrong with them or what is going to happen next. Sometimes patients bring a letter full of medical jargon for their GP to decipher. It is quite probable our patients forget what we say; it is hard to recall everything when you don't feel well or are in a strange environment such as a hospital. Doctors must give explanations and make plans with patients in a way that they will understand and be able to recall.

- **Being realistic**: Consultations have to be time-efficient for a doctor to be effective. There are other patients to see, and other urgent tasks to attend to. This is one of the reasons that structuring the consultation is important. Doctors need to be honest and realistic with their patients to be effective, and this includes being honest about the limits of their knowledge: knowing when to refer, to seek another's opinion or look something up.

Structuring a consultation (process and content)

All of these areas of the consultation are made effective by consultation skills; not just knowing *what* to cover (the **content**), but *how* to consult (the **process**).[6] We may remember to ask a patient with a cough about their smoking habit, but we need a different set of skills to persuade the patient to quit. It is the **process** of how doctors conduct consultations that helps them gain rapport with a patient, tell a patient bad news or encourage behaviour change. This is made more complex by the fact that all patients are different: no symptom exists in isolation. One patient with a cough will have entirely different ideas about its cause than another patient with almost identical symptoms. Different patients have different expectations of the consultation, depending on their beliefs, background, experiences and personality. There are similarities, too: patients tend to have similar desires, such as wanting to feel listened to and understood, wanting to understand what their symptoms mean and wanting relief from distress.

Consultation models

There is a lot of **content** a doctor can cover in each consultation, and they would be terribly ineffective if they tried to tackle it all. So, to know how to consult, a doctor needs to have an idea of how to structure their meetings with patients. A consultation model is a map of the consultation and helps provide this structure. Models describe what doctors need to *do* and *how* they can approach the consultation, and usually provide a logical sequence of events to follow. They help signpost where to go next, especially for trainees new to consulting. In an unfamiliar environment, we rely on maps to get us from A to B; with experience, we use the map less as we get to know our way around, and we experiment more comfortably by varying our route and speed as the situation demands. So it is with consultation models.

As with a map, we can turn to a consultation model to help us find our way when we get lost. When we learn to consult, we may be so busy gathering the information about the patient's problem that we forget what to do next. A model such as the Calgary Cambridge Guide[7] reminds us that after gathering information, we need to move to the next stage of explanation and planning with the patient. Models also give doctors a new way to think about the things that they already do. By embedding 'housekeeping' in a model, Neighbour[8] highlighted the importance of doctors attending to their own needs in order to get ready for the next patient.

Models are helpful in analysing and reflecting on consultations and developing skills. For example, a doctor might reflect that a patient didn't seem satisfied with an explanation they'd given them about a symptom. When they examine the steps of the consultation, they discover that they hadn't found out enough about the patient's perspective to tailor the explanation to their ideas, concerns or expectations.

All models have limitations, because they cannot be comprehensive enough to describe all the detail of real life (if they did, they wouldn't be models), and there is no 'one size fits all'. As Korzybski said, 'The map is not the territory'.[9] Models are useful as long as we are aware of their limitations and use them flexibly, adapting them to suit different situations. Table 2.1 outlines some well-known consultation models.

The next section looks at some of the specific skills in different areas of the consultation.

Preparing for the consultation

Consultations start before the patient enters the room, with the doctor preparing to see the patient:

- First, we need to prepare ourselves. Are we ready to concentrate on a new patient? Mistakes happen when we do not give a patient our full attention.
- First impressions count, so we must pay attention to our appearance and that of our room. We should clear up from the previous patient.
- We should reduce distractions. We might need a sip of water, to go to the toilet, to finish our notes from the previous patient, or to compose ourselves after a difficult consultation.
- Many doctors have rituals before they see a patient. These may be very subtle, and they may not even realise they engage in them – perhaps a stretch or a deep breath. Such rituals can help ground us, ready for a new consultation.
- We should check the information on the appointment screen: there may be a note next to the patient's name we need to be aware of, such as a visual or hearing impairment, or advice not to see the patient alone.
- We need to look at the notes from the last consultation and to think about why the patient might be coming. A patient will be unimpressed if they are returning for results and we haven't looked them up. Computerised note systems also remind us of other tasks that are due, such as taking the patient's blood pressure or reviewing medication.
- Recent correspondence and the medication list can be helpful. Is there any information from secondary care that we need to act on?
- Finally, we need to get our patient's name right. We should practise saying it out loud, or check with the patient if we're not sure.

Patients will have been doing preparations of their own. Before they see the doctor, they will have formed their own ideas about what is going on. They may have been worrying about the situation and might have sought the opinion of family, friends, colleagues and neighbours, or looked for advice online. Once they decided to make an appointment, they will also have formed expectations (or hopes) about what will happen. This is the patient's agenda. Sometimes patients hide serious issues from the doctor (intentionally or not) – the so-called **hidden agenda**. An example of this might be the patient who repeatedly attends with abdominal pain and headaches for which no cause can be found, but doesn't tell the doctor that they are experiencing domestic abuse (see Chapter 28).

Gaining rapport

Patients are often nervous about visiting the doctor. A warm, friendly start is important. In a seminal study of visits to a paediatric outpatient department in 1960s America, the doctor's lack of warmth and friendliness was strongly related to poor patient satisfaction and compliance.[10] We need to actively

Table 2.1 Consultation models.

Byrne and Long 1976[17] A GP and psychologist studied audiotapes of hundreds of GP consultations. Describes six stages to the consultation. Discusses considering the condition in conjunction with the patient. Sees illness as personal and unique to the patient.	1. The doctor establishes a relationship with the patient. 2. The doctor discovers (or attempts to) the reason why the patient attended. 3. The doctor takes a history, and possibly conducts an examination. 4. The doctor, in consultation with the patient, considers the condition. 5. The doctor and patient discuss treatment or further investigations. 6. The doctor brings the consultation to a close.
Stott and Davies 1979[18] Describes the potential of the GP consultation. Outlines four tasks that can be explored in any consultation.	1. Management of the patient's presenting problem. 2. Modification of help-seeking behaviours. 3. Management of continuing problems. 4. Opportunistic health promotion.
Pendleton 1984[19] David Pendleton was a psychologist who worked with a group of GPs. Identifies the patient's ***ideas, anxieties (concerns) and expectation (ICE)*** and the effects of the illness on the person as part of the patient's agenda.	1. Discover reason for attending: 　(a) nature and history of problem; 　(b) aetiology; 　(c) patient's ideas, anxieties, expectations; 　(d) effects of the problem. 2. Consider other problems (continuing problems/risk factors). 3. Choose an action for each problem. 4. Share understanding. 5. Involve patient in management, sharing appropriate responsibility. 6. Use time and resources appropriately. 7. Establish and maintain a positive relationship.
Neighbour 1986[8] Roger Neighbour (GP) described the GP consultation as five easy–to-remember tasks. Includes the health of the doctor.	1. Connecting with the patient and developing rapport and empathy. 2. 'Summarising' with the patient their reasons for attending: their feelings, concerns and expectations. 3. 'Handing over' or sharing with the patient an agreed management plan, which hands back control to the patient. 4. 'Safety-netting' or making contingency plans in case the clinician is wrong or something unexpected happens. 5. 'Housekeeping' or taking measures to ensure the clinician stays in good shape for the next patient.
Helman's folk model of illness 1981[20] Cecil Helman was a GP and medical anthropologist who suggested patients consult seeking the answers to six questions.	1. What has happened? 2. Why has it happened? 3. Why to me? 4. Why now? 5. What would happen if nothing were done about it? 6. What should I do about it?
Calgary Cambridge Guide 1996[21] A comprehensive patient-centred model, increasingly used to teach consultation skills to medical students. Includes skills such as building rapport and structuring the consultation while achieving tasks.	1. Initiate the session (establish rapport, identify reason(s) for consulting). 2. Gather information (explore problems: biomedical perspective, the patient's perspective). 3. Seek explanation (provide correct amount and type of information, aid accurate recall and understanding, achieve a shared understanding, incorporate the patient's perspective) and engage in planning (shared decision-making). 4. Close the session. **Throughout the consultation**: Build the relationship (develop rapport, involve patient) and provide structure to the consultation.

consider how we start our consultations and experiment to see what works for us (see Box 2.3). We should avoid traps such as asking a patient, 'What's brought you here today?', only to be told their neighbour drove them. Making assumptions about why patients are attending can also damage rapport.

In her book, *The Naked Consultation*,[11] Liz Moulton argues that any time we ask a patient a question, even a neutral one such as 'How are you today?', we risk crowding the patient's thoughts. Instead, we can gather a lot of information and help build rapport by letting the patient have space at the beginning

---

Box 2.3 Possible opening gambits

- 'Hello, I'm Dr White.'
- 'Mrs Green? Come in, have a seat.'
- 'What can I do for you today?'
- 'How can I help?'
- 'Thanks for waiting, I'm here for you now.'

Top tip: read the notes before you see the patient

A GP has just rushed late into surgery from a meeting. She switches on her computer and dives out to the waiting room to call in the first patient. Having never met this patient before, the GP makes friendly conversation as they enter the room. 'You've got a hoarse voice,' the doctor says. 'Have you got a cold?' If the GP had stopped to read the recent clinic notes and letters, she would have realised this patient has just been diagnosed with throat cancer. The patient, who has come for support and to talk through treatment options, loses faith in the GP and asks not to see her again.

Box 2.4 Active listening

We know when someone is really listening to us. They are likely to use the following skills:

- Giving their full attention to the speaker.
- Paying attention to their nonverbal communication: maintaining an open posture, nodding or smiling at appropriate points and making eye contact to show their focus is on the speaker.
- Using noises that facilitate social interaction (phatics), such as 'Uh-huh', 'Mmm' and 'I see', to encourage the speaker to continue.
- Checking understanding at appropriate points, without interrupting the speaker's flow, by clarifying questions or summarising.
- Picking up cues: 'Earlier you mentioned your father had something similar to what you are experiencing. Can you tell me more about that?'
- Reflecting on the speaker's nonverbal communication or the words they use with simple statements or questions: 'It's making you very upset.'
- Allowing silence when the speaker needs space to gather their thoughts and waiting with open attentiveness.

---

of a consultation so that they can control their story. This gives us a lot of information, as we listen not only to *what* they choose to say but also to *how* they say it. Other than a brief introduction, the doctor should be friendly but silent, and encourage the patient to speak with lots of nonverbal cues and active listening (see Box 2.4).

Agreeing on the purpose of the consultation

As we saw in Case study 2.1a, the primary reason a patient is attending may not be obvious; there can be multiple problems. Doctors may not identify the reason for a patient's attendance in up to 50% of consultations, and if asked separately after the consultation, doctors and patients disagree on the presenting problem in around 50% of cases.[12]

Consultations can be seen as a meeting between the patient and their doctor, with both parties having their own agendas. If the patient raises a lot of issues at the start, summarising these can help both the doctor and the patient prioritise what is most important. We need to stay flexible; rigidly sticking to an agenda can be counterproductive, especially if it is set too early. Patients do not always want to tell the GP everything at the start, and important interconnected problems or hidden agendas often require time to rise to the surface. We need to make space for these. When a patient tells us, 'I've got a sore throat', we must accept that while some patients just want an assessment and advice, others will have complex hidden issues, such as significant problem drinking. Remember that at any point, we can summarise and check progress with the patient. We might start by talking about a sore throat, but if a hidden agenda becomes apparent we have to reset the agenda and assess risk. Is this a problem we can make a plan to tackle another day, or something we need to deal with as a priority?

Gaining knowledge about the issues through questioning

Open and closed questions

How do we find out what we need to know about our patient's problems? When making diagnoses, the traditional clinical history-taking model is useful. For each symptom, there are a number of possible diagnoses, and we learn the questions needed to help us build up a better idea of which is more or less likely. In medical training, there is a lot of emphasis on learning the closed questions required for this deductive reasoning. For instance, when a patient presents with dysuria – pain on passing urine – we know this can be caused by a urine infection or by sexually transmitted infections such as chlamydia. We need to ask about other urinary symptoms, and also symptoms that are more associated with sexually transmitted infections and assess our patient's risk of sexually transmitted infections. We might ask questions like:

- 'Have you noticed a change to your urine? For example, is it smelly, cloudy or blood stained?'
- 'Are you passing urine more frequently?'

Case study 2.1b

Although Betty Bright's opening statement gave a few possible leads, Dr Meecham hasn't yet discovered Betty's main reason for attending and needs more information.

How could the doctor discover more about why Betty has come?
If Betty was given a little more time, she might become clearer about what she was hoping for. One study shows that, on average, doctors wait 23 seconds before interrupting a patient's opening statement.[13] Just 6 extra seconds would allow the patient to finish.

Another tactic is to summarise understanding of all the issues Betty has raised and ask her which is most important to deal with. Dr Meecham decides what to focus

on, but checks it out with Betty. He acknowledges the death of Betty's cat and how upset she must be, and then says, 'Today you want me to make sure you haven't got a chest infection, and if we've got time, you're hoping I could check out your knee. Have I got that right?'

Betty hesitates, and says that the knee can wait for another day. Actually, she's most worried about her mood: she thinks she's become very low and doesn't seem to be coping with things the way she normally does. Her cough has nearly gone, but she did want the doctor to check her chest is clear. Knowing what to focus on makes the consultation much more effective: it might have taken the whole consultation (or even several) for the doctor to discover the underlying problem. Getting Betty to open up is also about gaining rapport.

- 'Have you noticed any vaginal discharge or bleeding between your periods?' (Or penile discharge, if male.)
- 'Are you currently sexually active?'
- 'Have you had any new sexual partners in the last 6 months?'

These are 'closed' questions. In other words, they can be answered either with a brief answer or with a simple 'yes' or 'no'. Going through all the specific questions we need to ask like this can be time-consuming, and the onus is on the doctor to remember to ask everything on their list. Although these *are* important questions to get answered, if we invite the patient to elaborate on the problem, they may then tell us this information spontaneously – and much more, besides. We can then clarify any points that require it. Asking open questions should be accompanied by active listening skills (see Box 2.4).

Gaining knowledge about the patient through examination

We also gather knowledge about the patient's biomedical presentation through examination. In general practice, the examination tends to be system-specific and focussed on the presenting complaint or issues raised. The examination starts from the moment we first see our patient when we call them from the waiting room or they enter our room. Throughout the consultation, we are picking up information on the patient's body habitus, posture, gait, movements, facial expression and even skin tone. It is not unusual to detect a sign during the consultation that the patient hasn't noticed and doesn't mention, such as a suspicious-looking mole or mild jaundice.

It is important that we share our thinking about our examination findings with the patient. Usually, it is best to do this as part of our summary of the history and examination, but sometimes it is more appropriate to do it immediately after or even during an examination, particularly if the patient is anxious. For instance, if a patient has felt a breast lump and is showing us where it is, they will want immediate feedback that we can feel it too.

Gaining knowledge about the patient's perspective

An interesting thing about asking open questions is that we often discover aspects of our patient's perspective, in addition to their symptoms. A patient with a urinary tract infection (UTI) may erroneously believe that these are caused by poor hygiene. If we are truly listening, we can pick up on such cues and tailor our explanation to the patient and so reassure them. We can also provide written information. Linking explanations to the patient's understanding and addressing their concerns aids patient recall. If a patient and doctor disagree on an explanation, the patient remembers less of what they are told.

Ideas, concerns and expectations

Many patients see a GP because they are worried about a serious illness. If a patient is worried their symptoms may indicate cancer but the GP doesn't find this out and so doesn't address their concerns, we can imagine that the patient will not really know if the GP has considered cancer as an option or not. We can avoid this situation by considering the acronym 'ICE' (ideas, concerns and expectations) (see Table 2.1). What does the patient think is going on? What are they worried about? What are they hoping for from the consultation? Doctors are poor at guessing which patients expect antibiotics if they don't explicitly ask.[14] A consultation where a patient's beliefs and wishes are respected makes them a partner in their care; this makes them more likely to feel satisfied with the consultation and more likely to adhere to treatment[6] (see Chapter 4). After all, it is the patient (not the doctor) who has to go for the blood test, adopt lifestyle changes or take the medicine they have been prescribed.

This is what we mean by 'patient-centred practice'. In the most recent edition of *Good Medical Practice*,[15] the GMC says that doctors should 'work in partnership with patients' by listening and responding to their concerns and preferences, giving them 'the information they want and need in a way they can understand', respecting their right to be involved in decisions about their treatment and care and supporting them in their own efforts to 'improve and maintain their health'.

Gaining knowledge about the patient's context

There are many potential barriers to effective communication, including a patient's cultural background. Some aspects, such as their age or gender, might be obvious to us, but many others make up a person's 'culture' and may be less apparent, such as socioeconomic status, occupation, health and previous health experiences. Understanding the context of our patients' lives is important when making a diagnosis and helps us to tailor our explanations and management plan to the individual. We are more likely to consider tuberculosis (TB) as a differential diagnosis in a patient who is homeless or is living in (or recently moved from) an area where TB is endemic, than in an office worker with no known risk factors. Just as importantly, it may be reasonable to expect many of our patients to organise an X-ray and collect antibiotics if we give them the right form and a prescription, but this might prove difficult for a homeless patient or someone who has recently arrived in the country. Understanding our patient's background enables us to give them the right help and support. We can ask directly about their home or work situation, or find out this information by asking how their symptoms or illness are impacting on their life.

Understanding: what is going on and what do we do about it?

We have discussed the fact that in order to really understand our patients, we need to understand not only their symptoms, but their views on what has been happening, their fears, what

they are hoping for and their background and lives. To aid our understanding, we need to be curious and pay attention to the patient's words, demeanour and cues. We need to ask the right questions, and we can aid our understanding by summarising what we think we've heard and reflecting this back to our patients. At the end of this process, we hope we have a pretty good understanding of their situation.

Once we have all this information, how do we decide what to do? This is the shift in the consultation between finding out information and moving forwards to create a plan. First, we need to be sure about the nature of the problem and have a clear idea of a differential diagnosis (if the situation calls for one to be made), and then we can think about our options for what to do next. It is worth considering how many options are open to the GP (see Case study 2.1c).

The GP doesn't need to discuss all these options with the patient, but it is useful to be aware of the breadth of options in any situation. Sometimes, the options are around how to further investigate a problem. Sometimes there are a number of reasonable options, and it depends how the patient wants to proceed. At other times, the options are very limited; for example, if we think a patient has cancer, it is usually obvious they need urgent referral under a 2-week wait referral scheme, as long as the patient agrees.

The options a GP is likely to offer depend on the doctor's knowledge and experience. Some GPs have more experience than others in delivering brief psychological interventions in the consultation. The options also depend on medical evidence (e.g. there is less evidence for the benefit of antidepressants in a mild than in a moderate to severe depression; see Chapter 24). Options depend on resources and availability. The GP may be more likely to suggest counselling if they have easy access to this. On the other hand, in Case study 2.1c it would be

---

Case study 2.1c

When Dr Meecham asks Betty Bright more about her mood, Betty talks about how since retiring 2 years ago, she has been very lonely. After taking a history, Dr Meecham diagnoses mild depression. Betty had friends at work who've now stopped visiting, and she feels abandoned by them. Her cleaning work was quite active and she now feels unfit. She was looking forward to retirement and wants to make the most of it, but she has lost confidence.

What options are open to Dr Meecham?
- **Listening** may be all that is required; Betty may be able to come up with her own solutions if she has a supportive, understanding ear.
- **Counselling skills** might be employed to help Betty cope; perhaps the GP can help her reframe her expectations about her old friends at work. By 'reframe', we mean 'see an alternative perspective'.

- **Reassurance**: Betty may need to know that what she is experiencing is not unusual, or her fault, and that she can be helped to feel better.
- **Information**: Betty may need information about mood or bereavement. She may need information about local activities to get involved in.
- **Watchful waiting**: If Betty's symptoms are of recent onset, Dr Meecham might see how things go while keeping her under review.
- **Motivating**: Betty could be encouraged to engage with community activities, exercise or voluntary work.
- **Investigation**: Betty may need some investigations. If she is also tired, she may need blood tests to look for other underlying causes, such as anaemia, hypothyroidism or chronic renal failure.
- **Prescribing**: Betty may benefit from antidepressants.
- **Referral**: Betty may benefit from counselling or cognitive behavioural therapy (CBT), depending on local referral pathways.

clinically inappropriate and a waste of resources to refer Betty to a psychiatrist. The doctor will also draw on their experience of the patient and of what has helped patients in similar situations. Options can be combined: Dr Meecham might decide that Betty would best be helped by active listening, empathy and encouragement to get involved in community activities, while keeping her mood under review.

Reaching a shared decision and aiding the patient's understanding

Whatever options the doctor might have in mind, it is likely the patient has some ideas of their own. Some patients know exactly what they want; others may only know what they don't want. Before we discuss the management plan, we need to step back and share our thinking with the patient about the nature of the problem. This can include 'giving the diagnosis', but as discussed, GPs are not necessarily making diagnoses in every consultation. So we are aiming for both doctor and patient to agree on the nature of the issues. During the following steps, the doctor is often doing more talking than the patient, so we should keep the patient involved. The danger is that we overload the patient with information. We need to ask the patient what information they'd find helpful. We can aid our patient's understanding by the way we communicate information (see Box 2.5).

The doctor's perspective on the nature of the issues

Our patients need to know from us:
- Our understanding of what they have told us (a summary). 'What we've discussed today is…'
- Anything we have gleaned from the notes, results or hospital correspondence that ties in with the current issues. 'I can also see that you had a similar episode last year and had an MRI scan…'
- The examination findings and what these mean. 'When I checked your blood pressure, I found…'

- What we think the diagnosis or the nature of the issues is, and why. If we are not sure, we should share our uncertainty and discuss the possibilities.
- If we aren't certain about a diagnosis, we should share what we need to do to find out (e.g. further investigations or referral).

Explanations

A study of British general practice in the 1980s showed that patients placed more value on information about diagnosis, prognosis and causation than doctors assumed, and that doctors overestimated how much the patients wanted information about treatment.[16] The conclusion is that we need to find out what information our patients need. We can do so by asking. If we think back to Case study 2.1a, Dr Meecham thought Betty had mild depression. Before launching into an explanation, he tried to elicit what information Betty needed, and said, 'From everything we've discussed, I am wondering if you are somewhat depressed. Is this something you'd considered?' Betty explained that she had a few friends who had been diagnosed with depression, so it had crossed her mind. From this starting point, Dr Meecham could then explore Betty's understanding of what depression meant to her. Betty understood how depression could make people feel, but she didn't know what caused it to happen and was worried that she would need to take medication to feel better. Betty didn't really want to take tablets, as her friends had awful side effects. Dr Meecham was then able to clarify what information Betty did want. He explained that she wouldn't necessarily need medication to recover from depression, and was able to ask if she was interested in hearing a bit about other approaches that might help her feel better.

Making a plan in conjunction with the patient

Once we have all the information we need, and the patient understands what we are thinking and has had a chance to ask questions, we can form a management plan together.

Box 2.5 Aiding patients' understanding

- Use concise, clear English, avoid medical jargon and consider all of the words you use. For instance, 'X-ray' and 'scan' are more widely understood than 'imaging'.
- Use similar words and phrases to the patient.
- Use small amounts of information at a time, and make sure the patient understands each bit. Use the patient's response to guide movement forwards. In their book, *Skills for Communicating with Patients*,[7] Silverman, Kurtz and Draper call this 'chunking and checking' information.
- Organise information explicitly (e.g. 'There are three main things we need to discuss').

- Repeat and summarise to aid recall.
- Explain in different ways. Some patients understand visual information better than verbal explanations. Combine the use of pictures/written information, and, where appropriate, use visual decision-making aids
- Relate to the patient's illness framework. If a patient has mentioned a friend who had a similar illness, relate this to what they've told you in your explanation.
- Invite questions. Make it explicit early on that the patient can ask questions whenever they want to.
- Ask patients to repeat what you've told them or ask how they would explain what you've told them to a loved one.

We should make suggestions as to possible options and give information about them, including what they involve, pros and cons and any side effects or risks. We should then elicit the patient's reactions and preferences and discuss any concerns or anxieties. This way, we can work towards a plan that both doctor and patient agree with.

Before the patient leaves

We then need to decide a follow-up plan with the patient:
- Do they need to come back within a specific timeframe, or only if there is a problem?
- Does the patient know what to do if things don't go according to plan? For instance, if we don't give antibiotics to a patient who we think has a self-limiting viral illness, we need to consider what happens if a secondary bacterial infection develops. What are the signs that the patient should look out for?
- If we refer for tests, what should the patient expect? How will they get the results?

The patient should also be encouraged to ask questions.

We can end the consultation by getting the patient to summarise the plan, recap what has been discussed and, where appropriate, offer written information.

Reflecting on our consultation skills

When we think about consultations we've had with patients, we have a general sense of how they went. We might think, 'That was terrible' (many students' initial reaction to their performance in a consultation), or, 'That seemed ok', or even, 'What a great consultation'. Gut reactions are good starting points, but we want to know if they are correct and, if so, why. Observations from colleagues and patient satisfaction surveys can shed some light on how we are perceived in our consultations. Videotaping allows us see ourselves in action. Rarely is any one consultation all bad or all good, so we should focus on the things that went well as well as the aspects that might be improved.

We can use consultation models (see Table 2.1) to identify an area to focus on (e.g. sharing information: What did we explain to the patient? What reaction did they have? Did we allow them to ask questions? If so, what did they ask? What options did we share with the patient? Which did we hold back from offering, and why?)

We may gain more from our reflections if we discuss them with a colleague or write them down, rather than just thinking about them.

We see that there is no one 'correct' way to consult, but many ways to approach consultations, and that this is a lifelong learning process.

SUMMARY

GPs must communicate effectively with their patients; they need to be clear, honest and sensitive. They have to put the patient's best interests at the heart of what they do, and balance the patient's views and values with solid evidence-based and ethical practice. Although diagnosis and spotting serious illness are key tasks for the GP, there are many others, such as preventing ill health, signposting information and providing support, advocacy and continuity of care, that are essential for good patient management. The GP consultation is the forum in which the majority of this management happens; patients in general practice often bring unsorted problems that are a complex interplay between the biomedical, the psychological and the social. In the short time we have with each patient, we must make sense of these problems in a way that they can integrate into their frame of reference. We know that good relationships between doctors and patients gain better outcomes and more satisfaction for both patient and doctor. Reassuringly, there is good evidence that we can learn effective consultation skills. With reflective practice, we can continue to develop these skills throughout our medical careers.

 Now visit **wileyessential.com/primarycare** to test yourself on this chapter.

REFERENCES

1. General Medical Council. *Tomorrow's Doctors: Outcomes and Standards for Undergraduate Medical Education.* London: GMC; 2009.

2. Board of Medical Education. *Communication Skills Education for Doctors: An Update.* London: BMA; 2004.

3. Wilson T, Sheikh A. Enhancing public safety in primary care. *BMJ* 2002;**324**:584–7.

4. Baker R, Streatfield J. What type of general practice do patients prefer? Exploration of practice characteristics influencing patient satisfaction. *Br J Gen Pract* 1995;**45**:654–9.

5. Balint M. *The Doctor, His Patient and the Illness*, 2nd edn. London: Churchill Livingstone; 2000.

6. Kurtz S, Silverman J, Benson J, Draper J. Marrying content and process in clinical method teaching: enhancing the Calgary-Cambridge Guides. *Acad Med* 2003;**78**(8):802–9.

7. Silverman JD, Kurtz SM, Draper J. *Skills for Communicating with Patients*, 3rd edn. Oxford; Radcliffe Medical Press: 2013.

8. Neighbour R. *The Inner Consultation: How to Develop an Effective and Intuitive Consulting Style*, 2nd edn. Oxford: Radcliffe Medical Press; 2005.

9. Korzybski A. *Science and Sanity: An Introduction to Non-Aristotelian Systems and General Semantics*, 5th edn. New Jersey: Institute of General Semantics; 1995.

10. Korsch BM, Gozzi EK, Francis V. Gaps in doctor–patient communication: doctor patient interaction and patient satisfaction. *Pediatrics* 1968;**42**:855–71.

11. Moulton L. *The Naked Consultation*. Oxford: Blackwell; 2007.

12. Barry CA, Bradley CP, Britten N, et al. Patients' unvoiced agendas in general practice consultations: qualitative study. *BMJ* 2000;**320**:1246–50.

13. Marvel MK, Epstein RM, Flowers K, Beckman HB. Soliciting the patient's agenda: have we improved? *JAMA* 1999;**281**(3):283–7.

14. Cockburn J, Pit S. Prescribing behaviour in clinical practice: patients' expectations and doctors' perceptions of patients' expectations – a questionnaire study. *BMJ* 1997;**315**:520–3.

15. General Medical Council. *Good Medical Practice*. London; GMC; 2013.

16. Kindelan K, Kent G. Concordance between patients' information preferences and general practitioners' perceptions. *Psychol Health* 1987;**1**:399–409.

17. Byrne PS, Long BEL. *Doctors Talking to Patients*. London: Royal College of General Practitioners; 1984.

18. Stott NC, Davis RH. The exceptional potential in each primary care consultation. *Br J Gen Pract* 1979;**29**:201–5.

19. Pendleton D, Schofield T, Tate P, Havelock P. *The Consultation: An Approach to Teaching and Learning*. Oxford: Oxford Medical Publications; 1984.

20. Helman CG. Disease versus illness in general practice. *Br J Gen Pract* 1981;**31**:548–62.

21. Kurtz S, Silverman J. The Calgary-Cambridge Referenced Observation Guides: an aid to defining the curriculum and organizing the teaching in communication training programmes. *Medical Education* 1996;**30**(2):83–9.

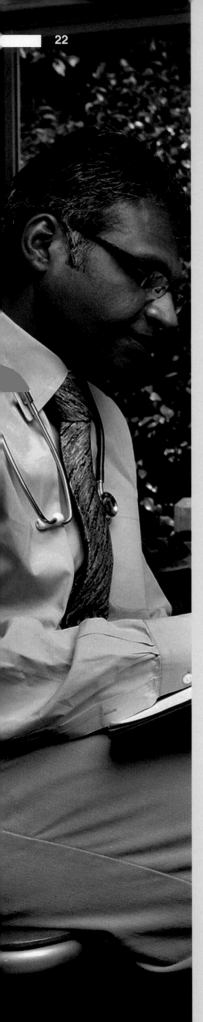

CHAPTER 3

Making a diagnosis

Barbara Laue

Senior Teaching Fellow in Primary Care, University of Bristol

Key topics

Learning objectives

- Be able to describe what is meant by 'diagnosis'.
- Be able to describe different types of diagnosis.
- Be able to recognise the different processes that are used when making a diagnosis.
- Be aware of the benefits and pitfalls of the different diagnostic processes.
- Be able to describe how diagnostic errors occur.

Essential Primary Care, First Edition. Edited by Andrew Blythe and Jessica Buchan.
© 2017 John Wiley & Sons, Ltd. Published 2017 by John Wiley & Sons, Ltd.
Companion website: www.wileyessential.com/primarycare

What is a diagnosis?

'Diagnosis' is a much-used word in medical practice and can be used to mean different things (see Table 3.1). According to the biomedical model of disease, 'diagnosis' is the name given to a problem with characteristic physical and pathological findings. However, ill health is often the product of more than just a physical pathology. Psychosocial factors are important too, and sometimes there is no underlying characteristic histology. This is why GPs talk of making a triple diagnosis: a physical, psychological and social diagnosis.

The diagnosis is an attempt to make sense of the 'story' that the patient tells us and to create some sort of order out of their experience. To continue the story-telling analogy, the diagnosis is the 'plot' which gives the framework to the narrative.[1] Patients come to their GP because they want answers to something they are experiencing: 'What is it?', 'What needs to be done?', 'What will happen?' Making a diagnosis helps the GP answer those questions. It guides investigations, management and prognosis, and can help to prevent complications. Some diagnoses may also lead to other family members being screened for the condition, such as in hyperlipidaemia. Making, recording and coding diagnoses accurately is important for disease surveillance, mortality statistics and research.

Science and art in diagnosis

There seems to be a simple and widespread view that the medical interviewer objectively observes and discovers 'what is there' and then develops a hypothesis or 'diagnosis' on the basis of that information. This view is reflected in how we talk about the medical interview: we 'take a history'.

In reality, it is more complex. We know from our current understanding of the scientific process that it is difficult or impossible to make observations completely objectively. Scientists bring perspectives and biases to the process that may affect their results. In the same way, medical interviewers bring knowledge and experience to their consultations which influence and guide what sense they are making of the patient's story.

It seems a good idea to have a closer look at history-taking at this point. Medical students often find that the patient's story seems to change when another person retakes the history after their initial clerking. This can make students feel inadequate or even cross with the patient.

With experience, we learn that patients' stories are often not completely formed when they present their symptoms. Through listening and responding, we are helping the patient to fashion their story. This implies a social-constructivist perspective of the history-taking process. Patients and their health professionals are together actively drafting and redrafting the patient's story during the consultation. In general practice, we often see patients early on in a condition, and jointly write the first draft. In the course of their journey through the healthcare system, patients may pick up on the vocabulary used by health professionals and gain in understanding, and then build this into the next draft of their story.

This is perhaps the point where science and art meet in the consultation. As health professionals, we need to be able to pick out key items of information to match to medical patterns in order to make medical sense and formulate hypotheses. Patients may find it difficult to express what they are experiencing, and their descriptions may not fit those in the textbooks. From our knowledge of the patient and their usual way of presenting, we may be able to decode what they are telling us.

Case study 3.1

Margaret Mather is in her early 70s, has hypertension and rarely consults for anything other than blood pressure checks. She presents in an anxious state to her GP, Dr Bethany Boyd. She has not been feeling right for a while. The only way she can describe what she is feeling is by saying, 'It feels like I have swallowed the wind'. She denies any cough or phlegm. She has been a lifelong heavy smoker.

From her knowledge of Mrs Mather and her understanding of the risks of smoking, Dr Boyd's first concern is that Mrs Mather has a serious lung condition. Unfortunately, an urgent CXR reveals a large central bronchial carcinoma.

Table 3.1 Examples to illustrate the use of the term 'diagnosis'.	
Recognition of a disease or condition by its outward signs and symptoms	Aortic stenosis: the patient may have a typical murmur and present with blackouts and shortness of breath on exertion Cold sore: typical cluster of blisters
Name for a physiological or biochemical abnormality leading to a distinct disease entity	Diabetes mellitus: sugar levels outside the normal range
A label/shorthand for a cluster of symptoms and signs	Fibromyalgia: history of widespread pain and multiple tender points on palpation
A framework for answering a patient's questions: 'What is wrong with me?', 'Is it serious?' and 'What can be done about it?'	Viral illness: patient presenting with slight sore throat and runny nose We usually don't know the exact virus causing it or whether it is indeed a virus, rather than, for example, an allergy

Diagnosis-making as 'labelling'

Making a diagnosis means giving a name to what the patient presents. This 'naming' can give the impression that we understand a condition more completely than we actually do. Very often, there is much uncertainty about the actual cause of a set of symptoms. In 25–50% of GP consultations, no disease-specific diagnosis is made.

When a cluster of signs and symptoms is seen repeatedly, it may be called a syndrome. When more is known, particularly when the aetiology is understood, it becomes a disease.

The labels we apply reflect the current understanding of a condition. For example, when the effects of human immunodeficiency virus (HIV) infection were first observed in the 1980s, it was postulated that the cause was immunodeficiency and the label 'acquired immunodeficiency syndrome' (AIDS) was applied. Research then identified the HIV virus as the causative agent. This was an essential discovery for the development of treatments and a preventive strategy.

'Labels' or diagnoses are essential for categorising signs and symptoms and matching them to what is known so that we can make a management plan and help the patient. They may also impair our thinking about conditions and stop us looking for alternative explanations. An example is duodenal ulcers. For many years, it was known that they occur in patients who produce an increased amount of acid in their stomach. It was also thought that gastric juices were too acidic to allow infective agents to grow. It was not until the 1980s that the bacterium *Helicobacter pylori* was discovered in the stomach and shown to be causally related to duodenal ulcers. The 'acid dogma' had blinded scientists to other causes.

Labels can reflect different perspectives. 'Illness' refers to the labels given by the patient or a lay person and is imbued with the person's emotions and cultural beliefs. 'Disease' reflects the medical interpretation. For example, the patient may say, 'I have a sore throat because I got cold and wet in the rain'. The doctor's summary might be, 'This is an upper respiratory tract infection due to a virus'.

Models of diagnosis-making

There are a number of ways in which we arrive at our diagnostic labels.

Cause-and-effect model

This is the traditional model that we commonly think of when we make a diagnosis. Something has gone wrong, there is a known cause for it and we are trying to find it. For example, when we diagnose someone with chickenpox, we are identifying the *Varicella zoster* virus as the cause of their illness.

Diagnosis based on histology

Some diagnoses are made on the basis of a typical histology or cytology. This is usually the case for cancer diagnoses. Being able to identify types and subtypes of specific cancers is essential for guiding research and targeting treatment. When treating cancer, we are aiming to destroy the cancerous cells, but we often also damage normal tissue in the process. If our understanding of a cancer is very detailed and specific, we have a better chance of developing treatments with less collateral damage.

End-of-distribution model

Many parameters that we measure are normally distributed (see Figure 3.1). We select a cut-off point at which we define a characteristic as abnormal and make the diagnosis. Examples are blood pressure measurements and glucose levels in the blood. The cut-off points are quite arbitrary and do not reflect a step change in risk. Our understanding of conditions, research findings and consensus in the medical community determines where on the continuum we make the diagnosis and when the treatment threshold is reached. Continually developing knowledge and understanding of conditions and their effects can lead to revision of the cut-off point. This is called 'diagnostic drift' (see Box 3.1).

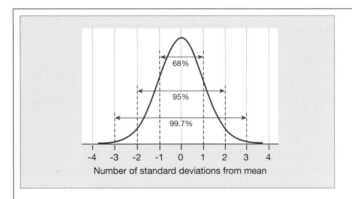

Figure 3.1 Normal distribution. *Source*: After http://www.marin.edu/~npsomas/Lectures/Ch_1/images/imageD5C.JPG (last accessed 6 October 2015).

Box 3.1 Example of diagnostic drift: blood pressure

In the past, the observation that blood pressure increases with age led to an acceptance of higher blood pressures in older people and thus less vigorous treatment. When research showed that older people benefit even more from good blood pressure control than younger people, this changed. More recent research has shown that strict blood pressure control helps to reduce the development of renal disease in patients with diabetes mellitus. This has resulted in blood pressure targets being set at a lower level for patients with diabetes mellitus.

Table 3.2 Examples of scoring systems used to make diagnoses.

Diagnosis	Scoring system
Depression	Patient Health Questionnaire-9 (PHQ-9)
Anxiety	Hospital Anxiety and Depression Scale (HADS)
Migraine	International Headache Society's diagnostic criteria
Fibromyalgia	http://www.arthritisresearchuk.org/ arthritis-information/conditions/fibromyalgia. aspx (last accessed 6 October 2015)
Irritable bowel syndrome	Manning criteria for diagnosing IBS

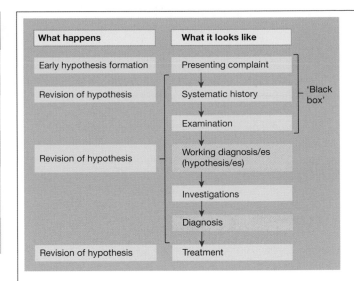

Figure 3.2 The diagnostic process used by an experienced clinician.

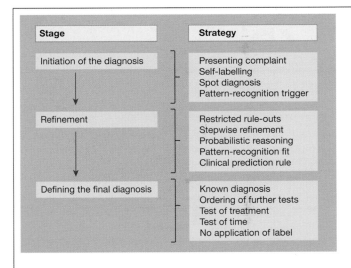

Figure 3.3 Heneghan's three stages to making a diagnosis.

There is a risk of overtreating and medicalising parameters that are near the cut-off point. Some of the drivers for this are increased understanding of certain conditions, reduced tolerance of uncertainty and new pharmacological developments. As well as critically examining their benefits, we also need to be alert to 'over-marketing' of drugs. An example would be the marketing campaign for treating 'low testosterone' with testosterone-replacement therapy, despite the lack of evidence of benefits.[2]

Empirical model

Some diagnoses cannot be identified by a causative agent, single measurement or typical histology. They are recognised as an entity through observation of typical clusters of signs and symptoms. Researchers try and make these cases more specific by introducing scoring systems for signs and symptoms (see Table 3.2).

Processes for reaching a diagnosis

To the untrained observer, the diagnostic process may seem like a 'black box'. The time-honoured sequence of history, examination and testing can make us think that the diagnosis only comes at the end of this process. Researchers in the 1970s showed that this is not how experienced clinicians actually operate. They found that clinicians formulate a hypothesis or diagnosis early on in the process and then shape and reshape it, and that this informs their actions throughout the process (see Figure 3.2).[3] Heneghan and colleagues characterised three distinct stages in this process: initiation of the diagnosis, refinement and definition of the final diagnosis. For each of these stages, they identified typical strategies (see Figure 3.3).[4]

The presenting complaint is often the starting point for the diagnostic process. In our early clinical days, we learn what symptoms are produced by particular body systems going wrong. There are an estimated 10 000 diagnoses, and we soon become aware that most symptoms are not highly specific for particular conditions. For example, shortness of breath is a common symptom that can be generated by different body systems and therefore has low specificity. This means we need

to look for patterns of signs and symptoms, time course and causal relationships.

Self-labelling

Sometimes patients present with a ready-made diagnosis: 'My haemorrhoids are bleeding again' or 'These statins are causing me terrible pains in my knees'. We need to be wary of this and gather more information. The patients may be wrong and might have inflammatory bowel disease or osteoarthritis of the knees.

Spot diagnosis and pattern recognition

These terms are often used interchangeably and refer to the instant recognition of a typical appearance, sound or cluster of symptoms and signs. Some patterns are familiar to everyone, such as the appearance of an adult with Down's syndrome. As we progress through medical school, we start to build an internal library of patient stories and images, referred to as 'illness scripts',[5] that we relate to certain diagnoses. Throughout our working lives, we add to this store of illness scripts. When we encounter new patients, we subconsciously look to see if their story matches one we have heard or seen before.[6] This process can accelerate the pathway to a diagnosis but runs the risk of missing a rare diagnosis that looks like something we have seen before.

Probabilistic reasoning

Symptoms are mostly not very specific for any condition, and yet we seem to be able to come up with manageable lists of differential diagnoses. This is possible because we use probabilistic reasoning, often on a subconscious level. We tend to have a wider understanding or 'feel' for the patient groups we care for, and take into account age, gender, ethnicity and what we know about the prevalence of conditions in these groups. For example, the probability of a cough being caused by tuberculosis (TB) is higher in an inner-city practice with a large Somali refugee population than in a settled affluent area.

Symptoms have a given sensitivity and specificity, but Bayes' theorem tells us that their predictive value depends on the prevalence of the condition in the population in which they are presenting. The following example shows how the prevalence of a condition in a given population alters the predictive value of symptoms.

Let us assume that symptom x has 80% sensitivity and 80% specificity for disease y, and explore the predictive value of this symptom in two populations with different prevalence for disease y. The sample size is 1000 in each of the examples (Table 3.3).

In practice, we do not make actual calculations, but instead use instinctive probabilistic reasoning based on our knowledge and experience. This serves as a filter to rule diagnoses in or out

with each additional piece of information. It also guides our actions. Some diagnoses may be less likely but more serious, and we therefore start investigating them even if the probability of their being correct is very low. An example is an acoustic neuroma, which has an incidence of around 17 in 1 000 000. Typical presenting symptoms for this tumour are unilateral deafness and tinnitus. Both these symptoms are common in general practice. This means that the probability of somebody who presents with unilateral deafness and tinnitus in general practice having this tumour is very low. However, since the condition is serious and eminently treatable, we would organise a magnetic resonance imaging (MRI) scan.

These examples illustrate how the setting affects the diagnosis. In a hospital clinic, the prevalence of the disease that is being considered is usually much higher than that in the general practice population. When a patient says to a GP, 'I am feeling really tired', the diagnoses at the top of the GP's list of possibilities will be depression and anaemia; Addison's disease will be way down the list. When an endocrinologist sees a patient complaining of tiredness, Addison's disease will be much higher up their list: all patients referred to the endocrinologist's clinic have been filtered such that 'tiredness' has a higher predictive value for Addison's disease than it does in the GP surgery.

Specificity of signs and symptoms

The nonspecificity of symptoms can make it very difficult to diagnose serious conditions such as cancer at an early stage. We know that early diagnosis improves cancer survival. Much research has thus been done to understand early presentations of cancers, by assessing the predictive value of symptoms. An example is a paper by Hamilton and colleagues on the presenting symptoms of ovarian cancer.[7] They found that persistent abdominal bloating was a significant symptom and that its predictive value was enhanced if it occurred in combination with other symptoms, such as nausea and abdominal pain.

Only a few symptoms and signs have very high specificity. We call them 'pathognomonic', as they almost certainly represent a specific condition. Table 3.4 gives a few examples of pathognomonic symptoms and signs.

Some symptoms, such as unintended weight loss, haemoptysis and hoarseness in someone who smokes, carry a higher risk of serious pathology. These are 'red-flag' symptoms: there is a high likelihood that the underlying condition is serious. Most of these are not very specific, and more information or further tests are needed to get to the diagnosis.

Table 3.3 Predictive value of symptoms by disease prevalence.

Population A: high prevalence of the disease (1 in 10)

	Disease present	Disease absent	Total
Symptom present	80	180	260
Symptom absent	20	720	740
Total	100	900	1000
Positive predictive value of the symptom = 80 out of 260 = **31%**			

Population B: low prevalence of the disease (1 in 100)

	Disease present	Disease absent	Total
Symptom present	8	198	206
Symptom absent	2	792	794
Total	10	990	1000
Positive predictive value of the symptom = 8 out of 206 = **4%**			

Table 3.4 Examples of pathognomonic symptoms and signs.

Virchow's node, a solitary lymph node in supraclavicular fossa	Stomach cancer
Koplik's spots: chalky-looking deposits on buccal mucosa opposite molars	Measles
Pain within minutes of drinking alcohol	Hodgkin's disease

Pitfalls of the diagnostic process

Errors in the diagnostic process are common. Some errors are system-related, such as test results getting lost and not being acted on. Others are cognitive. Balla and colleagues identified initiation and closure of the diagnostic process as the stages most vulnerable to cognitive errors.[8] Early on, when we set out the framework for further questioning, biases can creep in (e.g. using psychosocial labels, missing or ignoring red flags or attributing a symptom to the wrong condition). It is important to understand how these cognitive errors come about, so that we can develop an awareness of them and routines to guard against them. A range of diagnostic errors have been described.[9, 10]

Communication errors

These are an important cause of error. They may come about because we are rushed and interrupt patients in their initial statement, because we start off with closed questions or because we miss cues and fail to elicit the patient's ideas, concerns and expectations (ICE).

Anchoring errors

The patient may present a key symptom in the history, such as chest pain, that causes us to jump to an early conclusion, such as that the pain has a cardiac cause. We may then seek confirmation of this through further questioning, asking leading and closed questions and failing to consider other possible causes.

Availability errors

Availability errors occur when a symptom or story fits a diagnosis that we made recently, that we make commonly or that comes to our minds readily.

Attribution errors

Negative stereotyping can lead us to make snap judgements and close off other options.

Confirmation and framing errors

We can assemble elements that seem to support a favoured diagnosis, rather than build the diagnosis from all the evidence in front of us. We tend to give undue weight to the symptoms and signs that fit with our diagnosis and disregard those that don't.

Premature closure

We may fail to seek additional information after we have reached a working diagnosis. With growing expertise, we tend to put more weight on initial impressions. This places us at risk of curtailing the 'revision' and prematurely closing off further lines of inquiry.[13]

Failure of diagnostic revision

Underlying most of these errors is a general reluctance to review our first diagnosis and take a fresh look.

Case study 3.2

Neil Newman, age 55, is an overweight businessman with moderately severe asthma who stopped smoking 2 years ago. He presents to his GP, Dr Tom Thatcher, with left-sided chest pain. The pain has been there on and off since yesterday, but is a bit more severe today. Dr Thatcher sees him regularly for his asthma and knows that he is feeling stressed because he is working long hours and travelling long distances and that his asthma is often not well controlled. Today, Mr Newman appears anxious and a bit short of breath. He has a moderately reduced peak flow rate and a pulse rate of 96. Dr Thatcher is anxious not to miss a cardiac cause and refers him to the hospital for further assessment. Mr Newman has an electrocardiogram (ECG) and serum troponin; both of these are normal, and he is discharged with a diagnosis of musculoskeletal pain the same day.

A few days later, Mr Newman consults Dr Thatcher again with the same symptoms. The left-sided chest pain has continued and his chest still feels tight. Dr Thatcher remains concerned that this could be angina and re-refers the patient. On this occasion, one of the doctors at the hospital also considers pulmonary embolism as a potential diagnosis. A computed tomography (CT) pulmonary angiogram confirms this.

What types of cognitive error contributed to the delay in reaching the correct diagnosis of a pulmonary embolism?
- **Communication error:** Incomplete information-gathering. Dr Thatcher only took a limited history. This means he did not have the full story of the chest pain, which was not typical of angina.
- **Anchoring and framing:** Dr Thatcher immediately linked the symptom of chest pain to angina and did not broaden his questioning to explore the patient's breathing. He assumed that the patient's apparent shortness of breath related to his asthma not being controlled.
- **Availability:** Pulmonary emboli are less typical in their presentation than angina, and also less common. We are therefore more likely to consider angina as diagnosis.
- **Attribution:** The negative stereotype of an overweight stressed businessman who has been a smoker until recently tipped the diagnosis towards a cardiac cause.
- **Failure of diagnostic revision:** Dr Thatcher didn't give enough consideration to alternative diagnoses when the patient represented.

Preventing diagnostic errors

Failure to make the right diagnosis or to make it soon enough is a common reason for doctors being sued. How can we reduce the risk of making errors?

Table 3.5 gives some tips for reducing cognitive errors. At the top of this list are effective consultation skills (see Chapter 2).

John Murtagh, a professor of general practice in Australia, has developed a number of strategies or models for diagnosing that are helpful in avoiding errors.[13] He suggests that we ask ourselves five questions about the patient's presenting problem:

- What is the probable diagnosis?
- What serious disorder(s) must not be missed?
- What conditions can be missed in this situation? (pitfalls)
- Could the patient have one of the 'masquerades' commonly encountered?
- Is the patient trying to tell me something? (look for yellow flags)

To this list, it would be useful to add the mnemonic ICE from Chapter 2. We should always ask about the patient's ideas, concerns and expectations.

It is especially important that we do not fail to make a serious diagnosis. This is where 'red flags' have their value. Professor Murtagh recommends that a good history should include at least six key questions to pinpoint red flags:

- 'Tell me about your general health: do you have any tiredness, fatigue or weakness?'
- 'Do you have a fever or night sweats?'
- 'Have you lost any weight (unplanned)?'
- 'Have you noticed any unusual lumps?'

Table 3.5 Tips for avoiding cognitive errors.

Cognitive errors	Tips for avoiding error
Communication	Listen to the patient and give them time to tell their story Summarise, clarify and check what the patient has said Elicit the patient's ideas, concerns and expectations (ICE)
Anchoring	Do not focus on one prominent symptom too early Continue to ask open questions
Availability	Be aware of the limits of your knowledge Ask yourself: • What else could it be? • What must I not miss? • What fits and what doesn't fit this diagnosis?
Attribution	Ask yourself: • How am I feeling about this patient? • Do I have any prejudices (e.g. age, social status, gender, ethnicity)?

- 'Do you have persistent pain anywhere?'
- 'Have you noticed any unusual bleeding?'

There are also some informal clinical 'rules' or 'safety nets' that have grown out of clinical practice in a complex environment characterised by uncertainty. They are part of the medical discourse, passed on from one generation of doctors to the next, and provide some guidance when faced with uncertainty.

'Three strikes and you're out'

In general practice, we often use a 'wait and see' strategy when faced with undifferentiated and difficult-to-classify symptoms. Symptoms may resolve or become clearer when we see the patient again. This rule tells us to take action, investigate or seek a second opinion when a patient presents for a third time with the same problem and we still have not reached a diagnosis. It helps to guard against missing a serious problem that presents with atypical or innocuous symptoms.

'Common things are common' or 'If you hear hoofbeats, don't think zebras'

This rule encourages us to think of the common diagnoses first, before considering vanishingly rare conditions. It is grounded in knowledge of and a subconscious feel for Bayesian probabilities and clinical judgement. It may be at odds with the experience of medical students, who gain most of their clinical experience in secondary or tertiary referral centres, where unusual conditions are clustered.

'Rare things are common'

This rule seems to contradict itself. It refers to the fact that there are a lot of rare diseases and we are therefore likely to come across some of them but are very unlikely to see the same one twice in the course of our careers. If there is diagnostic uncertainty, it can be useful to think about 'zebras' differently: 'if you hear hoofbeats, think zebras'. It encourages us to keep our mind open to unusual possibilities.

'Uncommon presentations of common diseases are more common than unusual diseases'

This rule again reinforces the need to put common conditions at the top of our list of differential diagnoses. It encourages

---

Box 3.2 List of common conditions that often present in unexpected ways

Depression Diabetes Drugs: iatrogenic, OTC or self-abuse Anaemia Thyroid, Addison's and other endocrine disorders	Spinal dysfunction – pain syndrome Urinary tract infection (UTI) Prostate cancer Myeloma HIV infection

flexible thinking about conditions, rather than looking for stereotypes or rare conditions. Professor Murtagh has identified some common conditions that often present in unexpected ways, 'masquerading' as other things (see Box 3.2).

Learning to make a diagnosis

Proficiency and safety in making a diagnosis require practice, feedback and constant reflection. The more patients we see, the larger our bank of illness scripts becomes. Feedback from colleagues observing us and from replies to our referrals helps us to improve the efficiency of our information-gathering and reasoning skills. Every time a diagnosis is confirmed, we need to ask ourselves: Could I have made that diagnosis more quickly or more effectively? Are there questions that I should have asked or aspects of the patient's story that I should have given more credence to? Did I conduct an appropriate examination? Were all the tests that I did really necessary, or did I overlook tests that I should have done sooner?

SUMMARY

Diagnosing is a central activity in all consultations. Intuitively, we may think of a 'diagnosis' as being quite specific. In reality, many first consultations for a symptom result in a problem formulation that is imprecise. Problem formulation is the first step in making sense of the story and symptoms that a patient presents. It informs investigations, management and prognosis. Gathering more history and performing tests lead to a more precise diagnosis in many cases, but not all. Developing a hypothesis early in the consultation increases the chance of making a correct diagnosis. Doctors and other health professionals use a variety of cognitive processes to reach a diagnosis. The level of experience influences the relative contributions of hypothetico-deductive thinking and pattern recognition. These diagnostic processes have inherent benefits and pitfalls. We must be alert to cognitive errors. Misdiagnoses are relatively common, but strategies are available by which to prevent and identify them.

 Now visit **www.wileyessential.com/primarycare** to test yourself on this chapter.

REFERENCES

1. Hunter KM. *Doctors' Stories*. Princeton: Princeton University Press; 1991. pp. 44–47.
2. Kamerow D. Getting your 'T'up. *BMJ* 2014;**348**:g182.
3. Elstein AS, Kagan N, Shulman LS, et al. Methods and theory in the study of medical inquiry. *J Med Educ* 1972;**47**:85–92.
4. Heneghan C, Glasziou P, Thompson M, et al. Diagnostic strategies used in primary care. *BMJ* 2009;**338**:b946.
5. Barrows HS, Feltovitch PJ. The clinical reasoning process. *Med Educ* 1987;**21**:86–91.
6. Norman G. Research in clinical reasoning: past history and current trends. *Med Educ* 2005;**39**:418–27.
7. Hamilton W, Peters TJ, Bankhead C, Sharp D. Risk of ovarian cancer in woman with symptoms in primary care: population based control study. *BMJ* 2009; **339**:b2998.
8. Balla J, Heneghan C, Goyder C, Thompson M. Identifying early warning signs for diagnostic errors in primary care: a qualitative study. *BMJ Open* 2012;**2**: e001539. doi:10.1136/bmjopen-2012-001539.
9. Groopman J. *How Doctors Think*, 1st Mariner Book edn. New York: Houghton Mifflin; 2008.
10. Wellbery C. Flaws in clinical reasoning: a common cause of diagnostic error. *Am Fam Physician* 2011;**84**(9): 1042–8.
11. Elstein AS, Schwarz A. Evidence base of clinical diagnosis: clinical problem solving and diagnostic decision making: selective review of the cognitive literature. *BMJ* 2002;**324**:729–32.
12. Eva KW. Diagnostic error in medical education: where wrongs can make rights. *Adv Heath Sci Educ Theory Pract* 2009;**14**:71–81.
13. Murtagh J. *General Practice*. Roseville, Australia: McGraw-Hill; 1996.

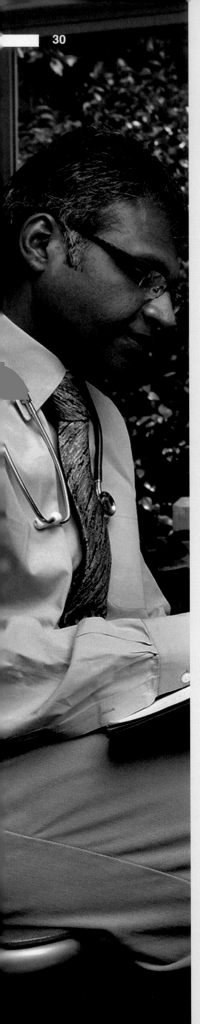

CHAPTER 4
Prescribing

Andrew Blythe
GP and Senior Teaching Fellow, University of Bristol

Key topics

Learning objectives

- Be able to describe the key steps to prescribing.
- Be able to describe how adherence with medication can be improved.
- Be able to describe common types of prescribing error.

Essential Primary Care, First Edition. Edited by Andrew Blythe and Jessica Buchan.
© 2017 John Wiley & Sons, Ltd. Published 2017 by John Wiley & Sons, Ltd.
Companion website: www.wileyessential.com/primarycare

Introduction

In the UK, most prescription-only medications are prescribed by doctors. With additional training, nurses and pharmacists can become independent prescribers. GPs can prescribe almost anything in the British National Formulary (BNF). This ability gives them considerable power, and with this power comes substantial responsibility. GPs must prescribe safely and according to the best available evidence. They must be confident that the benefit of anything they prescribe outweighs the potential harm. Some medicines are hazardous and require close monitoring. Medicines are also very expensive. Approximately 90% of all prescriptions are issued in primary care, so GPs carry the largest responsibility for controlling the drug budget of the NHS.

The pharmaceutical industry continues to generate new medicines, and as people live longer they accumulate chronic conditions, many of which require several different medicines for optimal control. And so the volume of prescribing in the UK continues to grow. The physical task of issuing and signing hundreds of prescriptions each day is a challenge for most practices. This was one of the drivers behind the computerisation of GP records. Computer systems can generate repeat prescriptions quickly and legibly, and can alert doctors to potential interactions between medications.

The cost of prescribing

Looking through the stacks of repeat prescriptions issued every day in a GP surgery, one can see that a large proportion are for a relatively small group of medicines:

- **Proton-pump inhibitors (PPIs):** Launched in the 1980s to control oesophageal reflux.
- **Antihypertensive medication:** Angiotensin-converting enzyme (ACE) inhibitors, calcium channel antagonists and diuretics.
- **Statins:** A class of cholesterol-lowering drugs released in the 1990s; 7 million people in the UK now take a statin.
- **Aspirin:** For the prevention and management of ischaemic heart disease.
- **Warfarin:** For the prevention of stroke.
- **Antidepressant medicines:** Mostly selective serotonin reuptake inhibitors (SSRIs), which in the 1990s replaced tricyclic antidepressants.
- **Inhalers:** For the control of asthma and chronic obstructive pulmonary disease (COPD).
- **Pain killers:** Paracetamol, codeine and nonsteroidal anti-inflammatory drugs (NSAIDs).
- **Medicines for diabetes:** Metformin, sulphonylureas and insulin.
- **Levothyroxine:** For the treatment of hypothyroidism.
- **Vitamin D**.

Most of these medicines regularly appear in the list of the top 20 net ingredients within the NHS drug budget.[1] Some other drugs, such as the new medicines for dementia and psychosis, make it into this list not because of the quantity in which they are prescribed but because of their cost. A year's supply of a new medicine for a single patient can cost hundreds of pounds. Some routinely prescribed medicines are surprisingly expensive, but some cost less than a pound for a month's supply.

Medicines tend to be most expensive when they are still under patent. This is the time when the pharmaceutical company can recoup the cost of research and development. When the patent expires, competitors can make the same medicine and the cost of the medicine falls. Some years later, if the medicine proves to have a good safety record, the manufacturers may apply for a licence to allow pharmacists to sell it without a prescription. Hence, omeprazole and ranitidine can be bought under the supervision of a pharmacist without a prescription, and sumitriptan can be bought for the treatment of migraine. When these drugs first came on the market, they revolutionised the treatment of reflux oesophagitis, peptic ulceration and migraine and were only available on prescription. Eventually, if a medicine proves to be exceptionally safe, it can be sold over the counter without a pharmacist's advice. Table 4.1 lists some of the commonly used medicines that can be purchased over the counter in the UK.

Within the UK, most people who are issued a prescription are able to get their medicine free of charge. Currently, in Wales and Scotland, all prescriptions are free. In England, there is a defined list of conditions and social circumstances that entitle people to free prescriptions (Table 4.2). These rules mean that most people do not pay for their prescription. There are some notable exceptions. Many common conditions are not exempt from prescription charges. This means that adults in work with, for example, asthma or hypertension have to pay for their medication. They have to pay a prescription charge for each item. This charge can be barrier to some people. GPs have to be aware that sometimes patients make a judgement about which prescription they can afford. Patients can buy a pre-payment certificate for about £100 a year, which is roughly the cost of 13 prescriptions. Many people don't know about this and are delighted to be told about it by their GP.

Adherence

How many medicines is it possible to take in a single day? Some people are prescribed more than a dozen different medicines to take daily. Some medicines can be taken in a single daily dose, but others, such as the safest and most widely prescribed painkiller, paracetamol, have to be taken four times a day. Some medicines have to be taken with food; others, like the antibiotic flucloxacillin, have to be taken an hour before food. Some tablets cannot be taken alongside certain foods. The cholesterol-lowering drug statin, for example, should not be taken with grapefruit juice. Iron tablets and most tetracyclines (a group of antibiotics used to treat acne, respiratory disease and bone infections) cannot be taken with milk. One of the most widely prescribed medicines for the treatment of osteoporosis has even more complicated instructions: patients have to take it with a glass of water before breakfast; they have to remain upright after taking the tablet (and not go back to bed); and they have to

Table 4.1 Medicines available over the counter.

Condition	Brand names	Generic name/active ingredients
Gastrointestinal		
Reflux	Gaviscon	Aluminium hydroxide, magnesium hydroxide, simeticone
Haemorrhoids	Anusol	Zinc oxide, bismuth oxide
Constipation	Dulcolax, Senna, Fybogel	Bisacodyl, senna, ispaghula
Diarrhoea	Imodium	Loperamide
Ears, nose, throat and eyes		
Hay fever	Benadryl	Cetirizine (antihistamine)
Dry eyes	Tears naturale	Hypromellose
Skin		
Acne	Panoxyl gel	Benzoyl peroxide
Eczema	Cetraben, E45, Doublebase, Dermol	Soft white paraffin, liquid paraffin, lanolin, glyceryl montearate, isopropyl myristate (all emollients)
Psoriasis	Alphosyl	Coal tar
Head lice	Hedrin, Derbac M, Lyclear,	Dimeticone, malathion, permethrin
Warts	Occlusal	Salicylic acid
Thrush	Canesten	Clotrimazole cream and pessaries
Other		
Anaemia	Iron tablets	Ferrous sulphate/gluconate
Pain relief	Panadol, Nurofen	Paracetamol, ibuprofen, codeine
	Ibuleve gel	Ibuprofen
Smoking cessation	Nicorette	Nicotine patches, inhalators, lozenges and gum
Depression	St John's Wort	St John's wort

Table 4.2 People who are exempt from prescription charges in England.

Qualifying groups
Patients over age 60 years
Pregnant women and women within 1 year of childbirth
All children under 16 and those in full-time education under 18
Patients in receipt of Employment Support Allowance, Income Support or Jobseeker's Allowance
Patients with one of the following specified conditions: • Diabetes requiring medication • Hypothyroidism • Addison's disease • Epilepsy requiring regular medication • Cancer: if on treatment for this or suffering from effects of treatment • Permanent fistula, such as colostomy or laryngostomy • Hypoparathyroidism • Myaesthenia gravis
Patients with any continuing physical disability which stops them from going out without the help of another person

wait at least 1 hour before having their breakfast. How closely do patients adhere to all these instructions?

It is possible to measure patients' adherence to their medication by supplying their medicines with electronic monitoring devices which record the time and date on which the container is opened. A review of studies on blood pressure-lowering medication using these devices showed that about half of all patients stop taking their medication within 1 year of starting it.[2] The drop off in adherence is most marked in the first 2 months.

What can we do to improve adherence?

The starting point should be a discussion with the patient about how the medicine might help and what side effects it might cause. If the patient is not convinced about the need for a medication then they may not even start it, let alone continue to take it.

Even if a patient and doctor are in agreement about the treatment regime, putting this into practice is a different matter. The practicalities of taking certain tablets may get in the way. The patient may simply forget to take an afternoon or evening dose, or the medicine may be too fiddly to use; patients with arthritic hands can find it difficult to unscrew bottles or use inhalers and sprays.

Simplifying the treatment regime, so that the patient takes fewer doses in the day, seems to be one of the best ways of improving adherence.[3] This is a challenge, however, because chronic diseases such as asthma and diabetes usually require more than one medication. As people accumulate chronic diseases, their list of medicines grows. In Germany, one-quarter of older people are on at least five different medicines.[4] The prescription of multiple medicines is referred to as ***polypharmacy*** (see Chapter 34).

Creating reminders for patients and improving packaging can improve adherence. Pharmacists can dispense weekly medication boxes with multiple compartments organised by day of week and time of day.

Side effects are another major obstacle to adherence. If a patient experiences a symptom after starting a new tablet, they are likely to blame the new tablet. They may contact their GP to ask what they should do, or they may simply stop taking the medicine in question.

Case study 4.1

Josephine Jenkins is a 79-year-old widow who was discharged from hospital 10 days ago. Her daughter phones the GP to request a home visit because she is becoming breathless and seems to be having difficulty getting around the house. Mrs Jenkins lives by herself in a house with one toilet at the top of the stairs. She has suffered from COPD for the last 10 years. She is on treatment for hypertension, had a myocardial infarction 5 years ago and has osteoarthritis of her hips. She uses a stick to walk and is able to get up and down the stairs because there is a hand rail on both sides.

Mrs Jenkins' discharge letter states that while she was in hospital, she was treated for an infective exacerbation of her COPD with a course of antibiotics and steroids. She had an echocardiogram, which showed mild to moderate left ventricular failure. During her admission, her amlodipine was stopped and she was started on furosemide. She was discharged with a month's supply of the following medication:

- Aspirin dispersible tablets 75 mg daily.
- Ramipril capsules 5 mg daily.
- Simvastatin tablets 40 mg at night.
- Seretide Accuhaler 500 (fluticasone proprionate 500 μg/ salmeterol 50 μg) one puff twice a day.
- Tiotropium bromide inhaler 18 μg daily.
- Salbutamol inhaler 100 μg per inhalation, two puffs when needed.
- Paracetamol 500 mg tablets, two tablets four times a day.
- Codeine phosphate tablets 30 mg, four times a day if needed.
- Furosemide tablets 40 mg daily (at 8 am).

What aspects of Mrs Jenkins' medication should the GP review during the home visit?

The GP should find out what medicines she is actually taking. On returning home, she may have reverted to taking her usual list of tablets, which doesn't include furosemide. It appears that she has been diagnosed with left ventricular failure; this accounts for some of her breathlessness. The furosemide has been prescribed to treat this and to help her breathlessness. Another possibility is that she has stopped the furosemide intentionally because it makes her go to the toilet often, which she finds difficult because it means going up and down the stairs frequently. She may not understand what the furosemide is for.

The GP should check her inhaler technique. Her breathlessness may be partly due to an inability to use the salbutamol inhaler. She might find it easier to use a spacer device with the inhaler.

Her worsening mobility may be because of the pain in her hips. The GP needs to check how often she is taking the paracetamol. Is she taking it four times a day? She has been prescribed codeine to take as top-up pain relief. This may be making her constipated. If so, she will need some sort of laxative. Fear of becoming constipated may be preventing her from taking the codeine.

Excluding the codeine, she is meant to take a total of 12 tablets/capsules a day. She might find it easier to remember to take all of these if they were put in a cassette with compartments for each day of the week.

Safe prescribing using the 10 steps

A perfect medicine would be one that worked for everyone with the same diagnosis, that reduced the morbidity and mortality attributed to that diagnosis and that did so without causing any side effects. Perfection eludes us, so we have to use our imperfect medicines with particular care. The British Pharmacological Society (BPS) encourages doctors to think about 10 steps when prescribing in order to optimise safety (see Table 4.3).

Making a diagnosis

The first step is to be confident about the diagnosis. Sometimes, however, GPs initiate a therapeutic trial, meaning they try a patient on a particular treatment to test out their working diagnosis.

Establishing the therapeutic goal

The second step is to decide upon the goal of treatment. Is it to provide immediate relief of a particular symptom? Is it to prevent flare-ups of a disease? Is it to prevent complications of the disease and reduce mortality?

Choosing the therapeutic approach

Medication may not be the best way of achieving this goal. For instance, for someone with early osteoarthritis of the knee, weight reduction may be a much better way of controlling the progression of the disease than taking a tablet.

Choosing the drug

If medication does look like the best way of achieving the goal, the next decision is what medication to use. For any particular goal, there may be more than one class of drug to choose from,

Table 4.3 10 stages of prescribing.

Stage	Task
1	Make a diagnosis
2	Establish the therapeutic goal
3	Choose the therapeutic approach
4	Choose the drug
5	Choose the dose, route and frequency
6	Choose the duration of therapy
7	Write a prescription
8	Inform the patient
9	Monitor drug effects
10	Review/alter the prescription

Source: Ross, S and Maxwell, S. Prescribing and the core curriculum for tomorrow's doctors: BPS curriculum in clinical pharmacology and prescribing for medical students. *Br J Clin Pharmacol* 2012: **74**; 644–61.

and within that class, there may be several different drugs made by competing manufacturers. To gain a licence for a new drug, a manufacturer has to demonstrate its effectiveness and safety, but the role for that drug within the armoury of treatments for a particular condition may only become clear with the passage of time, as evidence accumulates. Large randomised controlled trials (RCTs) which aim to measure meaningful end points such as the serious complications of a disease or mortality take years to conduct. And it can take years for rare serious side effects to come to light, which might necessitate withdrawal of a drug from the market. The National Institute for Health and Care Excellence (NICE) periodically reviews the evidence for treatments of particular conditions and publishes guidelines which recommend the use of particular drugs, taking into account their cost-effectiveness. Local clinical commissioning groups (CCGs) may also make recommendations on what drugs GPs should prescribe, principally to control costs. Some CCGs have created formularies that specify which medicine GPs should select from a particular class of drugs.

Some medicines can cause foetal abnormalities. Thalidomide, a drug prescribed in the 1960s for sickness in pregnancy, is the most notorious example of this; it caused deformities of limbs. So, when choosing a medicine for a woman of childbearing age, it is important to consider whether she might be pregnant. If so, the BNF should be consulted to find out about the risks of the drugs in question in pregnancy. Medicines have the potential to do greatest harm in the first 12 weeks of pregnancy. Therefore, if at all possible, it is best to avoid prescribing during this time. If the woman has a chronic disease that needs ongoing treatment then it's important to warn her of the risks before she gets pregnant, and if necessary to switch to a safer medicine.

Breast-feeding is another factor to consider. Most medicines taken by a mother find their way into her breast milk. Usually, the amount in the breast milk is too small to do any harm, but once again it is important to consult the BNF and balance the potential risks against the potential benefit.

Choosing the dose, route and frequency

The correct dose of a particular drug depends on the patient's age and weight. There is a separate BNF for children, which expresses the correct dose as milligrams per kilogram body weight. Older people often need lower doses of medication. The route by which a drug is metabolised can also have a bearing on the dose. For drugs that are excreted by the kidneys, the dose needs to be reduced if the patient's estimated glomerular filtration rate (eGFR) is low. Some medicines, such as the antiepileptic drugs phenytoin and carbamazepine, enhance the effect of certain hepatic enzymes, and this has the knock-on effect of reducing the plasma level of drugs that are metabolised by the liver. The combined oral contraceptive pill is an example of a drug that is metabolised by the liver. Therefore, an oestrogen-containing contraceptive pill would not be the best choice for a woman who is taking phenytoin or carbamazepine.

Most medicines come as tablets or capsules and as a liquid. Children and some frail elderly patients find liquid preparations easier to take. Some medicines come as suppositories, which can be helpful if a patient is vomiting or unable to take anything by mouth. Rectal diazepam, for example, is useful for stopping a prolonged epileptic fit. Injectable forms are also helpful when a patient is too ill to take medication by mouth and when a rapid onset of action is needed. Table 4.4 lists the different routes of administration of drugs.

The frequency with which a drug has to be taken is determined by its half life. In general, tablets have to be taken once, twice, three times or four times a day. Four times a day is six-hourly, and is generally interpreted as taking the medicine with each meal (e.g. 8 am, 1 pm and 7 pm) and at bedtime. Modified-release forms of certain medicines can help with compliance, because the medicines can then be taken just once a day. Propranolol, for example, is an effective drug for preventing migraine; in its ordinary form, it has to be taken twice a day, but as a modified-release preparation, it can be taken once a day. The frequency of administration may influence the choice of drug. An antibiotic that has to be taken twice a day is more likely to be taken than one that has to be taken four times a day.

Choosing the duration of therapy

When one gives a patient a prescription for antibiotics, they will often say, 'I assume I should finish the course?' Usually, the answer is yes, but for some antibiotics it is not clear how long that course should be: 3 days is probably sufficient for treating a simple urinary tract infection (UTI), but for epididymo-orchitis a 6-week course of antibiotics may be needed. When treating chronic diseases such as ischaemic heart disease, the treatment may be lifelong.

Writing a prescription

An NHS prescription issued by a GP has to be written on a special form. Like a cheque, it has a unique serial number. Figure 4.1 shows how this form should be completed.

Information identifying the patient is written at the top of the prescription. For infants and children, it is also worth writing their weight here. This makes it easier to check that the dose is correct.

The medicine itself can be written in generic form or as a particular brand. In general, it works out cheaper if a drug is prescribed generically, because then the pharmacist will select the brand that is cheapest. There are exceptions to this guidance, and in some cases it is preferable to prescribe by brand. Slow-release preparations of drugs are best prescribed by brand because, for the same total dose, the release characteristics may vary. For instance, if a patient's epilepsy is well controlled on one brand of slow-release carbamazepine, switching to an alternative brand might increase the risk of the patient having a fit.

The dose of the medicine can be indicated using a Latin abbreviation (Table 4.5). The pharmacist will translate this into plain English instructions when labelling the medicine container. It can be helpful if the GP writes the directions in a bit more detail. For instance, when prescribing a statin, instead of writing 'on' (omne nocte), they can write, 'Take one tablet at night to lower the cholesterol'. Reminding the patient what the drug is for might improve adherence.

GPs can also make things easier for patients by specifying the font size of the label. Patients with poor vision often struggle with labels and rely on the colour of the tablet or the packet. This is one reason why they complain when pharmacists

Table 4.4 Routes of administration of drugs.		
Route of administration	**Example drug**	**Example of condition that this drug is used for**
Mouth (tablet/capsule)	Amoxicillin capsule	Community-acquired chest infection
Mouth (liquid)	Amoxicillin suspension	Otitis media in child under 2 years
Mouth (sublingual)	Glyceryl trinitrate spray	Angina
Mouth (aerosol inhaler)	Salbutamol inhaler	Asthma
Subcutaneous injection	Insulin	Diabetes
Deep intramuscular injection	Prochlorperazine	Vomiting associated with renal colic
Intravenous injection	Furosemide	Acute left ventricular failure
Skin (patch)	Nicotine patch	Smoking cessation
Skin (cream/ointment)	Clobetasone ointment	Eczema
Ear (drops/spray)	Gentisone HC drops	Otitis externa
Nose (drops/spray)	Flixonase spray	Allergic rhinitis
Eye (drops/ointment)	Latanoprost	Glaucoma
Genital (pessary)	Clotrimazole pessary	Vaginal thrush
Rectal (suppository)	Diazepam	Status epilepticus

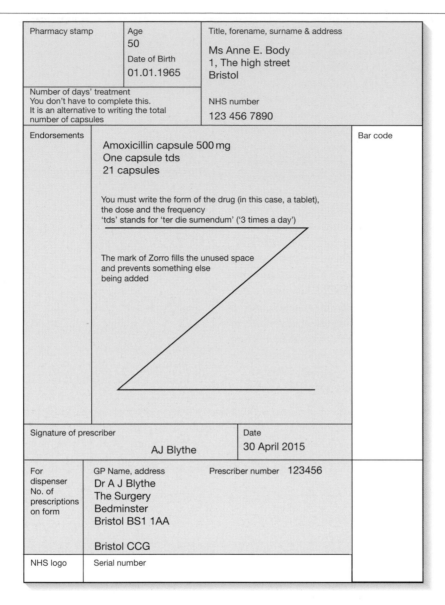

Figure 4.1 FP10 prescription form.

Table 4.5 Latin abbreviations commonly used on prescriptions.

Abbreviation	Latin	English translation
od	omne in die	every day
om	omne mane	every morning
on	omne nocte	every night
bd	bis in die	twice a day
tds	ter die sumendum	three times a day
qds	quater die sumendus	four times a day
prn	pro re nata	as needed
stat	statim	immediately

dispense a different brand of medicines from month to month. If a patient is known to have poor vision, the GP can write on the prescription, 'Please put instructions in large font'.

The GP can indicate the quantity of medicine to be issued in one of two ways: by writing the number of days that the medicine is to be taken for or by writing the total quantity. For controlled drugs (opiates and other drugs of abuse), the GP has to write the dose *and* the total quantity in both words and figures, so that there can be absolutely no doubt about the amount the pharmacist has to dispense.

Patients pay the same prescription charge regardless of the quantity that is written on the prescription. Thus, a patient has to pay the same for 7 antihistamine tablets as they do for 60. This puts some pressure on the GP to prescribe large quantities; in general, GPs prescribe 1 or 2 months' supply of a medication at a time.

Informing the patient

As the GP hands the prescription to the patient, it is worth their while reading it aloud. Doing so is a good way of checking that they have written what they intended and is an opportunity to reinforce the instructions that they have given the patient. Computers make prescribing quick, but being presented with a picking list can be hazardous. Type in 'Penicill…', planning to select Pencillin, and the computer will offer a list of drugs beginning with these letters. Amongst them will be penicillamine, a drug with lots of potential side effects that is used in the treatment of rheumatoid arthritis. In haste, it is all too easy to click on the wrong medicine in the options list, with potentially harmful results.

For some patients, it can be a good idea to write down some more detailed instructions on a separate sheet of paper or to issue them with an information sheet or a special card. Patients on a long course of steroids should not stop taking them abruptly, and in the event of illness they may need to increase their dose. For this reason, they should be issued with a card to carry in their wallet stating that they are on steroids.

Monitoring drug effects

Monitoring the response may mean reviewing the patient's symptoms, asking about potential side effects, measuring something such as their blood pressure or doing some investigations. The disease-modifying drugs that are used for patients with rheumatoid arthritis require particular care, and at the start require weekly or fortnightly blood tests to check for renal and hepatic toxicity. Table 4.6 lists some of the common and important medicines that need to be monitored with blood tests.

Patients may volunteer information about possible side effects, but sometimes they may be embarrassed to do so.

Table 4.6 Medicines that need monitoring with blood tests.

Medicines	Usage	Tests that have to be done	Frequency with which these tests have to be done	Potential side effects that may be identified
Warfarin	Stroke prevention in atrial fibrillation	INR	At least every 12 weeks, depending on stability of INR	Danger of haemorrhage as result of INR > 5
ACE inhibitors	Hypertension, heart failure	Urea and electrolytes (U&Es)	Before starting, 7–10 days after each dose, on increase in dose and every year	Worsening renal function
Diuretics	Heart failure	U&Es	At least once a year	Hypokalaemia
Digoxin	Atrial fibrillation, heart failure	U&Es	At least once a year	Hypokalaemia increases risk of digoxin toxicity
Statin	Hypercholesterolaemia	Liver function tests (LFTs)	Before starting, 3 months after starting and 1 year after starting	Hepatic toxicity (rise in ALT)
Lithium	Mania and bipolar disorders	Serum lithium (12 hours after last dose)	Weekly until on stable dose, then every 3 months	Lithium toxicity: ataxia, dysarthria, convulsions, nystagmus and tremor
		U&Es	6 months	Renal impairment
		Thyroid function tests (TFTs)	6 months	Hypothyroidism
Allopurinol	Gout	U&Es	1 year	Renal impairment
		Serum urate	After every change in dose and every year	Undertreatment
Sulfasalazine	Inflammatory bowel disease, rheumatoid arthritis	Full blood count (FBC)	Before starting, every month for first 3 months	Anaemia
		LFT		Hepatic toxicity
Methotrexate	Psoriasis, rheumatoid arthritis	U&Es	Before starting, every 1–2 weeks until treatment stabilised, then every 2–3 months	Renal impairment
		FBC		Bone marrow suppression: neutropenia and/or thrombocytopenia
		LFTs		Cirrhosis of liver

(Continued)

Table 4.6 (*Continued*)

Medicines	Usage	Tests that have to be done	Frequency with which these tests have to be done	Potential side effects that may be identified
Levothyroxine	Hypothyroidism	TFTs	2 months after any change in dose and every year	Under- or overtreatment
Nitrofurantoin	Prevention of UTI	LFT	Every year if on the drug for >1 year	Cholestatic jaundice, hepatitis

The SSRIs, for example, can affect people's ability to have an orgasm.

Reviewing and altering the prescription

If the patient is not responding as one would expect, or if the side effects are intolerable, then the dose must be altered or an alternative must be recommended. There are often no hard and fast rules about when it's best to increase the dose rather than stop and try something else. The patient's view may be crucial in deciding what to do.

Following these 10 steps will improve one's prescribing. Try to implement them for Case study 4.2.

Case study 4.2

A 40-year-old man has had a cough and fever for the last 48 hours. He is coughing up green sputum but has not coughed up any blood. He also has a mild headache, and when he coughs the centre of his chest hurts. As a child, he was given amoxicillin and came out in a rash. He doesn't take any regular medication. He smokes 20 cigarettes a day. He is a plumber and has not travelled abroad in recent months. On examination, he has a temperature of 38.5 °C. His oxygen saturation is 95% on air. The base of his left lung is dull to percussion, and you can hear coarse crackles in the same zone.

What would you prescribe for him?
- **Step 1:** The history of fever, headache and painful cough all point to a community-acquired lower respiratory tract infection (RTI) or pneumonia. His smoking makes him more susceptible to such an infection. The fact that he hasn't been abroad recently makes rare causes of pneumonia, like Legionella, less likely. The findings on examination are all consistent with a left lower lobe infection.
- **Step 2:** There are several goals of treatment: to make him feel better, prevent the complications of pneumonia, prevent hospitalisation and get him back to work.
- **Step 3:** Antibiotics offer the main hope of achieving these goals. Analgesic drugs such as paracetamol may be helpful, too. If he was older, physiotherapy might be helpful.
- **Step 4:** The most likely pathogen responsible for this infection is *Streptococcus pneumoniae*, a Gram-positive bacterium. This is sensitive to penicillin, so the first-line choice of antibiotic would be amoxicillin. However, the patient is allergic to penicillin. Some patients who are allergic to penicillin are also allergic to cephalosporins, so these should be avoided too. A macrolide antibiotic is therefore the preferred option.
- **Step 5:** There are four macrolides to choose from, but only two of them – clarithromycin and erythromycin – tend be used for community-acquired respiratory infections. Clarithromycin has to be taken twice a day, whereas erythromycin, which is a bit cheaper, has to be taken four times a day. Both these antibiotics are available in oral form. The standard dose of clarithromycin is 250 mg twice a day, but for pneumonia or severe infections like this, 500 mg twice a day is recommended. If the patient had severe renal impairment, you would have to decrease the dose.
- **Step 6:** The standard length of treatment for a respiratory infection is 1 week, but if the patient had bronchiectasis, you might consider giving a 2-week course.
- **Step 7:** When you write the prescription, run through these instructions with the patient.
- **Step 8:** Macrolides interact with some medicines, including the statins. This patient is not on any other medication. If he was on a statin, you would have to tell him to stop the statin temporarily. Macrolides can make people feel nauseated, so you should warn him about this. You should tell him to take the first dose as soon as possible and then the second dose about 12 hours later. If it's noon now, he should not wait until the evening to take his first dose.

- **Step 9:** It's important to give patients realistic expectations of treatment. The cough is unlikely to go completely for at least 2 weeks, but he should not be getting any worse in 2 days' time. If he feels that he is getting worse, he should return.

- **Step 10:** If he doesn't respond to this course of antibiotics, you should examine him again and consider investigations such as a chest X-ray. You might prescribe a different antibiotic and you might even have to consider admission to hospital.

Prescribing errors

For a long time, many newly qualified doctors have not felt confident about prescribing.[5] In their first year after qualification, doctors make errors on 8% of all prescriptions that they write, although most of these mistakes are spotted and corrected by hospital pharmacists before the medication is dispensed. In their second year after qualification, the error rate of doctors is even higher (10%), perhaps because they start to get complacent and do not check things in the BNF before prescribing.[6] In an attempt to ensure that all newly qualified doctors have acquired the minimum level of knowledge and skill required for safe prescribing, the Medical Schools Council and the BPS have collaborated on the development of new learning resources for prescribing and on the creation of a Prescribing Safety Assessment.[7] All medical students now have to sit and pass this exam or its equivalent before starting work as doctors.

Qualified GPs make prescribing errors, too. Research into the causes of prescribing errors in the community, commissioned by the General Medical Council (GMC), showed that over a 1-year period, prescriptions for one in eight patients contained an error.[8] Most errors were minor, such as writing insufficient information on the prescription or getting timing of doses wrong. But 1 in 550 prescription items contained a serious error, such as the prescription of a medicine for which the patient had a recorded drug allergy or contraindication. The study also showed that there were frequent failings to monitor medication.

The authors of the study conducted interviews with the GPs who had written the prescriptions in order to explore why errors occurred and what mechanisms were in place to minimise them. GPs talked about the pressure of time and having to make treatment decisions quickly during consultations. The signing and reviewing of prescriptions tended to be squeezed in between other activities during the day, often when there were many interruptions. The pressure on GPs' time was not the only issue. There was an increased risk of error if the standard dose needed adjustment because of the patient's age, weight or renal function. If the GP knew the patient well, there was a risk of them becoming complacent and failing to check the patient's notes for contraindications before prescribing a new drug.

Keeping up to date with new medicines and the new evidence that is published on old medicines is a cause of error. What might be considered good practice now may be viewed as a prescribing error in the future: 20 years ago, a beta blocker and a thiazide diuretic were often used together to treat hypertension; now, this combination is considered suboptimal, because of the increased risk of the recipient developing diabetes. Conversely, prescribing practices deemed inappropriate in the past can become acceptable. COPD was once considered an absolute contraindication to the use of beta blockers. Now, it is considered appropriate to start beta blockers if a patient has COPD and heart failure.

Several mechanisms exist for reducing the risk of prescribing errors. The pharmacists who dispense the medication can elaborate on the instructions to make them clearer for the patient. If a pharmacist is concerned about the dosage, they will try to contact the prescriber to check what was intended. Pharmacists are also encouraged to conduct medication usage reviews with patients. These reviews may reveal that the patient is not taking certain medicines or that there are potential harmful interactions between the different medicines that they are taking.

All GPs have systems in place for reviewing repeat prescriptions. Commonly, a limit of 6 months is put on a patient's list of repeat medications. If a patient requests any of their repeat medication after this time, this fact is brought to the attention of the GP, who can review the patient's notes and if necessary ask to see the patient. However, the importance of a medication review is not always clear to patients, and when they come to see the GP they often bring a list of other things that they want sorting out.

There are ongoing initiatives to monitor the safety of prescribing in general practice, based on the prevalence of certain prescribing errors.[9] Table 4.7 lists 23 key errors that pose a high or extreme risk to the patient.

	Table 4.7 Markers of dangerous/poor prescribing.	
	Indicator	**Increased risk of**
1	Prescription of aspirin or clopidogrel without PPI to someone who has had a peptic ulcer or gastrointestinal bleed	Gastrointestinal haemorrhage
2	Prescription of diltiazem or verapamil to patient with heart failure	Worsening cardiac function

(Continued)

Table 4.7 (Continued)

	Indicator	Increased risk of
3	Prescription of a beta blocker to someone with asthma who does not also have cardiac disease	Bronchospasm, worsening asthma
4	Prescription of an antipsychotic for >6 weeks to someone >65 years with dementia but without psychosis	Stroke
5	Prescription of mefloquine to a patient with a history of convulsions	Convulsions
6	Prescription of glitazone to a patient with heart failure	Heart failure
7	Prescription of metformin to a patient with eGFR < 30	Lactic acidosis
8	Prescription of oral prednisolone in a dose of 7.5 mg or more for >3 months, without osteoporosis-preventing treatment	Osteoporosis
9	Prescription of combined oral contraceptive pill to a woman with a body mass index (BMI) > 40	Thrombo-embolism
10	Prescription of a nonsteroidal anti-inflammatory drug (NSAID) without PPI to someone with a history of peptic ulcer	Gastrointestinal haemorrhage
11	Prescription of an NSAID to a patient with heart failure	Worsening heart failure
12	Prescription of an NSAID to a patient with eGFR < 45	Worsening renal function
13	Prescription of allopurinol at dose of >200 mg/day to at patient with eGFR < 30	Worsening renal function
14	Prescription of warfarin and aspirin in combination without gastric protection.	Gastrointestinal haemorrhage
15	Concurrent use of warfarin and any antibiotic without monitoring the INR within 5 days	Severe haemorrhage
16	Prescription of phosphodiesterase type-5 inhibitor (e.g. Viagra) to a patient who is on a nitrate or nicorandil	Severe hypotension
17	Prescription of a potassium sparing diuretic (e.g. spironolactone) to a patient who is also on an ACE inhibitor	Hyperkalaemia
18	Prescription of itraconazole with statin at dose of 80 mg or more	Myopathy
19	Prescription of trimethoprim for >7 days to someone who is on methotrexate	Haematological toxicity
20	Prescription of macrolide antibiotic to someone who is also taking a statin, with no evidence that they have been told to stop the statin temporarily	Myopathy
21	Patient aged >75 on loop diuretic who has not had their U&Es checked within the last 15 months	Hypokalaemia
22	Patient on an ACE inhibitor or angiotensin II receptor antagonist who has not had their U&Es checked within the last 15 months	Renal impairment
23	Patient on lithium who has not had their serum lithium level checked within the last 6 months	Lithium toxicity

Source: Adapted from Spencer et al. 2014.[9]

Reporting adverse drug reactions

If a patient is suspected to have had an adverse drug reaction, a Yellow Card (found at the back of the BNF) should be completed and sent to the Medicines and Healthcare products Regulatory Agency (MHRA). Doctors are encouraged to do this for any possible reaction to a new medicine or for any serious reaction to an established medicine. This is one of the main ways in which the safety of medicines is monitored in the UK.

The vast majority of prescribing takes place in primary care. There is a growing volume of medication that is issued on repeat prescription. Within this rising tide of medicines, wastage, nonadherence and prescription errors are common. When learning how to prescribe, it is important to get into good habits from the start. GPs can improve the quality of their prescribing by following guidelines and by putting in place systems to check for errors. GPs also have an important role in controlling the costs of prescribing.

SUMMARY

 Now visit **www.wileyessential.com/primarycare** to test yourself on this chapter.

REFERENCES

1. Health and Social Care Information Centre. Prescription Cost Analysis, England – 2014 [NS]. 8 April 2015. Available from: http://www.hscic.gov.uk/searchcatalogue?productid=17711&topics=0%2fPrescribing&sort=Relevance&size=10&page=1#top (last accessed 6 October 2015).

2. Vrigens B, Vincze G, Kristanto P, et al. Adherence to prescribed antihypertensive drug treatments: longitudinal study of electronically compiled dosing histories. *BMJ* 2008;**336**:1114.

3. Schroeder K, Fahey K, Ebrahim S. How can we improve adherence to blood pressure-lowering medication in ambulatory care? *Arch Intern Med* 2004;**164**:722–32.

4. Julius-Walker U, Theile G, Hummers-Pradier E. Prevalence and predictors of polypharmacy among older primary care patients in Germany. *Fam Pract* 2007;**24**(1):14–19.

5. Illing J, Peile E, Morrison J, et al. How Prepared are Medical Graduates to Begin Practice? A Comparison of Three Diverse UK Medical Schools. Final Summary and Conclusions for the GMC Education Committee. General Medical Council 2008. Available from: http://www.gmc-uk.org/FINAL_How_prepared_are_medical_graduates_to_begin_practice_September_08.pdf_29697834.pdf (last accessed 6 October 2015).

6. Dornan T, Ashcroft D, Heathfield H, et al. An in depth investigation into causes of prescribing errors by foundation trainees in relation to their medical education – EQUIP study. General Medical Council 2009. Available from: http://www.gmc-uk.org/FINAL_Report_prevalence_and_causes_of_prescribing_errors.pdf_28935150.pdf (last accessed 6 October 2015).

7. Maxwell SRJ. An agenda for UK clinical pharmacology. How should teaching of undergraduates in clinical pharmacology and therapeutics be delivered and assessed? *Br J Clin Pharmacol* 2012;**73**:6:893–9.

8. Avery T, Barber N, Ghaleb M, et al. Investigating the Prevalence and Causes of Prescribing Errors in General Practice: The PRACtICe Study. General Medical Council, 2 May 2012. Available from: http://www.gmc-uk.org/about/research/12996.asp (last accessed 6 October 2015).

9. Spencer RE, Bell B, Avery AJ, et al. Identification of an updated set of prescribing – safety indicators for GPs. *Br J Gen Pract* 2014;**64**(621):e181–90.

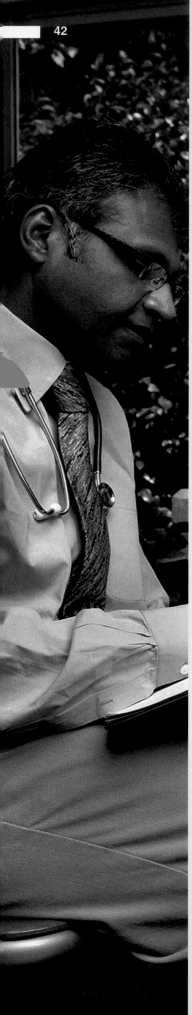

CHAPTER 5

The interface with secondary care

Sarah Jahfar
Teaching Fellow in Primary Care, University of Bristol

Key topics

Learning objectives

- Understand why referrals are made and what factors affect referral.
- Consider the advantages and disadvantages of the current referral system.
- Be aware of the '2-week-wait suspected cancer' referral system.
- Be aware of processes around admission to and discharge from hospital and the importance of communication between primary and secondary care.

Essential Primary Care, First Edition. Edited by Andrew Blythe and Jessica Buchan.
© 2017 John Wiley & Sons, Ltd. Published 2017 by John Wiley & Sons, Ltd.
Companion website: www.wileyessential.com/primarycare

Introduction

Effective communication between primary and secondary care is vital if we are to provide good-quality care.[1] GPs support patients on their journeys from primary to secondary care. This provides continuity of care during referrals and following admissions, helping patients with decision-making, treatment, recovery and, in some cases, end-of-life care; all of which can be an immensely rewarding part of our role.

Primary care interfaces with secondary care with regards to:

- referral of patients for hospital tests and admissions (either routine or emergency);
- discharge of patients from hospital;
- ongoing outpatient follow-up;
- verbal or written communication between GP and secondary care;
- continuing professional development for doctors.

Referring patients to secondary care

Making referrals is a major part of the GP's role.[2] Approximately 1 in 20 GP consultations results in a referral. This may involve a transfer of clinical responsibility from the GP to a wide range of professionals or a request for a diagnostic test unavailable in general practice. When deciding to refer, we have to balance many different and often competing factors, such as patient expectations, national and local clinical guidance and resource and cost implications.

Why do GPs refer?

Referrals are made for a variety of reasons:

- to establish or confirm a diagnosis;
- for treatment or an operation unavailable in primary care;
- for a specific test or investigation unavailable in primary care;
- for specialist advice on management of an established diagnosis;
- so that a specialist can take over management;
- reassurance for the GP;
- reassurance and/or a second opinion for the patient or their family;
- to manage the risk of litigation.

Factors which influence referral rates

There are wide variations in rates of referral. Evidence on why this should be the case is conflicting.[3] Variation in referral rates among GPs cannot be explained by inappropriate referrals.[4] Patient deprivation increases rates,[5] while GPs who have specialist training in an area of medicine may end up referring more in that area.[6] Taken together, patient factors (age, sex and social class) and practice characteristics (size, distance from the nearest hospital) only explain up to 50% of the observed variation.[7] Table 5.1 lists factors that have been found to affect the rate of GP referral.

Significance of referral rates

Inappropriate or excessive referral rates are expensive to the NHS and can be dangerous for patients and GPs. A referral may worsen the condition of a patient who is already over-somatising. Multiple referrals may create a 'collusion of anonymity'[8] – too many doctors are advising the patient and no one is taking overall responsibility. GPs who refer too often may become deskilled.

Low referral rates may also be a problem. GPs who rarely refer may be depriving their patients of a specialist opinion and the most up-to-date treatment, which could have a negative effect on a patient's health. The GP may think that they are delivering the best care but may be unaware of new interventions that might benefit their patients.

Table 5.1 Factors associated with referral rates.

GP or practice factors	Patient factors	Structural factors
GP beliefs or expectations about benefits of referral	Severity of symptoms	Distance to specialist service
GP age or experience	Desire for referral	Area deprivation
GP gender	Age	Availability or accessibility of specialist care
Degree of training in relevant specialty	Gender	
GP–patient relationship, congruence between GP's and patient's attitudes	Social class	Availability of community alternatives to specialist care
	Diagnosis	
GP relationship with specialist	Co-morbidities	Time available for consultation
Practice size	Help-seeking behaviour (delayed or prompt patient action around illness)	
Services available in practice		
GP psychological characteristics – for example, ability to tolerate uncertainty, concern that non-referral might damage patient relationships	Perception of the problem	
	Attitudes towards treatment	

Source: Armstrong et al. (1988, 1991); Ashworth et al. (2002).

Choose and Book

With the expansion of consultant numbers, changes in available services and the advent of 'Choose and Book' in England (a 'national electronic referral service which gives patients a choice of place, date and time for their first outpatient appointment in a hospital or clinic'[9]), referrals are usually generic, rather than personal to a specific consultant.

Quality of referrals

It is important for students and doctors to understand what constitutes a high-quality referral. It should contain all relevant information about the patient, their condition, what it is hoped will be achieved by the referral and an indication of the urgency.

Box 5.1 lists the essential features of a high-quality referral letter. A referral should be **necessary**, **timely** and **sent to the most appropriate specialist**. Although this seems obvious, it is not always clear to whom the referral should be sent. For example, if a patient with rheumatoid and osteoarthritis is struggling to walk and has pain in the hands, shoulders and knees, should the GP make a referral to a GP with a specialist interest (GPSI) in musculoskeletal problems or to a consultant rheumatologist, consultant orthopaedic surgeon, physiotherapist, occupational therapist or pain clinic? Box 5.2 lists the different people and agencies to which GPs can refer their patients. Ongoing communication between primary and secondary care is needed to maintain knowledge of referral pathways.

Increasingly, in an effort to reduce inappropriate or unnecessary referrals, to improve their quality, to ensure that patients

---

Case study 5.1a

Abdi Mohamed, age 36, has severe psoriasis which is unresponsive to maximal therapy. His GP, Dr Simpson, thinks that he will benefit from a dermatological opinion, with a view to possible treatment with PUVA (ultraviolet light therapy in conjunction with psoralen medication). Dr Simpson dictates a referral letter to dermatology (see Case study 5.1b) and her secretary sends this to the Choose and Book admin team. Mr Mohamed is advised that he will receive a letter with a password at his home address in a few days' time.

Mr Mohamed receives the letter and goes online to the Choose and Book website, rather than calling the appointments line. He inputs his password and is offered some appointments to choose from. Two of them are in the local hospital and another is in a community setting. Mr Mohamed opts to be seen at the hospital. In due course, he receives full confirmation of his appointment in the post.

Case study 5.1b

Dr Simpson's letter is on the GP practice's headed notepaper and includes the date, Mr Mohamed's full name, date of birth, address, telephone contact details and NHS number.

Dear Dermatology Colleagues,
Problem: Chronic widespread plaque psoriasis unresponsive to topical therapies
I would be grateful if you could see this 36-year-old man with severe psoriasis and advise regarding further treatment options.
Mr Mohamed has suffered from psoriasis for 10 years. It is usually well controlled with hydromol ointment for washing and as an emollient afterwards, calcipotriol ointment and occasional courses of Betnovate for flare-ups. He finds that his skin is worse in winter. It improved greatly when he spent 2 months in Africa last year. Mr Mohamed finds the plaques unsightly and embarrassing. Fortunately, he does not have any joint involvement. He has never seen a dermatologist, nor had any second-line treatments.
He moved to the UK from Somalia with his wife and three children 4 years ago and speaks good English. Mr Mohamed does not drink alcohol, smokes 20 cigarettes a day and works as a porter in the Royal Infirmary.

What else does the consultant team need to know?
The consultant needs to know if Mr Mohamed has any other significant illnesses, if he takes medication for anything other than psoriasis and if he has any allergies. Dr Simpson should explain what expectations Mr Mohamed has about this referral. Dr Simpson finishes the letter thus:

Mr Mohamed has a past history of hepatitis B.
He has no drug allergies and only uses the creams listed above.
Mr Mohamed is aware that you may offer him oral medication or consider him for PUVA. I have provided him with information from www.patient.co.uk and have restarted him on Betnovate ointment pending his appointment with you.
Yours faithfully,
Dr S Simpson

The history of hepatitis B is very important, as it could influence the dermatologist's decision with regards to oral immunosuppressant medication if it remains active. Omission of this past history could, in a worst-case scenario, endanger the patient's life.

Box 5.1 Essential content of a referral letter

- Intended destination of referral.
- Name of patient.
- Address and phone numbers.
- Date of birth.
- NHS number.
- Name of GP and practice.
- Address/contact details.
- Reason for referral, with history of condition, examination findings and tests thus far.
- GP thoughts and patient expectations for the referral.
- Past medical history.
- Current/past medication and allergies.
- Relevant family history.
- Relevant psychosocial history.
- Assessment of urgency.
- Information given to patient.

Box 5.2 Agencies to whom GPs can make referrals

- Another GP in the practice or a GPSI.
- Another member of the primary health care team (nurse, health care assistant (HCA), physiotherapist, counsellor, podiatrist).
- Consultants: NHS or private.
- Hospital departments: e.g. speech therapy, occupational therapy, orthotics.
- Social workers.
- Alternative/complementary therapists (usually non-NHS).
- Voluntary and charitable organisations.
- Psychologists.

are seen in the most convenient venue and to save the NHS money, clinical commissioning groups (CCGs) are setting up **referral reviews** in primary care. A clinician, such as a GPSI, vets all letters before they are sent. A small percentage of referrals are returned to the referring doctor with suggestions for management in primary care or use of an alternative pathway. As well as ensuring that referrals are timely and necessary, these referral reviews also have an educational role, as they allow case studies and information about management alternatives and other local pathways to be shared with GPs.

The GP as gatekeeper: advantages and disadvantages

Historically, GPs in the UK have acted as 'gatekeepers' to referrals. This means that patients cannot refer themselves directly to see a specialist, whether NHS or private, and must go through their GP first. A&E departments and sexual health clinics have always been exceptions to this rule; patients can go directly to

these services. Recently, some other services, such as psychology and physiotherapy, have started to offer direct access. As patients gain direct access to more services, our role is changing and we are becoming facilitators to referral, as well as gatekeepers.

Advantages

At the moment GPs still gate-keep referrals to the majority of secondary care and there are some good reasons in support of this. In making the referral, the GP learns how the patient is managing their health and is then in a good position to follow the patient up through the process of investigation and treatment. It is satisfying to support a patient throughout the course of their illness and the patient enjoys continuity. Observing the patient's journey can be a rich source of learning and keeps the GP's knowledge up to date. From the patient's perspective, the gatekeeper role relieves them of responsibility for deciding whether or not they need to see a specialist and, if so, of what type. This saves both the patient and the NHS money on unnecessary referrals or referrals to an inappropriate agency.

Disadvantages

The gatekeeper role places a lot of responsibility on the GP. Patients may feel that their access to health care is being restricted inappropriately and, if they are right, this restriction may lead to worse health outcomes. The GP may feel pressurised by some patients to refer inappropriately. The local funding organisation (CCG) may put pressure on GPs to save money by reducing referrals, which may not always be appropriate.

The 2-week referral system for suspected cancers

A special fast-track referral system exists for patients who may have cancer. This is known as the '2-week wait'. Under this system, the hospital must receive the GP's referral within 24 hours of the GP seeing the patient. In return, the hospital specialist must see the patient within 2 weeks.

Each area of the body (head and neck, lower gastrointestinal tract, etc.) has its own referral form, which lists the criteria for a 2-week-wait referral. These forms are a very useful resource and revision aid for medical students and doctors, and they remind us of the 'red flag' symptoms and signs that require urgent referral.

Patient access to referral letters

In 1999, a study investigated whether sending patients a copy of their referral letter might reduce non-attendance at outpatient departments. Its conclusion was that copy letters were ineffective in this regard.[10] There are other pros and cons to copying letters to patients. Giving patients copies of their referral letter may empower them. Patients want copies,[11] and refusing to provide such information, if they do, is denying their autonomy. Knowing that the patient will receive a copy may improve the letter's accuracy: accuracy levels are 63–95% when letters are assessed by doctors, 25–43% when assessed by patients.

An electronic health and medical record is vital if we are to develop an integrated NHS. Patients have a right to know what is being written about them. If such material is stored electronically, patients must be informed under the rules of the Data Protection Act and in accordance with the common law on confidentiality.

Clinicians are concerned that recording suspicions of serious disease or other background issues could be unnecessarily upsetting to patients, but this has not been shown to be a significant problem.[12]

The NHS plan states that all patients should be given copies of all letters about them. Patients are given this option when they attend hospitals, but not all GPs offer it systematically. Things are changing, and from April 2015 all practices in England have been obliged to offer patients online access to their GP records, although not in their entirety.[13] This is part of an NHS programme called 'Patient Online', which is designed to support GP practices in offering and promoting online services to patients, including access to records, online appointment booking and online repeat prescriptions. It will be interesting to see what effect this has on patients and doctors.

Admitting patients to hospital

Emergency admission

GPs frequently deal with emergencies, either in an 'on-call' clinic, during a home visit or in the occasional routine appointment. Once we have decided that urgent hospital care is required, we either call 999 – in acute conditions such as myocardial infarction or severe asthma – or ring the hospital to speak to the person responsible for admissions. Depending on the department, this may be a senior nurse in charge of an admissions unit, a GP working in the GP support unit (GPSU), an F1 or F2 doctor or a specialist trainee. We discuss the case and arrange the admission. Occasionally, the admitting nurse or doctor will suggest an alternative route which may be more suitable, such as an emergency outpatient clinic. We then write a referral letter for the patient to give to the admitting team. Depending on their clinical condition, the patient will be sent in by ambulance or taxi or driven by a friend or family member.

Increasing social deprivation and older age are strongly linked to higher rates of emergency admission.[14]

The number of emergency admissions to hospital peaks every winter. Part of the reason for this is the rise of influenza, which in a typical winter in the UK is responsible for about 12 500 deaths. There is some evidence that vaccinating against influenza reduces the number of emergency admissions due to respiratory illness, as well as attendances at A&E and GP surgeries.[15] Therefore, each year, GPs offer vaccination against influenza to all their patients over 65, to children (the age range is being extended every year) and to people under 65 who are in certain risk groups (see Table 5.2). There are many strains of influenza. Each year, a vaccine is prepared to offer protection

Table 5.2 Risk groups to whom influenza vaccine is offered every year.	
People with	**Includes**
Chronic respiratory disease	Those with asthma who are on regular inhaled steroid; everyone with COPD
Chronic cardiac disease	Those with heart failure or ischaemic heart disease
Chronic kidney disease	Stage 3, 4 or 5
Chronic liver disease	Those with alcoholic liver disease, hepatitis B or C
Chronic neurological disease	Those with multiple sclerosis, Parkinson's or a learning disability
Diabetes	
Those who are	
Immunosuppressed	Those with HIV or who are on cancer treatment
Pregnant	
Carers	
Frontline health professionals	Nurses, doctors

against the three strains which the WHO predicts are most likely to be in circulation. Adults are given an inactivated vaccine in a single subcutaneous injection. Children are given a live attenuated vaccine in a nasal spray.

Admission avoidance schemes

All areas of the UK have admission avoidance schemes, although they tend to differ according to local priorities and needs.[16, 17] Most patients and GPs are very keen to avoid admission – not only is it very expensive to the NHS, but patients know that they eat and sleep better and avoid the risk of hospital-acquired infections at home.

GPs have increasing access to investigations, such as blood tests, computed tomography (CT), magnetic resonance imaging (MRI) and ultrasound scans, which can be carried out on an urgent basis and may avoid admission. Sometimes, an admission seems like the only option because the patient's condition is deteriorating and the wait for an outpatient appointment is too long. To fill this gap in the service, hospitals have introduced *hot clinics*, in which patients are seen within 24 hours of referral. At the clinic appointment, the patient is assessed by a senior clinician and can have a battery of tests done at once. Usually, the patient can return home with a diagnosis and treatment plan, but occasionally the patient needs admission from clinic.

In England, all patients over the age of 75 now have a *named GP*. This offers better continuity of care, which is associated with reduced emergency department attendance and emergency hospital admissions.[18] Patients who have already had multiple admissions are given the option of having a *care plan*. This is a standardised form, reviewed regularly, which lists the patient's contact details, next of kin, usual state of health and ability to self-care, medication, preferred place of care (home, hospital, hospice, nursing home, etc.) and preferred place of death. We also discuss resuscitation status with the patient and their carer and mark the decision on the care plan. This then gets circulated, with the patient's consent, to the ambulance service, out-of-hours teams and district nurses. This should mean that, for example, terminally ill patients who wish to die at home can avoid an out-of-hours doctor calling an ambulance when they deteriorate.

Community matrons (CM) and *community nurses for older people (CNOP)* have their own caseload of patients at risk of admission, such as those with COPD or heart failure, and monitor their patients closely. In many parts of the country, *telehealth* has been introduced to help CMs and CNOPs monitor patients with chronic conditions. The patient's home is fitted with a base unit, which is connected to the telephone landline and a power socket or to a mobile phone. The base unit receives electronic signals from sensors positioned on equipment such as scales, a sphygmomanometer or a pulse oximeter, and the results are relayed to the monitoring centre. The CM or CNOP will be alerted to any significant change, which indicates a home visit is needed. Research evidence on the cost-effectiveness and benefits of telehealth have been variable.[19]

Some hospitals have a *GPSU*. This is situated within the hospital but is run by GPs. These GPs assess the patient,

discuss the case with the patient's own GP, have full access to hospital investigations and may be able to confirm or refute a diagnosis and send the patient home the same day. As this work-up is all done by a GP, it is not considered to be an admission and is both more convenient for the patient and cheaper for the NHS.

Community nursing, physiotherapy and occupational therapy teams, variously known as *rapid response* or *hospital at home*,[20] accept referrals from both GPs and secondary care. They can go into a patient's home up to four times a day, checking blood tests, making observations, conducting electrocardiograms (ECGs), administering oral or intramuscular medication and dressing wounds, thus avoiding the need for an admission. These teams also have access to 'safe haven' beds, usually in a local nursing home. Here, the patient will be safely looked after by nurses and treated in the community by a GP.

Discharge from hospital

Communication is crucial upon discharge, particularly in complicated cases or with vulnerable patients. A poor discharge can result in readmission and puts patients at serious risk. For example, if a patient's serum potassium level needs monitoring and the GP is unaware of this, the patient may end up being readmitted with hyperkalaemia.

The primary care team relies on a thorough hand-over from the hospital team, in the form of a discharge summary. In recent years, the quality of discharge summaries has hugely improved, as hospitals increasingly use pre-populated computerised forms.

Table 5.3 lists the essential details required for adequate communication from secondary to primary care on discharge.

Table 5.3 The discharge summary.

Essential discharge summary information	Clarification
Needs to be legible	Is print dark enough to fax/scan?
Surname and first name	All four of these identifiers are needed. Some patients have the same name and date of birth
Date of birth	
Address	
NHS number	
Name of consultant or team	The GP and patient need to know who to contact in the event of problems. Avoid abbreviations
Date of admission and date of discharge	
Key investigations carried out in hospital and a brief summary of the results	Resist the temptation to 'cut and paste' the whole report, as this makes it easy to overlook important findings
Key procedures, treatments, operations, events	What was done and why? If the patient was admitted for a routine operation but ended up on ITU, the GP needs to know!

(Continued)

Table 5.3 *(Continued)*

Essential discharge summary information	Clarification
Diagnosis	Without abbreviations – what seems obvious to you will not necessarily be so to the GP and patient
	Diagnoses are coded by staff. Incorrect coding can affect patient care and GP income. For example, does STI mean 'sexually transmitted infection' or 'soft tissue injury'? Is 'MI' 'myocardial infarction', 'minor illness' or 'mitral incompetence'?
What the patient and relatives have been told	Especially in serious illness, such as cancer
Medication stopped, started or changed	Explain rationale for any changes. How long should course continue?
Medication on discharge	Including name, dose, frequency, total number supplied
Future plans	Has outpatient appointment been arranged?
	Are any results outstanding or any further tests planned?
Special notes for primary care	Clarify whether the GP needs to review the patient proactively or to take any particular action
	(Tests instigated by secondary care should be followed up by secondary care)

SUMMARY

Throughout the course of some diseases and throughout most people's lives, medical care is transferred repeatedly from primary to secondary care and back again. Making the patient's 'journey' as smooth and as safe as possible requires excellent communication between primary and secondary care. It is useful to follow guidelines or templates when writing referral letters and hospital discharge letters, to ensure that important information is not overlooked. GPs have responsibility for deciding when patients need referral to hospital. Referral rates differ between GPs. The reasons for these variations are complex and are not fully understood. An emergency hospital admission is expensive, and in some cases can be avoided if GPs have access to sufficient resources in the community.

 Now visit **www.wileyessential.com/primarycare** to test yourself on this chapter.

REFERENCES

1. Kvamme OJ, Oleson F, Samuelsson M. Improving the interface between primary and secondary care: a statement from the European Working Party on Quality in Family Practice (EQuiP). *Qual Health Care* 2001;**10**(1):33–9.

2. Foot C, Naylor C, Imison C. The Quality of GP Diagnosis and Referral. King's Fund, 2010. Available from: http://www.kingsfund.org.uk/sites/files/kf/Diagnosis%20and%20referral.pdf (last accessed 6 October 2015).

3. McBride D, Hardoon S, Walters K, et al. Explaining variation in referral from primary to secondary care: cohort study. *BMJ* 2010;**341**:c6267.

4. Fertig A, Roland M, King H, Moore T. Understanding variation in rates of referral among general practitioners: are inappropriate referrals important and would guidelines help to reduce rates? *BMJ* 1993;**307**:1467–70.

5. Hippisley-Cox J, Hardy C, Pringle M, et al. The effect of deprivation on variations in general practitioners' referral rates: a cross sectional study of computerised data on new medical and surgical outpatient referrals in Nottinghamshire. *BMJ* 1997;**314**;1458–61.

6. Reynolds GA, Chitnis JG, Roland MO. General practitioner outpatient referrals: do good doctors refer more patients to hospital? *BMJ* 1991;**302**:1250.7.

7. O'Donnell CA. Variation in GP referral rates: what can we learn from the literature? *Family Practice* 2000;**17**:462–71.

8. Balint M. *The Doctor, His Patient and the Illness*. Pitman Paperbacks; 1968.

9. NHS Choose and Book. http://www.nhs.uk/choiceintheNHS/Yourchoices/appointment-booking/Pages/about-the-referral-system.aspx (last accessed 6 October 2015).

10. Hamilton W, Round A, Sharp D. Effect on hospital attendance rates of giving patients a copy of their referral letter: randomised controlled trial. *BMJ* 1999;**318**: 1392–5.

11. Hawary A, Sinclair A, Pearce I. Outpatient department correspondences: what are the urology patients' views? *Int J Pers Cent Med* 2012;**2**(3):468–72.

12. Jelley D, van Zwanenberg T. Copying general practitioner referral letters to patients: a study of patients' views. *Brit J Gen Pract* 2000;**50**:657–8.

13. NHS Patient Online. http://www.england.nhs.uk/ourwork/pe/patient-online/ (last accessed 6 October 2015).

14. Blunt I. Focus on Preventable Admissions. Trends in Emergency Admissions for Ambulatory Care Sensitive Conditions, 2001 to 2013. Nuffield Trust, October 2013. Available from: http://www.nuffieldtrust.org.uk/sites/files/nuffield/publication/131010_qualitywatch_focus_preventable_admissions_0.pdf (last accessed 6 October 2015).

15. Mangtani P, Cumberland P, Hodgson CR, et al. A cohort study of the effectiveness of influenza vaccine in older people, performed using the United Kingdom General Practice Research Database. *J Infect Dis* 2004;**190**:1–10.

16. Purdy S, Huntley A. Predicting and preventing avoidable hospital admissions: a review. *J R Coll Physicians Edinb* 2013;**43**:340–4.

17. Purdy S. Avoiding Hospital Admissions. What Does the Research Evidence Say? King's Fund Report. King's Fund, London, December 2010. Available from: http://www.kingsfund.org.uk/sites/files/kf/Avoiding-Hospital-Admissions-Sarah-Purdy-December2010_0.pdf (last accessed 6 October 2015).

18. Huntley A, Lasserson D, Wye L, et al. Which features of primary care affect unscheduled secondary care use? A systematic review. *BMJ Open* 2014;**4**:e004746. doi:10.1136/bmjopen-2013-004746.

19. Henderson C. Cost effectiveness of telehealth for patients with long term conditions (Whole Systems Demonstrator telehealth questionnaire study): nested economic evaluation in a pragmatic, cluster randomised controlled trial. *BMJ* 2013;**346**:f1035.

20. Shepperd S, Doll H, Angus RM, et al. Hospital admission through hospital at home programs: a systematic review and individual patient data meta-analysis. *CMAJ* 2009; **180**:175–82.

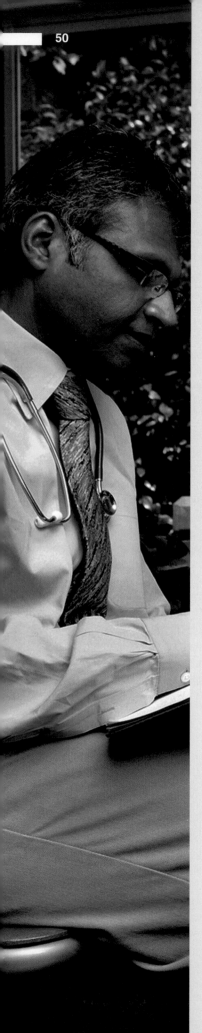

CHAPTER 6
The everyday ethics of primary care

Trevor Thompson

Reader in Healthcare Education, University of Bristol

Key topics

Learning objectives

- Be able to recall some of the key topics in medical ethics.
- Be able to recognise the core values of primary care.
- Be able to appreciate the wide range of responsibilities of the GP.
- Be able to structure one's approach to dealing with ethical issues.
- Be able to apply ethical reasoning to common clinical presentations.

Essential Primary Care, First Edition. Edited by Andrew Blythe and Jessica Buchan.
© 2017 John Wiley & Sons, Ltd. Published 2017 by John Wiley & Sons, Ltd.
Companion website: www.wileyessential.com/primarycare

Introduction

Doctors are well remunerated, have interesting and responsible work and are trusted more than any other professional group in the UK. High expectations for the professional behaviour of doctors are enshrined in the General Medical Council (GMC) publication *Good Medical Practice*.[1] For instance, doctors should keep up to date with medical knowledge, make accurate clinical records, communicate well, contribute to teaching and respond fully and promptly to complaints.

Despite these clear guidelines, the 'right thing to do' can be far from clear. In this chapter, we are going to explore the ethical tensions that emerge in everyday general practice. The problems we will meet are not the dramatic ones that often enliven ethical debate. No life-support machines will be turned off, no pregnancies brought to an untimely end. Rather, we are going to be looking at the ethical dimensions of routine situations that unfold in regular GP clinics.

Ethical issues emerge when values promote different or even opposing ends. For instance, 'continuity' (ongoing personal care by a particular doctor) sits in tension with 'easy access' (the ability to see a doctor quickly when a problem arises). Generally, the easier it is for a patient to get an immediate appointment, the less likely it is that this consultation will be with a doctor with personal knowledge of their clinical history.

The GP has responsibilities to a wide range of parties in the system in addition to the individual before them. Trying to meet the needs of different parties at the same time gives rise to interesting tensions. For instance, a patient may disclose an alcohol addiction and admit to regularly driving under the influence. The GP has loyalty to their patient, but also to the health of other road users – most of whom are not their patients – put in jeopardy by this risky behaviour.

Alas, there are (usually) no absolutely clear-cut solutions to the ethical quandaries presented here. However, by learning to recognise problems in practice, decipher the basis of conflicts and balance competing demands, we are more likely to make well-considered clinical decisions. We will also be in a stronger position to tackle the written tests of situational judgement that are an increasingly common aspect of career progression. First, some revision.

Concepts in medical ethics

Here is a reminder of a few of the more important concepts in medical ethics that come up regularly in practice, and which will inform our case analysis. The British Medical Association (BMA)'s Ethics Toolkit for Students is a free online handbook which covers these and other issues in an accessible format.[2]

- **Respect for autonomy:** Autonomy can be defined as the ability of a person to make their own decisions regarding care or participation in research.
- **Informed consent:** Leading from autonomy is the need for patients to understand and specifically agree to undergo a medical treatment. Consent can be formal or implicit.

Guidelines take account of special situations, such as emergencies and the treatment of children.

- **Mental capacity:** Capacity is the ability of a patient to understand the nature of their medical needs and any planned interventions, and therefore to give informed consent.
- **Confidentiality:** Dating back to the Hippocratic Oath, confidentiality is the obligation on doctors to keep secret certain types of information disclosed in clinical settings. Students may be asked to sign confidentiality agreements when on GP attachments.
- **Benefit and harm:** Often in medicine, good can only be achieved at the risk of harm. Medical interventions are ordinarily justified where the anticipated benefits exceed the harms.
- **Fairness or equity:** People should be treated fairly – people with equal needs should be given equal consideration – and should not be discriminated against in the provision of health services.

Core values in primary care

Values are the things we hold dear, the more or most important motivations for our actions. The values of primary care arise from a blend of virtue ethics (such as truthfulness), traditions (such as comprehensiveness) and more modern imperatives (such as being evidence-based).[3] What follows is a selection of values that will inform our case analyses:

- **Comprehensiveness:** GPs in the UK are the first port of call for all imaginable (and some unimaginable) ailments afflicting the human condition. In a single surgery, GPs will consult children, adults and elderly persons of both genders about problems of all bodily systems and a wide range of mental health and social problems. This is not the case in other countries, where, for instance, children are taken directly to paediatricians, women go directly to gynaecologists and so on (see Chapter 1 for more on comprehensive care).
- **Patient-centredness:** This value encompasses the impulse to try and discover the real concerns of the patient, to share with them the different options available and to seek, as appropriate, their input in making informed choices about their care. It also refers to the urge to engage patients in the design of services so that their needs are accurately accounted for. Of course, sometimes the patient wants the exact opposite, wishing the doctor to make the decision on their behalf.
- **Accessibility:** Probably the main dissatisfaction with contemporary medical services is over difficulties with getting timely care. There is no point in a great medical system if people cannot access it. Accessibility means having sufficient appointments, good disabled access, access to interpreter services and flexibility with appointment times and locations.
- **Continuity:** For most of the 20th century, patients in the UK enjoyed a personal relationship with 'their GP'. My mother had the same one for 40 years! Continuity implies the presence within the practice of a doctor or group of

doctors who are committed to long-term relationships with their patients, through 'thick and thin'. There are definite advantages, and some disadvantages, to such longitudinality. Continuity is on the wane in UK primary care.

- **Holism:** Holistic care implies care for more than the immediate presenting complaint. Holistic care seeks to put problems in context, to understand for instance the impact of work and family on the emotional life of the patient. It puts a high premium on a strong and trusting doctor–patient relationship and uses this leverage to promote lifestyle changes alongside pharmaceutical approaches.

- **Evidence-informed:** Although named 'evidence-based medicine' (EBM) only since the 1990s, good medical practice has always sought to be informed by evidence from research. GPs do not regularly consult original research, partly because there is insufficient time and partly because of the widespread availability of scholarly reviews and guidelines. Nonetheless, there is a very strong tradition of practice-based research in primary care, following pioneers such as James Mackenzie, Will Pickles, John Fry and Julian Tudor-Hart.[4]

These seem incontestable when viewed in abstract. However, as we shall soon see, our laudable values can easily fall into conflict with one another.

Responsibilities of the GP

At first glance, one might imagine that the GP's greatest responsibility is that to their patient. This is certainly the emphasis of *Good Medical Practice*, but, as the following analysis shows, the full range of responsibilities is wide and exacting.

- **Patients:** GPs spend most of their time with individual patients, dealing with their individual problems, and so this individual focus is understandable. There are various situations where special responsibilities arise, such as when caring for children or those with mental health problems or cognitive decline.

- **Partners and families:** Often, a problem presents that has major implications for those immediately connected to an individual patient. A good example is the needs of carers. If a GP refers a dependent patient for surgery, they have to think about how to meet the increased burden upon the patient's carer during the convalescence period.

- **The practice population:** GPs are often thinking about how best to organise their appointment system, improve access for special groups (such as teenagers) and improve their prescribing systems. As we shall see, sometimes the needs of the practice population can be in conflict with the needs of individual patients.

- **The wider public:** GPs are often involved in *commissioning* services for a geographical region. Although most GPs are actually not 'commissioners', they are all responsible for spending large amounts of the public purse, and most GPs

consider they have a responsibility not to waste public resources on unnecessary interventions.

- **The environment:** Health care uses a lot of resources and creates a lot of waste. Some medical waste creates particular environmental hazards (e.g. hormone medications that enter the water supply can disrupt endocrine systems in animals). Many doctors feel it is part of their duty to protect the global environment as much as possible from iatrogenic harm.[5]

- **Health care students:** Most GP practices are now involved in some aspect of medical education. Teaching is actually an explicit expectation of *Good Medical Practice* (para. 39).[1] Good teaching placements require considerable time and energy to organise, implement and review.

These are all worthy, outward-looking responsibilities. Meeting these diverse duties brings a lot of variety and satisfaction to the GP's work and creates interesting tensions.

In the reality of everyday practice, the GP has a parallel set of duties that relate not to patients and the community, but to the well being of the practice:

- **Self-care:** Being a GP is a demanding occupation. Many of us rather like the sense of being busy, of being in demand for our skills and of working intensively through the day. At times, though, the pressure can get too intense and our enjoyment and effectiveness can suffer. GPs have a duty to themselves, therefore, to avoid getting overstressed by taking adequate holidays, having interests outside of work and finding ways to talk about the difficult stuff.

- **Other doctors:** The relationship between GPs is a special aspect of UK primary care. A **_partnership_** depends on each partner being committed to the success of the practice and being willing to fairly share the workload, engage in decision-making and communicate openly about issues as they arise. GP income is not fixed but depends on the communal efforts of the practice, and hence GPs also have financial responsibilities to each other. Many GPs are employees, rather than partners, but they still share many of the same obligations.

- **Staff:** A GP practice of 8000 patients might employ 30 people, including doctors, nurses, managers, administrators, receptionists and cleaners. The GP therefore has major responsibilities as an employer to create a safe and pleasant work environment and ensure sustainable long-term employment.

So far, we have revisited some of the recurrent themes of clinical ethics, looked at some of the values that underpin primary care and examined some of the responsibilities of the GP – looking outward towards patient care and inward towards the healthy functioning of the practice. Unsurprisingly, these different values and responsibilities come into conflict in interesting ways. We are going to examine these conflicts through case studies. First, though, we will explore ways of approaching ethical conflicts when they emerge.

Approaching ethical issues

As a medical student, one can develop awareness of the ethics of everyday practice both as one 'sits in' on consultations and when conducting one's own consultations under supervision.[6] A challenge is that only the starkest issues may be flagged up by the GP as overtly 'ethical'. However, as we shall see, ethical issues lurk in many guises. Here are some strategies for approaching them:

1. **Be open to the ethical dimension:** Pay attention to any sense of *dissonance* in the consultation. By 'dissonance', we mean a mismatch between what we sense is right and what is unfolding in the consultation (e.g. a 10-year-old child translating the health problems of a non-English speaking parent somehow *feels* wrong). Where feasible, one should ask clarifying questions within the consultation. Any ethical issues should be recorded for later consideration; otherwise, they will easily get lost in the mayhem of clinical life. A good way to develop ethical sensitivity is to keep a place for the humanities in one's personal life. There are countless books, poems, films and works of art of relevance to medicine. Good art distils the essence of an ethical situation, and through this vicarious exposure we become better at appreciating them in the clinic. In Bristol, we have developed a curated and searchable online collection (www.outofourheads.net) – much of which tackles ethical issues (see Figures 6.1 to 6.3).

2. **Discuss ethical issues with colleagues:** It is very difficult to develop a nuanced ethical understanding on one's own. We seem to need to voice various perspectives in coming to a mature one. Most tutors will enjoy exploring ethical issues with students. When discussing with other students, it is important to scrupulously protect the anonymity of all parties. Senior input should always be sought if one finds oneself personally involved in an ethical issue.

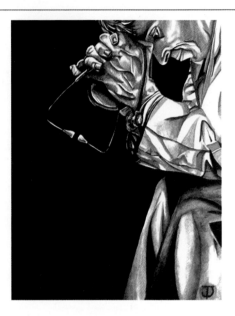

Figure 6.1 'Stress in Medical Practice' by Jack Day. Medical practice can be emotionally exacting, and we all need ways to nurture our emotional health as practitioners. *Source*: www.outofourheads.net. Reproduced with permission of Jack Day.

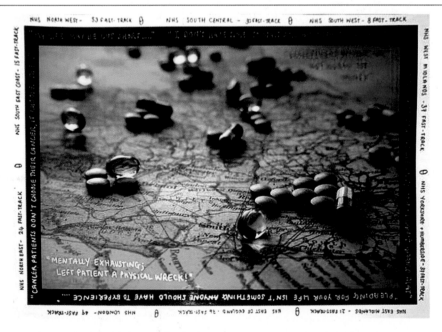

Figure 6.2 'Postcodes: Are They a Prescribing Destiny?' by Rachel Murphy. This artwork reflects on the differences in funding for fast-track cancer referrals in different UK regions – an artistic take on the principle of distributive justice. *Source*: www.outofourheads.net. Reproduced with permission of Rachel Murphy.

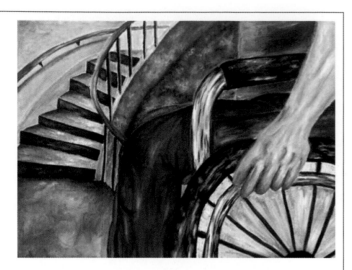

Figure 6.3 'Disability in Healthcare' by Fatima Rashed. Accessibility is a core value of general practice, and practices must take active steps to prevent a person's disability (seen or unseen) from blocking access to care. *Source*: www.outofourheads.net. Reproduced with permission of Fatima Rashed.

Table 6.1 The four-principles approach.

Principle	Obligation
Beneficence	To do what is in the patient's interests
Nonmaleficence	To not cause harm, and indeed to seek to prevent it
Autonomy	To respect the right of the individual to make choices about their own life
Justice	To treat patients and distribute resources fairly

3. **Aim for clarity on the ethical issues at stake:** Many readers will be familiar with the four-principles approach to identifying what is at stake in any given predicament (see Table 6.1). These principles focus mainly on the care of individual patients, but, as we have seen, the GP is called on to consider a wider constituency. However, they have proved their worth over time as a useful framework.[7] They are most interesting where they sit in tension – for instance, a patient may make a rational choice for a special intervention that will benefit them, but which comes at a cost that would deprive others of necessary care. In this chapter, we have set out values and responsibilities that sit in tension, such as when duties to an individual and duties to family, society and self collide. An understanding of these competing imperatives can greatly clarify the nature of conflicts.

4. **Consult formal guidelines:** These exist for many common presentations. For instance, the Fraser guidelines aid good practice in the provision of contraception services to under-16s without parental consent. We should also be aware of some key legislation, including the Mental Capacity Act (2005) and the Equality Act (2010), that has direct implications for medical practice. A related option is to contact one's defence organisation. GPs will often do this in order to get general advice and opinions. Such organisations can also clarify any legal issues.

5. **Find reasoned resolutions:** There is no 'right' response to a dilemma, but there can be a reasoned one. This often involves recognising the principles and parties at odds (e.g. maintaining confidentiality versus fulfilling duties to family members at risk) and striving for a reasonable compromise, or explaining why a certain position is an absolute that should not be compromised. For instance, one might argue that it is important to be both truthful and compassionate, and thus hold back certain information that, while true, would be unnecessarily distressing. But one might also argue it is always wrong to lie to a patient when they ask a direct (and clearly answerable) question about their health.

Five case studies in everyday ethics

We finish this chapter with a series of case studies. Read the presentation and identify the 'dissonances'. Then try and analyse the problem through the lens of ethical frameworks, values and responsibilities. Finally, decide on what you might actually 'do' to resolve the difficulties and how your decisions could be justified. There are various, nonspecialist resources to help you approach ethical issues, including those written for students and those specific to primary care.[6-8]

Case study 6.1

Presentation
A female patient is aggrieved because their GP revealed personal information in a letter to the council advising on her suitability to become a foster carer. The patient had difficulties in her marriage 2 years earlier, and the GP recorded 'couple rowing a lot at present'. The patient says she 'will never tell a doctor anything personal again'.

Analysis
Here, the conflict is between the doctor's duties to the patient and to wider society, and in particular to children who might be fostered by the patient. The patient feels that what was said in private has been revealed out of context (her marriage, she says, is now fine). The defensiveness of the patient rings some alarm bells for the GP. Confidentiality of medical records is relative, not absolute.

Resolution
A doctor must fairly report the medical record and not edit it at the request of the patient. The conflict can be mitigated by ensuring that the patient has a chance to see any report before it is sent, providing the opportunity to offer clarifications (this is standard practice). Patients should know that the doctor is *required* to make a record of consultations – but can show discretion. Patient and doctor should trust the fairness of the fostering assessment process – historical rows alone would not prevent fostering.

Case study 6.2

Presentation
A male GP is consulted when 'duty doctor' by a female patient with a complex query over her contraceptive medication. The GP advises the patient, but with a sense of dissonance – he knows he is not fully up to date with the latest contraceptive guidelines.

Analysis
Here, the imperative of competence is in tension with the values of accessibility, comprehensiveness and continuity. All practices offer urgent care. Any GP sees any problem. Some practices, which place particular value on continuity of care, operate 'personal lists', where a patient sees the same doctor for routine problems. Particularly with 'gendered' health problems, GPs can become deskilled in certain areas.

Resolution
Good Medical Practice requires GPs to be familiar with the latest guidelines. A good GP will keep a running list of topics they need to brush up on, by reading or going on a course. Here, the GP could check the guidelines after the clinic or discuss the situation informally with a GP colleague. If an error has been made, the GP should contact the patient promptly, explain the error, apologise and put matters right.

Case study 6.3

Presentation
A patient with schizophrenia turns up 20 minutes late for an appointment with the practice nurse for an injection of his 'depot' medication. The nurse, who is running late already, declines to see the patient. The patient then shouts personal abuse – including racial abuse – at the receptionist, who is very upset.

Analysis
Here, responsibility for the care of an individual patient is in conflict with the duty to create a safe environment for staff and other patients. If the patient did not have schizophrenia, this incident might be grounds to remove him from the list, but it is very likely that this behaviour is related to a medical diagnosis. However, if the behaviour is not challenged, the staff may feel that people can 'get away with anything'.

Resolution
Tricky. Practice policy should be reviewed, as in this particular case the patient should probably not have been turned away by the nurse. The receptionist must get support from the highest level in the practice. The patient should be contacted and asked to meet one of the partners to discuss the event and be given the opportunity to apologise. The mental health team should also be informed, and an alert should be placed on the patient's records.

Case study 6.4

Presentation
A GP has been in partnership for 6 years and in general loves her work. However, in the last 6 months, there have been several complaints from patients about her attitude, especially during busy on-call shifts, which she finds hard to accept. She has found herself sometimes resentful of other partners, who do not share the workload. She has noted her sleep is sometimes disturbed as she goes over the events of the day.

Analysis
This doctor is showing classical signs of stress and her happiness and performance are starting to suffer. If signals are ignored, things could develop into depression or 'burn-out'. Here, patient care is sitting in conflict with the duty of the doctor to care for themselves. The doctor's stress will also impact on the morale of the clinical and administrative team. The difficulty is in spotting the problem in oneself.

56 / Chapter 6: The everyday ethics of primary care

Resolution

A GP colleague may notice and feel able to share her observations. The problem may lie with the system and not the individual – perhaps the practice needs to employ some locums to relieve stress on appointments. There may also be significant issues boiling up in the home life of the doctor. She might benefit from confidential counselling and encouragement to 'have a life' outside of work. If the system is basically healthy, small changes can quickly bring positive results.

Case study 6.5

Presentation

A GP opens up his appointments screen and sees that the first case is a woman who brings multiple problems to the consultation, including regular requests for letters and referrals. Consultations invariably over-run, and what's more, the patient often arrives a few minutes late.

Analysis

Here, the value of patient-centredness is in conflict with the GP's duty to his practice population. He could easily be running 15 minutes behind after the first case. He could end up feeling stressed for the rest of the morning, and other patients (who often have work and childcare commitments) might also feel stressed and inconvenienced. Also, if the late-running doctor isn't able to take his full share of seeing 'extra' patients, then there is impact on his partners.

Resolution

The GP should be careful not to blame the patient for bringing many needs to the consultation. He could, however, legitimately explain that over-running is impacting on the care of other patients. Quite often, patients will not have thought of this. The GP could offer to deal with one problem and invite the patient to return to discuss the others. Rules over late arrival could be established. As the GP regains the initiative, he may find the patient feels rejected by him. This can be a necessary price to pay for sanity within our pressurised appointments system.

SUMMARY

Doing the right thing in general practice is not easy. GPs are pulled in various directions by the demands of patients, the need to keep their businesses viable and the expectations of the many regulators that oversee them. In modern practice, it is all the more important to have a moral compass to guide us to right action. Although this compass is to some extent 'in-built', the complexities of the medical environment mean we have to develop the skills to identify and juggle conflicting priorities. In this chapter, we have looked at the conflicts that can arise when applying the worthy values of primary care to the different groups we are asked to provide for. In every case, it seems the task is to find a wise compromise between competing demands. This ability will serve us very well in practice, and in any assessment of our ability to make judgements in clinical situations. General practice is an unparalleled environment in which to develop these skills – so get cracking!

REFERENCES

1. General Medical Council. *Good Medical Practice*. London; GMC; 2013.
2. British Medical Association. Ethics tool kit for students. Available from: http://bma.org.uk/practical-support-at-work/ethics/medical-students-ethics-tool-kit (last accessed 6 October 2015).
3. Pringle M. *Core Values in Primary Care*, 1st edn. New York: Wiley-Blackwell; 1998.
4. Green LA, Hickner J. A short history of primary care practice-based research networks: from concept to essential research laboratories. *J Am Board Fam Med.* 2006;**19**:1–10.
5. Schroeder K, Thompson T, Frith K, Pencheon D. *Sustainable Healthcare*. Oxford: Wiley-Blackwell; 2012.
6. Sheather J. Approaching ethical dilemmas. *Student BMJ* 2014;**22**:g4736.
7. Bowman D, Spicer J. *Primary Care Ethics*, 1st edn. Oxford, New York: Radcliffe Publishing; 2007.
8. Sugarman J. *20 Common Problems: Ethics in Primary Care.* New York: McGraw-Hill Medical; 2000.

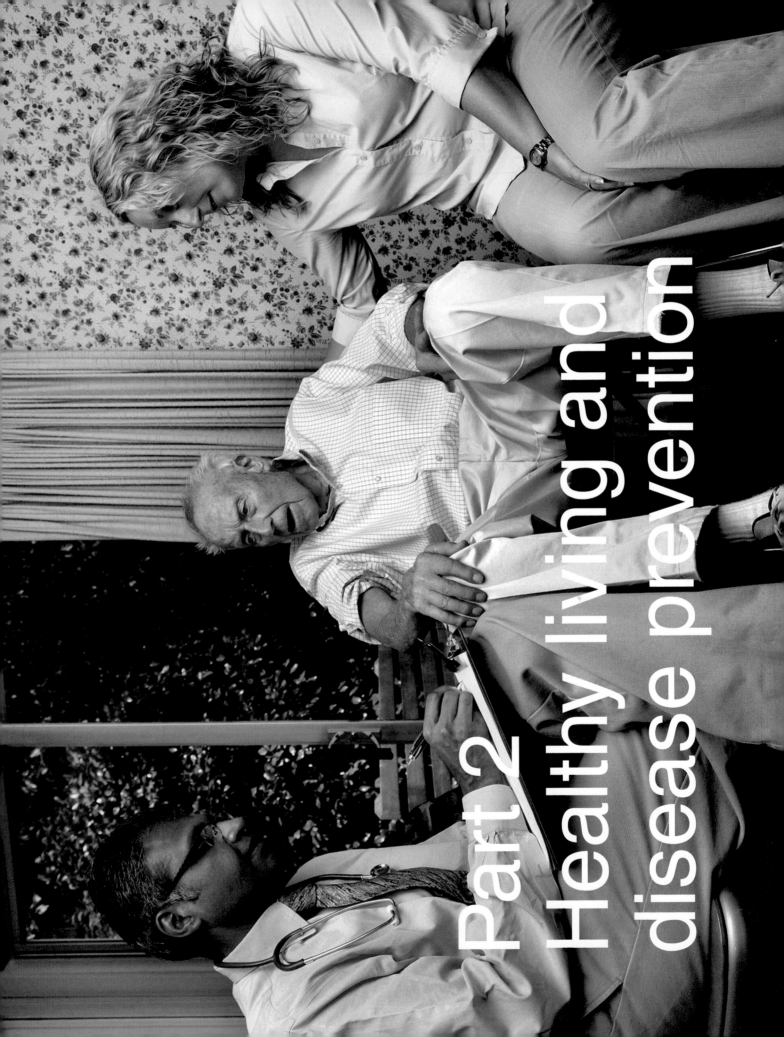

Part 2
Healthy living and disease prevention

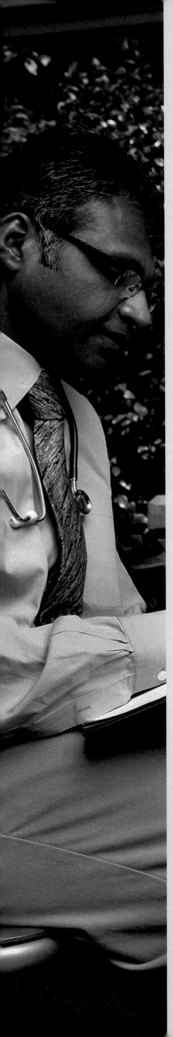

CHAPTER 7
Behaviour change

Jessica Buchan

GP and Teaching Fellow in Primary Care, University of Bristol

Key topics

Learning objectives

- Be able to understand the importance of addressing lifestyle issues with patients.
- Be able to assess a patient's readiness to change.
- Be able to demonstrate consultation skills that help, rather than hinder, behaviour change.
- Be able to assist patients in setting their own clear and achievable goals.

Essential Primary Care, First Edition. Edited by Andrew Blythe and Jessica Buchan.
© 2017 John Wiley & Sons, Ltd. Published 2017 by John Wiley & Sons, Ltd.
Companion website: www.wileyessential.com/primarycare

The role of the GP in health behaviour change

Health threatening behaviours are the commonest cause of premature illness and death in the developed world

Rollnick et al.[1]

Behaviour change is part of many GP consultations. Preventing illness is enormously cost-effective compared to treating illness. Doctors often see the devastating effects of preventable illness: half of all smokers will die from a smoking-related disease, and many of these will experience distressing symptoms for some time before they die.[2] Quitting at any age makes a difference to health: breathing symptoms and lung function improve within a matter of months. In the USA, beginning in the 1980s, the Physicians' Health Study looked at the health records of 20 000 male doctors and followed them up for 22 years. Among past smokers, the risks of dying from a stroke, heart attack or colorectal cancer fell to the same level as those of people who had never smoked within 10 years of quitting, and the risk of chronic obstructive pulmonary disease (COPD) fell to the same level within 20 years of quitting. The best outcomes were in those who quit before the age of 50.[3]

GPs are ideally placed to encourage health behaviour change in their patients, and this is one of our key tasks. Table 7.1 looks at the positive impact health behaviour change can have, while Table 7.2 outlines the common areas that result in health behaviour consultations.

GPs can:

- provide objective information;
- compare patients' behaviour with the normal or recommended behaviour;
- provide accurate information about risks and possible outcomes;
- give specific advice tailored to the patient;
- support and encourage change over time.

It can feel very frustrating when our well-meant advice appears to fall on deaf ears. Giving information about the negative

Table 7.1 Benefits of health behaviour change.

Areas of impact for health behaviour change	Example
Prevention of illness and premature death by tackling the root causes of health problems	Reduction of cardiovascular risk through stopping smoking and through healthy eating and exercise (see Chapter 9)
Improved prognosis and prevention or delay of the need for treatment	Tight glucose control in diabetes prevents complications
Improved self-esteem and general well–being, even where health problems are not directly caused by health-threatening behaviour	Diet and exercise improve general health in chronic conditions
Improved adherence with treatment	Taking new medicines (see Chapter 5) or sticking to a new diet (e.g. a gluten free diet in coeliac disease)
Benefit to families	Benefit to child health when parents quit smoking (see Chapter 12)
Benefit to communities	Reduction in drunk-driving where problem drinkers reduce intake
Benefit to society	Prevention is much more cost-effective for health service than treatment
Benefit to doctors and health care providers	Techniques of behavioural change doctors and health care providers can use on themselves to improve their own health and well-being

Table 7.2 Behaviour change consultations.

Areas that benefit from behaviour change consultations	New or changed behaviour GPs want patients to implement
Diet	Eating less, eating different foods, adjusting timing of meals (e.g. regular intake, not eating a large meal before bed)
Alcohol intake	Drinking less, abstaining, drinking differently (e.g. not binge-drinking)
Illicit drug use	Abstaining, reducing risk (e.g. not sharing needles)
Exercise	Increasing amount or type of exercise, doing specific exercises
Behaviour	Reducing risk-taking behaviour (e.g. using condoms to reduce sexually transmitted infection risk), trying new parenting techniques, attending appointments
Medication	Taking new medications, changing medications, adjusting format or timing
Self-monitoring	Interventional behaviour (e.g. monitoring glucose in diabetes) Diagnostic behaviour (e.g. peak flow monitoring in asthma, keeping a self-observation diary to look at patterns or triggers of symptoms)

effects of a patient's behaviour, such as their excess weight or alcohol intake, is not enough on its own to trigger change. GPs can even make behaviour more entrenched if they raise issues in a way that leads the patient to argue back with all the reasons why they can't change. GPs may be tempted to avoid difficult consultations, particularly when patients seem unwilling or unable to make lifestyle changes, and in a 10-minute consultation other issues may take priority. We shouldn't avoid raising the issues when necessary – we just need to raise them in the right way.

We can learn consultation skills that make our interventions more effective. Motivational interviewing[1,4] is a technique that was originally developed in the field of alcohol addiction. This technique has been adapted for use in the GP consultation as a brief intervention that encourages the patient to self-evaluate and problem-solve. In this type of consultation, the GP takes more of a facilitator role than the role of expert advisor, and accepts that behaviour change doesn't happen overnight, but is more of a process. This chapter aims to give an overview of some of the ways in which GPs can encourage behaviour change in their patients, and explains the potential pitfalls of this approach.

Barriers to health behaviour change

Knowing why health behaviour change is so important for our patients' health can make it hard for us to understand when patients don't change. We can feel helpless when we attend a home visit to an alcoholic who can no longer walk due to alcohol-induced peripheral neuropathy but who continues to drink, or when we consult with an obese patient with poorly controlled diabetes who complains about her non-healing leg ulcers, or even when we advise an otherwise healthy teenage smoker to stop, knowing she will ignore our warnings. It can also be confusing when our patients give us all the signals that they do want to implement change but don't actually go through with it.

What is going on? Let's first look at the obstacles to behaviour change so that we can understand which strategies can help. Case study 7.1 illustrates some reasons our patients don't do what we might think is best for them.

The patient perspective

To influence behaviour change, we must try and understand our patient's perspective. When we discover what drives our patients, we can make links between their behaviour and their priorities; this can help with denial and ambivalence.

The patient can feel that we are on their side when we listen to and acknowledge their difficulties. In their excellent and comprehensive book, *Health Behaviour Change*, Mason and Butler say it helps if we see ourselves less as a problem- and pathology-seeker and more as a facilitator of our patient's motivation.[4] Patients are experts in their own lives; they know what is important to them and what is possible. They have skills and experience to draw on. Our role is to help them clarify their goals and find their strengths.

Case study 7.1a

Barry Grant is 52. He owns a roofing firm. He works long hours. He finds it stressful running his own business, especially dealing with his young apprentices, who often don't turn up to work; he admits he has some 'anger-management issues' and thinks this is why his employees don't stick around. He struggles to make ends meet, as he can't work if the weather is poor. His social life revolves around the pub, where he goes every evening and weekend. His GP, Dr Sam Tower, calculates that Barry is consuming at least 40 units of alcohol each week. Dr Tower is concerned not only that Barry is putting his health at risk, but that his drinking is impacting on his mood. He also thinks Barry's finances and business could improve if Barry reduced his alcohol intake.

Barry has never seriously attempted to reduce his alcohol intake. What reasons could there be for this?

- **Unawareness:** Some patients are genuinely unaware of the health risks of their behaviour. Even if Barry does know some of the health risks of drinking too much,

he may not know how it could be affecting his mood. He may not be aware that his intake is above recommended limits – he's likely to see it as normal, due to the drinking culture of his social group.
- **Denial:** Even when patients are aware of the risks, they may ignore the evidence that their behaviour is causing them harm.
- **Priorities:** The GP's priority may be Barry's health or to help him manage his anger. This does not mean that these are Barry's priorities. Perhaps his social life is more important to him than his health.
- **Ambivalence:** Barry may have moments when he wants to cut back on his alcohol intake, but he may enjoy drinking and the social life it provides. The effect of this is an internal debate that keeps him in limbo, so that he never makes a commitment to change.
- **Change is hard:** It is much easier to keep doing something, even out of habit, than to change to a new behaviour. This is especially true if addiction is involved and change results in uncomfortable cravings or withdrawal symptoms.

Assessing readiness to change

Some patients, faced with the consequences of ill health, make major lifestyle changes with little or no further prompting. Others, on being advised to stop smoking, light up as they drive away. It is probable that these patients are at different 'stages of change'.

In the 1980s, Prochaska and DiClemente developed the Stages of Change Model,[5] which describes the process by which people make changes to their behaviour:

- **Precontemplative:** This is where a patient is not thinking about change. Barry (Case study 7.1) is likely to be at this stage. If his GP tried to discuss how Barry could cut back on his alcohol intake, the advice would very likely fall on deaf ears, as Barry is not ready to take action.
- **Contemplative:** This is where the patient is thinking about or planning to make a change to their behaviour. Rather than aim for Barry to stop drinking, his GP might try to move him to this stage by raising his awareness of the harm his drinking is causing.

- **Decision-making threshold:** This is the point at which a patient makes a decision to take action.
- **Action:** This is where a plan is enacted. Barry might cut back on his drinking or stop drinking altogether.
- **Maintenance:** This is the final stage. The model recognises that changing behaviour is not a one-off event. It is not enough to go without a cigarette or drink on one occasion: the patient has to keep sticking to their plan.
- **Relapse:** The patient returns to an earlier stage in the process: either the precontemplative or the contemplative stage.

As with any model, patients in real life show more complex behaviour than moving sequentially through the stages of change. They flit in and out of different stages at different times, perhaps spending a long time in one stage but moving quickly through another.

We can assess readiness to change by asking the patient directly, or by asking questions like those outlined in Tables 7.3 and 7.4 to explore their thinking. We must listen carefully to what we hear. Is there any resistance or ambivalence?

Table 7.3 Exploring reasons to change.	
Area to address	**Example**
Concerns	'What concerns do you have about your weight/drinking/smoking/stress levels?'
Importance	'In what ways is changing your weight/drinking/smoking/stress levels important to you?'
Pros and cons	Ask the patient to make a list of the pros and cons of their current behaviour
Scale questions	'On a scale of 0 to 10, where 0 is the lowest score you could give, and 10 the highest, how much do you want things to change? In assessing how much a person wants to change it can help to assign a numerical score and then explore why they scored themselves as they did. Be curious about would have to happen to increase their score.
Link between behaviour and the current issue	'You've had a lot of episodes of sinusitis. Have you ever wondered how smoking might be linked to this?'
Link between behaviour and other areas of the patient's life that are important to them	'You've mentioned your children. Can you think of any ways your drinking affects your relationship with them?'
What other people think	'What would your wife say about your stress if she were here with us?' 'In what ways do you agree or disagree with that?'
A different perspective	'If a friend was in your situation, what would you think about it/say to them? What advice would you give them?'
A future without change	'If things carried on as they are, how do you see your situation in 5 years time?' 'What might happen if you didn't change your weight/drinking/smoking/stress levels?'
A future with change	'If you imagine you've stopped smoking, what is it like for you?'
Self-observation	The patient can also be set 'homework'.[a] Having the patient monitor the behaviour over the course of a week and make comments on it can be used as a basis for discussion

[a] Given the tight timeframe of a GP consultation, many of these questions could be adapted for homework for the patient to think about/write answers to. The pros and cons list works well for this.

Area to address	Example
Ability	'How able do you feel to change your diet?'
Options	'If you decided to stop smoking, what would your options be?' 'How do you think you could reduce your stress levels?'
Other people's experiences	'Have you read about any ways/ do you know of any ways that have worked for other people?'
Past experience	'What did you learn from when you quit smoking before?'
Obstacles	'You sound very busy. How would you fit this into your life?' 'It can be hard not to drink in social situations. How would you handle this?'
Small changes	'What would be achievable for you right now?' 'What would have to happen to make it possible for you to increase your exercise at all?' 'Can you think of a change to your drinking that would feel possible, however small?'

Table 7.4 Enabling a patient to make changes.

Top tips: ways to raise sensitive behavioural topics with patients

- Talk in general terms (e.g. 'People often find that…', 'We know that…', 'Patients in similar situations to you…').
- Remain objective (e.g. 'The measurements we took show that, for your height, your ideal weight would be *x*. At the moment it is *y*.').
- Find ways to bring up the topic in relation to the patient's current condition (e.g. 'Some people find that exercise helps them manage their stress.').
- Reflect on any cues the patient gives about wanting to change. This can be in the form of an open-ended statement (e.g. 'So you have pain in your knees, you feel tired much of the time and you know you have put on quite a bit of weight recently. You are wondering if those things are related?' or 'You have some concerns about your weight/ smoking/diet?').

or ask them if they would like to know more about a topic (*elicit*).

2. Give information in a clear, neutral way (*provide*).
3. Crucially, end by assessing the impact of the information (e.g. 'What do you make of what we've discussed?') or ask how the patient thinks it applies to them (*elicit*).

Brief motivational interviewing

Precontemplative patients

If a patient is unaware of the risks of their current behaviour (see Chapter 8 for risks of drug and alcohol use and Chapter 9 for cardiovascular risk), we want to raise awareness by giving verbal, written or visual information, or by using a risk chart to demonstrate future projections of continuing a detrimental behaviour. A patient may not know that they have high cholesterol or that their drinking is over the recommended limits. They may not see themselves as being overweight – their weight may be normal for their family or culture. It's probably unusual for patients not to know that smoking carries health risks, but they may not appreciate the level of risk.

As we will see later, when we look at resistance, the way in which we raise awareness is important.

In Chapter 6 of their book *Health Behaviour Change*, Mason and Butler describe a technique for giving information to patients that avoids increasing resistance. They call it the elicit-provide-elicit model.

1. First, ask the patient to describe their behaviour (e.g. 'Would you mind describing to me what you eat in a typical day?')

Contemplative patients: increasing motivation

It's tempting to think that some of our patients are motivated people who find it easy to make changes to their lifestyle and some aren't. But work on behaviour change suggests that motivation is not a fixed trait, but something that fluctuates depending on the situation.[5] Some people are more motivated in one area of their life than others. Doctors may be motivated to study and learn, but may not fit exercise into their busy schedule or manage stress as well as they would like. The good news is that, if motivation is not a personality trait, it can be influenced. Athletes will have times when they don't feel motivated to train, but they learn ways to increase motivation, such as by raising the stakes (e.g. running for charity) or increasing their confidence that they can achieve their goal (e.g. having a manageable training schedule). We are all likely to fail to achieve a goal if it is not important to us, or if it is not feasible.

Using brief motivational interviewing techniques, we can encourage our patients to think about why a change in their behaviour is personally important to them. Even if change isn't very important yet, discussing our patient's priorities with them can boost motivation (see Table 7.3 for ways to do this). Next, we can get our patients to talk about how able they feel to make a change, even if they are not yet committed to change. (Table 7.4

Case study 7.2 Using brief motivational interviewing in the consultation

Stacey Stevens is 32. She has always been a little overweight, but since she got married 4 years ago her weight has gradually increased. She now weighs 72 kg, and is 1.52 m tall (body mass index (BMI): 31). She has a wardrobe full of clothes that don't fit and she is unhappy about her weight. She visits her GP, Dr Olivia Evans, to see if any medication might help. The doctor encourages her to try lifestyle changes.

Dr Evans first assesses Stacey's readiness to change by asking what she thinks about her weight.

STACEY   I'd really like to fit into my jeans again, but I'm wondering about trying for a baby soon and pregnancy makes you gain weight, so it might be a waste of time dieting now. Also, my mum's big, and she's happy – perhaps I should just accept that's who I am?

Dr Evans asks why losing weight has been on her mind? This helps the patient make an argument for change, rather than focus on the reasons not to.

STACEY   I've really lost confidence; I used to enjoy swimming but now I'm too self-conscious to be seen in a swimming costume.

DR EVANS   What would have to happen for it to become even more important for you to lose weight?

STACEY   If I couldn't get pregnant. My friend told me that being overweight can affect your chances. If that's true, I'd really want to shift some of this weight.

Dr Evans tells Stacey that her friend is correct and asks if she would like more information about this.

How ready do you think Stacey is to make the changes needed to lose weight?

She is contemplative. She is thinking about change but is pulled in two directions. We can see from the consultation that the GP is now better able to target information to Stacey's needs, and explain the reasons why reducing weight will improve her chances of a healthy pregnancy. Once she has done so, the GP can explore how Stacey might go about making lifestyle changes.

Outcome

Stacey leaves the surgery feeling more motivated, because she feels clearer about why weight loss is important to her, with some ideas of how she might go about it. She's not yet ready to start a diet, but she is going to read the information the GP has provided.

---

has questions we can ask to help our patients examine ways in which they can make change more realistic.)

Understanding resistance

A patient may experience a feeling of resistance when they feel they are being told or forced to do something, even if it's a change they were previously keen on making. Let's revisit Barry and see his reaction to his GP's advice (Case study 7.1b).

The decision threshold

There comes a point in the change process where thinking turns to action: the 'decision-making threshold'. It is at this point that patients may be more open to our advice, but we still want them to take responsibility for making change. It can be helpful to present a 'menu' of options that they can choose from.

Before launching into giving advice, ask the patient what they want (e.g. 'Have you thought about how you might go about changing your diet?' or 'Would you like to discuss some options?').

Then we can present a number of options that the patient can choose from: the menu. To prevent resistance, try and present a menu in general terms (e.g. 'Some people find the support from a slimming club helpful; others prefer to join an online programme. Some patients of mine have lost weight with a family member or friend' or 'Patients in similar situations

to you have found it easier to stop smoking altogether, rather than cut down').

(Finally we can help our patients make a decision. e.g. 'Do any of the options we've talked about appeal to you?' or 'If you decided to quit, what do you think you'd do?').

Patients know more about their lives than we do, so they need to make the decision about what will work for them. GPs have medical expertise, experience and local knowledge about services and support groups; we can't tell exactly what our patients need from us unless we ask them.

There is lots of specific information that patients can be directed towards to help them change behaviours when they have decided that they want to take action, be it to stop smoking, lose weight or reduce stress. The next part of this chapter covers general advice applicable to many areas of behaviour change.

Taking action: goal-setting

When patients are ready to make a change, it is helpful to ask them to set a goal, and to get a commitment. Ask what is the general outcome the patient wants to achieve, and why. Again, the patient should set their own outcome (e.g. 'I want to stop smoking'). Then ask them to list (write down) why it is important to them. They might list long-term health, being a good

Case study 7.1b

Barry and his GP, Dr Sam Tower, discuss the risks of consuming excess alcohol. Barry admits he's had concerns about his intake. Dr Tower tells Barry that he should stop drinking. Barry says he doesn't see how that's possible.

DR TOWER   Maybe you should stop going to the pub every night?

BARRY   I can't do that, the pub is my social life – I'd be lonely.

DR TOWER   Perhaps you could drink soft drinks?

BARRY   Yes, but...I'd look like a cheapskate – sitting there with a soda. I've got to pay my keep!

What is happening here?

Barry is expressing resistance. This can unearth strong feelings in our patients, such as, 'Why should I? You can't make me!' They may not directly express those feelings, but the consultation can quickly become confrontational, with the doctor arguing the case for change and the patient taking the opposing side. A sure sign this is happening is when our suggestions are met with, 'Yes, but...'

Resistance is not something we need to avoid completely, but it is a sign that we are pushing our patients too fast, or in the wrong direction. It can help to take a step back and see things from the patient's perspective. Dr Tower realises this is happening and tries to voice Barry's ambivalence:

DR TOWER   Hmmm, that's a problem. You've had some concerns about your drinking, and this morning we've discussed whether it could be worsening your mood and your finances. But your social life is important to you: you'd feel lonely if you didn't go to the pub.

BARRY   That's right. I suppose I could go later, rather than straight from work. I'd drink less that way.

The doctor made a reflective statement. This shows that he has listened and understood, and stops the consultation from becoming confrontational. Dr Tower phrases Barry's situation as a problem, but doesn't offer a solution. Barry now has a chance to hear and reflect on what the issues are and start working on his own solutions.

---

role model for their grandchildren and saving money; the list has to be personal to them. They can refer back to this when they need a motivational boost.

Setting SMART goals

Is the goal:

- **Specific?** 'I want to do 30 minutes of cardiovascular exercise five times a week.'
- **Measurable?** Is it something that can be recorded, so the patient knows if they've achieved it?
- **Attainable?** Is it within the patient's capability? The exercise has to be something they can physically do.
- **Realistic?** Has the patient considered how they are going to fit the exercise into their schedule?
- **Timed?** For someone who is sedentary, 30 minutes of exercise five times a week may not be immediately achievable, but it might be if it is built up to gradually over a 6-month period.

Being specific: look at the behaviours that lead to the outcome

Stopping smoking is a specific goal. Weight loss and stress reduction are not specific. A specific goal should be behaviour-related (e.g. setting a daily calorie intake or attending an aerobic class three times a week).

Measurable: write it down

There are two points in the behaviour change process where tracking behaviour is helpful:

- Before change occurs, we can ask our patients to keep a diary to see their behaviours more clearly. A patient may believe they don't eat very much and wonder why they are gaining weight; a food diary can reveal where the calories are being consumed.
- It also helps to track the change as it occurs. When it's going well, it can also act as a reward. Smokers may like to tick off each day they've not smoked on the calendar.

Attainable: make it easy

- Make the new behaviour easy to do and the old behaviour hard to do. Remove temptation from the house.
- Are small steps easier than leaping into change? It depends on the behaviour. Smokers may find it easier to quit than to cut down slowly, but exercise is best built up gradually.
- Medication can reduce withdrawal symptoms in some addictive behaviour, which makes the goal more attainable (e.g. nicotine replacement therapy for smokers).
- Pre-plan for temptation. Patients find temptation easier to handle if they already have a plan in place. A dieter may find it helpful to know that cravings tend to pass in a few minutes, and they may choose either a distraction or to replace unhealthy food with a healthy snack.

Realistic: link to existing behaviours

Many people struggle with making change if it is too hard. A young mum may want to lose weight but not have the time to cook different meals for herself and for her family. Adapting family meals to make them healthier makes her diet easier to achieve and benefits the whole family.

Timing and rewards

- Get a commitment. A patient who is really ready to take action knows how, when and why. GPs can help by asking the patient to outline their plan.
- Having timed goals allows patients to know when a particular goal has been reached.
- Be positive. Patients may find it helpful to give themselves material rewards when they have achieved a certain goal by a certain time, but a good feeling is also a reward. We can tap into this by praising patients for any progress they have made, even if it is learning from their relapse.

Relapse

We need to keep reminding ourselves that our patients are capable but change is hard. When patients relapse, we should avoid adopting the parental role of telling them off, which removes their power to take responsibility for their lifestyle and risks making them resistant to trying again. It may seem defeatist to end this chapter on the subject of relapse, but this is intentional. Our attitude to relapse tells us a lot about our attitude to change. Relapse is part of making change, not a failed attempt. We should aim to be encouraging, to explore what happened and what the patient has learnt and to support and motivate the patient to become ready to try again.

Case study 7.1c looks at relapse in Barry's case.

Case study 7.1c

With Dr Tower's support over a number of months, Barry decided to cut back on his drinking, and eventually quit drinking altogether. Barry lost weight, his mood improved and he met a new partner. His GP was so thrilled at this progress that he enlisted Barry to talk to medical students about the changes he had made. A year later, Barry presented at the surgery in a dishevelled state. It transpired that his relationship had broken down and he had turned back to alcohol. He was drinking more than ever, which resulted in the loss of his business. He had been ashamed to seek help as he felt he'd let Dr Tower down, as well as himself.

How should Dr Tower respond?
Much to Barry's surprise, Dr Tower did not think he'd failed or give him a telling off like he'd expected. Instead,

Dr Tower helped Barry see that change is a journey and that although he'd gone off course, he'd already come a long way. This helped Barry realise he needed ongoing support to tackle his drinking.

Outcome
Barry joined a local Alcoholics Anonymous group. A few years down the line, he is not drinking and has regular work. He had a couple of relapses in this time, but through the process of change he also realised he needed a better mechanism to handle stress. He took anger-management courses and now passes on his knowledge through voluntary work with young offenders. Barry has a renewed sense of purpose in life and tells people that although he set out to make one change in his life, the journey he has been on has resulted in a number of other positive changes.

SUMMARY

Behaviour change infiltrates every aspect of medical practice. According to the World Health Organization (WHO), noncommunicable disease is the leading cause of death globally, killing more people each year than all other causes combined. Such disease is caused, to a large degree, by modifiable behavioural risk factors, such as tobacco use, unhealthy diet, insufficient physical activity and the harmful use of alcohol.[6] There is also a marked difference in health outcomes for different sectors of society. To address these inequalities, we need strategies to help people change their behaviour. Changing behaviour is not easy for any of us. In trying to prevent illness, we are often asking patients to modify their lifestyle before they feel unwell. We expect patients to implement change in all kinds of consulations; we can't force them to alter their diet, take the medication we prescribe or do the exercises we recommend to recover from surgery or from a stroke. When we try to exert pressure, we risk increasing our patients' resistance, so we need to develop specific skills. If we can see our patients as experts in their own lives and encourage them to examine their priorities, make their own arguments for change and understand what hinders this process, then we can motivate them to make positive and lasting improvements, resulting in increased well-being and life expectancy.

Now visit **www.wileyessential.com/primarycare** to test yourself on this chapter.

REFERENCES

1. Rollnick S, Butler CC, McCambridge J, et al. Consultations about changing behaviour. *BMJ* 2005;**331**:961–3.

2. Aveyard P, West R. Managing smoking cessation. *BMJ* 2007;**335**:37–41.

3. Cao Y, Kenfield S, Song Y, et al. Cigarette smoking cessation and total and cause-specific mortality: a 22-year follow-up study among US male physicians. *Arch Intern Med* 2011;**171**(21):1956–9.

4. Mason P, Butler C. *Health Behaviour Change: A Guide for Practitioners*, 2nd edn. London: Churchill Livingstone Elsevier; 2010.

5. Prochaska JO, DiClemente CC. Stages and processes of self-change of smoking: toward an integrative model of change. *J Consult Clin Psychol* 1983;**51**:390–5.

6. World Health Organization. Global Status Report on Non-communicable Diseases. WHO. 2010. Available from: http://www.who.int/nmh/publications/ncd_report_full_en.pdf (last accessed 6 October 2015).

CHAPTER 8
Alcohol and drug misuse

Andrew Blythe
GP and Senior Teaching Fellow, University of Bristol

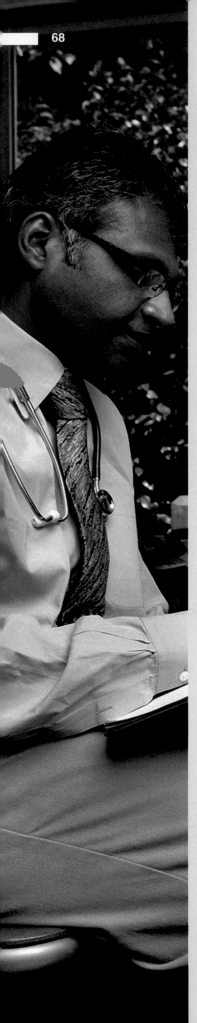

Key topics

Learning objectives

- Be able to identify someone whose level of drinking alcohol is harmful or hazardous.
- Be able to describe the effects of alcohol misuse on the patient and their family.
- Be able to offer help to someone whose alcohol consumption poses a risk to their health.
- Be able to make an assessment of someone who misuses drugs.

Essential Primary Care, First Edition. Edited by Andrew Blythe and Jessica Buchan.
© 2017 John Wiley & Sons, Ltd. Published 2017 by John Wiley & Sons, Ltd.
Companion website: www.wileyessential.com/primarycare

Identifying patients whose alcohol consumption is problematic

In Chapter 7, we discussed a patient who had a problem with drinking and we saw how GPs use motivational interviewing to help people alter their drinking habits. Alcohol misuse is extremely common in our society, but patients rarely go to their GP saying, 'I've got a drink problem – can you help me?' A family member or friend may bring them to seek help, but more commonly the patient presents alone with one or more of the complications of drinking (see Table 8.1). In a typical morning surgery, alcohol misuse may be a key factor underlying the problems of several patients.

Excessive consumption of alcohol can exacerbate many problems, including hypertension, depression and anxiety. The relationship between alcohol and mental illness is complex (see Figure 8.1), and it is sometimes difficult to decide which came first. Excessive drinking always makes depression and anxiety worse and negates the effect of antidepressant medication.

Alcohol has a particularly harmful effect on the liver, which metabolises it. Ultimately, it can cause cirrhosis of the liver. It is not the only cause of liver damage, and there is a risk that when someone's liver function is found to be abnormal, all the blame is attached to alcohol. Sometimes, liver disease is multi-factorial. Infection with hepatitis C and nonalcoholic fatty liver disease are two other conditions that ultimately can progress to cirrhosis.

By inducing liver enzymes, alcohol can increase the rate of metabolism of drugs that are processed by the liver. This is another way in which alcohol can exacerbate other problems. For example, it can increase the metabolism of antiepileptic drugs and thereby put patients at greater risk of having a fit.

Alcohol is an important cause of many cancers, particularly those of the oropharynx, oesophagus and liver. Amongst men, about one-third of all these cancers can be attributed to alcohol.[1] The risk of developing these cancers increases the more alcohol someone drinks, and is raised still higher if they smoke as well as drink.

If we suspect that someone might be drinking too much alcohol, we can use the 10-question AUDIT questionnaire[2] as a screening test. This questionnaire, developed by the World Health Organization (WHO), can be used in any setting. In primary care, where consultations are short, there

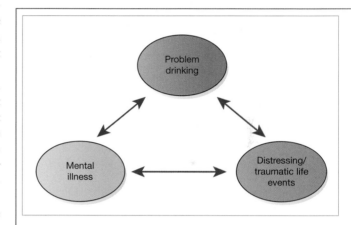

Figure 8.1 Interplay between alcohol, mental illness and life events.

Table 8.1	Problems caused by alcohol.	
Category	**System**	**Examples**
Mental	Neurosis	Anxiety, depression, phobia, increased risk of suicide
	Psychosis	Visual hallucinations
Physical	Effects of intoxication	Falls, fractures, head injuries
	Gastrointestinal	Cancer of mouth and oesophagus Gastritis and peptic ulceration Pancreatitis Enteropathy Colorectal cancer
	Liver	Cirrhosis of liver, portal hypertension, decompensated liver disease Liver cancer
	Cardiovascular	Stroke, ischaemic heart disease, cardiomyopathy, arrhythmia
	Breast	Breast cancer
	Neurological	Peripheral sensory neuropathy, proximal myopathy, cerebellar syndrome, Wernicke's encephalopathy
Social	Work	Absence, disciplinary action, loss of job
	Family	Marital breakup, domestic violence, adverse effect on children

is often not enough time to go through all 10 questions, so many GPs use AUDIT-C,[3] a validated screening tool consisting of the first three:

A How many days a week do you have a drink containing alcohol?

B How many drinks containing alcohol do you have on a typical day that you are drinking?

C How often have you drunk 6 or more units on a single occasion in the last year?

One unit of alcohol is 10 ml of ethanol. Not everyone has a good understanding of what a unit of alcohol is, so it is often better to ask a patient to describe what they drink and in what quantity. To calculate the number of units, for each type of drink, use this formula:

Units of alcohol = Volume (in litres) × Alcohol by volume (%)

Table 8.2 shows how to score the answers from the AUDIT-C questionnaire. If the patient scores more than 4, they may be drinking too much, and we should ask them the remaining seven questions from the AUDIT questionnaire, giving a score out of 40. The score from the full AUDIT questionnaire allows us to categorise the patient's drinking as low-risk, hazardous, harmful or dependent (see Table 8.3). Hazardous drinking is defined as drinking at a level which puts the patient at risk of experiencing physical or mental harm. Harmful drinking is defined as drinking at a level which is causing physical or mental harm.

Table 8.2 Scoring AUDIT-C.

	Question	Score 0	1	2	3	4
A	How often do you have a drink containing alcohol?	Never	Once a month or less	2–4 times a month	2–3 times a week	4 or more days a week
B	How many drinks containing alcohol do you have on a typical drinking day?	1–2	3–4	5–6	7–9	10 or more
C	How often do you drink 6 or more units on a single occasion?	Never	Less than once a month	Monthly	Weekly	Daily or almost daily

Total score: A + B + C

Source: Bush et al. 1998.[3]

Table 8.3 Interpreting the AUDIT questionnaire.

Score on full AUDIT	Level of risk	Recommended action
<8	Lowest risk	Give general advice. Reinforce safe limits
8–15	Hazardous	Give brief advice (10–15 minutes) in a single consultation
16–19	Harmful	Provide extended brief intervention: several appointments Undertake physical examination and blood tests Provide follow-up
20 or more	May be dependent	Refer to specialist services

Case study 8.1

Josephine Jakeman is 64 years old and was widowed a year ago. She is on medication for high blood pressure and has a routine blood pressure check done by the health care assistant (HCA) at her doctor's surgery. Her blood pressure is 158/96 mmHg (above target), so the HCA suggests she make an appointment to see the GP, Sonia Sanders. Dr Sanders checks her blood pressure again; it is about the same. In the past, Mrs Jakeman's blood pressure has been very well controlled, so Dr Sanders asks Mrs Jakeman if she can think of any reason why it's gone up.

MRS JAKEMAN	I've been findings things quite difficult since Michael died. I can't get to sleep and I lie awake at night worrying.
DR SANDERS	What do you do to help that?
MRS JAKEMAN	I've started having a glass of wine. That helps.

At this point, Dr Sanders asks the three questions from AUDIT-C and ascertains that Mrs Jakeman is drinking about two glasses of red wine (a third of a bottle) most nights of the week. She never has more than this.

What is her score for AUDIT-C?
She scores 5, so Dr Sanders continues with the rest of the AUDIT questions. Mrs Jakeman admits that a couple of months ago her daughter made a comment about her drinking, to the effect that she was drinking too much. Her full AUDIT score is 9, indicating that her level of drinking is hazardous.

What can Dr Sanders do to help?
She should feed back to Mrs Jakeman that this level of alcohol consumption might affect her health and is above the recommended limit. For women, the safe limit for drinking is 14 units a week, and no more than 2–3 units in a single day. The apparent discrepancy between these limits is accounted for by the fact that everyone should have at least 2 days a week with no alcohol, to allow their body to recover. For men, the safe limit is 21 units a week and 3–4 units a day.

Dr Sanders should explain to Mrs Jakeman what a unit is. Most bottles of wine are at least 12%, so a bottle (75 cl) contains 9 units of alcohol (0.75 × 12). She should also point out that alcohol makes people's blood pressure go up, so this may be why Mrs Jakeman's blood pressure is higher than normal.

Dr Sanders could suggest that Mrs Jakeman try to limit herself to just one glass of wine at night. Maybe she could do something different one night a week. Is she keeping in touch with her friends? She should consider the possibility that Mrs Jakeman may be depressed (see Chapter 24). She should give her some encouragement, too. Is there something that she's succeeded in changing in the past?

A brief intervention such as that in Case study 8.1 may be all that is needed for someone who demonstrates a hazardous level of drinking.[4] The components to this intervention are neatly encapsulated in the mnemonic 'FRAMES'.[5]

- **F = feedback:** Reflect back to the patient what they have told you about their drinking.
- **R = responsibility:** Put the responsibility for making changes in the patient's court.
- **A = advice:** Give the patient advice on what is a safe level of drinking.
- **M = menu:** Give the patient different options for making a positive change.
- **E = empathy:** Make clear that you understand what has led the patient to this position.
- **S = self efficacy:** Boost the patient's confidence in changing their behaviour.

If the GP supplements this brief intervention by issuing a leaflet, there is a one-in-three to one-in-four chance that the patient will reduce their alcohol intake.[6]

Helping people whose level of alcohol consumption is harmful

If we suspect that someone's level of drinking is harmful, we must make a thorough assessment. GPs usually do this over several consultations.

If the liver function tests (LFTs) are deranged, the patient's medication should be reviewed. Many medicines cause mild

Case study 8.2a

Neil Nolan is 44 and comes to see Dr Sanders to request a repeat prescription for omeprazole (a proton-pump inhibitor, PPI). He has just registered at the surgery and his previous GP notes have not arrived yet, so Dr Sanders asks him to tell her a bit more. He was prescribed a course of omeprazole 2 months ago because he had some epigastric pain. He's been without the omeprazole for a couple of weeks and the pain has returned; it does not spread elsewhere. In the mornings he feels nauseated, but he has never vomited anything resembling blood. His weight is steady and he has no difficulty swallowing.

This history suggests peptic ulcer disease or gastritis. Dr Sanders is suspicious that alcohol may be a factor in this and rapidly ascertains that Mr Nolan is drinking about 4 pints of strong lager (5%) every day; that's 70 units a week, giving him an AUDIT-C score of 8. Mr Nolan says he knows this is too much but that it's his way of relaxing after a hard day on the building site. He leads a team of construction workers and all the men go to the pub after work. He just wants a prescription to sort out his pain.

What should Dr Sanders do, apart from give a prescription for omeprazole?

Dr Sanders should:

1. Complete a full AUDIT questionnaire and gather some more background information about his previous medical problems and use of medication.
2. Examine him to:
   (a) check that there is no acute problem with his abdomen (such as evidence of a gastrointestinal haemorrhage) that might warrant admission; and
   (b) look for signs of alcoholic liver disease (see Figure 8.2).
3. Explain that there may be a link between Mr Nolan's drinking and his epigastric pain. She should explore Mr Nolan's view on this link and find out if he would like any help with reducing his alcohol consumption.
4. Seek Mr Nolan's consent to do some blood tests: serum urea and electrolytes (U&Es), liver function tests (LFTs) and a full blood count (FBC).
5. Arrange to see him again.

Either at this consultation or at the follow-up appointment, Dr Sanders should ask how things are at home. What's his mood like? How is he sleeping? Does he have a partner or any children?

Outcome

Mr Nolan's full AUDIT score is 17. He says he and his partner have one child. They are all getting along ok but he has difficulty sleeping some nights and he sometimes finds it difficult to control his temper when he's tired. 'I'd never hit anyone, though', he says. He feels a bit down sometimes, but denies any thoughts of suicide.

Mr Nolan is not jaundiced. His pulse is 88 and regular, and his blood pressure lying and standing is 138/88 mmHg. There are no stigmata of chronic liver disease, but he is tender on deep palpation of his epigastrium. There are no masses to feel in his abdomen and his liver is not palpable.

The results of his blood tests come back a few days later and show that his bilirubin is normal but his serum ALT is 132 IU/l (raised) and his mean cell volume is 102 fl (raised).

Everything points towards the fact that Mr Nolan's level of drinking is causing harm. He is suffering from insomnia; it's likely he has peptic ulcer disease or gastritis; and the results of his blood tests are consistent with alcoholic liver disease.

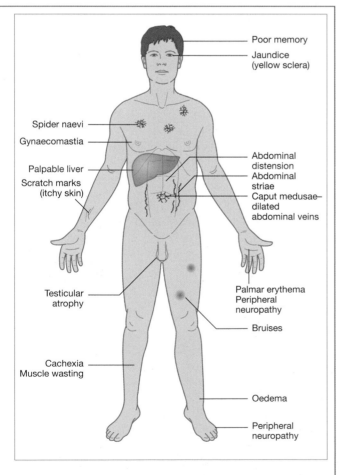

Poor memory
Jaundice (yellow sclera)
Spider naevi
Gynaecomastia
Palpable liver
Scratch marks (itchy skin)
Abdominal distension
Abdominal striae
Caput medusae–dilated abdominal veins
Testicular atrophy
Palmar erythema
Peripheral neuropathy
Bruises
Cachexia Muscle wasting
Oedema
Peripheral neuropathy

Figure 8.2 Signs of alcoholic liver disease.

inflammation of the liver. Statins, for example, commonly cause elevation of the serum alanine transferase (ALT) level, so it may be worthwhile stopping this for a while and then repeating the LFTs. If the LFTs remain abnormal, it is prudent to do a full liver screen (see Table 8.4). Remember, there may be other causes for the abnormal liver tests.

GPs must consider what effect the alcohol consumption is having on the patient's social functioning: the effect on their job and their family. People who drink too much are more likely to have accidents at work; they may face disciplinary proceedings because of lateness or unacceptable behaviour; and if caught over the legal limit for driving, they may lose their licence, which may in turn mean that they lose their job. Whenever we discover that someone is drinking in harmful quantities, we should always remind them that they should not drink and drive.

Alcohol damages families. If someone loses their job through drinking, they may find it difficult to get alternative work and so lose income for their family. This can put pressure on the patient's partner to work longer hours, which may affect any dependents, whether they be children or elderly parents. As someone's level of drinking increases, drinking becomes their priority, preventing them from fulfilling other duties and responsibilities; once again, the partner and dependents suffer. Alcohol also fuels domestic violence (see Chapter 28).

Having made an assessment of the harm that the alcohol has caused, the GP needs to work with the patient to help them cut down on their consumption and alleviate the harm. If there is evidence of chronic liver disease, the GP should refer the patient to a liver specialist, who will decide whether a liver biopsy is necessary.[7] Sometimes, the specialist will do a fibroscan first, because this is less invasive than a biopsy.

Table 8.4 Investigation of abnormal LFTs.

Test	Interpretation
Hepatitis A serology	Anti-hepatitis A virus IgM (Anti-HAV IgM) indicates recent infection
Hepatitis B serology	Hepatitis B surface antigen (HBsAg) positive suggests current infection
Hepatitis C serology	Anti-hepatitis C virus antibodies suggest infection. Ongoing infection is confirmed by an RNA polymerase test
Epstein–Barr virus (EBV) serology	Anti-EBV IgM indicates recent infection
Cytomegalovirus (CMV) serology	Raised anti-CMV IgM and IgG indicates recent infection
Autoimmune profile	Elevation of a variety of autoantibody levels suggests autoimmune hepatitis. Antimitochondrial antibody levels are raised in primary biliary cirrhosis
Serum immunoglobulins	Immunoglobulins are raised in many types of liver disease.
Serum ferritin	Very high level suggests haemochromatosis
Serum alpha-1 antitrypsin	Low level suggests alpha-1 antitrypsin deficiency
Alpha feto protein	Raised in hepatocellular carcinoma and some other cancers (stomach, biliary tract and pancreas)
Serum caeruloplasmin	Raised in Wilson's disease
Clotting screen	Prothrombin time raised in liver disease
Abdominal ultrasound scan	May show gallstones, evidence of fatty liver or carcinoma

The GP should give clear information about the benefits of reducing the level of drinking and should offer to refer the patient to a specialist alcohol advisory service for help with doing this. It may take time and several offers of referral before the patient feels ready to accept help. GPs shouldn't advise the patient to stop drinking abruptly, but in general it is safe to recommend that the patient reduce their intake by 10% in the first instance.

Detoxification and relapse

If someone is dependent on alcohol, they will experience withdrawal symptoms within about 12 hours of stopping drinking. In mild to moderate cases, these symptoms consist of anxiety, agitation, sweating, vomiting and diarrhoea. In severe cases, the patient can become confused and experience visual hallucinations (referred to as 'delirium tremens') and can have withdrawal seizures. Therefore, anyone who is at risk of withdrawal symptoms should be offered controlled detoxification using a 7–10-day course of a benzodiazepine, such as chlordiazepoxide.[7] In practice, this applies to anyone who drinks more than 15 units a day or who has an AUDIT score over 20.[8]

Detoxification, whether it is done at home or as an in-patient, always needs careful planning. During the period of withdrawal from alcohol, people are at increased risk of

---

Case study 8.2b

Dr Sanders refers Mr Nolan to a hepatologist. Mr Nolan has a fibroscan, which indicates he has a low risk of cirrhosis, so he does not have a liver biopsy. However, he does have an upper gastrointestinal endoscopy, which shows moderate gastritis but no ulcer and no evidence of oesophageal varices. A biopsy taken on endoscopy proves negative for *Helicobacter pylori*. The hepatologist suggests that he is followed up in clinic in 6 months' time.

Dr Sanders receives a letter from the hepatologist 7 months later, informing her that Mr Nolan has failed to attend his follow-up appointment. Mr Nolan's partner, Helen, brings him to see Dr Sanders 2 weeks later.

'Please can you help Neil stop drinking', she says. 'He's drinking more than ever. He's got to stop. He missed his hospital appointment because he overslept and his boss is threatening to fire him because he's been late so many times. I know he wants to stop. Can't you prescribe him something to help him stop?'

Dr Sanders speaks to Mr Nolan directly. Mr Nolan appears sober and confirms that his drinking has escalated; he's drinking at least 10 cans of strong lager a day now, and starts drinking at lunchtime.

Can Dr Sanders prescribe a home detox for Mr Nolan?
GPs can prescribe a home detox using chlordiazepoxide, but it is only safe for them to do so if the patient has never had delirium tremens or a withdrawal fit. Because Mr Nolan has not tried stopping drinking since his consumption escalated, there is a risk he might experience delirium tremens. So, in this situation, Dr Sanders should refer him to the local specialist alcohol advisory service for detoxification; this may have to be done as an in-patient.

developing Wernicke's encephalopathy due to a lack of thiamine. Therefore, a fortnight before the start of the detox regime, we prescribe oral thiamine. We also prescribe oral strong vitamin B.

People who are dependent on alcohol are used to drinking large volumes of sweet liquid, so we encourage them to stock up with soft drinks before an attempt at a home detox.

The patient should tell their friends and family that they are intending to stop drinking and request their support. This is often difficult, because people who drink heavily tend to socialise with people who are also heavy drinkers and lose contact with their other friends. If the patient has little or poor social support, in-patient detox is safer.

In the first days and weeks after completing a detox, the risk of relapse is high. To reduce this risk, the patient ideally needs daily support and encouragement. They can get this by attending Alcoholics Anonymous meetings, by attending an individual or group session at the local alcohol advisory service and by seeing their GP. There is evidence that prescribing acamprosate and naltrexone can reduce the risk of relapse.[8]

Once the patient is abstinent, their physical and mental health should start to improve, but it is common for people to suffer from a period of depression. If their mood does not lift within the first month of abstinence, an antidepressant should be considered.

Case study 8.2c

Outcome

Dr Sanders refers Mr Nolan to the local specialist advisory service. After careful assessment, the psychiatrist decides that Mr Nolan can complete a home detox but must attend the clinic every day. When Mr Nolan completes this detox, the psychiatrist starts him on acamprosate and asks the GP to continue to prescribe this, as well as strong vitamin B and thiamine. When Mr Nolan comes to see Dr Sanders about this, she re-refers him to the hepatologist so that he can be kept under review. His serum ALT falls to a near-normal level.

The role of the GP in helping people who misuse drugs

Drug misuse has many similarities to alcohol misuse. It has a profound deleterious effect on the physical, psychological and social well-being of the user and can present dangers to those around them. People who use drugs often misuse alcohol, too. They may take either substance in an attempt to 'self-medicate': to control the symptoms of mental illness or the effects of trauma, such as past sexual abuse. The prevalence of drug and alcohol misuse is particularly high amongst the prison population. For GPs who

work within the prison service, managing drug and alcohol misuse forms a large part of their work. But drug misuse is not confined to one sector of society. In the UK, about 0.8% of people between the ages of 15 and 65 inject heroin.[9] Heroin, crack cocaine and a huge variety of other substances, although illegal, are widely available. There are also a growing number of so-called 'legal highs': substances which give a sense of euphoria but which have not yet been named and classified in legislation.

GPs have a particular role to play in the care of people who use heroin and benzodiazepine. They can prescribe legal substitutes for maintenance or withdrawal therapy. There is a lot that GPs can do to reduce the harm from intravenous drug misuse, whatever the drug in question. The role of GPs in helping people who use other drugs, such as cannabis or cocaine, is less well defined. Sometimes, their main function is to make a referral to specialist services, many of them within the voluntary sector, for psychological therapy and social support. Even if GPs do not have the necessary skills to help people with every sort of drug addiction, they have a duty to provide general medical services to everyone. That means dealing with their chronic physical illnesses, such as asthma or psoriasis, managing their mental illness (which they have an above-average likelihood of having) and managing any acute illness that they may develop.

Doctors are well versed in asking patients about their consumption of tobacco and alcohol, but we often forget to ask about the use of drugs, which means that we can overlook possible explanations for symptoms. Ketamine, for example, can cause dysuria, and cocaine can cause panic attacks, anxiety and insomnia.

The risks of intravenous drug misuse

People who inject drugs have a much higher risk of death than the general population. Overdose, causing respiratory or cardiac arrest, is the commonest cause of death, followed by trauma and suicide.[10] People who inject drugs also run the risk of acquiring bloodborne viruses, notably human immunodeficiency virus (HIV), hepatitis B and hepatitis C. They acquire these infections by sharing equipment, and sometimes by having unprotected sex. People who misuse drugs often have to fund their addiction through prostitution or else engage in risky sexual behaviour, and this further increases their risk of acquiring HIV and hepatitis B. Therefore, GPs offer tests for these viruses to anyone who has a history of intravenous drug misuse. For those who have not had hepatitis B, GPs can provide a course of vaccinations. Needle-exchange programmes can also be provided in order to reduce the transmission of these viruses.

Intravenous drug misuse also runs the risk of causing cellulitis, abscesses, infective endocarditis and discitis. If someone who injects drugs develops a fever, the GP needs to take particular care to rule out these serious infections.

People who are dependent on opiates experience withdrawal symptoms if they stop taking them. These symptoms include agitation, insomnia, sweating, abdominal cramps, diarrhoea and aching muscles.

Opiate substitution therapy

Helping people to come off opiates is challenging and often takes years. The main method is to offer substitution with methadone or buprenorphine (a partial opiate agonist). Methadone comes in liquid form. Buprenorphine is prescribed as a tablet. If someone can be switched to either of these drugs, they can be stabilised, and the risks associated with their drug misuse can be reduced. Once on an opiate substitute, their dose can be reduced gradually until they are off it (withdrawal therapy) or they can be maintained on a constant dose (maintenance therapy). The hope in both cases is that mortality and criminal activity will be reduced. A meta-analysis of the published trials[11] revealed a reduction of both these end points in every case. Overall, however, this reduction was not significant, so we still can't be sure of the benefits of opiate substitution therapy.

In the UK, there has been a big expansion in the provision of opiate substitution therapy, mainly delivered in primary care, specialist centres and prisons. Despite this expansion, the number of deaths from heroin overdose has remained constant. Of greater concern is the fact that when someone is started on methadone, their risk of mortality actually increases for a while (particularly during the first 2 weeks).[12] This may be because they are prescribed too large a dose or because they continue to use opiates on top of the methadone. Only once they have been on methadone for a year does the crude mortality rate fall (see Table 8.5). Coming off methadone therapy is also a risky time. During the first month off therapy, the crude mortality rate is eight to nine times higher than the mortality rate on treatment. This may reflect the fact that the patient has lost their tolerance to opiates: if they relapse and take the dose of heroin that they used to take before going on methadone, it may prove to be a fatal overdose.

Opiate substitution therapy is associated with a reduction in the incidence of HIV.[13] This may be because the patient stops injecting or injects less often. It may also be because people who go on opiate substitution therapy represent the most motivated users, who are willing to stop sharing needles.

Knowing all of this, how should GPs go about prescribing opiate substitution therapy? With caution, is the short answer.

When someone asks a GP to go on opiate substitution therapy, the GP can feel pressured to prescribe immediately, but they must ensure that this is a safe course of action. First, the GP needs to find out what drugs the patient is taking, how much and how often. Patients may lie about this in order to obtain drugs that they can sell on, so the GP has to get confirmation. In the UK, GPs do this by requesting a urine sample, which can be tested for opiates, methadone, benzodiazepines, cocaine and amphetamine. Before prescribing methadone substitution therapy, the GP needs to receive a lab report stating that the urine contains opiates and does not contain methadone (which would suggest the patient is buying this on the black market or receiving opiate substitution therapy from elsewhere). The courts in England tend to monitor a criminal's drug misuse by testing a sample of hair.

As part of the initial assessment, the GP also needs to ask about alcohol use, find out about the patient's general physical and mental health and conduct an examination to look for evidence of problems caused by the drug misuse, such as abscesses.

It is essential to ask who the patient lives with and cares for. There have been tragic cases in the UK where children have died as a result of taking methadone prescribed to a parent. If there are children in the house, methadone should be dispensed daily and consumed at the pharmacy under supervision (see Chapter 12 for more information about protecting children). If the patient is pregnant, the GP should refer them urgently to a specialist drug clinic.

The GP needs to check the patient's HIV and hepatitis status. This doesn't have to be done before starting opiate substitution therapy.

To minimise the risks of overdose when starting therapy, GPs start patients on a low dose of methadone (usually around 30 mg a day). They write the prescription on a special form that allows them to specify that the methadone must be dispensed daily under the supervision of the pharmacist. This means that the patient cannot store up the methadone at home and take a larger dose than intended.

If the patient does not feel controlled on the starting dose of methadone and is still using opiates on top of it, then the GP can gradually increase the dose to a maximum of 80 mg daily. The GP can check the patient's compliance by requesting urine samples, which should show methadone but no opiate.

Prescribing opiate substitution therapy by itself is not sufficient to return a patient to a drug-free life. Patients also need psychological and practical support. This is normally provided by specialist drug misuse support workers, who often run clinics within the GP practice.

People who misuse drugs often lead chaotic lives and may miss appointments. This adds to the challenge of prescribing them with opiate substitution therapy. If they fail to collect their methadone or buprenorphine therapy from the pharmacy for 3 days or more, it is not safe for them to continue with the same dose, because they may have lost their tolerance. Pharmacists and GPs have to work closely to manage situations such as this. If a patient has failed to collect their prescription for the third consecutive day, the pharmacist must inform the

Table 8.5 Crude death rates before, during and after opiate substitution therapy.

	Crude mortality rate (deaths per 100 person years)
Off treatment	1.3
First 2 weeks on treatment	1.7
On established treatment	0.7
Weeks 1–2 off treatment	4.8
Weeks 3–4 off treatment	4.3

GP, and if the patient reappears, the GP must make a fresh assessment and recommence opiate therapy at a lower dose.

A note of caution

Patients who misuse drugs or alcohol, or both, need support from their GP over a period of years. When they do succeed in coming off the substance, there is a high chance that they will relapse. This can be frustrating for everyone, but it is important to keep offering support and to recognise that harm reduction rather than cure is sometimes the only realistic goal. The GP must consider the safety not just of the patient who is misusing drugs or alcohol, but also of those around them. If the GP feels that the safety of a child or dependent is compromised by the patient's substance misuse, they must take positive action to protect the vulnerable person. In practice, this may mean informing social services.

SUMMARY

Alcohol and drug misuse have a lot in common. They cause considerable physical, mental and social harm to the user and to those around them. Alcohol misuse is the most common. Approximately 5% of the adult UK population drinks to a harmful level. The AUDIT-C questionnaire is a good screening test by which to identify these people. Those who are drinking to a harmful level need a thorough assessment. In many cases, GPs can help patients to cut down on their drinking by giving them feedback, advice and a list of options. Some patients are dependent on alcohol or drugs and can't stop without experiencing withdrawal symptoms. These patients will need additional support and, in some cases, controlled detox. Patients in high-risk groups need referral to a specialist service for detox. Despite the widespread provision of opiate substitution therapy in primary care, the evidence that it helps people to come off drugs is lacking, although it may help to reduce harm.

 Now visit **www.wileyessential.com/primarycare** to test yourself on this chapter.

REFERENCES

1. Schütze M, Boeing H, Pischon T, et al. Alcohol attributable burden of incidence of cancer in eight European countries based on results from prospective cohort study. *BMJ* 2011;**342**:d1584.

2. Saunders JB, Aasland OG, Babor TF, et al. Development of the alcohol use disorders identification test (AUDIT): WHO collaborative project on early detection of persons with harmful alcohol consumption II. *Addiction* 1993;**88**(6):791–804.

3. Bush K, Kivlahan DR, McDonell MB, et al. The AUDIT Alcohol Consumption Questions (AUDIT-C): an effective brief screening test for problem drinking. *Arch Intern Med* 1998;**158**:1789–95.

4. NICE. Alcohol-use disorders: preventing harmful drinking. NICE Public Health Guideline 24. 2010. Available from: https://www.nice.org.uk/guidance/ph24 (last accessed 6 October 2015).

5. Miller WR, Sanchez VC. Motivating young adults for treatment and lifestyle changes. In: Howard G (ed.) *Issues in Alcohol Use and Misuse in Young Adults.* Notre Dame, IN: University of Notre Dame Press; 1993.

6. Austoker J. Cancer prevention in primary care: reducing alcohol intake. *BMJ* 1994;**308**:1549.

7. NICE. Alcohol-use disorders: diagnosis and clinical management of alcohol-related physical complications. NICE Clinical Guideline 100. 2010. Available from: http://www.nice.org.uk/guidance/cg100 (last accessed 6 October 2015).

8. NICE. Alcohol-use disorders: diagnosis, assessment and management of harmful drinking and alcohol dependence. NICE Clinical Guideline 115. 2011. Available from: http://www.nice.org.uk/guidance/CG115 (last accessed 6 October 2015).

9. Hay G, Gannon M, Macdougall J, et al. Capture-recapture and anchored prevalence estimation of injecting drug users in England: national and regional estimates. *Stat Methods Med Res* 2009;**18**:323–39.

10. Degenhardt L, Bucello C, Mathers B, et al. Mortality among regular or dependent users of heroin and other opioids: a systematic review and meta-analysis of cohort studies. *Addiction* 2010;**106**:32–51.

11. Mattick RP, Breen C, Kimber J, Davoli M. Methadone maintenance therapy versus no opioid replacement therapy for opioid dependence (review). *Cochrane Database Syst Rev* 2009 Jul 8;(3):CD002209. Doi: 10.1002/14651858. CD002209.pub2.

12. Cornish R, Macleod J, Strang J, et al. Risk of death during and after opiate substitution treatment in primary care: prospective observational study in UK General Practice Research Database. *BMJ* 2010;**341**:c5475.

13. MacArthur GJ, Minozzi, S, Martin N, et al. Opiate substitution treatment and HIV transmission in people who inject drugs: systematic review and meta-analysis. *BMJ* 2012;**345**:e5945.

CHAPTER 9

Preventing cardiovascular disease

Andrew Blythe

GP and Senior Teaching Fellow, University of Bristol

Key topics

Learning objectives

- Be able to estimate a person's risk of developing cardiovascular disease over the next 10 years.
- Be able to describe ways in which people can reduce their risk of developing cardiovascular disease.

Essential Primary Care, First Edition. Edited by Andrew Blythe and Jessica Buchan.
© 2017 John Wiley & Sons, Ltd. Published 2017 by John Wiley & Sons, Ltd.
Companion website: www.wileyessential.com/primarycare

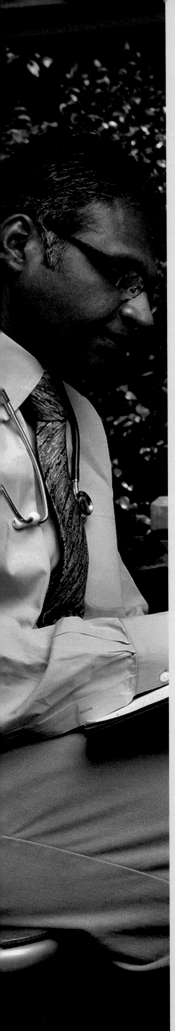

The burden of cardiovascular disease

GPs spent a large part of their time trying to prevent patients from developing cardiovascular disease (CVD) (*primary prevention*) or trying to prevent patients with established CVD from getting worse and having another major event (*secondary prevention*). A lot of the medicines that GPs prescribe are aimed at reducing this risk, such as antihypertensive and cholesterol-lowering medicines and smoking-cessation therapies.

CVD includes:

- coronary heart disease (myocardial infarction and angina);
- cerebrovascular disease (transient ischaemic attacks and stroke);
- peripheral vascular disease.

CVD is also a common cause of chronic kidney disease.

In keeping with the trend in most developed countries, over the last 40 years the incidence of CVD in the UK has declined. However, it is still the second most common cause of death after cancer. As the prevalence of obesity and type 2 diabetes increases in the UK, it is possible that the incidence of CVD will rise again.

The incidence of CVD increases with age, and it is three times more common in men than in women. Approximately 640 000 men and 275 000 women in the UK have had a myocardial infarction. Angina is more common: approximately 1.3 million people in the UK are living with angina. These data come from an analysis of validated computer records held in primary care.[1]

CVD is particularly common in people with chronic and severe mental illness. This is partly because of the high rate of smoking in this group of patients and the tendency for antipsychotic drugs to make people gain weight and increase their risk of diabetes. As we will discuss in other chapters, CVD is also more common amongst people with other illnesses, such as psoriasis.

Estimating the risk of a patient developing cardiovascular disease

Several factors increase the risk of an individual developing CVD. They include:

- smoking;
- high blood pressure;
- adverse lipid profile;
- diabetes;
- older age;
- male gender;
- family history;
- Indian subcontinent or Afro-Caribbean ethnic group.

The challenge for GPs is to successfully identify those patients most at risk and to work with them to reduce that risk. A patient's smoking status, blood pressure and serum cholesterol are the only modifiable risk factors, so these are the things that GPs focus on.

The most established method of estimating the risk of a person developing CVD is an algorithm derived from the Framingham data,[2] which may be familiar to many readers as a set of tables at the back of the British National Formulary (BNF). Framingham is a town in Massachusetts, USA. It is the setting of a prospective cohort study that began in 1948, with the aim of identifying risk factors for the development of CVD.

The Framingham tables enable one to estimate the risk of an individual developing CVD over the next 10 years on the basis of their age, sex, smoking status, systolic blood pressure and total cholesterol : HDL cholesterol ratio. There used to be two sets of tables in the BNF: one for patients with diabetes and one for those without diabetes. But the risk of a patient with diabetes over the age of 40 developing CVD is so high that the tables for diabetic patients are no longer considered useful.

There is good evidence that, in the UK, cardiovascular risk calculators which are based upon the Framingham data overestimate the risk of CVD in communities where the observed incidence of coronary heart disease is low (mostly affluent communities) and underestimate the risk in communities where the observed incidence is high (poorer communities).[3] GPs are guided in their prescribing of antihypertensive and cholesterol-lowering medication by an individual's 10-year risk of developing CVD. If this estimate of risk is biased in favour of the wealthy then this is a good example of Julian Tudor Hart's Inverse Care Law, which states that 'the availability of good medical care tends to vary inversely with the need of the population served'.[4]

Within the UK, an alternative method of estimating a person's risk, derived from data collected in the UK, has now replaced the Framingham tables. The new risk calculator is called QRISK2[5] and is recommended by the National Institute for Health and Care Excellence (NICE).[6] The QRISK2 calculator can be found at www.qrisk.org. It takes more risk factors into account than the Framingham tables, including:

- level of deprivation (a person's postcode is used as a proxy);
- body mass index (BMI);
- ethnicity (people from the Indian subcontinent are at increased risk of CVD);
- family history (if someone has a first-degree relative who developed CVD before the age of 60, this is significant).

If the Framingham tables are used for someone who has a significant family history of CVD or someone from the Indian subcontinent, a multiplier must be applied to the risk. Another advantage of QRISK2 is that it allows us to calculate the 10-year risk of developing CVD for a person who is already on antihypertensive medication. The Framingham tables can be used only for patients who are not on treatment for high blood pressure.

For several years, NICE recommended that all those whose risk of developing CVD over the next 10 years was more than 20% should take a statin and an antihypertensive drug if their blood pressure was greater than 140/90 mmHg. This strategy targeted prevention at the people who were at highest risk of developing CVD. However, these people form a minority of the population. In absolute terms, more cases of CVD occur in the majority of the population with average or low risk.[7] This is what Geoffrey Rose calls the 'prevention paradox'.[8] In 2014, amid considerable debate within the profession, NICE reduced the threshold for offering statins for primary prevention to a risk of more than 10% over the next 10 years.[6] This means that many more people in the UK (millions) can now be prescribed a statin. It remains to be seen how many doctors and patients embrace this. Meanwhile, the threshold for deciding if antihypertensive therapy should be offered to someone whose blood pressure is over 140/90 mmHg remains at a risk of 20% over the next 10 years.

In the coming years, guidelines may be based on people's lifetime risk (not their 10-year risk) of developing CVD.

Smoking cessation

In the UK, the prevalence of smoking is falling slowly, and the UK is now the second best country in Europe for its nonsmoking rates. But approximately one in four people in the UK still smokes. Smoking is commonest in young people. The life expectancy of smokers is 10 years less than that of nonsmokers. People who smoke have a one in two chance of dying as a result of their smoking.

People can be persuaded to stop smoking by personal advice from their GP or another health care professional, or by national campaigns such as bans on advertising and prohibition of smoking in the workplace. Before advising someone on how to stop smoking, we need to ask them a few questions:

1. **Would you like to stop smoking?** If the answer is yes then it is worthwhile pursuing the matter. If the answer is no then prolonged discussion may not be appropriate, although the GP should still explain why they asked this question, make clear the link between the patient's smoking habit and the problem that they are addressing and remind them that if they would like to stop smoking in the future, there is help that the GP can offer.
2. **Have you tried to stop smoking before?** If the answer is yes then the GP needs to find out what they tried last time and how they got on with it.
3. **Is there any particular way of stopping smoking that you have heard about and would like to try?**

Almost all GP surgeries offer Quit Smoking clinics. At these clinics, patients can obtain prescriptions for medication to help them stop smoking, providing they attend once a fortnight for counselling. Their compliance with cessation can be checked using a carbon monoxide meter.

Nicotine replacement therapy

Nicotine replacement therapy doubles a smoker's chance of quitting and is most effective if it is prescribed alongside some sort of counselling. It is available in the form of patches, gum and inhalators. The starting dose for a patch (which releases nicotine over the course of a day) depends on how much a person smokes. Someone who lights up a cigarette as soon as they wake up usually needs a high starting dose. There are no absolute contraindications to nicotine replacement therapy. Sometimes people benefit from using a combination of patches and gum.

Bupropion

Bupropion (Zyban) was invented as an antidepressant but is also effective at helping people to stop smoking. It is taken as an 8-week course, and patients are advised to stop smoking on the eighth day of treatment. It is contraindicated in those with epilepsy, bipolar affective disorders and eating disorders. It should not be taken while breast-feeding. The commonest side effects are a dry mouth and sleeping problems. If taken while receiving counselling from a Quit Smoking counsellor, it is more effective than nicotine replacement therapy at helping people to stop smoking.

Varenicline

Varenicline (Champix) is a partial agonist of a subtype of nicotinic acetylcholine receptors. It is even more effective than bupropion, but has more side effects and is prescribed less often.

Case study 9.1

Robert Rutherford, age 52, is diagnosed with hypertension and would like to stop smoking. He tried stopping 9 years ago with the help of nicotine patches that he bought from the chemist. He succeeded in stopping smoking for 3 months but then started again when he began a new job. He smokes 20 cigarettes a day now.

What advice should his GP give him about smoking cessation?

His GP should encourage him to give up smoking and explore his reasons for wanting to stop now. His GP should advise him that most smokers have to make several attempts at stopping before they finally succeed. Stopping smoking will substantially reduce his risk of developing heart disease in the future. He could try nicotine patches again and have them on prescription. If he attends a Quit Smoking clinic for counselling once a fortnight, his chances of stopping smoking will be much better. He might also want to consider some of the other therapies, such as bupropion or varenicline. His GP should ask him if he has heard about these things and offer him some information about them, perhaps by directing him to the NHS website (www.nhs.uk).

Blood pressure

This is a continuous variable. It is not a disease. It is one of many risk factors for CVD, second only to smoking in its importance. Blood pressure varies within a given individual over the course of a day.

Measuring blood pressure

Measuring blood pressure is the practical procedure that GPs and practice nurses carry out most often, so it is worthwhile spending some time focussing on it.

Traditionally, blood pressure is measured in a patient's right arm when they are at rest (seated). In practice, this means that we don't check their blood pressure the minute they sit down in the consulting room, but 5 minutes later.

A range of devices are available for measuring blood pressure (see Figure 9.1). Mercury sphygmomanometers were once the most commonly used. They remain the gold standard, but today anaeroid sphygmomanometers and automatic devices are used more often.

Obtaining an accurate reading of the systolic and diastolic blood pressure requires an understanding of the Korotkoff sounds.

The first Korotkoff sounds are the repetitive, tapping sounds that one hears when one deflates the bladder in the blood pressure cuff. The systolic blood pressure is the highest pressure at which these sounds are heard over two consecutive heart beats. Sometimes, these sounds are faint. As one deflates the cuff further, theses sounds may disappear. The point at which they disappear is referred to as the second Korotkoff sound. Further deflation of the cuff leads to reappearance of the sounds; the point at which they reappear is referred to as the third Korotkoff sound. If the cuff has not been inflated to a high enough level at the start, then the third Korotkoff sounds may be mistaken for the first. This is one way in which someone's blood pressure can be underestimated.

To measure the diastolic blood pressure, we have to keep deflating the cuff. Sometimes the sounds suddenly disappear; sometimes they become muffled and never disappear; and sometimes they become muffled, then disappear at a lower pressure. The point of muffling is referred to as the fourth Korotkoff sound. The point at which the sounds disappear is known as the fifth Korotkoff sound. The diastolic blood pressure is the pressure at which the fifth Korotkoff sound is heard. In pregnancy, the sounds may never disappear, in which case the fourth Korotkoff sounds should be used as a measure of diastolic blood pressure, with this caveat recorded in the patient's notes.

Figure 9.2 explains the key steps in measuring blood pressure.

Diagnosing hypertension

What level of blood pressure is high?

NICE defines hypertension as anything consistently over 140/90 mmHg measured in a clinic setting (the GP surgery or hospital).[9] Readings taken on a single day are not sufficient to make a

(a)

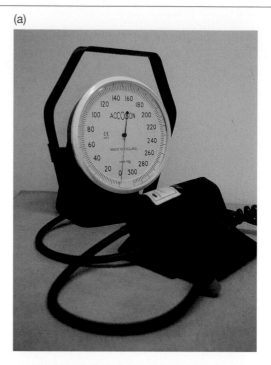

(b)

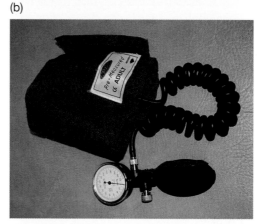

(c)

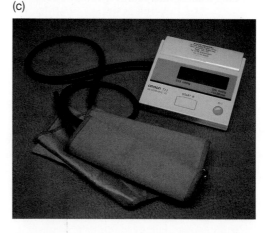

Figure 9.1 Devices for measuring blood pressure: (a) desktop anaeroid sphygmanometer; (b) portable anaeroid device; (c) automatic device.

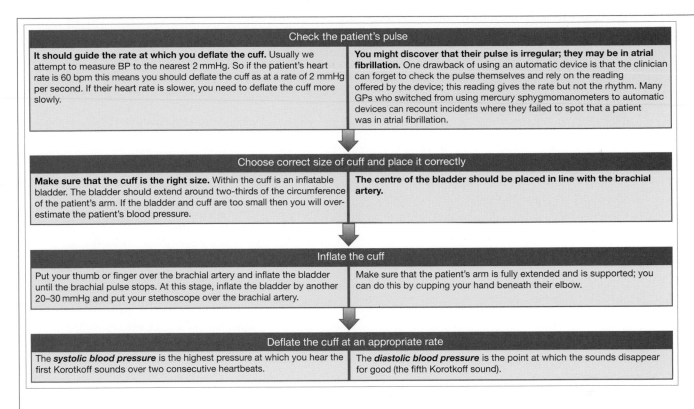

Check the patient's pulse

It should guide the rate at which you deflate the cuff. Usually we attempt to measure BP to the nearest 2 mmHg. So if the patient's heart rate is 60 bpm this means you should deflate the cuff as at a rate of 2 mmHg per second. If their heart rate is slower, you need to deflate the cuff more slowly.	**You might discover that their pulse is irregular; they may be in atrial fibrillation.** One drawback of using an automatic device is that the clinician can forget to check the pulse themselves and rely on the reading offered by the device; this reading gives the rate but not the rhythm. Many GPs who switched from using mercury sphygmomanometers to automatic devices can recount incidents where they failed to spot that a patient was in atrial fibrillation.

Choose correct size of cuff and place it correctly

Make sure that the cuff is the right size. Within the cuff is an inflatable bladder. The bladder should extend around two-thirds of the circumference of the patient's arm. If the bladder and cuff are too small then you will over-estimate the patient's blood pressure.	**The centre of the bladder should be placed in line with the brachial artery.**

Inflate the cuff

Put your thumb or finger over the brachial artery and inflate the bladder until the brachial pulse stops. At this stage, inflate the bladder by another 20–30 mmHg and put your stethoscope over the brachial artery.	Make sure that the patient's arm is fully extended and is supported; you can do this by cupping your hand beneath their elbow.

Deflate the cuff at an appropriate rate

The *systolic blood pressure* is the highest pressure at which you hear the first Korotkoff sounds over two consecutive heartbeats.	The *diastolic blood pressure* is the point at which the sounds disappear for good (the fifth Korotkoff sound).

Figure 9.2 Key steps in measuring blood pressure.

diagnosis of hypertension. If, on a single clinic visit, a patient has two consecutive blood pressure readings equal to or greater than 140/90 mmHg, they should have ambulatory blood pressure measurement (ABPM) or home blood pressure measurements to confirm or refute the diagnosis of hypertension.

Ambulatory blood pressure readings and home blood pressure measurements are lower than those obtained in a clinic. On average, ambulatory systolic blood pressure readings are 10 mmHg lower than those in clinic and ambulatory diastolic blood pressure readings are 5 mmHg lower. The normal ABPM for adults is less than 135/85 mmHg during the day and less than 120/75 mmHg at night. The lack of a nocturnal dip is a bad prognostic sign and is associated strongly with end organ damage.

Step 1: First visit to clinic

If blood pressure is >140/90, take a second reading.

If the second reading is >140/90, proceed to ABPM or home monitoring.

If the second reading is substantially lower than the first, take a third reading and record the lowest of the second and third readings.

Step 2: Ambulatory blood pressure measurement

The monitor should take two readings per hour and at least 14 readings over the course of the day, during waking hours. Take the average of all these readings.

Step 3 (alternative): Home blood pressure measurement

On two occasions during the day, the patient should sit down and take two readings, 1 minute apart. The patient should do this for at least 4 days, then discard the readings from the first day and calculate the average of all the other readings.

If the average blood pressure is >135/85 mmHg then the diagnosis of hypertension is confirmed.

What investigation is necessary?

Once it has been established that a patient has hypertension, a further assessment is needed. We need to make sure that they do not already have CVD. This involves taking a history, examining their cardiovascular system and obtaining an electrocardiogram (ECG). An irregular pulse may be the result of atrial fibrillation, a displaced apex beat may indicate left ventricular hypertrophy and an abnormal ECG may also show evidence of left ventricular hypertrophy. If the voltage criteria for left ventricular hypertrophy are met, an echocardiogram should be requested. There may be clues on examination to suggest other risk factors for CVD, such as xanthomas, a feature of hypercholesterolaemia.

In order to calculate the patient's 10-year risk of developing CVD, their total cholesterol and high-density lipoprotein and their fasting glucose or glycosylated haemoglobin must be requested to determine whether they have diabetes. Before starting them on medication, a baseline measurement of their

Table 9.1 Summary of antihypertensive medication.

	Drug	Contraindications	Side effects
A	ACE inhibitor (ramipril)	Pregnancy Renovascular disease	Cough First-dose hypotension Taste disturbance Angio-oedema
B	Beta blocker (atenolol)	Asthma Heart block Peripheral vascular disease Dyslipidaemia	Fatigue Insomnia Cold peripheries Bradycardia
C	Calcium channel antagonist (amlodipine)	Myocardial infarction Heart failure	Constipation Peripheral oedema Flushing Headache
D	Thiazide-like diuretic (indapamide)	Gout Dyslipidaemia Urinary incontinence	Hypokalaemia Hyponatraemia Sexual dysfunction Gout Glucose intolerance

renal function must be obtained, so their serum urea and electrolytes (U&Es) should be checked and their urine should be tested for blood and protein.

Lowering blood pressure

We do not start by prescribing medication, but start instead with lifestyle advice.

Lifestyle advice

- Stop smoking.
- Increase exercise. Aim for 30 minutes of exercise a day. This need not be all in one stretch.
- Reduce salt intake to less than 6 g/day.
- Restrict alcohol consumption to a moderate level. Aim for less than 21 units/week for men and less than 14 units a week for women.

This lifestyle advice must be reinforced periodically.

Antihypertensive medication

We can consider starting antihypertensive medication immediately (before ABPM or home readings) if the reading in clinic is above 180/110 mmHg.

Medication should be started if:

- Blood pressure >160/100 mmHg (clinic) or >150/95 mmHg (ABPM), regardless of the patient's 10-year risk of developing CVD.

- Blood pressure >140/90 mmHg (clinic) or >135/85 mmHg (ABPM) and the patient's risk of developing CVD over the next 10 years is >20%. This includes all patients with diabetes.
- Blood pressure >140/90 mmHg (clinic) or >135/85 mmHg (ABPM) and there is evidence of end organ damage.

The aim is reduce blood pressure to:

- <140/90 mmHg (clinic) for patients under 80 years old.
- <150/90 mmHg (clinic) for patients over 80 years old.

Clinic blood pressure measurements can be used to monitor treatment, unless the patient is thought to suffer from 'white coat hypertension'.

Lower targets are advised for people who have chronic kidney disease or diabetes.

There are several different classes of drug to choose from:

1. ACE inhibitors (e.g. ramipril) or angiotensin II receptor blockers (e.g. candestartan);
2. beta blockers (e.g. atenolol);
3. dihydropyridine calcium channel antagonists (e.g. amlodipine);
4. thiazide-like diuretics (e.g. indapamide).

The contraindications and common side effects of these drugs are listed in Table 9.1. Certain ethnic groups respond better to different drugs. NICE recommends the following strategy for deciding which drug to use:[9]

Age >55, or black of any age

- start with C (or D);
- add A if second drug is needed.

Age <55

- start with A;
- offer angiotensin receptor blocker if patient doesn't tolerate ACE inhibitor;
- add C or D if second drug is needed.

If triple therapy is needed, use A + C + D.

The combination of a beta blocker and a thiazide diuretic (B + D) should be avoided because of the increased risk of developing diabetes.

Do not combine ACE inhibitors and angiotensin II receptor blockers when treating hypertension.

If the patient is on a conventional thiazide diuretic (e.g. bendroflumethiazide) and their blood pressure is controlled, leave them on this.

Beta blockers are fourth-line therapy except:

- for those with established CVD;
- in women of child-bearing age;
- in young patients who are unable to tolerate ACE inhibitors.

Alpha blockers can be used when triple therapy has been tried or when other drugs are contraindicated.

Most patients need more than one drug to lower their blood pressure. In practice, patients end up on a particular combination of drugs because the other drugs haven't worked (they haven't lowered the blood pressure), the other drugs are contraindicated or the other drugs have caused side effects.

Cholesterol reduction

Lipid-lowering drugs cost the NHS more than any other category of drug, but they are getting cheaper. In the UK, approximately 2 million prescriptions for statins (HMG CoA reductase inhibitors) are issued every month, and each year the number of people on statins rises. GPs are encouraged to prescribe statins not only to those whose 10-year risk of developing CVD is greater than 10% but also to everyone with chronic kidney disease stage 3 or worse and those with diabetes who are over the age of 40. Statins are also available over the counter, without a prescription.

Side effects of statins

The commonest side effect of statins is gastrointestinal upset. Statins can cause myopathy, and very rarely rhabdomyolysis. They can also have an adverse effect on the liver. Before starting someone on a statin, their liver function tests (LFTs) should be checked. Their creatine kinase (CK) should be checked if they complain of muscle aching. Their LFTs should be checked again 1–3 months after starting the statin, 6 months later, and then again at 1 year. The statin must be stopped if:

- CK rises above five times the normal level; or if
- alanine transferase (ALT) rises above three times the normal level.

Familial hypercholesterolaemia

Approximately 110 000 people in the UK have familial hypercholesterolaemia. Their fasting cholesterol levels are very high, and they are at high risk of premature death as the result of CVD. If a GP discovers that someone's total cholesterol is more than 7.5 mmol/l, they must consider the possibility that the person has familial hypercholesterolaemia and take a detailed family history. If a first-degree relative has suffered from coronary heart disease before the age of 50, referral to a specialist lipid clinic is prudent. People with familial hypercholesterolaemia need high doses of statins, and their family members should have their lipid profiles checked.

Other causes of high serum cholesterol levels include hypothyroidism and a diet rich in saturated fat.

SUMMARY

The term 'cardiovascular disease' includes angina, myocardial infarction, stroke, transient ischaemic attacks and peripheral vascular disease. Preventing and treating CVD forms a large part of any GP's work. It is possible to estimate the risk of an individual developing CVD using tools such as QRISK2. The risk can be reduced by stopping smoking, lowering blood pressure and lowering cholesterol.

 Now visit **www.wileyessential.com/primarycare** to test yourself on this chapter.

REFERENCES

1. British Heart Foundation. Cardiovascular Disease Statistics 2014. Available from; http://www.bhf.org.uk/publications/statistics/cardiovascular-disease-statistics-2014 (last accessed 6 October 2015).

2. Anderson KV, Odell PM, Wilson PWF, Kannel WB. Cardiovascular disease risk profiles. *Am Heart J* 1991; **121**:293–8.

3. Brindle PM, McConnachie A, Upton MN, et al. The accuracy of the Framingham risk-score in different socio-economic groups: a prospective study. *Br J Gen Pract* 2005;**55**(520):838–45.

4. Tudor Hart J. The inverse care law. *Lancet* 1971;**297**:405–12.

5. Hippisley-Cox J, Coupland C, Vinogradova Y, et al. Predicting cardiovascular risk in England and Wales: prospective derivation and validation of QRISK2. *BMJ* 2008;**336**:1475.

6. NICE. Lipid modification: cardiovascular risk assessment and the modification of blood lipids for the primary and secondary prevention of cardiovascular disease. NICE Clinical Guideline 181. July 2014. Available from: http://www.nice.org.uk/guidance/cg181 (last accessed 6 October 2015).

7. Jackson R, Marshall R, Kerr A, et al. QRISK or Framingham for predicting cardiovascular risk? *BMJ* 2009;**339**:b2673.

8. Rose G. Strategy of prevention: lesson from cardiovascular disease. *BMJ* 1981;**282**:1847–51.

9. NICE. Hypertension: clinical management of primary hypertension in adults. NICE Clinical Guideline 127. August 2011. Available from: http://www.nice.org.uk/guidance/cg127 (last accessed 6 October 2015).

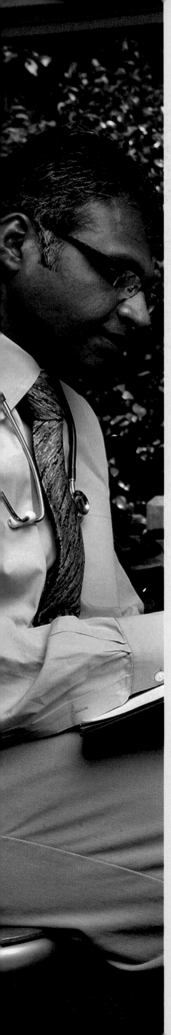

CHAPTER 10

Caring for people with learning disabilities

Andrew Blythe

GP and Senior Teaching Fellow, University of Bristol

Key topics

Learning objectives

- Be able to describe the different causes of learning disability.
- Be able to discuss the key findings of reports on the health of people with a learning disability.
- Be able to describe techniques that promote effective communication with someone who has a learning disability.
- Be able to conduct a health check on someone with a learning disability.

Essential Primary Care, First Edition. Edited by Andrew Blythe and Jessica Buchan.
© 2017 John Wiley & Sons, Ltd. Published 2017 by John Wiley & Sons, Ltd.
Companion website: www.wileyessential.com/primarycare

Types of learning disability

A learning disability is a lifelong condition in which intellectual impairment makes it difficult for the affected person to perform the basic tasks of everyday life. Roughly 1 in 200 adults in the UK has a learning disability, but this figure depends on where the line is drawn for a mild learning disability. As a rough rule of thumb, a learning disability can be categorised according to a person's IQ:

- IQ 50–70 indicates a mild disability.
- IQ 30–50 indicates a moderate disability.
- IQ <30 indicates a severe disability.

When people with learning disabilities lived in large institutions, their health care was provided by health professionals who worked onsite. Now that they live in the community, people with a learning disability are registered with a GP. Those who have a moderate to severe learning disability are also kept under review by the local community learning disability team.

In many cases, the cause of the learning disability remains elusive, but amongst those where a cause is identifiable, genetic defects provide the commonest explanation (see Table 10.1).

Down's syndrome

Most cases of Down's syndrome are the result of the affected individual having three rather than two versions of chromosome 21. In the UK, Down's syndrome is usually identified before birth by screening offered to all pregnant women. The screening test, based on an ultrasound scan and blood tests, does not give a diagnosis, it simply refines the risk. Pregnant women in their 20s have a background risk of having a child with Down's syndrome somewhere in the region of 1 in 2000. The risk increases with maternal age. If the screening test produces a revised risk of more than 1 in 150, then the woman is offered the option of having a definitive test, such as chorionic villous sampling or amniocentesis, both of which have a small risk of miscarriage. Knowing that the foetus has Down's syndrome, some women opt for termination, and as a result the incidence of Down's syndrome in the UK is less than it would be otherwise.

Most children born with Down's syndrome have a moderate learning disability. They have a characteristic appearance, as shown in Figure 10.1. There is not usually any noticeable delay in their development during the first year of life, but their development of speech is often slow. People with Down's syndrome are more likely to have certain physical problems (see Table 10.2).

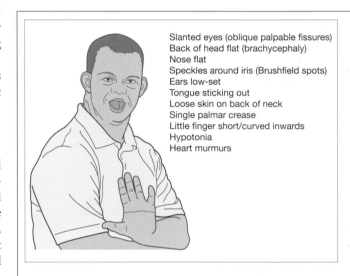

Slanted eyes (oblique palpable fissures)
Back of head flat (brachycephaly)
Nose flat
Speckles around iris (Brushfield spots)
Ears low-set
Tongue sticking out
Loose skin on back of neck
Single palmar crease
Little finger short/curved inwards
Hypotonia
Heart murmurs

Figure 10.1 Physical characteristic linked to Down's syndrome.

Table 10.1 Causes of learning disability.

Cause	Example	Antenatal screening in UK
Unknown		
Genetic/chromosomal		
Trisomy	Down's syndrome	Yes (nuchal translucency scan + blood test)
Sex-linked	Fragile X	No
Sequence deletion	Cri du chat	No
Metabolic	Phenylketonuria	Yes (heel-prick blood test)
Hormone deficiency	Hypothyroidism	Yes (heel-prick blood test)
Nutritional deficiency	Iodine deficiency in pregnancy	
Intrauterine infection	Rubella	Antenatal blood test done to confirm immunity
Birth trauma and anoxia		
Brain abnormalities	Tuberous sclerosis, neurofibromatosis	
Poisoning	Lead, alcohol	

Table 10.2 Physical problems that are more common in people with Down's syndrome.

Problem	Types
Hearing loss	Glue ear, perforations due to chronic otitis media in childhood, build-up of wax blocking tympanic membranes (people with Down's syndrome are more likely to have narrow auditory canals), early age-related hearing loss
Visual problems	Refractive errors, cataracts, congenital glaucoma, keratoconus, nystagmus
Congenital heart disease	Ventricular septal defects, patent ductus arteriosus, Fallot's tetralogy
Acquired heart disease	Mitral valve prolapse, aortic regurgitation
Endocrine problems	Hypothyroidism
Autoimmune conditions	Coeliac disease
Dementia	Early-onset Alzheimer's
Cancer	Childhood leukaemia
Musculoskeletal problems	Foot deformities, dislocated patella, dislocated hip, scoliosis, atlanto-axial instability

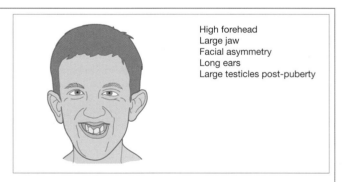

High forehead
Large jaw
Facial asymmetry
Long ears
Large testicles post-puberty

Figure 10.2 Physical characteristics linked to Fragile X syndrome.

Fragile X

Fragile X syndrome is the commonest inherited cause of learning disability. It is usually diagnosed in the first year of life, and affects about 1 in 4000 individuals. It occurs when a sequence of nucleotides is repeated too many times within a particular gene on the X chromosome. Female carriers can have a mild learning difficulty, but males are affected more severely. Affected individuals are more likely to have an obsessive and anxious personality and may have difficulty concentrating and sleeping. Their speech may be hampered by the tendency to repeat words. The physical characteristics which are linked with the Fragile X syndrome are shown in Figure 10.2. People with Fragile X syndrome can be identified by a blood test.

Inequalities of health experienced by those with a learning disability

GPs need to pay special attention to the health of people with a learning disability, because they find it difficult to access health services and they are more likely to have physical illnesses. Repeated studies have shown that people with a learning disability are less likely to receive satisfactory health care compared to the general population, and are more likely to die at a young age.

In 2007, Mencap, the UK's leading charity supporting those with learning disabilities, published the report Death by Indifference,[1] in which it presented case studies of six people with learning disabilities, each of whom died prematurely. The report does not make comfortable reading. Its authors called for a confidential inquiry into the deaths of people with learning disabilities. This inquiry was conducted, and its findings were published in 2013.[2]

The confidential inquiry studied the deaths of 247 people in the southwest of England who had a learning disability and compared them to 58 people without a learning disability. It found that people with a learning disability died earlier than the rest of the population. The median age of death in men with a learning disability was 65 years, compared to 78 for all men; the median age in women with a learning disability was 63, compared to 83 for all women. In part, this difference may be explained by the fact that people with a learning disability are more likely to have congenital malformations that have an adverse effect on their health. People with Down's syndrome, for example, have a much higher incidence of congenital heart disease. The inquiry matched the two groups for age, sex and cause of death, but it did not match for socioeconomic status or congenital abnormalities. However, it seems that other factors contributed to the disparity in life expectancy. Amongst people with a learning disability, 37% of deaths were judged to have been preventable, compared to just 13% of deaths in the general population.

The investigators concluded that people with a learning disability were more likely to die prematurely because their symptoms were not investigated adequately, diagnoses were missed or they were not started on the right treatment.

The carers of people with learning disabilities did not feel listened to. False assumptions were made about the quality of life experienced by people with learning disabilities, and because of this they were sometimes put on palliative care pathways inappropriately. Sometimes, care was not delivered in accordance with the Mental Capacity Act.

Social factors also contributed to premature death. Some people were in inappropriate accommodation. Many people with learning difficulties spent their entire lives in large institutions as recently as 30 years ago. When these institutions were closed down, their residents were transferred to houses or flats in the community, with varying degrees of onsite support.

Despite the findings of the 2013 confidential inquiry,[2] there is some cause for optimism. The life expectancy of people with Down's syndrome has improved considerably over the last 50 years. In the 1960s, the life expectancy was around 18 years – now it is over 60 years.

How can GPs improve the health of those with a learning disability?

As with any patient, the role of the GP is to provide treatment for acute and chronic problems, to offer screening and to provide health promotion. Health promotion is particularly important for those with a learning disability, because they are more likely to be over- or under-weight. Historically, people with learning disabilities have been much less likely to participate in national screening programmes, such as cervical screening.[3] This may be because they have not been encouraged to participate and have not received information about such programmes in a format that they can understand.

Conducting a consultation with someone who has a learning disability

The Disability Discrimination Act 2005 requires health professionals to make reasonable adjustments to their provision of health care to accommodate the specific needs of people with a disability. In the case of people with a learning disability, the main adjustment that needs to be made is to offer a longer consultation. Information gathering, examination and explanation all take more time when the patient has a learning disability.

People with a learning disability often come to see the GP with a support worker or family member. This person will have important information and should not be ignored, but the GP should start by making the patient the focus of their attention. For the consultation to be fruitful, they need to win the patient's trust. The first few exchanges are crucial to setting the tone and building a relationship. The GP should establish how the patient likes to be addressed, tell them their name (first and surname) and find out a bit about them. From their answers, the GP will be able to gauge the level of their disability.

Coming to see a GP can provoke anxiety in anyone, but for someone with a learning disability it can be very frightening. So the GP should take care to explain what they are going to do in the consultation (e.g. 'First, I'm going to ask you some questions about your problem. Then I might need to look at the bit that hurts. After that, I'll explain what I can do to help. Is there anything you want to ask me before I start?'). They should use short words and short sentences, breaking up their questioning into chunks with pauses. Medical jargon should be avoided (as in all consultations).

Throughout the consultation, the GP should check the patient's understanding. They can't rely on just asking them if they understand, because someone with a learning disability will often say, 'yes' whether they understand or not. The GP can check their understanding by rephrasing the question and seeing if they get the same response, or by asking them to repeat the important information. As a final check, it's worth asking the patient what they will tell a friend or support worker about the consultation.

Under the Mental Capacity Act, everyone is assumed to have the capacity to make a decision on their health care until it is proven that they do not. Capacity is decision- and time-specific. In other words, a person may have the capacity to decide if they want an operation to correct a bunion but not to decide on the details of their will. To confirm someone's capacity to make a particular decision, we must be confident that they can understand the necessary information, retain that information, weigh up the options and communicate their decision. In order to maximise the patient's capacity, a doctor should do everything possible to facilitate their understanding and assist with communication. Often, this means repeating information and using pictures.

Leaflets tailored to the needs of those with learning disability are available for many common conditions. These leaflets contain small amounts of text, accompanied by pictures that reinforce the key messages. The website www.easyhealth. org.uk has an excellent collection of leaflets and short videos. The Royal College of Psychiatrists also produces a good series of booklets, titled Books Beyond Words, as well as leaflets on mental health problems for those with a learning disability.[4]

When referring someone with a learning difficulty to another health care professional, their learning difficulty should be highlighted in the same way that a visual or hearing impairment would be highlighted, so that the recipient can make reasonable adjustments when offering the appointment.

Diagnostic overshadowing

Sometimes, patients with a learning disability are brought to see their GP by a carer or support worker because that person has noticed a change in their behaviour. This presents a particular challenge because there are so many possible causes, and there is a danger of falling into the trap of *diagnostic overshadowing*. This is a term used to describe the mistake of falsely attributing a new symptom to an existing condition. In this case, the risk is that a change in the patient's behaviour, such as a reluctance to go to their regular swimming session, will be attributed to their learning disability when it is actually due to depression, fatigue due to hypothyroidism or a musculoskeletal injury (see Case study 10.1).

The General Medical Council (GMC) has an excellent online education resource to help doctors consult more effectively with people who have a learning disability.[5]

Case study 10.1

Andrew Appleby is 67. He has a mild learning disability and lives alone. He doesn't do much cooking for himself, but usually goes to his local café for lunch. In the evening, he makes himself a sandwich. He smokes 20 cigarettes a day and doesn't drink any alcohol. He has chronic obstructive pulmonary disease (COPD), for which he has a salbutamol inhaler, and he suffers from recurrent mild depression, for which he has been on medication in the past.

Mr Appleby comes to see the practice nurse for his annual flu vaccine. The nurse notices that he appears to have lost a bit of weight since she saw him last and asks if she can weigh him. It transpires that he has lost 3 kg over the last 4 months. He says this is because he hasn't felt like going to the café as often recently and that he doesn't think there is anything wrong. But the nurse is worried and asks the GP to see him.

What should the GP ask Mr Appleby?

The GP should explore with Mr Appleby how he has been feeling recently and ask if anything has changed. He should ask him what he eats in a typical day and find out how he is managing generally. Has he got enough money to go the café? What is his mood like? How is he sleeping? What is he spending his time doing? The GP should also ask Mr Appleby if he has any new physical symptoms, particularly those that might suggest lung or bowel cancer.

Outcome

Mr Appleby admits to feeling a bit low most days and says that the reason he's not going to the café is that he can't be bothered. He hasn't been going out for walks as often because he feels tired. He doesn't sleep very well at night. He doesn't have a cough but he has been using his salbutamol inhaler a bit more frequently; he attributes this to his smoking. He doesn't have any pain in his chest or abdomen and has no difficulty swallowing his food. He opens his bowels once a day, he doesn't have to strain on the toilet and hasn't seen any blood in his stool or urine.

At this stage, it would be easy to attribute Mr Appleby's weight loss to his lack of self-care and a recurrence of his depression. This is the trap of diagnostic overshadowing. The GP pauses to summarise the evidence before him. Mr Appleby is a smoker, is clearly feeling tired and is losing weight. The possibility of cancer still needs to be excluded, so the GP requests a chest X-ray and a batch of blood tests. The chest X-ray shows some background scarring compatible with COPD but no focal lung lesion. The blood tests reveal a microcytic anaemia (haemoglobin 115 g/l). This anaemia raises the possibility of a gastrointestinal malignancy. After lengthy discussion with Mr Appleby, the GP refers him urgently for a colonoscopy and upper gastrointestinal endoscopy. Unfortunately, the colonoscopy reveals a tumour in the sigmoid colon.

Common problems in people with a learning disability

People with a learning disability are more likely to suffer from mental illness. Depression and anxiety are more common, as is psychosis. The presentation of these illnesses may be different in someone who has a learning disability, and so the GP often needs to seek help from the community learning disability team. This team includes psychologists and consultant psychiatrists who specialise in the care of people with learning disabilities.

Early-onset dementia is more common in people with learning disabilities. If someone over 40 with a learning disability is having difficulty remembering, communicating or executing tasks, it's worth asking a family member or carer who knows them well if they used to be able to do a particular task a few years ago. Don't fall into the trap of diagnostic overshadowing and automatically attribute the difficulty to their learning disability; they may have dementia. If a GP suspects dementia, they will need to involve the local community learning disability team, who can conduct a detailed psychological assessment.

People with learning difficulties are more likely to succumb to respiratory tract infections (RTIs), so the GP should use their clinical judgement when interpreting guidelines for prescribing antibiotics. Respiratory disease is the leading cause of death in people with learning disabilities.

Epilepsy is much more common. In the 'Confidential Inquiry into Premature Deaths of People with Learning Disability',[2] 43% suffered from epilepsy. Uncontrolled epilepsy is a recognised cause of premature death, and antiepileptic medication can cause a long list of side effects. So it is particularly important for the GP to review the management of epilepsy in everyone with a learning disability (see Chapter 23).

Some syndromes, such as Down's syndrome, are associated with particular health problems and need specific annual tests. People with Down's syndrome should have their vision and hearing checked regularly and their thyroid function checked once a year. They are also more likely to develop coeliac disease, so routine testing for this may be recommended soon.

Annual health checks for people with a learning disability

In 2004, Mencap produced a report, Treat Me Right!,[6] which suggested that the health of people with learning disabilities could be improved if GPs offered them annual health checks.

Table 10.3 Things to cover in an annual health check.

Advice on healthy living	Contraception and sexual health	Common problems to look out for	Engagement with national screening programmes	Review of chronic diseases
Diet Smoking Alcohol Exercise	Contraception STI check	Obesity: measure body mass index (BMI) Vision: record visual acuity Hearing: ask if the patient has problems and inspect their auditory canals Blood pressure Heart valve disorders Joint problems Incontinence Diabetes: check fasting glucose Hypothyroidism: check thyroid function tests (TFTs) Depression and/or anxiety Dementia: start GPCOG[a] screening from age 40 Communication problems	Cervical smears Mammography Bowel cancer screening Abdominal aortic aneurysm screening	Epilepsy Asthma Eczema/psoriasis

[a] GPCOG: General Practitioner assessment of Cognition.

Since then, a study in Australia has demonstrated that conducting annual health checks dramatically improves the detection of visual and hearing impairment, increases the uptake of cervical screening and results in a modest increase in the detection of new diseases.[7] This study used cluster randomisation to assign people with learning disabilities to usual care or annual health checks with their GP using a 21-page booklet.[8] Carers were asked to complete the first section of this booklet before accompanying the patient to an appointment with the GP. During this appointment, the GP asked questions and conducted a focused examination. The booklet reminded the GP to ask about common and sometimes overlooked conditions in people with learning disabilities. The appointment ended with the production of a health action plan. Both groups of patients were followed up for 1 year. The group that had the health check was 6 times more likely to have a visual impairment detected and 30 times more likely to receive a hearing test.

Annual health checks for people with learning disabilities are now offered in most GP surgeries in the UK. Usually, the checks are conducted jointly by a nurse and a GP who has developed a special interest in this area. The aims of an annual health check are to:

- give advice on healthy living;
- give advice on contraception and sexual health;
- screen for common problems, including poor eyesight, hearing loss, dental problems, dementia, diabetes and hypothyroidism;
- review any behavioural problems and mental health;
- review any chronic diseases, especially epilepsy;
- review communication with all other health professionals;
- review all the medications that the patient is prescribed.

Table 10.3 lists all the things that should be checked once a year. The individual components of the health check are all fairly basic, but it is often very straightforward things such as visual and hearing tests that get overlooked. Behavioural problems may be aggravated by poor hearing, caused by impacted ear wax, and falls may simply occur because the patient needs spectacles.

If the patient is over 40, blood should be taken to check their fasting glucose and lipid profile, and this information should be used to calculate their risk of developing cardiovascular disease (CVD) (see Chapter 9).

The end result of an annual health check should be the production of a health action plan.

Another benefit of conducting annual health checks is that the patient gets used to coming to the GP surgery and builds up a relationship with the GP. This makes it less likely that they will be frightened of coming to the GP when they are ill.

Case study 10.2

Michelle Mitchell has Down's syndrome. She is 32 and lives with her parents, who are in their late 60s. She has a part-time job working in a garden centre. She has asthma and is on treatment for hypothyroidism. She finds it difficult to manage her medication and her money, so her parents have to help with both these things. Her medication consists of a steroid inhaler (beclometasone 100 µg/inhalation, two puffs twice a day), a salbutamol inhaler when required and levothyroxine (150 µg once a day).

Miss Mitchell attends the GP surgery for an annual health check. Her parents are concerned that she is putting on weight. She says that her foot hurts. The nurse weighs and measures her, and finds that her body mass index (BMI) has increased from 28 last year to 31. Her blood pressure is 136/70 mmHg.

What particular things should the GP ask about?
The GP might start by asking Miss Mitchell about her job. This is something that Miss Mitchell might find easy to talk about, and the discussion might reveal more information about the foot pain and how it is affecting her. Next, the GP could explore the various causes of her weight gain: Has there been any change in her diet or amount of exercise? Is she taking the levothyroxine every day? What about the possibility of pregnancy? Is she having regular periods? Is she sexually active, and if so, is she using any contraception? The GP should ask Miss Mitchell if she would like to discuss any of these issues on her own, without her parents being present. Only once the GP has gathered all this information and gained Miss Mitchell's trust should he examine her foot. The GP also needs to review her asthma, although this might be a bit too much for one consultation.

Outcome
Miss Mitchell says she used to belong to a walking club but stopped going because it made her foot pain worse. She is taking her levothyroxine every day. She has regular periods, roughly every 4 weeks. Her last period was a fortnight ago. She tells the GP that she has a boyfriend,

Jack, who she met at the club which she goes to once a week. Jack also has Down's syndrome. She says that they have not had sex but she thinks that this might happen in the future. She doesn't want to have a baby, so she would like to come back to see the GP another time, by herself, to talk about contraception.

Examination reveals a hallux valgus with a bunion. The GP explains to Miss Mitchell and her parents that the deformity of her big toe could be corrected by an operation and that this might relieve the pain. Miss Mitchell says that she would like to see a surgeon to talk more about this.

The GP also finds out that it is over a year since Miss Mitchell went to a dentist and 2 years since she went to an optician. Her asthma seems under control; she uses the salbutamol inhaler just once or twice week and is not bothered by her breathing at night.

The health action plan looks like this:
- Refer to orthopaedic surgeon for correction of hallux valgus.
- Give easy-to-read leaflet on contraception and make appointment to discuss contraception.
- Make appointment to see the dentist and optician.
- Have annual flu vaccination (because she has asthma and is on an inhaled steroid).
- Have blood test to check thyroid function (to ensure she is on correct dose of levothyroxine).
- Have smaller helping of pudding at lunchtime.

A year later, Miss Mitchell has had the operation to correct her hallux valgus and, because her foot is no longer painful, she is doing more walking again and has lost weight. She has a contraceptive implant and is spending more time with Jack now. She's been to the optician too, and has glasses now.

Supporting carers

The carers of people with learning disabilities often need support from the GP. As in the case of Miss Mitchell (Case Study 10.2), it is often the parents who are the main carers, and they worry what will happen to their son or daughter if they get ill themselves or die. Plans need to put in place for this eventuality, with the help of the community learning disability team. Carers may be eligible for benefits, such as the carer's allowance, and should have an annual flu vaccination.

People who have a learning disability are more likely to have particular physical and mental health problems than the general population. Historically, they have been less likely to participate in health screening programmes and they have found it difficult to access health care. People with learning disabilities have a significantly shorter life expectancy than the general population, and some of this premature mortality is preventable. GPs can improve the health of people with learning disabilities by providing annual health checks that look for common problems and review chronic illness. Consulting with someone who has a learning disability takes extra time. The capacity of someone with a learning disability to make a decision about their health can be maximised by careful explanation.

SUMMARY

Now visit **www.wileyessential.com/primarycare** to test yourself on this chapter.

REFERENCES

1. Mencap. *Death by Indifference*. London: Mencap; 2007.

2. Heslop P, Blair P, Fleming P, et al. The Confidential Inquiry into premature deaths of people with intellectual disabilities in the UK: a population based study. *Lancet* 2014;**383**:880–95.

3. Pearson V, Davis C, Ruoff C, Dyer J. Letter: only one quarter of women with learning disability in Exeter have had cervical screening. *BMJ* 1998;**316**:1979.

4. Royal College of Psychiatrists. Information for People with Learning Disability and Their Carers. Available from: http://www.rcpsych.ac.uk/healthadvice/problemsdisorders/learningdisabilities.aspx (last accessed 6 October 2015).

5. GMC. Learning Disabilities. Available from: http://www.gmc-uk.org/learningdisabilities/default.aspx (last accessed 6 October 2015).

6. Mencap. Treat Me Right! Available from: https://www.mencap.org.uk/node/5880 (last accessed 6 October 2015).

7. Lennnox N, Bain C, Rey-Conde T, et al. Effects of a comprehensive health assessment programme for Australian adults with intellectual disability: a cluster randomised trial. *Int J Epidemiol* 2007;**36**:139–46.

8. Lennox NG, Green M, Diggens J, Ugoni A. Audit and comprehensive health assessment programme in the primary healthcare of adults with intellectual disability: a pilot study. *J Intellect Disabil Res* 2001;**45**:226–32.

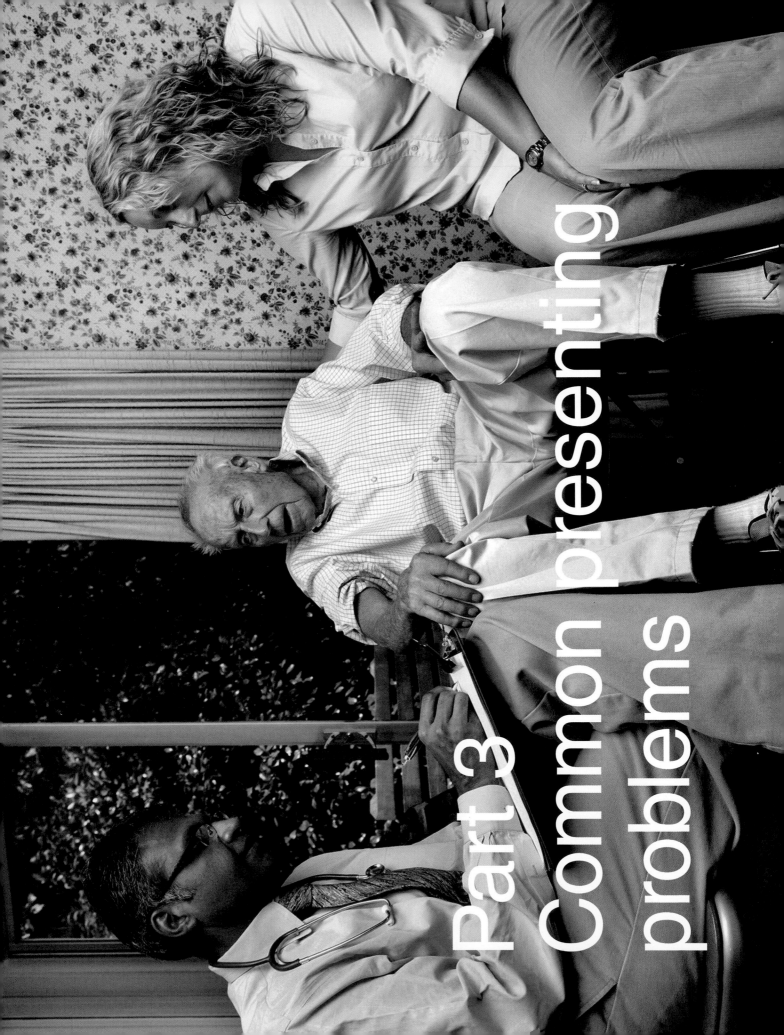

Part 3 Common presenting problems

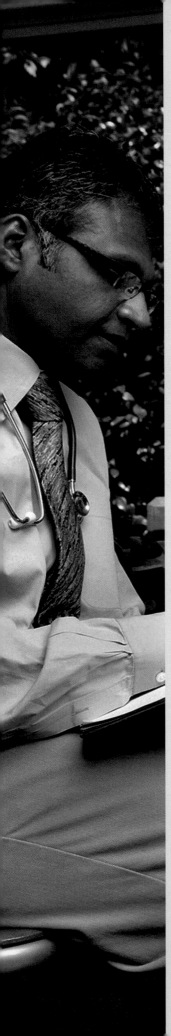

CHAPTER 11
Tiredness

Andrew Blythe
GP and Senior Teaching Fellow, University of Bristol

Key topics

Learning objectives

- Be able to take a focused history from someone who complains of feeling tired all the time.
- Be able to diagnose and treat hypothyroidism.
- Be able to diagnose type 2 diabetes and explain this diagnosis to a patient.
- Be able to conduct an annual review of someone with type 2 diabetes.
- Be able to investigate a person who is found to be anaemic.

Essential Primary Care, First Edition. Edited by Andrew Blythe and Jessica Buchan.
© 2017 John Wiley & Sons, Ltd. Published 2017 by John Wiley & Sons, Ltd.
Companion website: www.wileyessential.com/primarycare

Tired all the time

Feeling tired is one of the commonest reasons for consulting a GP, and it probably has the longest list of possible explanations of any symptom. It's convenient to categorise the causes into social, psychological and physical, but often there is a combination of causes at play. Table 11.1 lists some of the most common and important causes that a GP must consider when a patient presents with tiredness. The likelihood of these underlying diagnoses varies according to the age of the patient. A person in their 20s who says that they feel tired all the time is most likely to be suffering from mild to moderate depression, whereas someone in their 70s or 80s is more likely to have a serious underlying physical explanation.

Unravelling the causes of someone's tiredness is one of the diagnostic challenges that in some ways defines the uniqueness of general practice. Tiredness isn't a symptom that is related to any particular hospital speciality; it requires a holistic approach. The priority must always be to exclude serious physical pathology, but psychological and social causes are more common, and sometimes no satisfactory explanation is found.

When a patient presents with tiredness, start with some open questions, such as, 'Can you tell me a bit more?' and 'What effect is this having on you at home and at work?' Ask if anything else has changed. This might prompt the patient to mention another symptom or it might provide them with the opportunity to talk about major events in their life that may have a bearing on things, like the death of someone close to them or problems at work.

Have they ever felt like this before? This is a useful question in any consultation, but is often particularly useful in the context

Table 11.1 Causes of tiredness.

	Causes	Examination	Investigation
Physical	Anaemia	Pulse. Are nails and conjunctivae pale?	Full blood count (FBC)
	Hypothyroidism	Neck exam. Is there a goitre?	TFT
	Diabetes	Body mass index (BMI). Look for tinea	Fasting glucose or HbA1c
	Early pregnancy		Urinary human chorionic gonadotrophin (HCG)
	Renal failure	Blood pressure	Serum creatinine, urea and electrolytes (U&Es)
	Hepatitis C		Liver function tests (LFTs), then hepatitis serology
	Cancer (particularly in elderly)	Look for clubbing, lymph nodes, breast lumps and abdominal masses	Consider CXR, upper and lower endoscopy and abdominal ultrasound scan
	Heart failure	Check JVP and position of apex beat. Any basal crackles?	Electrocardiogram (ECG), then echocardiogram
	Hypo/hypercalcaemia	Chovstek's sign	Serum calcium
	Coeliac disease		Tissue transglutaminase (tTG)
	Addison's disease	Blood pressure	Serum electrolytes, then serum cortisol level
	Chronic fatigue syndrome		
Psychological	Depression		PHQ-9
	Stress		
Social	Overwork		
	Shift work (night work)		
	Looking after someone who needs care around the clock (baby or disabled person)		
	Other things that prevent sleep, e.g. noisy neighbours		

of tiredness. The patient might reply, 'It's a bit like last time I was anaemic', or, 'It feels like the time when I got depressed'.

Ask about their diet, drinking and weight. Vegetarians are at risk of anaemia. Excess alcohol consumption is linked to a variety of mental health problems, particularly depression and anxiety. Weight loss is a worrying symptom; think about hyperthyroidism, cancer and depression. Weight gain might indicate hypothyroidism or an increased risk of type 2 diabetes.

For women of fertile age, always consider the possibility of pregnancy and ask when their last period was.

Once we have a bit more information about the problem, we can ask the patient if there is anything in particular that they are worried might be causing their tiredness. Is there anyone in their family who has an illness that presented in this way? Thyroid disease and pernicious anaemia have a strong genetic component.

Have in mind the common causes of tiredness – depression, hypothyroidism, anaemia and diabetes – and ask some specific questions in order to evaluate their likelihood. For depression, ask if they have felt bothered by feeling down, depressed or hopeless, and ask if they have felt bothered by not having interest in things (these are referred to as the Whooley screening questions; see also Chapter 24). For hypothyroidism, ask about bowel habit and achiness. For diabetes, ask about urine output, thirst, vision and skin infections. For anaemia, ask about blood loss (menstrual periods and the presence of blood in the stool or urine).

What examination should be done in someone who complains of tiredness?

Taking a good history is the key to finding a cause for tiredness.[1] A physical examination often yields very little information. However, there are some things we do need to do. Check the person's pulse and blood pressure. A tachycardia should raise the alarm (anaemia, heart failure and hyperthyroidism are possibilities) and hypotension raises the possibility of hypoadrenalism (Addison's disease). Look at the neck to see if there is a goitre, and feel for lymph nodes. Examination beyond this is determined by the history. If there is a possibility of heart failure, look for the jugular venous pressure (JVP), feel for the apex beat and listen to the heart and the lung bases. In an elderly person, or if cancer is a possibility, do a full examination; but in a young person, further examination may not be warranted.

Case study 11.1

Lisa Lowry is 27 years old. She works in a call centre and comes to see her GP because she is feeling tired and hasn't felt well enough to go to work this week. She suffered from depression when she went to university and didn't complete her degree. She has had a variety of jobs since then. She also suffers from irritable bowel syndrome (IBS), which can make her feel bloated and gives her an erratic bowel habit. She was issued with a prescription for a 6-month supply of the progestogen-only contraceptive pill 3 months ago. She used to take mebeverine (an antispasmodic) for her irritable bowel, but hasn't had a prescription for this for over a year. Her mother takes thyroid tablets, and she is worried that she might have a thyroid problem.

What questions should the GP ask?
Several possible causes for tiredness should be going through the GP's mind:

1. **Depression:** Is she feeling low? What are her concentration and memory like? Has there been any change in her appetite or her weight? If the answers to these questions suggest she is depressed, the GP should ask if she has any thoughts of suicide.
2. **Stresses at work:** Is there a problem at work? Employees of call centres often have to work to strict targets, and this pressure can make problems like IBS worse. The GP should ask how she feels about work. Does she enjoy it?
3. **Thyroid disease:** Thyroid disease often runs down the female line of a family and is 10 times more common in women than in men, so the possibility of thyroid disease (hypo- or hyperthyroidism) is significant. The GP should ask about her bowels. Persistent diarrhoea might suggest hyperthyroidism and constipation might suggest hypothyroidism, but a bowel habit that alternates between the two in this age group is more likely to be the result of IBS.
4. **Early pregnancy:** Could she be pregnant? Is she still taking the progestogen-only pill? Has she missed any doses?

Outcome
Lisa says she isn't feeling down, it's just that she doesn't seem to have much energy. She admits that the call centre is a stressful environment, but she likes the team of people she works with. She feels a bit bloated a lot of the time and puts this down to her irritable bowel. She's opening her bowels once or twice a day at present. She stopped taking the progesterone about 2 months ago, around the time she split up with the boyfriend (she didn't mention this event to start with). When the GP asks her to clarify if she's had sex since stopping the pill, she can't be sure. The last time she had sex was with her ex-boyfriend, about 2 months ago. She didn't have any bleeds when she was on the pill and hasn't had a period since stopping it.

The GP decides that before doing anything else, they should do a pregnancy test. Lisa produces a urine sample and the test is positive. This is a shock, but provides the explanation for her tiredness. Tiredness is one of the main symptoms of early pregnancy.

What investigations should be conducted?

All GPs have a standard batch of blood tests that they request for someone who complains of feeling tired all the time. This always includes a full blood count (FBC), serum urea and electrolytes (U&Es), liver function thyroid function and a test to exclude diabetes (a fasting glucose or glycosylated haemoglobin). Some GPs add to this list measurement of the serum calcium level, tissue transglutaminase and plasma viscosity. Table 11.1 lists the reasons for doing these tests.

The point of doing an examination and of doing a batch of blood tests is to exclude a treatable physical cause. A lot of the time, the tests all come back normal, which leaves the patient either feeling relieved or wondering why they still feel tired. Patients are more likely than their doctors to think that their tiredness has a physical cause,[2] and often need to be guided by their GP in making the link between their tiredness and their psychosocial problems. This is referred to as the *reattribution of symptoms*.

Thyroid disease

Hypothyroidism

Diagnosis

Hypothyroidism (an underactive thyroid gland) is a satisfyingly treatable cause of tiredness that is managed almost entirely in primary care. Hypothyroidism is so common (its prevalence is around 2–3% of the general population[3]) that doctors tend to check people's thyroid function almost anytime they are requesting other blood tests. As a result, the diagnosis of hypothyroidism is often stumbled upon unexpectedly when an abnormal thyroid function test (TFT) is reported amongst a batch of blood tests.

The classical symptoms of hypothyroidism are illustrated in Figure 11.1. With this constellation of symptoms, one would have thought that the diagnosis would be easy to make, but not everyone presents with all of these symptoms, and quite often the symptoms develop so gradually that the patient and their GP fail to spot them. Often, it takes a fresh pair of eyes (not those of the patient's regular GP) to spot the clues.

There are some signs associated with hypothyroidism, but these often develop at quite a late stage; they include bradycardia, pleural and pericardial effusions, nonpitting oedema of the legs and slow relaxing reflexes. Other clues can come from the results of a variety of blood tests. Hypothyroidism can cause the serum cholesterol and mean cell volume to rise and the serum sodium level to fall. Severe hypothyroidism can also cause anaemia.

When a doctor suspects thyroid disease and requests TFTs, the first test to be done in the laboratory is a measurement of the thyroid stimulating hormone (TSH). If this is normal, then no further tests are done. If the TSH is low or high, then the free T4 level is measured. A diagnosis of hypothyroidism is

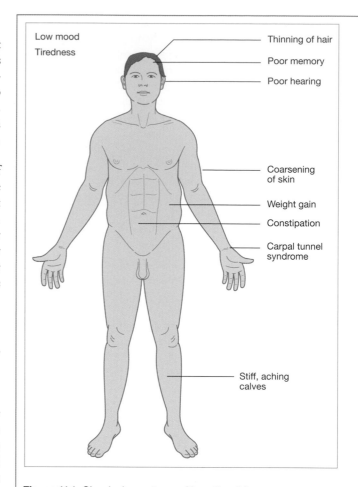

Figure 11.1 Classical symptoms of hypothyroidism.

confirmed when the TSH level is above 10 IU/l and the free T4 level is below normal range.[4]

Most cases of hypothyroidism are due to autoimmune disease: Hashimoto's thyroiditis or atrophic thyroiditis. There is a strong link with other autoimmune diseases – type 1 diabetes, pernicious anaemia, vitiligo and coeliac disease – so, in patients with these conditions, it is worthwhile checking thyroid function. If the patient's TSH is raised but their free T4 is normal then their thyroid autoantibodies should be checked. If they have a positive autoantibody test then they are at significant risk of developing autoimmune hypothyroidism and their TFTs should be checked every year. If their antibody test is negative, their TFTs should be checked every 3 years.

Hypothyroidism can also be caused by a number of drugs, notably lithium (used for treating bipolar affective disorder) and amiodarone (used for treating arrhythmias), so GPs have to ensure that all their patients on these particular drugs have their TFTs checked at least once a year. Box 11.1 lists all other groups that should have their TFTs checked regularly.

When they are 10 days old, all babies in the UK have their TSH checked in order to screen for congenital hypothyroidism.

Treatment

Hypothyroidism is a satisfying diagnosis to make because, with a simple daily dose of levothyroxine, given in tablet form, the patient feels back to normal. Once they are established on treatment, they often say to their GP that they hadn't realised how ill they were beforehand. Providing the GP monitors the dose of levothyroxine, it is very safe. The major risk is that treating hypothyroidism may unmask ischaemic heart disease. Also, overtreatment may precipitate atrial fibrillation and cause osteoporosis.

A patient under the age of 50 can be started on at least 50 µg of levothyroxine daily.[4] An older patient or a patient with ischaemic heart disease should be started on the lower dose: 25 µg daily. The full treatment dose for a large adult may be up to 300 µg daily, but usually it is around 100–125 µg daily. Levothyroxine has a long half life, so the dose has to be built up gradually, in 25 µg increments. TFTs should be checked 2–3 months after each increase:[5] if the patient's TSH is still above the normal range, the dose of levothyroxine should be increased by another 25 µg. The aim is to bring the TSH within the normal range – ideally in the lower half of this range. Once the patient is on the correct dose, they need to have their TSH checked once a year.

Hyperthyroidism

Hyperthyroidism is less common than hypothyroidism. Someone with hyperthyroidism may present to their GP with a cluster of classical symptoms (irritability, weight loss, diarrhoea, sweating and difficulty sleeping), but sometimes the symptoms are vaguer and the patient just says they feel tired or unwell. The GP makes the diagnosis on the basis of a suppressed TSH and a raised free T4 and then, in most cases, refers the patient to an endocrinologist. Usually, the endocrinologist will advise starting carbimazole (or propylthiouracil, if the patient is pregnant) together with a beta blocker for symptomatic relief. Ultimately, the patient may need treatment with radioactive iodine or a thyroidectomy. Either of these treatments can make the patient hypothyroid, but even if they are rendered euthyroid, they are at greater risk of developing hypothyroidism later in life, which is something the GP needs to be alert to.

Type 2 diabetes mellitus

Type 2 diabetes mellitus is a largely preventable disease, linked to an unhealthy lifestyle. As the UK population has consumed more sugary and fatty foods, we have got fatter as a nation, and the prevalence of type 2 diabetes has increased from 2% 2 decades ago to somewhere in the region of 6% today.

Case study 11.2a

Malcolm MacDonald is 56 and is a lorry driver. He comes to see his GP, Dr Mary Muir, because he is feeling tired. When Dr Muir asks if there is anything else that's bothering him, he mentions a 'sweat rash' in his groins; this is red and itchy. Dr Muir notes that Mr MacDonald is overweight. Mr MacDonald is not on any regular medication and has no medical history of note. Dr Muir suspects type 2 diabetes and asks a few specific questions about this.

- **Has he noticed any change in his vision?** Sometimes his vision is a bit blurry, but he puts this down to being tired.
- **Has he noticed any change in his thirst?** Yes, he does get very thirsty in the afternoon.
- **Has he noticed any change in the frequency with which he is passing urine?** A bit, but he puts this down to the volume that he drinks. He only gets up once at night to pass urine; more often at the weekend, if he's been to the pub the night before.

What test should Dr Muir do to confirm the diagnosis of diabetes?
Dr Muir could request a urine sample and test this for glucose. A positive result would make the diagnosis more

likely, but to make a firm diagnosis Dr Muir should either check Mr MacDonald's fasting blood glucose or measure his glycosylated haemoglobin level (HbA1c).

A fasting blood test means that the patient should not have anything to eat or drink other than water for 8 hours before the test. In practice, this means making an appointment to come before having breakfast one morning.

Mr MacDonald has several symptoms of diabetes: tiredness, a fungal rash, thirstiness and visual disturbance. So, a fasting blood glucose reading ≥7.0 mmol/l or an HbA1c reading ≥48 mmol/mol would confirm the diagnosis of diabetes. To make a diagnosis of type 2 diabetes in the absence of any symptoms requires two fasting plasma glucose readings ≥7.0 mmol/l.

Diabetes is sometimes picked up as the result of routine urinalysis that shows glucose in the urine. Most of the time, it is diagnosed when patients present with one or more of the following symptoms: tiredness, skin infections (boils and fungal infections), increased urine output (polyuria), increased thirst (polydipsia), urine infections or blurring of vision.

Three pathological changes contribute to the development of type 2 diabetes:

1. a decrease in the production of insulin;
2. an increase in the manufacture of glucose by the liver; and
3. an increased resistance to insulin in the peripheral tissues.

All these changes occur as an individual becomes more obese.

How should the diagnosis of diabetes be explained to a patient?

Start by asking the patient what they know about diabetes already – they are likely to know someone with diabetes, and this will colour their view of the condition. Some misunderstandings they have about the condition may need to be corrected. Without scaring the patient, the fact that diabetes is a serious and lifelong condition should be explained. It cannot be cured, but it can be controlled. The main problem in diabetes is that the level of sugar in the blood is too high. Over time, this sweetness in the blood can damage the eyes, the kidneys and the nerves, leading to loss of feeling in the feet and hands. People with diabetes often have high blood pressure too, and this contributes to the damage to the kidneys, eyes and heart. The good news is that by reducing the patient's level of sugar and by controlling their blood pressure, we can prevent this damage.

A person with diabetes has to learn to manage this condition for the rest of their life. They will attend the surgery, and sometimes the hospital, for regular check-ups, but these check-ups will usually amount to less than 2 hours a year. The other 8758 hours of the year, the patient has to manage their diabetes by themselves. It is thus very important that they receive adequate instruction on how to do so. The National Institute for Health and Care Excellence (NICE) recommends that all patients with newly diagnosed diabetes are referred to an education programme.[6] The GP starts this process of education with their initial explanation of the condition, then gives the patient a folder of information. The patient's partner and children need education too, particularly if they are the ones who prepare the family meal.

Adopting a healthier lifestyle – eating less sugary food, losing weight and doing more exercise – is the key to controlling diabetes. However, people find it difficult to make these changes, and most people with type 2 diabetes end up on medication. In the UK Prospective Diabetes Study, 9 years after diagnosis less than 9% of patients achieved satisfactory glycaemic control when they were treated with diet alone.[7]

Case study 11.2b

Mr MacDonald's fasting plasma glucose is 9.2 mmol/mol, so Dr Muir makes a diagnosis of type 2 diabetes and imparts this bad news to him. This is not a complete surprise to Mr MacDonald. When his GP asks what he knows about diabetes, he recalls a fellow lorry driver who had to stop driving because the diabetes affected his vision; he had insulin injections.

Dr Muir asks Mr MacDonald to describe what he eats and drinks in a typical day. What did he have yesterday, for example? He started the day with a cup of tea (with two teaspoons of sugar) and toast topped with butter and jam; then he stopped at a café for a fried breakfast with another cup of tea. For lunch, he had a sandwich (white bread and egg mayonnaise), a packet of crisps and a bottle of cola. In the evening, he had two pork chops, mash and carrots, then a slice of apple pie and a cup of tea.

He doesn't do any regular exercise. He doesn't smoke and only drinks at the weekend, because he drives for a living.

Mr MacDonald weighs 98 kg and his height is 176 cm.

What is his body mass index?

$$\text{Body mass index (BMI)} = \frac{Mass\ (kg)}{Height^2\ (m)}$$
$$= \frac{98}{1.76 \times 1.76} = 31.6\ kg/m^2$$

This puts him in the obese category. A healthy BMI is 19–25 kg/m². A BMI of 25–30 is classified as being overweight, and a BMI above 30 defines someone as being obese.

What advice should Dr Muir give Mr MacDonald about his diet?

There are several things that Mr MacDonald could do to bring his diabetes under control and improve his symptoms of tiredness, thirst and blurred vision.

1. He could eat smaller portions of food, with the aim of losing weight. At the same time, he could do some regular exercise.
2. He could replace his sugary drinks with water or take his tea without sugar.
3. He could have fewer fried breakfasts – but he shouldn't replace them with sweet cereals.
4. He could replace apple pie with fresh fruit.
5. He could replace some of the meat in his evening meal with more vegetables.
6. He could have fish instead of pork chops.
7. He could make his own sandwiches, with wholemeal bread and a low-fat filling.

It is important that Dr Muir talks to Mr MacDonald in specific terms like this about what things he could do, and that they agree on some of these as a first step. To review the strategies for helping people to make behaviour change such as this, look at Chapter 7. The principles underlying this dietary advice are listed in Table 11.2.

What other things should Dr Muir do during her first consultation with Mr MacDonald?

Dr Muir should explain how the fluctuating and high sugar level can cause blurring of vision. She should recommend that that Mr Macdonald makes an appointment to see an optician, but he shouldn't get spectacles immediately because his acuity may change when his blood sugar level falls. Dr Muir should explain that diabetes can cause permanent damage to vision (like it did to Mr MacDonald's colleague), but that the good news is that this can be prevented by bringing the sugar level and blood pressure under control. Dr Muir should ensure that Mr MacDonald is invited to have yearly photographs of the back of his eye (retinal screening) to look for early signs of damage. It is unlikely that he will need to go on insulin, but he may well need to take tablets as well as making changes to his diet.

There is a danger of overloading Mr MacDonald with information on his first consultation about diabetes. With this in mind, Dr Muir's next step is probably to request a further batch of blood tests prior to seeing Mr MacDonald, or having a practice nurse see him, for a full review of his diabetes.

Table 11.2 Principles behind dietary advice for someone with type 2 diabetes.

Principle	Comment
Reduce consumption of sugary foods	This includes ready meals, processed food and sweet snacks
Limit fatty foods to <30% of the total daily calorie intake	
Limit saturated fats to <10% of the total daily calorie intake	This means limiting the intake of pastries, biscuits and hard cheese
Increase the intake of dietary fibre	Wholemeal bread, brown rice and vegetables are good sources of fibre
Reduce consumption of sugary drinks	This doesn't just mean cutting out soft drinks: alcoholic drinks contain a lot of sugar and calories

Reviewing patients with type 2 diabetes

It is important to review patients with type 2 diabetes to see how well their diabetes is controlled, to look for evidence of complications and to target all their risk factors for cardiovascular disease (CVD). Searching for complications needs to begin at the time of diagnosis, because some people already have serious complications then.[8] Although it takes 10 years for diabetic retinopathy to develop, some patients might have diabetes for this long before it is diagnosed.

The annual review of someone with diabetes is an important opportunity to educate them about diabetes and give them general advice on health promotion. Doing regular exercise is terribly important, but patients with diabetes report that they receive vague advice about exercise from health care professionals.[9] Patients often encounter barriers to increasing their level of physical activity (such as lack of time or money, or physical problems such as arthritis), and they find it difficult to maintain exercise regimes. Everyone should aim to do at least 30 minutes of moderate physical activity at least 5 days a week, and if someone with type 2 diabetes is trying to lose weight, they should be aiming for 60 minutes of moderate activity a day. In order to sustain this level of physical activity, the exercise needs to be incorporated into the patient's daily routine. Walking is one form of exercise that people with diabetes are able to sustain. Having a reason for walking every day, like owning a dog, acts as an added incentive.[9]

As with many chronic diseases, people with diabetes are at high risk of developing depression,[10] so it worthwhile enquiring

Table 11.3 Annual review of a patient with type 2 diabetes.

	History	Examination	Investigation
Checking adherence	Diet, exercise and medication	BMI	
Blood glucose control	Any hypos? Any home glucose readings?		HbA1c
Cardiovascular complications	Any problems with erectile function?	Pulse, blood pressure	Lipid profile
Renal		Blood pressure	Serum urea, creatinine and electrolytes Urinary albumin: creatinine ratio
Feet	Do they check their feet for cuts and calluses? Are their shoes in a good state of repair?	Inspection Pedal pulses Sensation: 10 g monofilament and vibration sense	Doppler studies if pedal pulses not palpable
Eyes	Have they noticed any change in their vision? When did they last go to the optician? Date of retinal screening	Visual acuity Visual fields Fundoscopy	
Mood	Whooley questions		
Complications of therapy			B12
Associated conditions			Thyroid function tests (TFTs)

about their mood at the time of review. If the patient is suffering from depression, this has a knock-on effect on their diabetes: it hinders their ability to stick to dietary and exercise regimes and degrades their quality of life.

A full review should be done at least once a year. Table 11.3 summarises the essential components of the diabetes review. The outcome of this review may be a referral to an ophthalmologist, to a diabetic foot clinic or vascular surgeon, or to a renal physician. It should also include an action plan for the patient.

Controlling the blood glucose level

There is a growing range of medicines available to help reduce the blood sugar level of people with diabetes. The mechanisms of action and side effects of these medicines are listed in Table 11.4. The main problem with some of them is that they make people gain weight. Metformin doesn't make people gain weight, and there is strong evidence that it reduces morbidity and mortality from diabetes, so except in people who have a normal or low BMI (rare amongst those with type 2 diabetes), metformin is first-line drug therapy when dietary measures alone have failed. Metformin commonly causes gastrointestinal disturbance, so patients need to build up the dose gradually while they get used to it.

If a person with newly diagnosed diabetes has symptoms or if their HbA1c is very high, metformin may be started immediately, rather than waiting to assess the impact of dietary measures. In general, however, dietary measures should be tried alone for 6 weeks before starting drug therapy.

Patients often need more than one drug to control their blood glucose level. Figure 11.2 illustrates the options available, as recommended by NICE.[6] Ultimately, some patients require insulin – either a twice-daily dose of a mixture of different types of insulins or a once-daily dose of a long-acting insulin. Whatever drug therapy is recommended, the patient should be reminded that it is not a substitute for sticking to a healthier diet; drug therapy is just an additional measure.

We can monitor the success of blood glucose-lowering therapy by checking the patient's level of glycosylated haemoglobin (HbA1c), expressed in mmol/mol, every 3 months. In general, we aim for a target range of 48–58 mmol/mol. Tight control of the patient's blood glucose level reduces the risk of the complications of diabetes, but it also increases the chances of the patient becoming hypoglycaemic, and the dangers of hypoglycaemia are considerable. If someone becomes hypoglycaemic while they are driving, they may crash their car. Hypoglycaemia can also cause falls, which in turn may result in fractures. Some people get little warning, if any, that they are becoming hypoglycaemic. Elderly people, those who drink too much alcohol and those with cognitive impairment are at particularly high risk of developing hypoglycaemia. For all these reasons, doctors need to tailor the tightness of blood pressure control to the patient's particular circumstances. Sometimes, having a more relaxed target is safer.

Table 11.4 Medicines for lowering blood glucose.

Drug	Route of administration	Mechanism of action	Side effects
Biguanide: metformin	Tablet	Reduces hepatic gluconeogensis Increases sensitivity to insulin Reduces absorption of carbohydrate from gut	Gastrointestinal disturbance Lactic acidosis B12 deficiency
Sulphonylurea: gliclazide	Tablet	Increases endogenous insulin production	Hypoglycaemia Weight gain
Thiazolidinediones (glitizones): pioglitazone	Tablet	Increases tissue sensitivity to insulin	Increased risk of fragility fracture in women May cause fluid retention: don't use in those with left ventricular impairment Weight gain Increased risk of bladder cancer
DPP-4 inhibitors (gliptins): sitagliptin	Tablet	Delays clearance of natural incretins	Nausea, diarrhoea
Incretin mimetics: exanatide, liraglutide	Subcutaneous injection	Increases release of endogenous insulin following carbohydrate ingestion	Nausea, diarrhoea
Prandial glucose regulators: nateglinide, repaglinide	Tablet	Boosts insulin production	Symptoms of hypoglycaemia
Sodium glucose co-transporter 2 blockers	Injection	Results in excretion of glucose in urine	Urinary tract infections (UTIs)

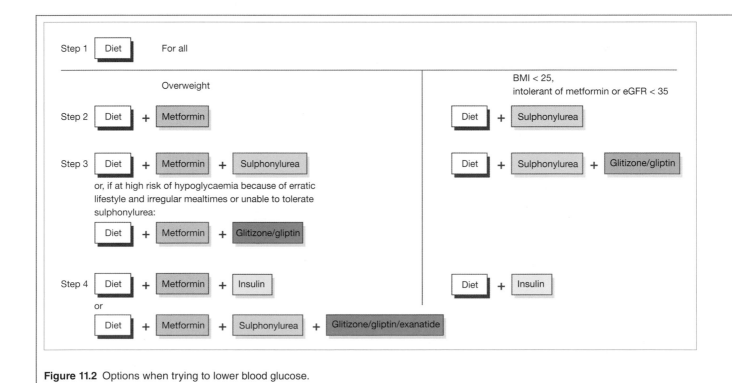

Figure 11.2 Options when trying to lower blood glucose.

Top tip

If someone has diabetes, ask them if they drive. If they take a sulphonylurea, they are at risk of hypoglycaemia. Advise them to check their blood glucose level before starting a car journey, and every 2 hours during a long journey.

Controlling blood pressure and other cardiovascular risk factors

To prevent the vascular complications of diabetes, controlling blood pressure is just as important as controlling the blood sugar level. If someone with type 2 diabetes has kidney, eye or cerebrovascular disease, the target for their blood pressure should be lower than the usual: a blood pressure under 130/80 mmHg should be aimed for. Angiotensin-converting enzyme (ACE) inhibitors are the first-line antihypertensive drug of choice, except for women of fertile age (calcium channel antagonists are safer for them) and for those of Afro-Caribbean family origin. A statin is recommended for anyone with diabetes whose 10-year risk of developing cardiovascular disease is over 10% (see Chapter 9).

Anaemia

When patients come to their GP feeling tired, they often worry that they might be anaemic. Certainly, anaemia is common. Women who have heavy periods are at high risk of developing iron-deficiency anaemia, and pernicious anaemia, caused by vitamin B12 deficiency, is very common in the elderly. Table 11.5 lists the common causes of anaemia.

Tiredness is not the only way that anaemia can present. The other common presentations include breathlessness, angina, a feeling of weakness, giddy spells, faints and falls. Severe anaemia causes a tachycardia, and the patient's conjunctivae and nails look pale, but a mild anaemia is difficult to detect on examination. If anaemia is suspected, an FBC must be

Table 11.5 The common and important causes of anaemia.

Children	Dietary iron deficiency anaemia Coeliac disease Inherited blood disorders, e.g. sickle cell disease, thalassaemia Leukaemia
Young adults	Menorrhagia (women) Coeliac disease Inflammatory bowel disease Bleed from peptic ulcer Bleed from oesophageal varices Leukaemia
Middle age–old age	Anaemia of chronic disease Nonsteroidal anti-inflammatory drug (NSAID)-induced gastritis/ulcer Bleed from oesophageal varices Stomach cancer Bowel cancer Renal tract cancer Renal failure Pernicious anaemia Dietary folate deficiency Myelodysplasia Chronic lymphatic leukaemia Haemolytic anaemia Drug-induced anaemia

---

Case 11.2c

Outcome

Mr MacDonald's optician reports that his visual acuity is 6/6 in each eye, with no evidence of retinopathy. Mr MacDonald has another batch of blood tests and submits a sample of urine; the results are:

- HbA1c 63 mmol/mol;
- total cholesterol : HDL ratio 5.2;
- renal function, liver function, FBC and TSH: all normal;
- urine albumin : creatinine 0.8 mg/mmol (normal).

When Mr MacDonald goes to see the practice nurse for his first diabetes review, the nurse explains these results and examines him. His blood pressure is 146/92 mmHg. His feet look in good condition, apart from a small patch of tinea (Athlete's foot) between his fourth and fifth toes. His pedal pulses are intact, and testing with a 10 g monofilament reveals normal sensation, which means that he is at low risk of diabetic foot damage.

Mr MacDonald is not optimistic about his ability to increase his amount of exercise but is keen to try to lose weight by having smaller portion sizes. The nurse talks about the benefit of making the other dietary changes suggested by Dr Muir. She supplies him with a home blood pressure monitor and asks Dr Muir to supply a prescription for an antifungal cream for his tinea.

Mr MacDonald still feels tired 6 weeks later and has not succeeded in losing any weight. He comes to see Dr Muir with his home blood pressure readings; the average reading is 144/86 mmHg. At this stage, Dr Muir recommends he starts taking metformin. His 10-year risk of developing CVD is 21%, so Dr Muir also recommends that he starts an ACE inhibitor to lower his blood pressure and a statin for his cholesterol.

Table 11.6 Causes of microcytic, normocytic and macrocytic anaemia.

Microcytic	Normocytic	Macrocytic
Iron deficiency	Chronic disease	B12 deficiency
Thalasseamia	Renal failure	Folate deficiency
Chronic disease	Gastrointestinal bleed	Hypothyroidism (rare)
	Haemolysis	Medication: anticonvulsant therapy, antiretroviral therapy, azathioprine
		Liver disease

obtained. The normal values for the haemoglobin level are different for children and adults; they are lower in adult women than in men, and are even lower in pregnant women because of the dilution effect.

If a GP receives a result revealing that a patient is anaemic, what should they do?

The GP's first response is to study the FBC in more detail. If the anaemia is severe (<70 g/l), the patient needs urgent assessment, and if there is evidence to suggest that this is an acute problem then usually the GP will send the patient to hospital for transfusion and further investigation; the patient may have had a gastrointestinal bleed. If the anaemia is severe but chronic then the patient will have adjusted to this and is unlikely to be at immediate risk, so it may be possible to avoid admission.

It's important to look at the white cell count and platelet count to see if there is a general problem with blood cell production due to a haematological malignancy or suppression of the bone marrow.

The mean cell volume gives us a lot of information. Table 11.6 shows the causes of anaemia, classified according to mean cell volume. The commonest cause of a microcytic anaemia (low mean cell volume) is an iron-deficiency anaemia. In a woman of fertile age, this is most likely to be the result of menorrhagia, but in a man or a post-menopausal woman, a cause needs to be sought. In particular, it is essential to investigate the upper and lower gastrointestinal tract, because an iron-deficiency anaemia may be the first indicator that the patient has a stomach or bowel cancer. Having reviewed the patient' symptoms, an examination needs to be undertaken (palpate their abdomen and do a digital rectal examination) and an upper gastrointestinal endoscopy and a colonoscopy or barium enema requested.

Pernicious anaemia and folate deficiency are the commonest causes of a macrocytic anaemia and usually do not require investigation in hospital unless there are neurological complications. People with pernicious anaemia are more likely to have stomach cancer, so it is important to check for symptoms that might indicate stomach cancer, and if necessary refer for gastroscopy.

Table 11.7 lists the basic tests that it is useful to request when investigating anaemia.

Table 11.7 Tests to use when investigating the cause of anaemia.

Test	Interpretation
Blood film	Shape of blood cells may indicate cause, e.g. large oval cells with hypersegmented nuclei seen in B12 and folate deficiency
Reticulocyte count	Raised reticulocyte count indicates bleeding or haemolysis
Serum ferritin	Reduced ferritin indicates chronic blood loss. Very low serum ferritin is seen in thalassaemia
Serum B12	Reduced B12 may be caused by pernicious anaemia or dietary deficiency
Anti-intrinsic factor antibody level	Raised antibody level has high specificity but poor sensitivity for diagnosing pernicious anaemia. Antibody level is raised in 50% of patients with pernicious anaemia
Serum folate	Low red cell folate may be caused by dietary deficiency, malabsorption, malignancy or certain medicines, e.g. methotrexate
TFTs	Severe hypothyroidism causes anaemia
LFTs	Alcoholic liver disease can cause anaemia as the result of gastrointestinal bleeding or vitamin/folate deficiency. Serum bilirubin is raised in haemolytic anaemia
Urinanalysis	Nonvisible haematuria and/or proteinuria suggests renal disease

Treating anaemia

Once a cause for iron-deficiency anaemia has been established, the usual treatment is a 3-month course of oral iron (ferrous fumarate or ferrous sulphate). This makes the stool turn black and often causes constipation, and the patient should be warned of this.

If someone is anaemic and has a low serum B12 level and a raised anti-intrinsic factor antibody level it's reasonable to assume that they have pernicious anaemia. Pernicious anaemia can't be treated orally, because the underlying problem is an inability to absorb vitamin B12 from the small bowel. GPs thus prescribe six loading doses of hydroxocobalamin, given by intramuscular injection over the course of a fortnight, then one injection every 3 months for life. However, if the B12 deficiency is due to a poor diet (this is a less common scenario), then oral vitamin B12 supplements are satisfactory.

Folate deficiency is treated with a daily dose of oral folic acid, usually for 4 months. If someone is on a drug known to cause folate deficiency, it is usual to prescribe folic acid as long as they are on that drug. Folate deficiency and vitamin B12 deficiency can coexist. If one deficiency is treated but not the other, there is a risk that irreversible neurological damage may occur.

Chronic fatigue syndrome

Some patients who complain of tiredness end up being diagnosed with chronic fatigue syndrome, also known as myalgic encephalomyelitis (ME). There is no test for this syndrome, but there are a number of diagnostic criteria that must be met.[11] First, all other causes of tiredness need to be explored thoroughly. If examination and investigation do not yield any cause, and if the tiredness has persisted for more than 4 months (or 3 months in a child), then the GP may start to consider a diagnosis of chronic fatigue syndrome. Features that point towards a diagnosis of chronic fatigue syndrome include tiredness that comes on after activity, muscle and joint pains, difficulty sleeping and difficulty concentrating.

Treatment for chronic fatigue syndrome is supportive: this means giving advice on sleep hygiene, healthy diet and pacing activity levels. Children should always be referred for expert help, and most adults require specialist input, too. Under the supervision of a specialist, cognitive behavioural therapy (CBT), graded exercise therapy and activity management can be helpful.

Top tip

It's common for people to feel tired a few weeks after an infection, particularly after glandular fever or a chest infection. This is not what is meant by chronic fatigue syndrome.

SUMMARY

Tiredness is a common reason for a patient to consult their GP, and has many causes. The GP must always seek a physical cause, but in the majority of cases the cause turns out to be psychological or social. Type 2 diabetes, hypothyroidism and anaemia are probably the commonest physical causes of tiredness seen in general practice. Reflecting the rise in sedentary lifestyles and obesity, type 2 diabetes continues to get more common. GPs manage type 2 diabetes by helping patients to modify their lifestyle and by prescribing medication to reduce blood glucose, blood pressure and cholesterol. At the same time, GPs monitor their patients for the development of complications caused by diabetes. Hypothyroidism is a completely treatable cause of tiredness that is managed entirely in primary care. Anaemia requires careful investigation by GPs. Iron-deficiency anaemia in men and post-menopausal bleeding in women are two ways in which bowel or stomach cancer may present.

 Now visit **www.wileyessential.com/primarycare** to test yourself on this chapter.

REFERENCES

1. Ridsdale L, Evans A, Jerrett W, et al. Patients who consult with tiredness: frequency of consultation, perceived causes of tiredness and its association with psychological distress. *Br J Gen Pract* 1994:**44**;413–16.

2. Moncrieff G, Fletcher J. 10-minute consultation: tiredness. *BMJ* 2007;**334**:1221.

3. Tunbridge WMG, Evered DC, Hall R, et al. The spectrum of thyroid disease in a community: the Whickham survey. *Clinical Endocrinol* 1977;**7**:481–93.

4. Vaidya B, Pearce HS. Management of hypothyroidism in adults. *BMJ* 2008;**337**:a801.

5. Association for Clinical Biochemistry, British Thyroid Association, British Thyroid Foundation. UK Guidelines for the Use of Thyroid Function Tests. Available from: http://www.british-thyroid-association.org/info-for-patients/Docs/TFT_guideline_final_version_July_2006.pdf (last accessed 6 October 2015).

6. NICE. Type 2 diabetes: the management of type 2 diabetes. NICE Clinical Guideline 87. May 2009. Available from: http://www.nice.org.uk/guidance/cg87 (last accessed 6 October 2015).

7. Turner RC, Cull CA, Frighi V, Holman RR. Glycaemic control with diet, sulfonyluea, metformin, or insulin in patients with type 2 diabetes mellitus: progressive requirement

for multiple therapies (UKPDS 49). UK Prospective Diabetes Study Group. *JAMA* 1999;**281**:2005–12.

8. UK Prospective Diabetes Study 6. Complications in newly diagnosed type 2 diabetic patients and their association with different clinical and biochemical risk factors. *Diabetes Res* 1990;**13**:1–11.

9. Peel E, Douglas M, Parry O, Lawton J. Type 2 diabetes and dog walking: patients' longitudinal perspectives about implementing and sustaining physical activity. *Br J Gen Pract* 2010:**60**;572–7.

10. Chew-Graham C, Sartorius N, Cimino, LC, Gask L. Diabetes and depression in general practice: meeting the challenge of managing co-morbidity. *Br J Gen Pract* 2014;**64**:386–7.

11. NICE. Chronic fatigue syndrome/myalgic encephalomyelitis: diagnosis and management of CFS/ME in adults and children. NICE Clinical Guideline 53. August 2007. Available from: http://www.nice.org.uk/guidance/cg53/chapter/1-guidance#presentation (last accessed 6 October 2015).

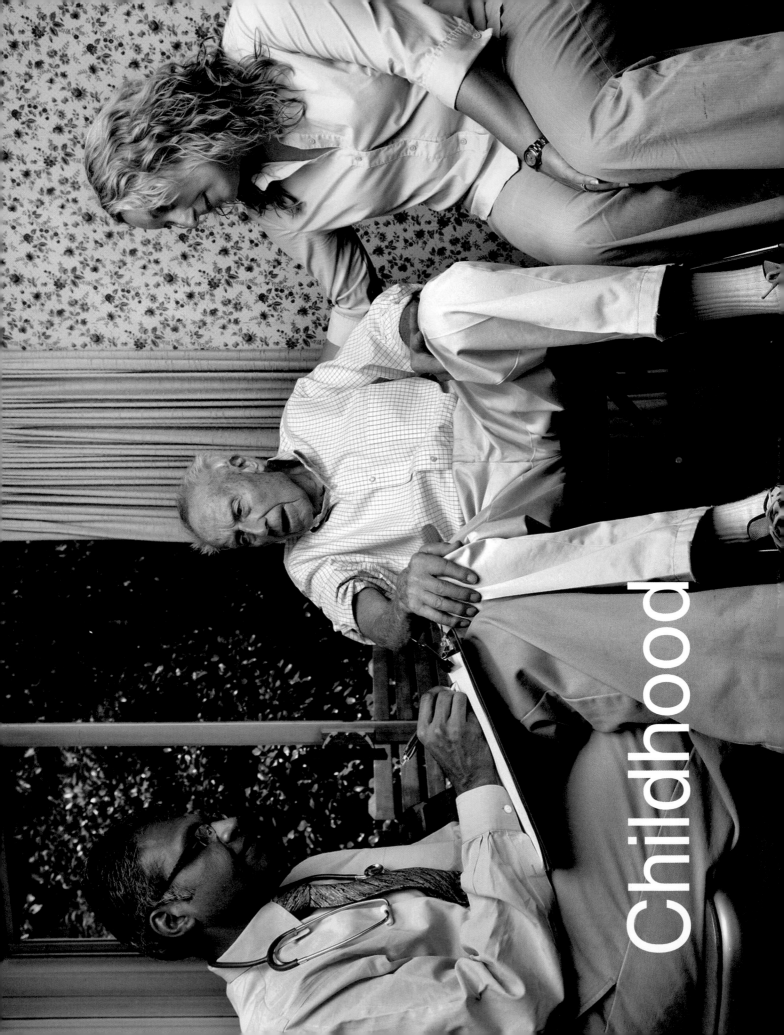

Childhood

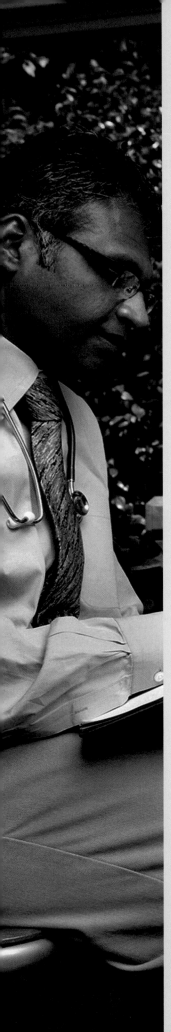

CHAPTER 12

Child health in primary care

Jessica Buchan
GP and Teaching Fellow in Primary Care, University of Bristol

Key topics

Learning objectives

- Be able to recognise the role of the GP in child health promotion.
- Be able to understand the purpose of developmental reviews in children.
- Be able to outline the approach to the 6–8-week check in primary care.
- Be able to describe the UK's screening and vaccination programme in children and young people.
- Be able to appreciate the particular skills required to consult with children and parents.
- Be able to identify children at risk of abuse and describe strategies to protect them.

For simplicity, in these child health chapters the term 'parent' encompasses any adult who has a parental role and is regularly caring for children; the term 'child' means any person from birth to the age of 18.

Essential Primary Care, First Edition. Edited by Andrew Blythe and Jessica Buchan.
© 2017 John Wiley & Sons, Ltd. Published 2017 by John Wiley & Sons, Ltd.
Companion website: www.wileyessential.com/primarycare

The healthy child

The parental role in raising children

To be healthy, children need safe water, nutritious food, physical activity, clothing appropriate for the environment and clean, comfortable living conditions free from toxins such as tobacco smoke. A child should also be able to explore and learn in an environment that is safe. When young, children should be supervised by an adult who can predict risks and protect them from physical hazards. As they grow, they need age-appropriate opportunities to develop their independence.

Perhaps above all, children need to be loved. They need a strong bond with an adult who makes them feel valued, is interested in them as an individual and treats them with respect and warmth. These aspects of parenting are considered to be protective against the adverse health and social outcomes that can result from social disadvantage. GPs have a role in both advising and educating parents in providing this care, and act as advocates for vulnerable children whose parenting or environment falls short of these basic needs.

The role of the GP in the well-being of the child

Every consultation with a child and their carers is an important opportunity for the GP to promote the well-being of the whole child. The doctor's role is often seen as spotting illness or developmental abnormality in children, but for the many children attending with self-limiting illness who are developing normally, the doctor's role is to reassure and educate their parents. Consultations enable the doctor to find out about, and build a relationship with, the family. This is especially the case in routine child health development checks, where the well-being of the parents and the child's social circumstances are part of the assessment. Consultations about child accidents or injuries are an opportunity to explore the circumstances and discuss injury prevention.

The Healthy Child Programme is a public health strategy[1] in the UK that outlines the child health services that primary health care teams should provide. It covers:

- screening tests;
- immunisations;
- developmental reviews;
- information for parents on parenting;
- information for parents on keeping children safe and healthy;
- parental support.

Screening and developmental reviews

Neonatal screening

In the UK, neonates are checked at birth, and should have a full physical check within 72 hours. This is similar to the check done by GPs at 6–8 weeks. Newborns also have their hearing screened using the automated oto-acoustic emission test in the first few weeks of life. This is often done prior to discharge if the child is born in a hospital. If hearing loss goes unrecognised, the child will have impaired speech; communication difficulties can impact learning and behaviour. In the first 5–8 days of life, babies also have a blood test, known as the 'heel-prick test.' A drop of blood is taken from the heel to screen for:[2]

- **Phenylketonuria:** Untreated, this results in severe neurological impairment, which can be prevented by a phenylalanine-restricted diet.
- **Congenital hypothyroidism:** A preventable cause of mental impairment and growth retardation.
- **Sickle cell disease:** Diagnosis increases awareness, so that crises can be avoided or treated promptly.
- **Cystic fibrosis:** Early diagnosis improves access to treatment and reduces tissue damage.
- **Medium-chain acyl-CoA dehydrogenase deficiency:** A treatable cause of sudden infant death.

Developmental reviews

We decide what normal development is by comparison with the normal ranges and patterns. Different children attain developmental milestones at different ages and in different ways. All normal babies learn to walk; a quarter will do so at 11 months, 90% by 15 months. 18 months is a cut-off point for referral for a child who isn't walking. Over this limit, some children will still attain normal walking, but an underlying condition such as mild cerebral palsy becomes more likely. The GP will refer a child who isn't walking earlier than 18 months if there are additional concerns about their development or social situation.

Babies do not all learn to walk in the same way: some crawl on all fours first; others do a 'commando' crawl, with their stomach on the floor; some mobilise initially by sitting upright and 'shuffling' on their bottoms. Variation is seen in other areas, such as language acquisition and social skills. A child may reach some milestones at an early age but be late with others.

A developmental review should cover:

- Any parental concerns about the child or their ability to care for it.
- Assessment of a family's needs and risks.
- Health promotion (e.g. discuss parental smoking, check and record the results of screening tests and check that the immunisation record is up to date).
- Assessment of growth and physical and emotional development. Growth is an important indicator of a child's health and well-being.
- Detection of developmental and physical abnormalities: gross and fine motor skills, behaviour and social skills, hearing, vision and language.

The 6–8-week check

It is usually the GP who undertakes the 6–8-week check, which is a full external physical review (see Tables 12.1 and 12.2). The main physical abnormalities that the 6–8-week check looks for are: congenital cataract, congenital heart disease, congenital

Table 12.1 Taking the history at the 6–8-week check.

Current health and immediate issues	• Is the mother well? • Is the baby well? If unwell, postpone the check and vaccinations and assess the child • Concerns the parents want to raise, e.g. feeding/sleeping • Any problems looking after the baby? • How is the baby being fed?
Problems in pregnancy/ family history	• Maternal or foetal issues in pregnancy, e.g. diabetes/IUGR • Family history, especially cardiac, hip and eye problems
The birth	• Prematurity or post-term? Interventional delivery? • Issues during or after birth, e.g. was mother or baby hospitalised for any reason?
Screening	• Has the baby had heel prick test? Are the results known? • Has the baby had neonatal hearing screen? • Has an ultrasound of the hips been done, if indicated?
Growth	• Have the parents any concerns about growth?
Development history	• Is there a responsive smile (8 weeks)? • Can the baby's eyes fix and follow on an object, e.g. a face. Do both eyes move together at 6 weeks? • Does the baby respond to sound, e.g. startle at loud noise or pause at start of prolonged noise?

Table 12.2 The physical examination in the 6–8-week check.[4]

• A systematic approach is helpful, e.g. head to toe (some GPs start at the feet).
• Be flexible: take the opportunity to listen to the heart and lungs when the baby is quiet.
• Have a warm room: the baby needs to be fully undressed.
• Get permission from the parents to undress the baby for the examination: this helps assess tone and handling.
• Be prepared: babies often urinate when the nappy is removed, so loosen the sides and place it back over the genitals.
• Talk through the examination as you go to involve the parents.

Growth	• **Measure weight, length and head circumference:** Record results on centile charts based on World Health Organization (WHO) standards.[3]
General inspection	• **Skin:** Colour, e.g. jaundice, rashes, and birthmarks. • **Social interaction:** Eye contact and social smile. • **Position and movement:** Head and limbs. • **Symmetry and proportion:** Limbs, face and head. • **Dysmorphic features.**
Handling	• **Normal tone:** Neither tense nor floppy. • **Head control:** A 6-week-old baby lying prone should be able to briefly lift its head. A baby held ventral suspension (the examiner's hand under the chest and abdomen) will briefly lift its head in line with the trunk.
Systems	• **Head and neck:** Check fontanelles, head shape, palate, presence of clavicles. • **Musculoskeletal:** Check joints, limbs and spine. A mark, tuft of hair or dimpling over the lower spine needs further assessment for spina bifida. • **Respiratory:** Chest movements, breathing rate, lung fields. • **Abdomen and anus:** Organomegaly, hernias. An umbilical hernia often resolves – refer for repair if it doesn't close in the first year.
Congential heart disease	• Check for cyanosis, respiratory and heart rate, apex beat, heart sounds and femoral pulses. • Murmurs are common but need assessment. • Innocent murmurs are soft and only occur in a small area of the precordium. If the baby is thriving, refer to paediatric out-patients. • Refer immediately if there is a murmur associated with failure to thrive, breathlessness, cyanosis or absent femoral pulses.

(Continued)

Table 12.2 (*Continued*)

Congenital dislocation of the hip	• Compare leg length and groin creases. • Barlow and Ortolani tests (see Figure 12.1). • Refer for an urgent ultrasound if there are any abnormalities found.
Assessing the eyes	• **Visual:** Does the baby make eye contact and fix and follow? At 6 weeks, a baby's eyes should fix on an object in the midline and follow it to the side. • **External appearance:** Check for obvious squint. One eye bigger than the other may indicate glaucoma. • **Corneal light reflection:** The light from the ophthalmoscope directed at the face should reflect at an equal spot in both eyes, unless there is a squint. • **Red reflex:** Light from the ophthalmoscope should have an unobstructed path to the back of the eye and the eyes should appear to glow a uniform red or orange, like the 'red eye' in a photograph taken with the flash on. Dark spots indicate cataracts or corneal or vitreous abnormalities. A white or pale reflex can mean congenital cataracts or retinoblastoma. If the latter is suspected, same-day referral can be vision- and life-saving.
Assessing the genitals	• Can both testes be palpated in the scrotal sac? If not, are they retractile, incompletely descended or absent? Incompletely descended testes may descend, examine again when the baby is 3 months old, refer if concerns persist. Orchidopexy is usually done by the age of one. Bilateral absent testes need urgent referral. • Retractile testes can be felt in the upper part of the scrotum and manipulated down, and parents can feel them when the child is in a warm bath. No treatment is needed, but there is a higher risk of ascent, so follow up until puberty. • Unusual and pronounced genitalia in girls indicate congenital adrenal hyperplasia (likely to have presented earlier than 6 weeks).

The baby lies on its back. Each hip is tested in turn. The hips and knees should be flexed. The doctor stabilises the pelvis on one side, and tests the other side by placing the thumb on the medial thigh and index finger over the greater trochanter.

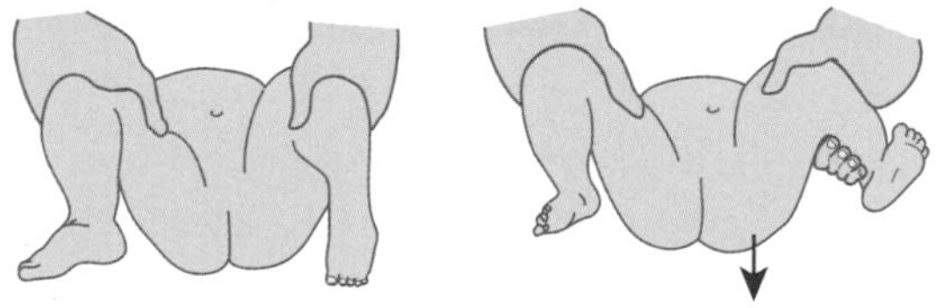

Barlow's test assesses whether the hip is dislocatable. The hip is flexed and adducted, and gentle pressure is applied posteriorly (as if pushing the femur into the couch). A 'clunk' can be felt if the femur slips out of the acetabulum.

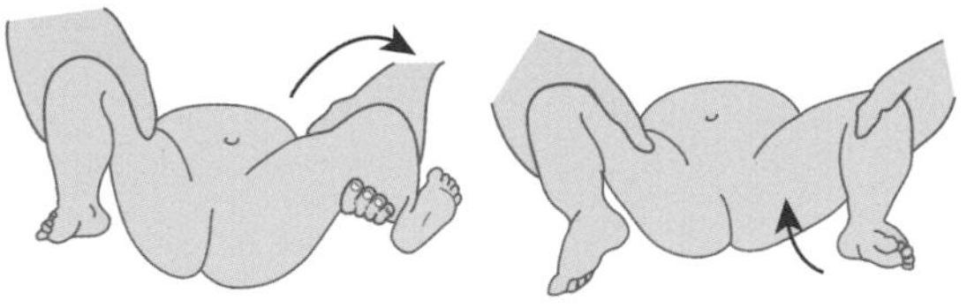

Ortolani's test attempts to relocate a dislocated hip by gently abducting the flexed hip then using the index finger to attempt to lift the femoral head back into the acetabulum.

Figure 12.1 Assessing for congenital dislocation of the hips.

dysplasia of the hip (see Figure 12.1) and undescended testes.[4] The 6–8-week check is also a good opportunity to promote child health, immunisations and accident prevention.

Further developmental reviews

Health visitors review a child's development at around 1 year of age, and again between 2 and 2.5 years old. A school entry hearing and vision check is performed, and eye tests are free to children under 16 in the UK. Where problems are detected, parents and children should be referred to the appropriate early-years services: either community support services or secondary care, or both.

Immunisations

At first, a neonate has passive immunity from the maternal antibodies that cross the placenta. This immunity wears off over time, and children are vaccinated so that they develop active immunity to specific diseases. The time at which passive immunity declines is different for different infectious illnesses, which dictates the schedule for vaccines. Passive immunity against measles, mumps and rubella lasts up to a year, so the vaccine is given at this age. There are also some infectious diseases that are less serious as the child gets older. *Haemophilus influenzae* type b (Hib) can cause pneumonia or meningitis in infants. The risks associated with contracting haemophilus influenza are much less in children over 4 years old, so older children do not need a catch-up dose if they have missed the Hib vaccination.[5]

Vaccination against common communicable diseases has had a major positive impact on child health and well-being; diseases such as diphtheria and polio are now rare in the Western world. Parents in the UK are invited to have their children vaccinated according to the current immunisation schedule (see Table 12.3), but it is not currently mandatory for them to do so. In the 1990s, there were claims of a link between autism and the measles, mumps, and rubella (MMR) vaccine. The claims have not been backed up by evidence, but they resulted in national immunisation coverage falling by around 10%. The situation put many children at risk, because measles is highly infectious, so coverage needs to be high to control outbreaks.

Table 12.3 UK childhood immunisation schedule.

Age	Immunisation	Route
2, 3 and 4 months	*DTaP/IPV(polio)/Hib* (diphtheria, tetanus, pertussis (whooping cough), polio, and *Haemophilus influenzae* type b)	Injection (combined)
Also at 2 and 3 months	Rotavirus gastroenteritis vaccine	Oral
Also at 2 and 4 months	*PCV* (pneumococcal conjugate vaccine) *MenB* (meningitis B vaccine)	Injections (separate)
Also at 3 months	*MenC* (meningitis C vaccine)	Injection (single vaccine)
0–12 months (or older) Offered to children who are close contacts of someone with tuberculosis (TB) or who emigrate from a country with high incidence	*BCG (bacillus Calmette-Guerin)* TB vaccination	Injection
1 year	*Hib* 4th dose *MenC* 2nd dose *MenB* 3rd dose *MMR* (measles, mumps and rubella) *PCV* 3rd dose	Hib and MenC combined MMR combined PCV single vaccine MenB single vaccine
Phased roll-out programme (to cover children aged 2–17) Offered to eligible age group and children at risk from flu, e.g. those with chronic health conditions	*LAIV* (live attenuated influenza vaccine)	Annual nasal spray
Preschool booster (3 years 4 months to 5 years)	*DTaP/IPV* *MMR* 2nd dose	DTaP/IPV combined MMR combined
Between 12–13 years (girls)	*HPV* (human papillomavirus types 16 and 18) (Gardasil)	Two injections 6–24 months apart
13–18 years booster	*Td /IPV* (diphtheria, tetanus and polio vaccine) *Men ACWY*	Td/IPV combined Men ACWY vaccine

There is good evidence for the safety of childhood vaccines. It is common for children to have a mild fever following some immunisations, but serious allergic reactions are rare. Children should not be given a vaccine in general practice if they have had a proven anaphylactic reaction to the vaccine or a component of the vaccine before; specialist advice should be sought. In the UK, Public Health England produces 'The Green Book',[5] which has all the latest information on vaccines and vaccination schedules and procedures.

Consulting with children

Consulting with children requires special skills. We tailor our consultation style to the age of the child: we may need to allow a toddler to 'warm up' to us while we talk to the parent, whereas a 13-year-old may feel ignored and misunderstood if we don't involve them enough. Information also needs to be tailored to the child's level of understanding.

Box 12.1 General tips

- **Know who you are consulting with:** Don't presume the adult with the child is their parent. Check names, including what the child likes to be called.
- **Introduce yourself to everyone who attends:** Occasional eye contact and a smile can help reassure older siblings or another family member that they are not being ignored.
- **Listen and don't dismiss what parents tell you:** Parents are astute observers of their children.
- **Be approachable:** For younger children, be playful but gentle. Get down to their level. For the older child, show interest in what they are telling you.
- **Reassure the child:** Tell them what you are going to do before you do it. If possible, show them, too: in a young

- child, a cursory check of their parent's temperature or throat, or their toy's abdomen or chest, can provide reassurance before you examine them.
- **Be flexible in your examination:** Babies can be examined on a couch, with the parent next to them. Toddlers may feel more reassured being examined on their parent's knee. A mobile child may initially need to be examined while playing.

- **Leave less pleasant procedures until last:** Using a tongue depressor to examine a child's throat is not painful, but it is not pleasant, and it is best left until the end of an examination. Build up to examinations starting at the periphery: taking a temperature or feeling a pulse can reassure a child before you launch into listening to their chest or feeling their abdomen.

Acting in a child's best interests

We need good negotiating skills, and to know what situations we are competent to handle and when to seek specialist advice; decisions about children can be complex. We are helped by listening carefully to, and respecting the views of, the children we consult with. But sometimes we need to override parent or child confidentiality in the best interests of the child.

The General Medical Council (GMC)'s 'Principles for Protecting Children and Young People' say that 'The "best interests" of a child or young person should be the guiding principle in all decisions that may affect them. Assessing a child's or young person's best interests will include what is clinically indicated in a particular case.'[6] The welfare of the child overrides other considerations, such as consent, confidentiality and the parent's wishes. However, a best interest is not always easy to ascertain, especially if a doctor believes it should override the parent's or child's wishes, so it is important that GPs know their limits. Decisions about what is in the child's best interests should, and usually do, involve sharing information with other professionals. The degree to which other professionals are involved varies according to the situation, from a GP's seeking advice from a child protection lead about breaking confidentiality, to a court case when a parent or child refuses life-saving treatment.

Child health promotion

Obesity

Children who are obese in childhood are likely to remain so into adulthood. Obese adults are at increased risk of cardiovascular disease (CVD), stroke and diabetes. Obese children can suffer direct health consequences, such as worsening of asthma, but the most immediate problem is psychosocial, with increased rates of bullying and low self-esteem. The prevalence of childhood obesity is increasing.[7] The Avon Longitudinal Study of Parents and Children (ALSPAC)[8] recruited around 14 000 pregnant women with estimated dates of delivery in 1991 and 1992. The children have been followed up ever since, making it one of the largest epidemiological studies of children to date. Results so far show that maternal education has an inverse association with child obesity, with a threefold risk increase in the least-educated group. Increased TV viewing and decreased duration of sleep are associated with an increased risk of obesity. Breastfeeding and late introduction of solids appear to be protective, but the effect disappears when adjusted for other confounders.

Parents of overweight children tend to be overweight or obese themselves, so it's important to take a whole-family approach. General recommendations for all children are that they should be moderately to vigorously active for at least an hour a day; this can be broken into smaller chunks of time. Preschool children who are mobile should be active for at least 3 hours a day. Processed, fatty and sugary food should be avoided.

Accident prevention

Accidents are the second biggest cause of child death, and every year 100 000 children are admitted to hospital following serious injury.[9] Primary care has a role in identifying which children are at risk of injury. This includes knowing the disadvantaged children in a community, but also being aware of the stage of development of children so that advice can be targeted. There are many 'teachable moments' in a consultation with children. A newborn may not be able to roll over, but their wriggling can move them a surprising distance, so they should never be left unattended on a raised surface. Consultations with babies can be an opportunity to reinforce this message. NICE has produced specific guidance to reduce unintentional injury, based on good evidence that GPs can help parents improve home safety.[10] The NHS Choices website (www.nhs.uk) provides clear guidance to parents on preventing accidents.

GPs also have a surveillance role. GPs receive reports on their patients from out-of-hours and accident and emergency departments. These need to be reviewed to make sure significant or recurrent injuries are followed up. In some situations, it is appropriate for the GP to review the child or share information with health visitors. All injuries should be correctly coded and recorded on the notes.

Smoking

The dangers of passive smoking are well known. In the infant, exposure to cigarette smoke increases the risk of sudden infant death, and for all children it increases the risk of respiratory disease, such as asthma, and makes colds and middle-ear infections more likely.[11] Cigarettes contain numerous toxic chemicals that are linked to cancer. Cigarette smoke leaves behind toxic residue on clothes, furniture and carpets, and children can be harmed by this 'thirdhand' smoke. Ventilating rooms and staying in one room are ineffective: smoke from one cigarette was found to linger in the room for up to 2.5 hours, even with a window open.[11] If a child sees one of their parents smoke, this normalises smoking for them, and they are more likely to take up smoking themselves.

Vulnerable families and children at risk

There are many parents in our communities who raise children without enough money to make ends meet, who have little or no social support and who struggle with their own physical or mental health issues. The Healthy Child Programme[1] says that 'Poverty is one of the biggest risk factors linked to poorer health outcomes. Poorer children are less likely to be breastfed, more likely to be exposed to tobacco smoke, and more likely to be injured at home and on the roads.'

Multiple disadvantages increase the risk of poor health and social outcomes for children, including developmental and behavioural problems, teenage parenthood, offending behaviour, substance abuse, mental illness and poor educational attainment. GPs need to be aware of families that are vulnerable or under significant stress so that support can be offered.

Child abuse

Most parents want the best for their children. Tragically, some parents harm the children in their care. Whether the harm is intentional or a result of the parent's ignorance or poor health, the results are just as devastating. Abuse is categorised as emotional, physical, sexual or neglect.[12] Emotional abuse can be hard to identify and takes a number of different forms. The parent can cause the child to feel fearful or unloved or be excessively controlling; their expectations of their child may be inappropriate for the child's age. Physical abuse is harming the child by shaking, burning, poisoning or hitting them. The parent may fabricate illness, which can result in physical harm. Sexual abuse can either be direct sexual contact with the child, taking indecent images or exposing the child to inappropriate sexual material. Neglect is when the child's physical and emotional

---

Case study 12.1

Ricky Riley, aged 3, is brought to see his GP, Dr Malcom Brewer, by his father. Dr Brewer observes Ricky and his father in the waiting room when he calls Ricky in. When Ricky doesn't look up from the toys he is playing with, Ricky's father suddenly grabs Ricky's wrist and pulls him abruptly away from the toys, while shouting at him and calling him a 'brat'.

Mr Riley explains that Ricky has a sore throat and couldn't attend nursery, so he's had to take a day off work. Ricky is quiet and withdrawn during the consultation. Ricky is coryzal, with visible thick green nasal discharge, a raised temperature of 37.9 °C and pharyngitis. On exposure of Ricky's chest, Dr Brewer notices bruising consistent with adult finger marks on Ricky's upper left arm. Mr Riley says these were from a fight Ricky got into at nursery with another child. Dr Brewer finds a circular scab on Ricky's lower back. Mr Riley says this injury was sustained when Ricky ran into the end of his cigarette.

Dr Brewer had already looked at Ricky's medical records and the family medical record. Ricky has a younger brother aged 18 months. The children have not been subject to a child protection plan in the past (this should be recorded in medical notes, but we can also check with social services). The GP records show Ricky is up to date with immunisations, but there are a number of missed scheduled appointments recorded. There are a few letters from the emergency department at the local hospital, where Ricky has presented with minor injuries. Ricky's mother is known to have anxiety and to have suffered with postnatal depression.

What should Dr Brewer do?
Any GP who suspects child abuse has a duty to act. Having a serious concern is enough; the GP does not need proof. Dr Brewer should ask himself:
- Why am I worried?
- What is the level of risk?
- What are the implications of doing nothing or deferring action?
- What should I do right now?

What are the concerning features of this case?
Dr Brewer is concerned by Ricky's father's aggressive behaviour (physical and verbal) towards his son. Ricky has two injuries that are not consistent with the story his father gives: adult finger marks are unlikely to have been sustained in a fight at nursery; a cigarette burn is abuse until proven otherwise. It is normal for a child to become quiet and withdrawn during illness, but in this context it raises suspicion that the child is frightened of his father. The letters from the emergency department record minor injuries. Each incident alone may not have been indicative of abuse, but suspicions are raised when there are several injuries.

Outcome
Dr Brewer is concerned about physical abuse. He speaks to the named paediatrician for child protection. Ricky is transferred to the local hospital emergency department for an urgent specialist assessment. Ricky, his mother and his younger brother are thought to be at risk of ongoing physical abuse from Mr Riley. They are removed to a place of safety while a child protection plan is put in place.

Table 12.4 Recognising child abuse.

Alert presentations in child

Suspect if	• The child has unexplained or multiple injuries, or a story doesn't 'fit' or changes • A nonmobile child has an injury that would require them to be mobile • The child's explanation different from the caregiver's • There child shows signs of injury known to be associated with abuse (e.g. cigarette burns, genital, anal or perianal injury, symmetrical scalding, bruising on an unusual site, e.g. abdomen) • The child shows frozen watchfulness: they appear afraid of the carer • The child is thin/malnourished or shows visible signs of social deprivation • The child shows overly sexualised behaviour • The child reveals sexual intercourse under the age of 13 (when they are unable to consent to sex by law) • A teenager reveals sexual intercourse with imbalance of power (e.g. partner is not of similar age/maturity)
Consider when	• The child shows depression, anxiety or behavioural issues • The child shows failure to thrive/developmental delay

Alert presentations in carer

Suspect if	• The carer shows behaviour of concern (e.g. acting in a threatening manner towards the child or obviously not coping) • Presentation of injury is delayed
Consider when	• The carer makes multiple presentations • The carer fails to attend on multiple occasions

needs are not met. The parent may not adequately clothe, feed or supervise their child, or may fail to seek appropriate medical care. The current child protection legislation is based on the Children Act 1989.[13] Section 17 of the act defines the phrase 'a child in need' as any child whose vulnerability is such that they are unlikely to reach or maintain a satisfactory level of health or development, or whose health and development will be significantly impaired without the provision of services. It also includes children who are disabled. 'Harm' is defined as ill treatment or the impairment of health or development. 'Harm' also includes seeing or hearing the ill treatment of others, so it encompasses children who witness domestic abuse in the home. The act describes the duties and powers that children's social care teams have towards children.

Table 12.4 outlines presentations of child maltreatment. Not all of these presentations signify abuse, but abuse is under-reported and underdiagnosed, and can be fatal. We should always ask, 'What is a child really experiencing?' GPs need to recognise the possibility of abuse, make enquiries and gather enough information to refer for a specialist assessment. Gaps in a medical record may be easily explained, but they may also indicate neglect. Communication about even minor concerns is vital; often, the true picture will only emerge when a number of concerns are put together from different sources.

The British Medical Association (BMA) provides a free-to-access toolkit for doctors, covering specific areas in examining and treating children in the UK based on existing guidelines.[14]

SUMMARY

The health and experiences of children and young people have a lifetime effect. GPs have opportunities in every consultation with families to promote child health and identify vulnerable children. GPs should know what constitutes normal development and behaviour, monitor children's well-being and take part in delivering national child health screening and vaccination programmes, such as those outlined in the Department of Health's Healthy Child Programme. The 6–8-week check is a review that screens for abnormalities, but is also an opportunity to build relationships between GPs and the families they care for. GPs must recognise and respond to the needs of children, which can be masked by the needs of their parents and caregivers. They must be competent in dealing with safeguarding issues and act quickly and effectively if they suspect abuse.

 Now visit **www.wileyessential.com/primarycare** to test yourself on this chapter.

REFERENCES

1. Department of Health. *Healthy Child Programme: Pregnancy and the First Five Years of Life*. DOH: London; 2009.

2. Public Health England. Newborn Blood Spot Screening Programme: Supporting Publications. Available from: http://newbornbloodspot.screening.nhs.uk/professionals (last accessed 6 October 2015).

3. Royal College of Paediatrics and Child Health. UK-WHO growth charts, 0–18 years. Available from: http://www.rcpch.ac.uk/Research/UK-WHO-Growth-Charts (last accessed 6 October 2015).

4. NICE. Postnatal care: routine postnatal care of women and their babies. NICE Clinical Guideline 37. October 2006 (updated December 2014). Available from: https://www.nice.org.uk/guidance/cg37 (last accessed 6 October 2015).

5. Public Health England. *Immunisation against Infectious Disease: 'The Green Book'*. Public Health England: London; 2013.

6. General Medical Council. *Good Medical Practice: Protecting Children and Young People: The Responsibilities of all Doctors*. GMC: London; 2013.

7. Health & Social Care Information Centre. Statistics on Obesity, Physical Activity and Diet. Available from: http://www.hscic.gov.uk/catalogue/PUB16988/obes-phys-acti-diet-eng-2015.pdf (last accessed 6 October 2015).

8. Ness AR. The Avon Longitudinal Study of Parents and Children (ALSPAC) – a resource for the study of the environmental determinants of childhood obesity. *Eur J Endocrinol* 2004;**151:**U141–9.

9. Kendrick D, Hayes M, Ward H, Mytton J. Preventing unintentional injuries: what does NICE guidance mean for primary care? *Br J Gen Pract* 2012;**62**(595):62–3.

10. NICE. Preventing unintentional injuries among children and young people aged under 15. NICE Public Health Guideline 31. November 2010. Available from: https://www.nice.org.uk/guidance/ph31 (last accessed 6 October 2015).

11. ASH. Secondhand smoke: the impact on children. Available from: http://www.ash.org.uk/information/facts-and-stats/fact-sheets (last accessed 6 October 2015).

12. NICE. When to suspect child maltreatment. NICE Clinical Guideline 89. July 2009. Available from: https://www.nice.org.uk/guidance/cg89 (last accessed 6 October 2015).

13. The Children's Act 1989. Available from: http://www.legislation.gov.uk/ukpga/1989/41/contents (last accessed 6 October 2015).

14. British Medical Association. Children and young people toolkit. Available from; http://www.bma.org.uk/practical-support-at-work/ethics/children/children-and-young-people-tool-kit (last accessed 6 October 2015).

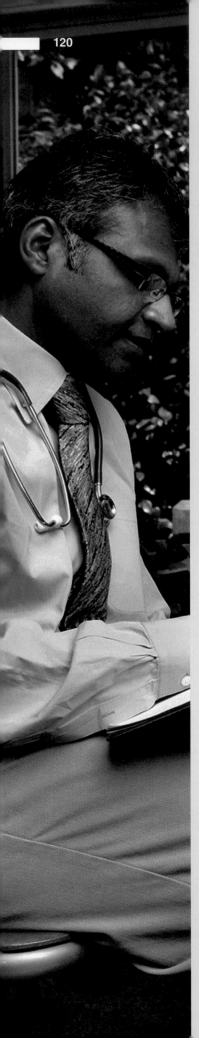

CHAPTER 13

Managing the feverish and ill child in primary care

Alastair Hay[1], Lucy Jenkins[2] and Jessica Buchan[2]
[1]Professor of Primary Care, University of Bristol
[2]Teaching Fellow in Primary Care, University of Bristol

Key topics

Learning objectives

- Be able to assess the risk of serious illness in children, including assessment of fever and dehydration.
- Be able to advise parents on the conservative management of fever.
- Be able to assess a child with a suspected febrile fit.
- Be able to discuss the pros and cons of antibiotic use in common childhood infections.
- Be able to discuss the management of urinary tract infections in children.
- Be able to recognise symptoms and signs in a child that might indicate cancer.

For simplicity, in these child health chapters the term 'parent' encompasses any adult who has a parental role and is regularly caring for children; the term 'child' means any person from birth to the age of 18.

Essential Primary Care, First Edition. Edited by Andrew Blythe and Jessica Buchan.
© 2017 John Wiley & Sons, Ltd. Published 2017 by John Wiley & Sons, Ltd.
Companion website: www.wileyessential.com/primarycare

Assessment of the ill child in primary care

It may be that the initial assessment of a child is done over the telephone. In this case, a detailed history and parental concerns are especially important. If simple home treatment is advised, the GP must be sure to 'safety-net'. If the GP is uncertain or the parent is concerned, it is always best to see the child and assess in person. Children with symptoms suggesting a high risk of serious illness should have a face-to-face assessment within 2 hours.

Chapter 12 discussed a general approach to consulting with children. Parents know their children very well, so it is essential to take their concerns seriously. When a child is ill or in pain, there may be particular challenges if they are crying or reluctant to be examined.

Table 13.1 summarises the key topics to cover when taking a history from the parents of an ill child. Figure 13.1 presents an overview of the examination. The objective measures listed in Table 13.2 are particularly useful to record in the notes, so that comparisons can be made when an ill child is reviewed.

Red flags and assessing the likelihood of serious illness

To identify serious illness in children, a thorough assessment of the child's activity levels, colour and vital signs, respiratory and circulatory systems should be made. This has been formalised in an approach known as the ***traffic-light system***, aimed at helping identify the likelihood of serious illness in children under 5 years old with fever, but which also applies to other childhood illnesses.[1] A rapid heart rate increases the risk of serious bacterial infection.[2]

> **Top tips**
>
> - Children <3 months with a temperature of 38 °C or higher are at high risk for serious illness.
> - Children aged 3–6 months with a temperature of 39 °C or higher are at high risk for serious illness.

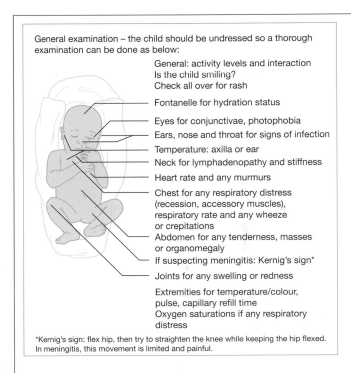

General examination – the child should be undressed so a thorough examination can be done as below:

General: activity levels and interaction
Is the child smiling?
Check all over for rash

Fontanelle for hydration status

Eyes for conjunctivae, photophobia

Ears, nose and throat for signs of infection

Temperature: axilla or ear

Neck for lymphadenopathy and stiffness

Heart rate and any murmurs

Chest for any respiratory distress (recession, accessory muscles), respiratory rate and any wheeze or crepitations

Abdomen for any tenderness, masses or organomegaly

If suspecting meningitis: Kernig's sign*

Joints for any swelling or redness

Extremities for temperature/colour, pulse, capillary refill time
Oxygen saturations if any respiratory distress

*Kernig's sign: flex hip, then try to straighten the knee while keeping the hip flexed. In meningitis, this movement is limited and painful.

Figure 13.1 Examination of the unwell child.

Table 13.1 History in the unwell child.

History of presenting complaint	Other important features of history
Duration and degree of fever	**Past medical history** Including conditions which predispose to infections, e.g. sickle cell disease, primary immunodeficiency, nephrotic syndrome
Is the child feeding normally?	
Localising symptoms: • coryza • sore throat • earache • headache or photophobia • abdominal pains • cough or breathing problems • diarrhoea and vomiting • joint pain • rash	Any known **infection contact** or illness in family members and recent travel
	Immunisation status
	Regular **medications** and known drug allergies
	Social history It is important to have an idea of the child's home circumstances, as this may influence management
Urinary output	
Behaviour – irritable or drowsy	

Table 13.2 Vital signs to check in an unwell child.

Vital sign	Normal values by age in years				
	<1	1–2	2–5	5–12	>12
Heart rate (beats/minute)	110–160	110–150	95–140	80–120	60–100
Respiratory rate (breaths/minute)	30–40	25–35	25–30	20–25	15–20
Temperature	A normal temperature is 36.5–37.2 °C. Under 5, a fever is >37.5 °C.			Over 5 years, a fever is >38 °C.	
Oxygen saturations	Normal for all ages is >95% in air				
Capillary refill time (CRT)	Press for 5 seconds on the big toe, finger or sternum and count the seconds it takes for the colour to return. Normal is <2 seconds				
Signs of dehydration	Prolonged CRT, abnormal skin turgor, abnormal respiratory pattern, weak pulse, cool extremities				

Table 13.3 Identifying serious illness in infants.

Parental concern	Parents may describe the following in their baby: • Twitches, jitters or fits • Sleepy and difficult to wake for feeds • Feeding poorly • Unusual cry • Unusual breathing or history of apnoea • History of head injury
Specific symptoms	Vomiting: progressive, projectile or bilious (can indicate bowel obstruction) Dehydration: poor urine output (should have a wet nappy every 4 hours) Jaundice: progressive or with other signs of illness, or pale stools and dark urine Blood in stools: a description of 'redcurrant jelly' can indicate intussusception or *E coli* gastroenteritis
General examination	Drowsy, reduced tone or jittery and rigid Pallor or obvious jaundice Cyanosis or cold peripheries Dehydration: sunken eyes, sunken fontanelle, reduced skin turgor Measurements: tachycardia, reduced CRT, pyrexia or hypothermia
Specific examination	Petechial rash Bruising or not moving all four limbs Joint swelling or unusual position of limb Abdominal distension with tinkling bowel sounds (bowel obstruction)

'High-risk' symptoms and signs indicate serious infection and should prompt assessment by a paediatric specialist. A child who is pale, mottled, ashen or blue needs immediate assessment. In any unwell child, the GP should consider:

- **Pneumonia:** Suggested by respiratory symptoms and signs. Tachypnoea, nasal flaring, intercostal recession, cyanosis and low saturations are signs of intermediate risk of serious disease. Grunting and severe recession are high-risk signs.
- **Urinary tract infection (UTI):** The child may be systemically unwell, with unexplained fever
- **Appendicitis:** Typically, abdominal pain starts centrally then localises to the right iliac fossa with anorexia, fever and vomiting. If suspected, refer promptly to the surgical team for assessment.
- **Septicaemia:** Limb pain, cold hands and feet have been shown to be specific signs.
- **Septic arthritis:** Presents with a painful swollen joint.

- **Meningococcal disease:** Fever with headache, photophobia and rash. Check vital signs, neck stiffness and Kernig's sign. Neurological signs are high risk. If suspected, urgent hospital transfer should be arranged and intramuscular benzylpenicillin administered.[3]
- **Herpes simplex encephalitis:** An uncommon but serious illness causing reduced level of consciousness, focal neurological signs and sometimes seizures.

Top tip: consider UTI in unexplained fever

A child with an unexplained fever of 38 °C or higher lasting for 24 hours or more should have a urine sample tested.

A urine sample is not necessary if an alternative focus of infection has been found, but it should be considered after 24 hours if the child remains ill.[4]

In infants, serious illness can present with nonspecific symptoms such as irritability, lethargy and poor feeding. Infants may have few localising signs, or their only sign of illness may be a change from their normal behaviour. Table 13.3 outlines features in the history or examination that indicate serious illness in infants.

No single feature has been shown to rule out serious infection. Doctor and parental instinct are important. It may be hard to define a gut feeling that there is something seriously wrong with a patient, but this has been shown to be a diagnostic red flag regardless of the level of the doctor's experience.[5] This feeling should act as a prompt for thorough assessment, referral (if needed) and clear safety-netting. Gut feeling has been found to be influenced by parental concern that this illness is different: parents know their children very well, and parental concern is 14 times more likely in a child with a serious infection.[6]

Top tip: Spotting the Sick Child

- **www.spottingthesickchild.com** This is an interactive online tool developed by the UK Department of Health for use by all health care professionals and medical students.

Childhood fever

Fever is the result of a complex physiological response to infection. Prostaglandins mediate a rise in temperature, creating a hostile environment for viruses and bacteria. On average, a child is seen by their GP for a febrile illness 3.7 times a year.[7] Most febrile illnesses are not serious, but fever is the second most common reason for a child to be admitted to hospital in the UK. Worldwide, infectious disease is still the largest cause of child mortality. Improvements in sanitation and hygiene and medical advances, notably immunisation and antibiotics, mean that this is not the case in the UK, but there are still a number of serious and life-threatening infections that present with fever.

Causes of fever

Viral infections are very common; the majority of these are upper respiratory tract infections (RTIs), including tonsillitis and otitis media. Other common viral infections, which often cause rashes, are detailed in Table 13.4. A mild fever after routine childhood vaccinations is fairly common. Fever should not be blamed on teething.

Persistent fever or recurrent serious illness should always be taken seriously. Table 13.5 outlines some of the important causes. A travel and contact history is important, especially in children with recurrent fevers. A referral to secondary care for further specialist investigation would be indicated at this stage.

Top tip: advice for parents on managing fever

- Tepid sponging is not recommended.
- Do not over- or underdress a child with fever.
- Treat the child, not the temperature: paracetamol and/or ibuprofen can be given to relieve a child's distress. These medications do not affect the natural history of the illness and does not reduce the risk of febrile convulsions.[1,8]

Table 13.4 Viruses and rashes.			
Virus and incubation period	**Symptoms and signs (as well as fever)**	**Possible complications**	**Usual duration of illness**
Chicken pox (varicella zoster virus) 14–16 days	Mild malaise, sore throat and headache can occur Crops of red spots, then blisters, which dry out and crust over. The rash has a centripetal spread: the first spots tend to appear on the head and neck, then spread to the trunk	Otitis media and pneumonia (most common) Secondary bacterial skin infection Eczema herpeticum Encephalitis (rare)	14 days

(Continued)

Table 13.4 (*Continued*)

Virus and incubation period	Symptoms and signs (as well as fever)	Possible complications	Usual duration of illness
Measles (RNA morbillivirus) 10–14 days	Prodrome: miserable, coryzal child with cough and conjunctivitis (which can be key to the diagnosis) Widespread maculopapular rash develops after 4 days Koplik's spots: tiny white spots on reddened background on inside of cheeks	Otitis media Pneumonia Encephalitis	10 days
Mumps 16–21 days	General malaise can occur, but mild or subclinical infections are common Tender enlargement of parotid/submandibular glands, which is usually unilateral	Aseptic meningitis Epididymo-orchitis Pancreatitis	
Rubella (rubella rubivirus) 14–21 days	Often subclinical Lymphadenopathy and pink maculopapular rash, first appears on head and neck	Arthritis	10 days
Hand, foot and mouth (coxsackie virus) 3–5 days	Rash with painful non-itchy vesicles on hands and feet and blisters/ulcers in the mouth Upper RTI and cough, but child often fairly well	Reduced eating due to oral pain (teething gels can help)	5–7 days
Erythema infectiosum/ fifth disease (parvovirus) 4–14 days	Red maculopapular rash starting in the face, causing 'slapped cheek' appearance and lacy rash, which comes and goes on rest of body. Occasional arthralgia. Otherwise, systemic symptoms are uncommon	Rare	4–7 days
Roseola infantum 10–15 days	High fever with sore throat, then maculopapular rash appearing when fever reduces	Rare	3–6 days

Source: Images within table from: Blundell, A & Harrison, R (2013) *OSCEs at a Glance*, 2nd edn. Reproduced with permission of John Wiley & Sons, Ltd.

Table 13.5 Causes of persistent or recurrent fever in children.

Malaria	Nonspecific presentation is typical in children, so a travel history is essential
Respiratory symptoms **Cystic fibrosis** **Nonresolving chest infection – possible aspiration pneumonia** **Tuberculosis**	Recurrent chest infections and failure to thrive Ask about history of inhaled foreign body Suspect if haemoptysis and night sweats. Ask about contacts and check immunisation status
Infective endocarditis	This is rare. Suspect in children with congenital heart disease or history of cardiac surgery, or a new murmur
Kawasaki's disease	Fever lasting >5 days and at least four of the following: conjunctival redness, red throat/tongue, peeling skin on hands, rash, cervical lymphadenopathy
Urinary tract reflux	May present with recurrent UTI
Immunological deficiencies (congenital or specific diseases such as HIV)	Recurrent, severe or unusual infections, often with associated failure to thrive
Neoplasm	Leukaemia and lymphoma are the most common
Systemic juvenile chronic arthritis	Persistent fever with musculoskeletal symptoms
Occult abscess	May have few localising signs
Factitious fever	A fever that is deliberately feigned or faked by a carer or child

The PITCH study showed that combined ibuprofen and paracetamol was slightly better in reducing the temperature in the first 24 hours than using one agent alone, although there was no difference in relief of distress at 48 hours.[9] The GP should thus advise the parent to use the agent of their choice and add in a second if one treatment alone does not relieve distress (but not to give both together, as this increases the risk of dosing errors).

Febrile seizures (fits)

The aetiology is not completely understood, but febrile fits are thought to be caused by the temperature rising rapidly early in an infection (usually viral) in a child's immature brain. By definition, a febrile fit is one without any underlying central nervous system (CNS) infection, neurological or metabolic abnormality or drug toxicity. Febrile fits run in families.

Febrile seizures are quite common: 3% of children between the age of 6 months and 6 years will have a fit, usually due to viral infections such as colds and ear infections. A typical presentation is an uncomplicated tonic clonic fit with loss of consciousness, associated with a temperature >37.8 °C. The child should recover quickly; they may be drowsy for a short time afterwards, and will be fully recovered within an hour. The GP must establish if this was a fit and if further investigation or referral is needed. A clear and detailed witness history is essential, with particular focus on exactly what happened, any associated symptoms (tongue biting or incontinence), duration and how the child was afterwards. A full examination should include the neurological system.

Referral[10] is indicated if:
- It is a child's first seizure.
- The diagnosis is unclear.

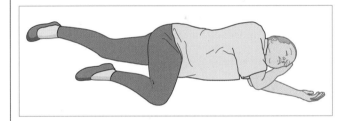

Figure 13.2 The recovery position.

- The child is having febrile fits that are frequent, severe or complex (lasting more than 15 minutes, focal or recurring in the same illness, or if the child is not recovering within an hour).
- The parents are very worried or request specialist review.
- The child is at increased risk of epilepsy (e.g. due to positive family history or coexisting neurological conditions).

If the GP is confident about the diagnosis, referral and further investigations are not indicated. A fit may be upsetting for a child, but will always be distressing for a parent. The parents will need a clear explanation and advice. Parents should be advised that if the child has a further seizure, they should be protected from injury and put in the recovery position (see Figure 13.2). The child should not be restrained and not have anything put into their mouth. Parents should dial 999 if the seizure lasts more than 5 minutes. Studies following up children after simple febrile fits have shown that there is no impairment of intelligence, academic performance or behaviour.[11]

Table 13.6 Assessing and managing a dehydrated child.

Degree and signs of dehydration	Management
None or mild	
Dry mouth Otherwise fairly well	Home management: offer fluids frequently and in small amounts; avoid juice and fizzy drinks Continue breastfeeding and other milk feeds Offer rehydration solution to high-risk children Observe closely: review any deterioration **General advice:** • Diarrhoea usually lasts 5–7 days; vomiting usually lasts 3 days • Careful hygiene at home is essential • Stay out of childcare/school until 48 hours after last episode of diarrhoea or vomiting
Moderate	
Dry mouth Reduced urine output Lethargy Tachycardia Sunken eyes and fontanelle Prolonged CRT Reduced skin turgor	Consider **admission** **If home management:** • Offer oral rehydration solution 5–10 ml every few minutes (50 ml/kg over 4 hours) • Observe closely and monitor fluids in and out – review any deterioration • GP should arrange early review
Severe	
As for moderate No urine output for 12 hours May be irritable or comatose Hypotension	**Admit** as emergency

Dehydration in children

Children are particularly susceptible to dehydration and can decompensate quickly as a result of dehydration caused by diarrhoea, vomiting or febrile illness. All babies in the UK are now offered vaccination against rotavirus, a leading cause of diarrhoeal illness in infants. Bloody diarrhoea suggests a bacterial cause; some such causes have serious complications, such as haemolytic uraemic syndrome with *Escherichia coli*. Dehydration may also result from reduced oral intake with oral pain (such as in tonsillitis).

Top tip: new presentation of type 1 diabetes

Always ask about polyuria, thirst and weight loss in a child with dehydration with no clear cause. This may be a first presentation of type 1 diabetes mellitus with ketoacidosis. These children can deteriorate rapidly, so immediate referral is indicated.

Capillary refill time (CRT), skin turgor and abnormal breathing patterns are the most useful individual signs for predicting moderate dehydration in children, but the overall picture is most useful.[12] Children at higher risk of dehydration and admission include those under 12 months, those with more than six loose stools or three vomits in 24 hours and those not taking any oral feeds.[13] All these children should have a face-to-face assessment and close observation. Those with severe dehydration are at risk of shock and should be admitted. See Table 13.6 for an outline of the assessment and management of the dehydrated child.

Top tip: when to send a stool sample to the lab

A stool sample for microscopy, culture and sensitivities should be sent if diarrhoea lasts more than 7 days, or sooner if the diarrhoea is bloody, the child is immunocompromised or very ill or there is recent foreign travel.[14]

Antibiotic use and parental expectations

Alexander Fleming is credited as being the first to observe what he called 'penicillium' inhibiting the growth of a *Staphylococcus* in 1928. However, it was Howard Florey who carried out the first clinical trials of penicillin in 1941, on a postmaster from Wolvercote, near Oxford. Florey worked with Ernst Chain to discover penicillin's therapeutic action and its chemical composition. Together, these three received the Nobel Prize in 1945.

By the end of World War 2, penicillin was in widespread use, with 'miraculous' effects. Unsurprisingly, patients and doctors saw its potential for a broader and broader range of decreasingly severe infections, leading to huge growth in the use of antibiotics.

Table 13.7 When should antibiotics be used?[17]		
Delayed prescription[a] or no antibiotics	'Immediate' antibiotic	'Immediate' antibiotic and/or consideration of hospital referral
Acute otitis media (AOM)	Bilateral AOM in children under 2 years	Systemically very unwell
Acute sore throat/tonsillitis/ pharyngitis	AOM with otorrhoea	Child has symptoms and signs suggestive of serious illness and/or complications
Common cold/acute rhinosinusitis	Acute sore throat/acute pharyngitis/acute tonsillitis when three or more Centor criteria (Chapter 17) are present	Pneumonia, mastoiditis, peritonsillar abscess, peritonsillar cellulitis, intraorbital and intracranial complications
Acute cough/bronchitis		Pre-existing comorbidity, e.g. significant heart, lung, renal, liver or neuromuscular disease, immunosuppression, cystic fibrosis and prematurity

[a]See the section on Reducing Unnecessary Antibiotic Prescribing in the Consultation for a definition of delayed prescribing.

Antibiotics should not be given for a fever with no clear source. Unnecessary prescribing increases antimicrobial resistance, encourages future consultations for similar symptoms, risks side effects and has cost implications. In primary care, when antibiotics are given for RTIs, the benefit is only modest, often amounting to no more than 1 day of reduced symptoms in illnesses that typically last 2 or 3 weeks. The vast majority of all antibiotic prescribing occurs in primary care. However, there is considerable variation in prescribing; a study comparing 26 countries in Europe found a threefold variation in antibiotic prescribing between nations, and a study of antibiotic prescribing in UK primary care found a fourfold variation between GP practices.[15] A lack of evidence that this variation is associated with clinical outcomes suggests a significant proportion of antibiotic prescribing is unnecessary. There is widespread concern that antibiotic prescribing in UK primary care increased by 17% between 2002 and 2012.[16] These variations in antibiotic prescribing between countries[14] and individual practices[15] have been directly linked to antimicrobial resistance.

When should antibiotics be used?

Antibiotics undoubtedly save lives in severe infections such as pneumonia, pyelonephritis, meningitis and septicaemia. While it is not possible to give firm 'rules' for when antibiotics should be used in all infections, the National Institute for Health and Care Excellence (NICE) has made recommendations about which groups of children with RTIs may not need an antibiotic at first presentation, and who should receive an 'immediate' antibiotic and/or hospital referral[17] (see Table 13.7).

Do parents expect antibiotics?

Some parents (and adults) clearly want an antibiotic when they make an appointment to see a primary care nurse or GP. We have known for over 20 years that when a clinician perceives a parent wants an antibiotic, they are more likely to prescribe them.[18] However, we also know that clinicians are frequently incorrect in their assumptions regarding which patients are expecting antibiotics.[19]

Reducing unnecessary antibiotic prescribing in the consultation

- Ask about parental expectations.
- After taking a history, say something like, 'I am about to examine your child and I have a few ideas about what we might do next, but I was wondering if there was anything you hoped I would do today?', or, 'And were you hoping I would prescribe an antibiotic?'
- NICE recommends[17] that parents:
  - are reassured that antibiotics are not needed immediately because they are likely to make little difference to symptoms and may have side effects;
  - reattend for clinical review if their child's condition worsens or becomes prolonged;
  - are given advice about the usual natural history of the infection, including the average total length of the illness (before and after seeing the doctor):
    - acute otitis media (AOM): 4 days (a recent study suggests this should be longer[20]);
    - acute sore throat/acute pharyngitis/acute tonsillitis: 7 days;
    - common cold: 10 days;
    - acute rhinosinusitis: 18 days;
    - acute cough/acute bronchitis: 21 days;
  - are given advice about managing symptoms, including fever (particularly analgesics and antipyretics).
- It is less helpful to label less severe infections as 'viral'. Clinically, it is virtually impossible to distinguish viral from bacterial infection in primary care.
- Consider offering a 'delayed prescription', where the parent is advised to cash the prescription only if the child's symptoms do not settle or their condition worsens.
- Make sure the parents understand the side effects of antibiotics, such as diarrhoea, vomiting, rashes and allergy, including anaphylaxis.
- Offer written information to parents about the natural history of infections, safety-netting information about the symptoms and signs warranting reconsultation and advice

on how best to manage symptoms at home. This has been shown to reduce antibiotic prescribing without reducing parent consultation satisfaction.[21]

Coughs, colds and influenza

RTIs are the most common problem managed in primary care internationally, and present most frequently at the extremes of age, including in preschool children. In the first 5 years of life, preschool children universally experience at least one episode of runny nose, cough, earache, fever or rash,[22] with most children thought to experience between six and eight RTI episodes per annum. Within any given illness episode, around 30% of children with these sorts of symptoms are brought to primary care, most commonly for coughs, colds, rashes, fever and wheeze.[22] See Table 13.8 for commonly implicated microbes in upper RTIs.

Diagnosing influenza ('flu') can be difficult, since young children are not able to report symptoms such as aching limbs. Flu is often more severe than other RTIs, with higher rates of complications (such as pneumonia and AOM). Children with chronic lung, heart, kidney, liver and neurological diseases and children with diabetes and immunosuppression are at particular risk of influenza complications and should be vaccinated. Annual vaccination against flu is being rolled out for all children in the UK from the age of 2 to 17. Chapter 12 outlined the current childhood vaccination schedule.

Table 13.8 Commonly implicated microbes in common RTIs.

Common cold	Pharyngitis/ tonsillitis	Sinusitis	AOM	Croup	Acute bronchitis
Rhinovirus Parainfluenza Respiratory syncytial virus (RSV) Coronavirus	*Strep. pyogenes* Adenoviruses Influenza A and B Parainfluenza 1, 2 and 3 Epstein–Barr virus Enteroviruses *Mycoplasma pneumonia*	*Haemophilus influenzae* *Strep. pneumoniae* *Moraxella catarrhalis* *Staph. aureas* *Strep. pyogenes*	*Strep. pneumonia* *Haemophilus influenzae* *Moraxella catarrhalis*	Parainfluenza Influenza Adenoviruses	Adenovirus Influenza Parainfluenza RSV

Case study 13.1

Request for medical advice
It is 11.00 on a Monday morning in February. Mrs Kumar requests telephone advice about Sanjay, her 18-month-old son. The message from the GP's receptionist says: 'Fever and cough for 5 days, now wheezy and breathless'.

Before phoning Mrs Kumar, the GP checks Sanjay's medical record and establish he has been seen four times already this winter and received three courses of antibiotics. He appears to be otherwise well, with no other significant past medical history, and he is up to date with his immunisations.

What is the most likely diagnosis?
The time of year and child's history fit with RSV bronchiolitis, but other diagnoses (e.g. croup or pneumonia) are possible, and further assessment is necessary to determine how unwell Sanjay is. Given high recent antibiotic use, it is likely Sanjay's mother will be expecting antibiotic treatment for this illness, too.

Telephone consultation
Although the GP has already decided she wants to see Sanjay, she telephones Mrs Kumar to check Sanjay does not require an immediate ambulance. Sanjay is a little breathless and wheezy, but his lips and tongue are pink, he has been able to take three-quarters of his morning milk and Mrs Kumar reports he was smiling while watching his older sibling play a few minutes earlier.

Face-to-face consultation
History: From the history, the GP learns that Sanjay's nappies have been wet, he has not vomited or had diarrhoea, his cough has not been 'barking' and he has felt a 'little warm' to touch. Mrs Kumar does not own a thermometer. There is no history of asthma, but his older sibling and father have mild eczema. As the GP completes the history, she asks Mrs Kumar about her expectations; Mrs Kumar is concerned Sanjay may have 'another chest infection' and that 'previous similar illnesses have responded well to antibiotics'. The GP asks how she feels about using antibiotics and Mrs Kumar replies that she 'only really wants to use them when they are necessary' as she has heard the concerns about antibiotic resistance in the news.

Examination: Sanjay appears comfortable and smiles as the GP asks Mrs Kumar to undress him. His temperature is 38.2 °C. The GP counts his respiratory rate over 30 seconds and calculates it is mildly elevated at 20 breaths per minute. He has very slight subcostal recession on inspiration, but no intercostal recession or tracheal tug. The paediatric pulse oximeter reports heart rates of 150 beats per minute (which the GP determines, using published data,[23] is normal for his age and temperature) and oxygen saturation of 99%. His peripheries are pink and his CRT is less than 2 seconds. Auscultation reveals widespread, bilateral expiratory wheeze with good air entry. No crackles or bronchial breathing are heard.

What is the most likely diagnosis?
Mild to moderate RSV bronchiolitis is most likely with a mother who may have been 'medicalised' by previous antibiotic use, but may be willing to use a 'delayed' or no antibiotic strategy because of antibiotic resistance concerns.

How should the GP approach treatment?
The GP decides not to talk about 'viruses and bacteria' because she has heard this confuses some parents.[24] Instead, she advises Mrs Kumar that Sanjay does have a chest infection and uses the consultation as an opportunity to teach Mrs Kumar how to recognise if Sanjay's illness deteriorates. She shows Mrs Kumar Sanjay's chest and how his breathing is a little faster than usual, but that he is comfortable. She advises Mrs Kumar to purchase a thermometer.

Signs of deterioration would include: withdrawal from social interaction, a temperature repeatedly rising above 39 °C, the appearance of breathlessness with even more rapid breathing and indrawing of soft tissues, bottle/fluid refusal and drier-than-usual nappies. The GP advises Mrs Kumar that if any of these signs occur, the practice would be happy to review Sanjay the same day. She also advises that a cough is a healthy, protective mechanism by which Sanjay is clearing the infected phlegm from his chest, that the infection is causing a temporary narrowing of Sanjay's airways (causing him to wheeze) and that Mrs Kumar should expect the cough to last another 14–21 days (against a background of other, gradually improving symptoms).

Mrs Kumar is still concerned that the GP is not prescribing antibiotics. What should she do?
The GP thinks Sanjay has a chest infection. She advises that she doesn't think antibiotics will help and that they could give Sanjay diarrhoea or vomiting, but that a 'delayed antibiotic' would be a reasonable compromise – but that it is only to be used if Sanjay's symptoms *worsen* over the next few days (not if symptoms persist, as this is what the GP is expecting). She books Sanjay in for a telephone review the next day, so that she can 'hear how he is getting on'.

Finally, she records the details of the consultation, including Sanjay's vital sign measurements, in case he is reassessed when she is not in the surgery, so that the next clinician has some objective evidence to help them decide if Sanjay's infection is worsening.

Sore throat in children

Young children can have difficulty localising pain or finding the right word to describe its location, so they may complain of ear or neck pain when they actually have a sore throat. Very young children may present as generally unwell or refusing food. Parents may have noticed crying on swallowing, a hoarse-sounding cry, white spots on the tonsils or that the child's breath smells. Children with tonsillitis, glandular fever or enlarged lymph nodes can also complain primarily of abdominal pain.

For uncomplicated sore throat, most children recover within a week with hydration and simple analgesia. If the child is unwell, or the sore throat persists, the Centor criteria (see Chapter 17) can help us decide if we should use antibiotics. In areas of the world where rheumatic fever is prevalent, throat swabs looking for group A β-haemolytic *Streptococci* (GABHS) can be helpful, but in the UK these are not used, as up to 10% of patients can asymptomatically carry the bacteria in their throat.

Glandular fever can have a very similar presentation to bacterial tonsillitis, so is often initially treated with antibiotics, and only investigated when symptoms persist. Serological tests have a high false-negative rate in the early stages of the illness. Ampicillin or amoxicillin can cause a widespread itchy maculopapular rash if glandular fever is present. This is not an allergic reaction but can be mistaken for one, and the child can be falsely labelled as penicillin-allergic, which affects their future medical care.

Recurrent tonsillitis

Tonsillitis is unpleasant for children and, if recurrent, can impact on their education and on family life. Tonsillectomy is not without risk, and children can still get episodes of pharyngitis following tonsillectomy. Children tend to get fewer episodes of tonsillitis as they get older, without having to resort to surgery. We need to strike the balance between a watch-and-wait approach and denying surgery for children who would benefit. The Scottish Intercollegiate Guidelines Network (SIGN) has produced guidance that recommends referring children with seven or more significant episodes in the preceding year, or five in the each of the preceding 2 years.[25] Suspected sleep apnoea causing daytime sleepiness or failure to thrive needs urgent referral.

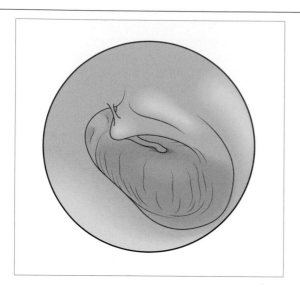

Figure 13.3 Acute otitis media (AOM): an inflamed eardrum. *Source*: Clarke, R (2014) *Lecture Notes: Diseases of the Ear, Nose and Throat*, 11th edn. Reproduced with permission of John Wiley & Sons, Ltd.

Earache in children

Young children with an infection in the middle ear (otitis media) may present as miserable and generally unwell, with a fever and/or vomiting. Parents may notice the child rubbing their ear or a red pinna. Pain from teething can refer to the ear. Otitis media is a complication of a cold, as the normally air-filled space behind the eardrum fills with mucus and can become infected. On examination, the eardrum is red and bulging (see Figure 13.3). If the eardrum has perforated, there is often creamy discharge, and it may not be possible to see the tympanic membrane at all. Analgesia is helpful. Table 13.7 outlines when antibiotics are indicated. Children with a perforated eardrum or otorrhoea should be followed up to check that healing has occurred and that signs of infection, such as discharge, do not persist.

Urinary tract infections in children

Once children acquire the verbal skills to explain their symptoms, diagnosing a UTI becomes relatively straightforward, with many of the symptoms overlapping with those of young adults, such as dysuria, frequency, loin pain and fever. Making the diagnosis in preverbal children, especially in young infants, is more challenging, and this is compounded by the difficulties of obtaining a clean, uncontaminated urine specimen.

Clinicians need to identify the preschool children at highest risk of UTI from among all the acutely unwell children presenting to primary care. The 2007 NICE guidelines[4] recommend collection of a urine sample for microbiological confirmation of UTI in children under 5 years with unexplained fever, vomiting, lethargy, irritability, poor feeding, abdominal pain, offensive urine, haematuria, frequency or dysuria; but the guidelines also acknowledge a lack of evidence to support the diagnostic utility of these symptoms and signs, and uncertainty regarding the role of dipstick testing.

Diagnosis and appropriate prompt treatment of a UTI are essential to avoiding renal scarring, which can lead to hypertension and renal impairment in adulthood. A clean-catch urine sample should be sent, but this should not delay treatment. Treatment should be based on local antibiotic sensitivities. Local policies vary, but in general children under 6 months or those with severe, atypical or recurrent UTIs should be referred for further investigations.

Top tips: obtaining a urine sample in children

Ideally, this is a midstream, clean-catch sample, with the genital area wiped clean beforehand.

For toilet-trained children, sit the child on a bowl sterilised with boiling water. Allow the urine to cool, then decant into the laboratory container.

For children in nappies, first ask the parent to clean (with nonbactericidal soap) and dry the nappy area, and then sit with the child on their knee with the bowl placed under the perineum to collect the urine.

An alternative method is the bladder-stimulation technique.[26] This involves tapping over the symphysis pubis every second for 1 minute, for alternate minutes. This is not uncomfortable for the child and usually gives fairly quick results.

Syringing the urine out of pads or urine collection bags stuck on to the child's perineum is sometimes used, but can contaminate the sample.

Suspected cancer in children

Childhood cancers are relatively rare, so most GPs will only identify one or two in their career. Understandably, parents are upset if a cancer is not spotted quickly. Textbooks describe the symptoms of cancer when a child is first seen in secondary care. GPs cannot rely on these textbook descriptions and must be on the lookout for all possible red-flag symptoms and signs. Studies have shown that presentation is varied: at first consultation, most children later diagnosed with a cancer had only a few symptoms, and often these were nonspecific.[27] Examination of all children is essential. The challenge is balancing our own and parents' anxieties about missing a serious diagnosis against overinvestigation of common and usually benign symptoms. A diagnosis (or potential diagnosis) of a childhood cancer is devastating, so care and time should be taken to develop a good supportive relationship with the parents and child from the beginning. The prognosis is variable, depending on the type of cancer and stage at diagnosis.

Table 13.9 Childhood cancers in primary care.

Average number of cases per year in the UK and age affected[29]	Presenting symptoms and signs
Leukaemia 406/year Peak 2–5 years	80% acute lymphoblastic leukaemia Short history is common: malaise, anaemia, oral infections, bruising, bone pain Examination may reveal organ infiltration, lymphadenopathy, hepatosplenomegaly or bone pain
CNS and brain tumours 405/year All ages	Signs of raised intracranial pressure: headache, nausea and vomiting, visual disturbance (blurred vision, squint, ataxia, nystagmus), seizures, lethargy, personality/behavioural change Endocrine symptoms of slow growth or delayed puberty in teenagers
Lymphoma (Hodgkin's disease and non-Hodgkin's lymphoma) 165/year	Lymphadenopathy: non-tender in Hodgkin's – long history Non-Hodgkin's lymphoma (more rapid progression) may present with breathlessness or symptoms of mediastinal mass
Neuroblastoma 90/year Usually under 4 years old	Nonspecific malaise, flushing, weight loss, fever, pallor, diarrhoea, abdominal mass Bone pain, breathlessness, periorbital bruising and skin nodules are signs of metastatic disease
Sarcoma: soft tissue (85) and **bone** (55) Usually affects teenagers	Bone pain, swelling, mass, fracture Consider sarcoma in an unusual location if local symptoms are related to a mass (e.g. urinary retention)
Wilms' tumour (nephroblastoma) 80/year Usually under 5 years	Renal mass (usually painless) Progressive abdominal distension Can cause hypertension and haematuria 10% have metastases to liver and lung at diagnosis
Retinoblastoma 45/year Usually under 2 years	White pupillary reflex: parents may identify on photographs or at 6–8-week postnatal review Squint or change in acuity Consider if family history

The remaining 135 childhood cancers that occur each year are as follows: germ cell (55), skin (25), liver (20) and other (35). Any unusual symptoms should be referred for specialist paediatric opinion.

Top tip

Consider urgent referral if a child makes three or more presentations with the same problem and there is no clear diagnosis.[28]

1500 children are diagnosed with cancer each year in Great Britain.[29] Table 13.9 details the incidence and red-flag symptoms for these and other less common childhood cancers.[27,28] Acute symptoms or ill children may require immediate referral (e.g. if there are signs of raised intracranial pressure or sepsis). GPs can arrange bloods, such as full blood count (FBC), for some symptoms, but if cancer is suspected, these should not delay urgent referral for specialist review and imaging under the 2-week wait. It is important to be aware that certain syndromes are associated with an increased risk of childhood cancers (e.g. children with Down's syndrome have an increased risk of childhood leukaemia).

The prognosis is good for most childhood cancers (70–80% 5-year survival rate). These are children who will require increased GP care and support for the rest of their lives.

GPs may be involved in prescribing medications and vaccinations, and in supporting family members. Children who survive cancers are at higher risk of further cancers and often have long-term sequelae of treatment. These include problems with growth and puberty, endocrine dysfunction causing fertility problems in adulthood and long-term complications of chemotherapy.

Top tip: lymphadenopathy in children

Lymphadenopathy is common in children, as upper RTIs are so common.

Refer if lymph nodes are:

- unexplained;
- persisting >6 weeks;
- increasing in size;
- >2 cm in size;
- widespread.

Also refer if there are other associated red-flag symptoms (weight loss, night sweats, unexplained fevers, abdominal mass or hepatosplenomegaly).[27]

SUMMARY

The ill child is a common presentation; the GP may be speaking to parents on the phone, assessing a child in the surgery or advising nursing colleagues. The majority will have a self-limiting illness, and often parental explanation, reassurance and management advice is all that is needed. However, bacterial infections like meningitis can be life-threatening, so prompt identification and treatment are essential. A thorough history and examination are necessary for all childhood illnesses. These may need to be done more quickly in an ill child where urgent treatment or referral is needed. In addition, the child or parent may be distressed, and young children often manifest few localising signs. Measurement of vital signs is useful, and there is ongoing research into red-flag symptoms and decision-making aids. Gut instinct and parental concerns have also been shown to have an important role. In sore throat, cough, ear infections and UTIs, GPs need to be able to assess whether there is an indication for antibiotics and to be able to discuss with parents the pros and cons of their use. The ill child can be a first presentation of childhood cancer. Although cancer in children is not common, it is important that GPs recognise presentations needing urgent specialist assessment.

 Now visit **www.wileyessential.com/primarycare** to test yourself on this chapter.

REFERENCES

1. NICE. Feverish illness in children: assessment and initial management in children younger than 5 years. NICE Clinical Guideline 160. May 2013. Available from: https://www.nice.org.uk/guidance/cg160 (last accessed 6 October 2015).

2. Brent AJ, Lakhanpaul M, Ninis N, et al. Evaluation of temperature-pulse centile charts in identifying serious bacterial illness: observational cohort study. *Arch Dis Child* 2011;**96**(4):368–73.

3. Meningitis Research Council. Meningococcal meningitis and septicaemia: guidance notes. Diagnosis and treatment in general practice. 2011. Available from: http://www.meningitis.org/assets/x/50631 (last accessed 6 October 2015).

4. NICE. Urinary tract infection in children: diagnosis, treatment and long-term management. NICE Clinical Guideline 54. August 2007. Available from: https://www.nice.org.uk/guidance/cg54 (last accessed 6 October 2015).

5. Van de Bruel A, Thompsom M, Buntinx F, et al. Clinicians' gut feeling about serious illness in children: an observational study. *BMJ* 2012;**345**:e6144.

6. Van den Bruel A, Aertgeerts B, Bruynickkx R, et al. Signs and symptoms for diagnosis of serious infections in children: a prospective study in primary care. *Br J Gen Pract* 2007;**57**:538–46.

7. Behjati S, FitzSimons JJ. Fever in children: how to assess and manage this condition. *Student BMJ* 2009;**17**:b159.

8. Reese C, Graves MD, Oehler K, Tingle LE. Febrile seizures: risks, evaluation, and prognosis. *Am Fam Physician* 2012;**85**(2):149–53.

9. Hay AD, Costelloe C, Redmond NM, et al. Paracetamol plus ibuprofen for the treatment of fever in children (PITCH): randomised controlled trial. *BMJ* 2008;**337**:a1302.

10. NICE. Scenario: management after a febrile seizure. NICE Clinical Knowledge Summaries. October 2013. Available from: http://cks.nice.org.uk/febrile-seizure (last accessed 6 October 2015).

11. Chang YC, Guo NW, Huang CC, et al. Neurocognitive attention and behaviour outcome of school-age children with a history of febrile convulsions: a population study. *Epilepsia* 2000;**41**(4):412–20.

12. Colletti JE, Brown KM, Sharieff GQ, et al. The management of children with gastroenteritis and dehydration in the emergency department. *J Emerg Med* 2010;**38**(5):686–98.

13. NICE. Diarrhoea and vomiting in children. NICE Clinical Guideline 84. April 2009. Available from: https://www.nice.org.uk/guidance/cg84 (last accessed 6 October 2015).

14. Goossens H, Ferech M, Vander Stichele R, et al. Outpatient antibiotic use in Europe and association with resistance: a cross-national database study. *Lancet* 2005;**365**:579–87.

15. Ashworth M, Charlton J, Ballard K, et al. Variations in antibiotic prescribing and consultation rates for acute respiratory infection in UK practices 1995–2000. *Br J Gen Pract* 2005;**55**:603–8.

16. Public Health England. English surveillance programme for antimicrobial utilisation and resistance (ESPAUR). Report 2014. Available from: https://www.gov.uk/government/uploads/system/uploads/attachment_data/file/362374/ESPAUR_Report_2014__3_.pdf (last accessed 6 October 2015).

17. NICE. Respiratory tract infections: prescribing of antibiotics for self-limiting respiratory tract infections in adults and children in primary care. NICE Clinical Guideline 69. July 2008. Available from: https://www.nice.org.uk/guidance/cg69 (last accessed 6 October 2015).

18. Vinson DC, Lutz LJ. The effect of parental expectations on treatment of children with a cough: a report from ASPN. *J Fam Pract* 1993;**37**(1):23–7.

19. Britten N, Ukoumunne O. The influence of patients' hopes of receiving a prescription on doctors' perceptions and the decision to prescribe: a questionnaire survey [see comments]. *BMJ* 1997;**315**(7121):1506–10.

20. Thompson M, Vodicka TA, Blair PS, et al. Duration of symptoms of respiratory tract infections in children: systematic review. *BMJ* 2013;**347**:F7027.

21. Francis NA, Butler CC, Hood K, et al. Effect of using an interactive booklet about childhood respiratory tract infections in primary care consultations on reconsulting and antibiotic prescribing: a cluster randomised controlled trial. *BMJ* 2009;**339**:b2885.

22. Hay AD, Heron J, Ness A, et al. The prevalence of symptoms and consultations in pre-school children in the Avon Longitudinal Study of Parents and Children (ALSPAC): a prospective cohort study. *Fam Pract* 2005;**22**(4):367–74.

23. Thompson M, Harnden A, Perera R, et al. Deriving temperature and age appropriate heart rate centiles for children with acute infections. *Arch Dis Child* 2009;**94**(5):361–5.

24. Cabral C, Ingram J, Hay AD, et al. 'They just say everything's a virus' – parent's judgment of the credibility of clinician communication in primary care consultations for respiratory tract infections in children: a qualitative study. *Patient Educ Couns* 2014;**94**:248–53.

25. SIGN. Management of sore throat and indications for tonsillectomy. Scottish Intercollegiate Guideline 117. April 2010. Available from: http://www.sign.ac.uk/pdf/sign117.pdf (last accessed 6 October 2015).

26. Herreros Fernández ML, González Merino N, Tagarro García A, et al. A new technique for fast and safe collection of urine in newborns. *Arc Dis Child* 2012;**98**:27–9.

27. Ahrensberg JM, Hansen RP, Olesen F, et al. Presenting symptoms of children with cancer: a primary-care population-based study. *Br J Gen Pract* 2012;**62**:e458–65.

28. NICE. Referral guidelines for suspected cancer. NICE Clinical Guideline 27. June 2005. Available from: https://www.nice.org.uk/guidance/cg27 (last accessed 6 October 2015).

29. Cancer Research UK. Childhood cancer statistics. 2015. Available from: http://www.cancerresearchuk.org/cancer-info/cancerstats/childhoodcancer/ (last accessed 6 October 2015).

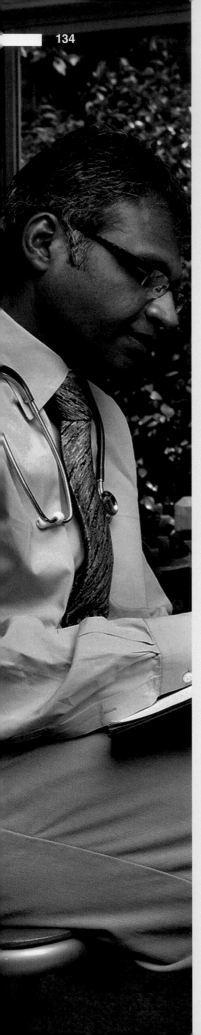

CHAPTER 14
Managing common conditions in infancy

Jessica Buchan

GP and Teaching Fellow in Primary Care, University of Bristol

Key topics

Learning objectives

- Be able to recognise and give parents advice on managing common conditions presenting in babies in the first few weeks of life.
- Be able to identify signs and symptoms in an infant that indicate an underlying abnormality, and when to refer on for further assessment.

For simplicity, in these child health chapters the term 'parent' encompasses any adult who has a parental role and is regularly caring for children; the term 'child' means any person from birth to the age of 18.

Essential Primary Care, First Edition. Edited by Andrew Blythe and Jessica Buchan.
© 2017 John Wiley & Sons, Ltd. Published 2017 by John Wiley & Sons, Ltd.
Companion website: www.wileyessential.com/primarycare

Introduction

The term 'infant' describes a child under the age of 1. The first year covers a period of rapid growth and development. At the newborn stage, the baby is wholly dependent on its caregivers and has a limited means of communication. By the end of the first year, the infant is mobile to varying degrees, and able to demonstrate and vocalise a range of needs and wants.

Assessing growth in infants

Across babies, growth and development follow a predictable pattern, but a range of factors, including genetic and environmental influences, can affect them differently in individual children. The UK-WHO growth charts[1] enable doctors to plot a child's height, weight and head circumference over time and compare a baby's rate of growth to optimal growth based on data from healthy breastfed babies. There are specific charts for prematurity, very low-birth-weight babies and babies with Down's and Turner's syndromes.

Growth is a good marker of health in infants. Newborn babies can lose up to 10% of their birth weight in the first few days, but should regain this by 2 weeks. *Failure to thrive* is when the baby's rate of weight gain slows. Weight loss crossing two centiles is considered severe. Failure to thrive indicates an underlying cause for concern (see Table 14.1).

Children on the low end of the centile charts may be constitutionally small (by definition, 1 in 250 children is below the 0.4% centile), but they are more likely than those on the 75th centile to have an underlying abnormality, so a cause for their low weight should be investigated. GPs also use growth charts to check that one parameter (such as head circumference) is not out of proportion with the others (such as weight and length).

Rashes, jaundice and skin problems

Rashes in the newborn are common. Toxic erythema of the newborn is a frequently occurring, self-limiting rash typified by flat red patches with a small central papule or pustule.

Table 14.1 Underlying causes of failure to thrive.

Pregnancy	Prematurity with complications Maternal ill health, e.g. drug addiction, foetal alcohol syndrome or maternal malnutrition Foetal chromosome abnormalities
Physical difficulty feeding	Poor milk supply: stress or maternal malnutrition Poor latch in a baby with cleft palate or tongue tie Vomiting due to reflux or cow's milk intolerance Difficulty sucking in prematurity or muscular disorders
Malabsorption	Inborn errors of metabolism Gut disorders, e.g. coeliac disease Endocrine, e.g. diabetes or hypothyroidism
Increased metabolism	Hyperthyroidism
Environmental	Inadequate parenting or neglect Maternal mental disorders

Each lesion resolves within 24 hours, and new lesions appear on other areas of the trunk. The baby is systemically well, and the rash resolves over several days. Milia are tiny white spots appearing on the face, especially the nose. They are blocked pores and resolve over the first month. They are commonly known as 'milk spots'. Crusted lesions are of more concern, and may indicate a staphylococcal skin infection requiring antibiotics. A vesicular rash can indicate a late presentation of neonatal herpes simplex, which can have serious consequences and needs urgent admission for assessment. If a baby is unwell with a rash, it is prudent to involve paediatricians.

Case study 14.1

Dr Rosie Gerard sees Edith Brown, 21 days old, in her morning surgery. Edith's mum says that Edith has been more sleepy than usual for the last few hours; she had to be woken for feeds but would then fall asleep on the breast. Her mum now thinks she's looking 'a bit yellow again'. Edith was a normal vaginal delivery at term, after an uneventful pregnancy. At day 3, Edith developed jaundice. She had phototherapy and the jaundice had resolved.

Is jaundice a cause for concern in babies?
60% of babies become jaundiced after birth. Unconjugated hyperbilirubinaemia is often physiological; red blood cells

break down after birth and the immature liver is less efficient at processing bilirubin. High levels of bilirubin can cause neurotoxicity. Jaundice can also indicate infection, underlying haemolytic condition or metabolic condition, such as G6PD deficiency.

Jaundice is of concern if it:
- started in the first 24 hours of life;
- is increasing;
- is conjugated hyperbilirubinaemia;
- occurs in a baby who is jittery or shows signs of being unwell (see Chapter 13);
- lasts for more than 2 weeks (although jaundice can be prolonged in breastfed babies);

- is associated with pale stools and yellow urine – this indicates biliary atresia, a surgical emergency.

What should Dr Gerard do next?
Dr Gerard examines Edith. She seems sleepy but opens her eyes in response to stimuli. Her skin has a faint yellow tinge to it and her sclera are yellow. Edith has normal tone, with a temperature of 37.6 °C and a heart rate of 150 bpm. Dr. Gerard is aware that jaundice can be prolonged in

breastfed babies, but she is concerned because in this case the jaundice had resolved and now is increasing. Edith is also drowsy and not feeding well. Dr Gerard suspects there is an underlying infection or other cause for her jaundice and admits her urgently for specialist review.

Outcome
Edith is diagnosed with a urinary tract infection (UTI) and found to have vesico-ureteric reflux.

Nappy rash

Almost all babies get a degree of nappy rash at some point, due to a reaction of the sensitive skin to the urine and faeces. Most parents are aware of the advice to change the nappy frequently, keep the area clean and dry and use barrier creams. Parents seek the advice of the GP when these measures are not helping or the rash is severe. Infection with bacteria or candida should be considered if the rash is inflamed or worsening. A rash with 'satellite' lesions – red spots separate from the rash – may indicate candidal infection and responds to topical antifungals. Seborrhoeic dermatitis can cause a pale pink rash in skin folds or a bright red nappy rash. Although it is not an infection, there is a link to skin yeasts. It is usually self-limiting but can be helped by emollients and topical antifungals.

Cradle cap

Seborrhoeic dermatitis causes cradle cap, a nonserious, common condition where yellow greasy crusts form on the scalp. Parents can be advised to soften cradle cap scales with oil and wash the scalp regularly with baby shampoo; a soft brush can loosen scales.

Umbilical granuloma

When the umbilical cord falls off, the healing umbilicus can overgrow and cause a red fleshy lump to appear. If left untreated, it can continue to weep. GPs used to cauterise this with silver nitrate, but this is now not recommended. A safe and effective treatment is to advise the parents to sprinkle a pinch of table salt on to the area and rinse with warm water after 10–20 minutes twice daily for 2–3 days.

Sticky eyes

Conjunctivitis in the first 28 days of life can be caused by bacteria, including those transmitted from the mother's genital tract, such as group A β-haemolytic *Streptococci* (GABH), *Chlamydia trachomatis* and *Neisseria gonorrhoeae*. Red eyes with sticky discharge should be swabbed and the risk of sexually transmitted infection in the mother should be considered. Much the commonest reason for sticky eyes in infants presenting to primary

care is nasolacrimal duct obstruction. The eyes are watery because the tears are unable to drain away. The duct usually opens up by 10 months of age and rarely needs surgery.

Feeding, vomiting and crying

Feeding

A baby born at term needs approximately 120–150 ml/kg of milk per day, or commonly 8–10 breastfeeds. The World Health Organization (WHO) recommends exclusive breastfeeding for the first 6 months of a child's life and supplementary breast feeding for up to 2 years.[2] The health benefits[3] include reduced rates of infections such as gastroenteritis and upper respiratory tract infections (RTIs). Breastfeeding is also protective against sudden infant death syndrome (SIDS),[4] childhood asthma[5] and the development of diabetes. Breastfeeding provides the baby with antibodies, is convenient and doesn't require the preparation of bottles. The foremilk (the first milk the baby gets when feeding) is watery and the hindmilk richer and more calorie-dense. Breastfeeding naturally adapts to meet the baby's changing requirements. If the baby needs more calories, it feeds more, stimulating further milk production.

A baby crying after feeds, fussing frequently or pulling off from the breast can indicate feeding difficulties. If the position is incorrect or the baby is not able to latch on properly, the mother may report sore nipples, clicking noises when the baby feeds, excessive feeds (more than 12 in 24 hours) or prolonged feeding. GPs can refer to health visitors for assessment and there are often local groups women can attend that provide breastfeeding support.

Other than women with human immunodeficiency virus (HIV) or on toxic medication such as chemotherapy, most women are able to breastfeed, but it is not always straightforward for them to do so. Feeding difficulties can be very demoralising for women who want to breastfeed. When feeding is being established, cracked and sore nipples are common. Bacteria such as *Staphylococcus aureus* can enter and cause mastitis (an infection of the breast tissue) or an abscess. Many women worry they have inadequate milk supply. Frequent feeds, rest and hydration often help. If the baby is falling off their growth centiles, underlying causes of failure to thrive must be looked for (see Table 14.1).

Tongue tie

This is where the lingual frenulum under the tongue is short and 'anchors' the tongue down. It can prevent the baby latching on properly to breastfeed. The midwife or health visitor often picks this up in the first few weeks of life and arranges for the frenulum to be snipped – a simple, quick procedure. Mild cases of tongue tie may be missed and present with feeding difficulties, sore nipples or recurrent mastitis.

Vomiting

Effortless vomiting (posseting) after feeding is common. It can result from overfeeding or from the baby's swallowing air during feeds. Feeding position should be assessed. Posseting does not distress babies.

Progressive vomiting or vomiting with failure to thrive can result from milk intolerance or gastrooesophageal reflux.

Acute vomiting in a baby that was previously well can indicate sepsis or serious illness (see Chapter 13). Bilious vomiting can indicate bowel obstruction. Projectile or large amounts of vomiting after feeding can suggest pyloric stenosis, especially if the vomiting is worsening. Weight loss or dehydration is a late presentation. If pyloric stenosis is suspected, the baby needs to be assessed as soon as possible by the on-call paediatric surgical team.

Crying

It is quite normal for healthy newborn babies to cry periodically, sometimes for no obvious reason; comforting or feeding doesn't always settle them. Babies with 'colic' are well in between episodes. Their growth and development are normal and they show no signs of illness, infection or injury. Parents often attribute colic to bowel-related pain, but the underlying cause of periodic crying is unknown, and likely to be multifactorial and neurodevelopmental in part. Parents may seek advice both to help them manage and because they are concerned by their baby's distress.

GPs should assess the infant and perform a thorough examination. It is important to ask about home circumstances, support networks and maternal mood. Presentations may indicate maternal depression or psychosocial difficulties. The GP should sensitively assess whether the baby is at risk of nonaccidental injury. A study asking parents retrospectively about their behaviour when their babies cried found that 6% reported abusive behavior.[6]

Babies' crying usually reduces by 12–16 weeks. Friends and family can help give parents a break. Parents are often advised to try various methods to soothe their baby: burping the baby after feeds, holding the baby upright, playing white noise (such as from a washing machine), avoiding maternal ingestion of caffeine in breastfed babies, avoiding overstimulation, putting the baby in a warm bath or gently rubbing the back or abdomen. It is acceptable to leave a baby to cry for a short time, as long as the baby is not unwell and in a safe place (on their back in their cot). If parents are finding it difficult to cope, health visitors can make a more detailed assessment in the home environment and work with the GP to provide support. Cry-sis (www.cry-sis.org.uk) is a charity that supports parents with babies who cry excessively or don't sleep well.

Medication for colic and gastrooesophageal reflux in babies

There is little evidence for medication in colic. A week's trial of simeticone drops added to the feed is safe.

Crying or fussing after feeding in a thriving baby does not mean the baby has reflux,[7] and for mild symptoms treatment is not needed as it tends to resolve. If a baby becomes distressed after feeds, vomits, arches its back or is not gaining weight at the expected rate, the GP may suggest a trial of an alginate, such as Gaviscon, before feeds. However, severe symptoms and faltering weight should be assessed by a paediatrician. Endoscopy may be required. If reflux is diagnosed, the baby may be tried on an H2 receptor antagonist or a proton-pump inhibitor (PPI). GPs are not advised to prescribe PPIs for mild symptoms: there have been links to infection.[8]

Babies with persistent crying who have severe eczema, rashes, perianal redness or faltering weight might have cow's milk allergy. GPs may suggest a trial of hydrolysed formula for a 2-week period or advise elimination of cow's milk from the mother's diet.[9]

Sleep and preventing sudden infant death

In the first few weeks of life, babies tend to sleep for at least 16 out of 24 hours. They have more rapid sleep cycles than adults, and wake to feed every few hours. They slowly establish more of a pattern, but this varies throughout infancy. Teething, illness or a change in nutritional requirements can all alter a previously established sleep pattern.

Sudden infant death: the Back to Sleep Campaign

The Back to Sleep Campaign, launched in 1991, has reduced the incidence of sudden infant death. The campaign was based on findings from a large Avon and Somerset population-based case control study in 1990, which identified that babies sleeping on their front had an increased risk of sudden infant death.[10] Parental smoking, overheating and co-sleeping (especially on a sofa or armchair) all increase the risk. Breastfeeding is protective. Parents should be advised about safe sleeping positions and environments for their babies.

Prematurity

Prematurity is classed as being born under 37 weeks' gestation. There are specific risks of prematurity, such as an increased risk of respiratory infections and cognitive and neuromotor impairment. The level of risk depends on the gestation, the birth weight and the underlying cause of prematurity. Babies born under 33 weeks, babies whose birth weight is under 1.5 kg and babies from a pregnancy complicated by intrauterine growth retardation or infection are at significant risk of complications. Babies born at 34–36 weeks may just be slow to feed compared to a baby born at term. Growth should be carefully monitored using a growth chart adjusted for age for the first year. For instance, at 8 weeks after birth, a baby born at 35 weeks' gestation will have a corrected age of 3 weeks. This is not the case for vaccinations, which are given according to the chronological age. Premature babies are at risk of retinopathy of prematurity, in which there is abnormal development of blood vessels in the retina. Babies under 32 weeks are at particular risk and should have had a specialist assessment.

SUMMARY

Parents of young infants often turn to the GP for advice on caring for their baby. GPs need to be able to assess the situation and give evidence-based advice to parents on all aspects of care, from promoting and supporting breastfeeding to managing minor conditions such as nappy rash. This needs to be done in a way that builds parental confidence in their ability to look after their baby. GPs also need to understand the range of normal growth and development, and to recognise the infant who is not thriving or reaching their expected milestones.

Now visit **www.wileyessential.com/primarycare** to test yourself on this chapter.

REFERENCES

1. RCPCH. UK-WHO growth charts, 0–18 years. Available from: http://www.rcpch.ac.uk/Research/UK-WHO-Growth-Charts (last accessed 6 October 2015).

2. World Health Organization. *Global Strategy for Infant and Young Child Feeding*. Geneva; WHO UNICEF: 2003.

3. Ip S, Cheung M, Raman G, et al. *Breastfeeding and Maternal and Infant Health Outcomes in Developed Countries. Evidence Report/Technology Assessment 153*. Rockville, MD: Agency for Healthcare Research and Quality; 2007.

4. Chen A, Rogan WJ. Breastfeeding and the risk of post-neonatal death in the United States. *Pediatrics* 2004;**113**:e435–9.

5. Sonnenschein-van der Voort AM, Duijts L. Breastfeeding is protective against early childhood asthma. *Evid Based Med* 2013;**18**(4):156–7.

6. Reijneveld SA, van der Wal M, Brugman E, et al. Infant crying and abuse. *Lancet* 2004;**364**:1340–2.

7. Sherman P, Hassall E, Fagundes-Neto U, et al. A global, evidence-based consensus on the definition of gastroesophageal reflux disease in the pediatric population. *Am J Gastroenterol* 2009;**104**:1278–95.

8. Orenstein S, Hassall E, Furmaga-Jablonska W, et al. Multicenter, double-blind, randomized, placebo-controlled trial assessing the efficacy and safety of proton pump inhibitor lansoprazole in infants with symptoms of gastroesophageal reflux disease. *J Pediatr* 2009;**154**:514–20.

9. Douglas P, Hill P. Clinical review: managing infants who cry excessively in the first few months of life. *BMJ* 2011;**343**:d7772.

10. Fleming PJ, Gilbert R, Azaz Y, et al. Interaction between bedding and sleeping position in the sudden infant death syndrome: a population-based case-control study. *BMJ* 1990;**301**:85–9.

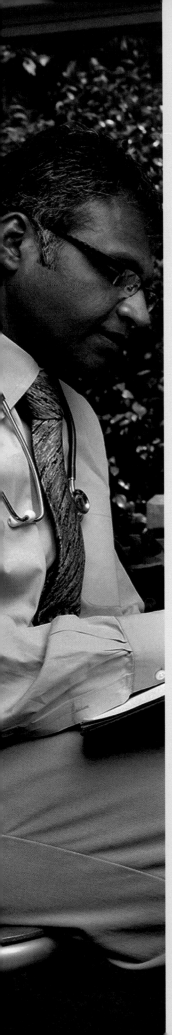

CHAPTER 15

Managing chronic conditions in childhood

Lucy Jenkins[1], Alastair Hay[2], Matthew Ridd[3] and Jessica Buchan[1]
[1] GP and Teaching Fellow in Primary Care, University of Bristol
[2] GP and Professor of Primary Care, University of Bristol
[3] GP and Consultant Senior Lecturer in Primary Care, University of Bristol

Key topics

Learning objectives

- Be able to diagnose asthma in children.
- Be able to describe how to manage acute asthma in children.
- Be able to manage eczema in children.
- Be able to manage chronic otitis media.
- Be able to evaluate the factors that result in recurrent abdominal pain and constipation in children and have a strategy for management.
- Be able to assess a child with bedwetting and advise the parents on management options.
- Be able to assess a child with behavioural problems.

For simplicity, in these child health chapters the term 'parent' encompasses any adult who has a parental role and is regularly caring for children; the term 'child' means any person from birth to the age of 18.

Essential Primary Care, First Edition. Edited by Andrew Blythe and Jessica Buchan.
© 2017 John Wiley & Sons, Ltd. Published 2017 by John Wiley & Sons, Ltd.
Companion website: www.wileyessential.com/primarycare

Recurrent wheeze and asthma

Wheeze is a common symptom, with parents reporting its presence at least once per year in around a quarter of preschool children.[1] In children under 18 months, many winter episodes associated with coryza, fever, cough and shortness of breath are thought to be caused by respiratory syncytial virus (RSV) bronchiolitis. The Scottish Intercollegiate Guidelines Network (SIGN)/British Thoracic Society (BTS) asthma guidelines[2] state that there is no standardised method for diagnosing asthma but suggest asthma should be considered in preschool children in the presence of recurrent:

- wheeze;
- cough;
- difficulty breathing; and/or
- chest tightness.

These symptoms are often associated with upper respiratory tract infections (RTIs), and in many young children these episodes will resolve by the time they start school. Children with more than one of these symptoms, multiple triggers for symptoms of wheeze or chest tightness, a personal or family history of atopy or widespread wheeze heard on auscultation may be more likely to become asthmatic. Asthma is also suggested by a history of improvement in symptoms or lung function in response to adequate therapy. Objective evidence of reversible obstruction using spirometry or peak-flow readings is often possible from the age of 5 years.

One group of commentators[3] has reviewed the evidence and suggests there are two patterns of wheeze:

- **Episodic viral wheeze:** The wheeze is triggered by RTIs with associated fever, coryza and cough. Children are asymptomatic between episodes. This is not a risk factor for developing asthma, and no treatment has been shown to be disease-modifying (i.e. to change the natural history by reducing episodes or preventing progression to asthma). Therefore, treatment, such as inhaled β_2 agonist as required, should be used only to relieve symptoms, and just for the duration of symptoms.
- **Multiple-trigger wheeze:** As well as being triggered by RTIs, the wheeze is triggered by exercise, smoke and allergens. This can be treated by a defined 4–8-week course of a leukotriene receptor antagonist or inhaled corticosteroid. If the symptoms recur after completing this course, restart the treatment and reduce to the lowest possible controlling dose. The child should be referred if not responding.

Parents of children with asthma and wheeze often ask about diet and prevention. The SIGN and BTS asthma guidelines[2] state there is currently insufficient evidence to recommend the use of modified infant formulae, fish oils, selenium, vitamin E or dietary probiotics to prevent or treat asthma. They also recommend that parents should avoid exposing children to tobacco smoke and should accept all immunisations as recommended by national immunisation programmes.

Acute asthma in children

Asthma can present with acute exacerbations that can be serious and life-threatening. In 2011–12, there were 25 073 emergency hospital admissions in the UK for asthma in children under 14, and 14 deaths, some of which might have been preventable.[4] The ability of a GP and their team to confidently mange acute asthma is essential and may save children's lives.

Case study 15.1 describes how to assess and manage acute asthma in children. Important differential diagnoses to consider

---

Case study 15.1

A receptionist tells the duty doctor, Dr Cathy Blunt, that she has just spoken to the mother of Susie Simmonds, age 4, who says that Susie has had a flare-up of her asthma and is quite wheezy. She needs her blue inhaler much more than usual. The receptionist told Susie's mum to bring her straight down.

How can the GP prepare for this appointment?
An asthma attack can be potentially life-threatening. Dr Blunt reviews Susie's medical notes to assess her risk. Important factors are:

- Current treatment – higher risk if on three or more asthma medications.
- High beta agonist usage.
- Number and severity of past exacerbations. Did these require hospital admission or intensive care?

Dr Blunt reviews the BTS and SIGN guidlines on management of asthma, which give clear guidance regarding signs of asthma severity and management for children.[2] Dr Blunt also alerts the practice nurses that a potentially ill asthmatic child is coming in and their help may be needed.

The notes state that Susie is on twice-daily inhaled, low-dose corticosteroid and a β_2 agonist as required. She had two courses of oral steroids last winter but has never been admitted to hospital.

How should the GP assess Susie?
Dr Blunt makes a rapid initial assessment of Susie's colour, level of distress and ability to talk. Dr Blunt knows that a calm and reassuring manner is essential; an asthma attack can be very frightening for the patient and parents.

Dr Blunt records and documents Susie's heart, respiratory rate and oxygen saturations and listens to her chest. If Susie was older, a peak flow reading might be possible.

Susie's mum says that Susie developed a cold 5 days ago, and for the last few days she has been coughing more. She has been wheezy and breathless in the last 24 hours. Her parents have doubled up her twice-daily steroid inhaler and have been giving her two puffs of her salbutamol every 4 hours but she is not improving. She last had the salbutamol 2 hours ago.

Susie is a bit breathless and tired, but her colour is normal and she is not distressed. On gentle probing and getting down to her level, she is able to say in a full sentence what she had for lunch. Her examination findings are: respiratory rate 36, heart rate 130, oxygen saturations 97%. Auscultation reveals widespread expiratory wheeze but no crackles.

What treatment does Susie need?
Susie's examination findings support a moderately severe exacerbation of her asthma. She needs immediate treatment to open up her airways: 6–10 puffs of salbutamol via a spacer with facemask. She can be given another two puffs every 2 minutes, depending on her response.

Susie responds well to this but remains quite wheezy. Therefore, Dr Blunt decides to give her soluble prednisolone from practice stocks (1 mg/kg, up to a total of 20 mg for those aged 5 years or under and up to 40 mg for older children).

Does she need to be admitted to hospital?
The BTS/SIGN guidlines[2] give clear guidance about this, including for children who are not responding to treatment. Not every child fits neatly into a box on a guideline table. If a child has signs across categories, treatment should be given according to the most severe features. Dr Blunt should also consider the home circumstances and parental coping abilities. She may lower her threshold for admission if it is late in the day.

Susie's mum is happy that things are much improved. Dr Blunt advises her to continue giving Susie the salbutamol as needed (up to every 4 hours) and another two daily doses of oral steroid, making it a 3-day course. Dr Blunt also gives Susie's mum clear guidance on the signs of deterioration and when to seek urgent review. Dr Blunt phones Susie's mum that afternoon. She remains well, so follow-up in the surgery is organised within the week.

What should happen at her review appointment?
At follow-up, it is important to ensure that her symptoms have resolved. This is an opportunity to look into any avoidable precipitants of the recent exacerbation and review her asthma treatment. This may involve reviewing inhaler technique and treatment devices. It is important that her parents feel confident about stepping treatment up and down. They need a written personalised asthma care plan for Susie. Parental smoking, pets and immunisations may also be discussed.

Top tip: life-threatening asthma

The following suggest very poor respiratory effort:
- silent chest (indicates almost no air movement);
- fatigue;
- oxygen saturations <92%;
- agitation;
- altered consciousness;
- cyanosis.

These are all signs of life-threatening asthma and require immediate hospital transfer by calling 999. These children should be treated with β_2 agonist via oxygen-driven nebuliser or oral/intravenous steroid and observed closely until the ambulance arrives.

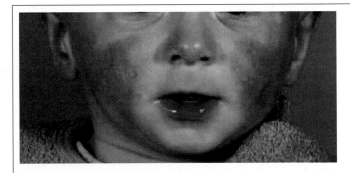

Figure 15.1 Facial atopic dermatitis. *Source*: Morris-Jones, R (ed.) (2014) *ABC of Dermatology*, 6th edn. Reproduced with permission of John Wiley & Sons, Ltd.

Eczema in children

Atopic eczema or atopic dermatitis, characterised by dry, itchy skin, is very common in preschool children, affecting around 20% in this group. Figure 15.1 shows a child with facial atopic dermatitis. For most (85%) children, it is relatively mild. However, some have severe disease. It is easy to underestimate

in a breathless child include upper airway obstruction (foreign body, epiglottitis or croup), lower respiratory disease (pneumonia or a viral wheeze, such as with bronchiolitis), cardiac failure and drug ingestion.

Table 15.1 Eczema treatment escalator for increasing severity of disease.

Mild	Moderate	Severe
Emollients and soap substitutes	Emollients and soap substitutes	Emollients and soap substitutes
Mild potency corticosteroids	Moderate potency corticosteroids	Potent topical corticosteroids
	Topical calcineurin inhibitors	Topical calcineurin inhibitors
	Bandages	Bandages
		Phototherapy
		Systemic treatment

the impact of the condition; disturbed sleep from itching, avoidance of certain activities and the need to apply treatments to the skin throughout the day can affect the whole family.

The mainstay of treatment is the regular use of emollients to moisturise the skin – even when the skin appears 'clear'. Many different types are available to prescribe and to buy over the counter, which vary significantly in their greasiness, from lotions, which are watery, through to ointments, which are thick and heavy. The former are usually more cosmetically acceptable, but the latter may be required in more severe disease. Eczema 'flares' (worsening itch, redness of the skin) require treatment with topical anti-inflammatory agents, usually corticosteroids. These vary in strength from mild to very potent.

The strength of steroid cream used should be matched to the severity of the flare, but special caution has to be taken with more delicate skin (face, genitals and axillae). Nonmedical measures which can help include keeping the nails short (to reduce damage from scratching), wearing cotton clothing, keeping the bedroom cool and avoiding perfumed products and bubble baths, which can irritate sensitive skin.

A key message to get across to families is that management of the condition is one of 'control' rather than 'cure'. Specialist referral is indicated in more severe disease, when dermatologists may advise additional treatments (see Table 15.1). Children commonly improve as they get older, yet a significant proportion will go on to have persistent disease, often accompanied by the other 'atopic' conditions of asthma and hay fever.

Glue ear (chronic otitis media)

Fluid can accumulate behind the eardrum in children, resulting in conductive hearing loss. On examination the eardrum has a dull appearance, with an absence of the normal light reflex, but is not red or inflamed. Chronic otitis media is commonest in children under 5 years old, boys, children exposed to tobacco smoke and children in childcare. An effusion can persist for some weeks after a cold, but 90% resolve in 3 months, so active observation[5] is recommended with audiometry. GPs ask about the impact on home and school life. Persistent, significant hearing loss can result in behavioural problems, difficulties with educational attainment or delay in language acquisition. There is no role for medication, but small ventilation tubes

(grommets) inserted into the eardrum can improve hearing in the short term, although the benefits tail off after 6 months. Hearing aids are an alternative management strategy. Children with glue ear and documented hearing loss that has persisted for 3 months or more should be referred, as should children with glue ear with educational or developmental delay or recurrent otitis media (e.g. more than three or four episodes in 6 months).

Recurrent abdominal pain and constipation

Children with acute abdominal pain need urgent assessment, and admission if a serious cause is suspected. Harder to manage in primary care can be recurrent abdominal pain, which is thought to affect around 10% of children. Episodic stomach pains can interfere with childrens' education and usual activities. The cause can be multifactorial, and most cases (over 90%) are 'functional', by which we mean there isn't a pathological explanation, but rather a complex relationship between all the contributing factors.[6] Abdominal migraine falls into this category. In this condition, the child has at least two episodes of severe periumbilical pain lasting at least an hour, with two symptoms of anorexia, nausea, vomiting, headache, photophobia or pallor. A careful history (see Table 15.2) and examination to assess for organic disease are more important than giving a precise diagnosis. The following features indicate a serious underlying cause of abdominal pain in children:

- weight loss, growth failure or slowing growth;
- unexplained fever;
- chronic severe diarrhoea or significant vomiting;
- gastrointestinal bleeding;
- family history of inflammatory bowel disease;
- persistent chronic right iliac fossa or right upper quadrant pain.

It can take more than one consultation to assess recurrent abdominal pain

Constipation

Childhood constipation may account for up to a third of referrals to a paediatric gastroenterologist from primary care.[7] Functional constipation (no underlying organic disease) often presents with a degree of faecal incontinence. Rather than saying their child is constipated, parents may report staining of the child's underwear

Table 15.2 Assessing functional abdominal pain.

Functional recurrent abdominal pain can be linked to

Anxiety disorders
Bullying
School refusal
Sexual abuse

It is important to assess

The family and social situation
Any concerns about the child's welfare
The school situation
Any obvious triggers

Further assessment

Consider asking parents to keep a diary of symptoms and possible triggers

Table 15.3 Diagnosing and managing functional constipation in children.

History

In the previous 2 months, has the child had:
- passage of stool two or fewer times each week?
- one or more episode of soiling or incontinence each week?
- behaviour suggesting they are avoiding opening their bowels?
- painful or hard bowel movements?
- large stools that might obstruct the toilet?

Intervention in functional constipation	Example
Assess for triggers	Emotional factors, e.g. bullying or a toilet phobia
Advise on good toileting habits	Encourage the child to sit comfortably on the toilet for 5 minutes after eating (a footstool and a favourite book can help)
Give dietary advice	Eat dietary fibre, fresh fruit and vegetables and drink plenty of water
Prevent pain and faecal impaction	Magrocol osmotic laxatives are used first-line in constipation that has persisted several days, continued for a few weeks until a regular bowel habit is regained. Higher doses of laxatives are used to treat impaction if there is a history of soiling
Monitor progress	A symptom diary, using a visual guide to stool consistency such as the Bristol stool chart,[8] can be helpful, allowing the parents to identify when constipation is worsening
Keep the child under regular review	Stimulant laxatives can be added if osmotic laxatives are not enough on their own

or bedclothes despite their being toilet trained. Constipation in children can start after a febrile illness, dehydration, a change in circumstances, abuse or emotional factors such as bullying, parental separation or a toilet phobia. Studies have shown that some children seem to have a delayed colonic transit time,[7] which GPs may describe to parents as a sluggish bowel. Whatever the initial trigger, the problem can easily become a vicious cycle; impacted stool can stretch the rectum, which desensitises it so that the child has difficulty clearing the stool. Hard stool causes pain and reluctance to open the bowels. The aim of treatment is to regulate the bowel and, if impaction is present, to clear it. Parents can be helped to adjust medication by monitoring the frequency and consistency of their child's stool using pictorial charts,[8] aiming for a regular passage of smooth, formed stool. We should ask about the presence of blood; anal fissures may occur and cause painful defecation and fresh blood on wiping.

Children with constipation should be referred to secondary care if the constipation is associated with:
- rectal bleeding;
- failure to thrive;
- significant behavioural or developmental disorders;
- a suspected underlying cause such as cow's milk allergy or suspected coeliac disease.

Table 15.3 outlines an approach to managing constipation in primary care.

Bedwetting

Primary nocturnal enuresis is bedwetting at night in children over 5 years of age who have never consistently been dry. By the age of 8, most children are dry at night. Urgency and frequency of urination during the day suggest the possibility of overactive bladder, which can cause nighttime wetting. Bedwetting is common in general developmental delay. Enuresis is a rare presentation of an underlying neurological problem such as spina bifida or cerebral palsy, but in these cases children are more likely to also have daytime symptoms, encopresis (soiling) and other neurological signs.

Secondary nocturnal enuresis is bedwetting that occurs after the child has been dry for 6 months or more, and is more likely to be due to an underlying condition, such as bullying, abuse or other stressors. If the onset is recent, we should assess for diabetes mellitus or a urinary tract infection (UTI).

A watch-and-wait policy is the best management if the child is under 5 and there is no suggestion of an underlying cause or significant daytime wetting. After the age of 5, the following may help:
- Encourage adequate (but not excess) daytime fluids.
- Avoid caffeine (in some fizzy drinks) and chocolate.
- Encourage emptying the bladder before bed.
- Offer rewards (e.g. star chart for dry nights or for using the toilet if they wake).
- Do not punish bedwetting.

For children distressed by wetting, alarms that wake them at night when they pass urine have been shown to be effective and to result in long-term dryness.

Desmopressin reduces the amount of urine the kidneys produce and is useful for quick control of night-time wetting, such as when sleeping at a friend's house or as a regular second-line treatment if an alarm fails.

Behavioural issues in children

There is a plethora of advice available on everything relating to children's behaviour, from managing a toddler's tantrums to coping with teenage mood swings. Parents will have often sought advice (including from friends and family) before they present to the GP. Therefore, parents' concerns about their child's behaviour should never be dismissed. It may be that the advice they've already received is conflicting and they just need to talk things through. Sometimes, the severity and impact of the child's behaviour is more than the parents can manage without additional support, or there may be an underlying condition or developmental delay that needs specialist diagnosis and management. The role of the GP is to make an initial assessment (see Table 15.4), support the parents, signpost information and support and refer appropriately. In managing behavioural issues that arise in childhood, GPs work closely with health visitors.

Hyperactivity

About 5 in 100 children in the UK are thought to suffer from attention deficit hyperactivity disorder (ADHD). It is commoner in boys.[9] ADHD can cause problems with social, psychological and intellectual development, and makes anxiety, depression and conduct disorders more likely. The cause is not fully understood, but genetic factors, exposure to alcohol, smoking and drugs in the antenatal period, anoxia at birth or very low birth weight and severe neglect make the condition more likely. Normal children fidget, find it hard to sit still and have difficulty concentrating, especially if they are of preschool age. For ADHD to be diagnosed, the behaviour needs to be greater than expected for a child of the patient's age (see Table 15.5).

If we suspect ADHD, a specialist assessment is needed. Treatment includes parenting programmes and medication such as methylphenidate (Ritalin) to improve impulse control and concentration. About half of children with ADHD grow out of it by adulthood.[9] If symptoms persist, cognitive behavioural therapy (CBT) may be tried.

Autism and Asperger's syndrome

The psychiatrist Lorna Wing[10] coined the term 'autistic spectrum disorder'. There is a wide range of disability on this spectrum, from children with severe learning difficulties and no meaningful communication to high-functioning children with normal or high IQ with Asperger's. Autistic children may find interacting with others difficult; they may not make eye contact, and social smiling is rare. Autistic children struggle with imaginative play and social communication, but also throw tantrums more often than children of the same age and can have difficulty with coordination. They feel more comfortable with routine, which (unlike in other children) doesn't improve as they get older. Many parents of a preschool autistic child have concerns that they don't participate in social interaction skills such as smiling, waving

Table 15.4 Assessing children's behaviour.

Aspect	Area of investigation	Comments
Timescale	When behaviour started Pattern of behaviour, e.g. fluctuates/worsening	Is behaviour normal for expected stage of development?
Triggers	Noticeable *change* to behaviour Possible triggers, e.g. starting school Situational	Seemingly innocuous events can upset a child who is sensitive or prone to worry
Consistency	Is the behaviour consistent across different settings and different people?	Behaviour related to an underlying condition tends to occur in multiple settings
Severity	How frequent? Is anyone at risk (e.g. of being physically hurt)?	Severity has a different focus from impact. A child's anxiety about new situations may be severe but, if they are rarely in new situations, have little impact
Impact	Effect on the child Activities the child can't do or finds difficult Effect on relationships/schoolwork/other siblings/parents	Is the child avoiding activities that they want to do or would benefit from doing?

This is not an exhaustive list, but an overview of the areas to cover. It is often useful to get a collaborative history from other caregivers and settings, such as a report from the child's teacher.

Table 15.5 Diagnosing ADHD.[9]

History

Age-inappropriate behaviour that affects the child's life and:
- started before 12 years of age
- has persisted for 6 months or more
- is apparent in more than one setting
- is not better explained by another mental disorder

Features of hyperactive– impulsive subtype	Features of inattention subtype
The child does the following excessively or when inappropriate: • fidgets • runs around • has difficulty playing quietly • talks excessively • interrupts others • has difficulty waiting their turn	The child: • has trouble concentrating and paying attention • makes careless mistakes and does not listen to, or follow through on, instructions • is easily distracted • is forgetful in daily activities and loses essential items, such as school books or toys • has trouble organising activities

and imitating and lack interest in others. Skills can also regress, so language and play skills that the child has gained can be lost. Such difficulties are less apparent at the high-functioning end of the spectrum. Asperger's syndrome may not be apparent until the school years, or even adulthood.

Other medical problems, such as seizures, hearing and visual impairment, can be associated with autism. The Checklist for Autism in Toddlers (CHAT) is a screening tool that can be used by health visitors at the 18-months development check. This covers areas such as imaginative play (e.g. whether the child pretends to make a cup of tea), whether the child points at objects of interest and whether the child enjoys social games like peek-a-boo.

Specialist diagnosis is needed. The mainstay of treatment is educational support and behavioural therapy. Sometimes, medication is used to help with aggression or anxiety.

SUMMARY

Parents of the under-5s consult a GP about their child on average six times a year. Many presentations are for self-limiting illnesses that resolve without specific treatment. GPs also help families manage chronic and recurrent conditions. Of these, asthma is the most common chronic illness in childhood, but it can present with acute exacerbations that can be serious and life-threatening. Eczema is usually managed in the community; hospital input is rarely needed, so the GP must be able to educate parents and review treatment. Abdominal pain in children is often benign, but GPs have to be astute at picking up serious underlying causes. Constipation can be managed in primary care but needs early diagnosis and treatment to prevent chronicity. The impact of behavioural problems can be reduced with parental support and input from childcare and educational settings, but GPs also need to know when specialist assessment and management is required.

Now visit **www.wileyessential.com/primarycare** to test yourself on this chapter.

REFERENCES

1. Hay AD, Heron J, Ness A, et al. The prevalence of symptoms and consultations in pre-school children in the Avon Longitudinal Study of Parents and Children (ALSPAC): a prospective cohort study. *Fam Pract* 2005;**22**(4):367–74.

2. British Thoracic Society and Scottish Intercollegiate Guidelines Network. *British Guideline on the Management of Asthma*. SIGN 141. October 2014.

3. Bush A, Grigg J, Saglani S. Managing wheeze in preschool children. *BMJ* 2014;**348**:g15.

4. Asthma UK. Asthma facts and FAQs. Available from: http://www.asthma.org.uk/asthma-facts-and-statistics (last accessed 6 October 2015).

5. NICE. Surgical management of otitis media with effusion in children. NICE Clinical Guideline 60. February 2008.

Available from: https://www.nice.org.uk/guidance/cg60 (last accessed 6 October 2015).

6. Berger MY, Gieteling MJ, Benninga MA. Clinical review: chronic abdominal pain in children. *BMJ* 2007;**334**(7601):997–1002.

7. Auth M, Vora R, Farrelly P, Baillie C. Clinical review: childhood constipation *BMJ* 2012;**345**:e7309.

8. Lewis SJ, Heaton KW. Stool form scale as a useful guide to intestinal transit time. *Scan J Gastroenterol* 1997;**32**(9):920–4.

9. Guevara J, Stein M. Clinical review: evidence based management of attention deficit hyperactivity disorder. *BMJ* 2001;**323**:1232.

10. Gulland A. Obituary: Lorna Wing. *BMJ* 2014;**349**:4529.

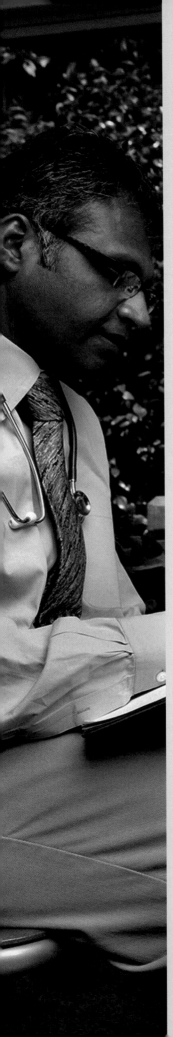

CHAPTER 16

Teenage and young-adult health

Jessica Buchan[1] and David Kessler[2]

[1] GP and Teaching Fellow in Primary Care, University of Bristol

[2] GP and Reader in Primary Care Mental Health, University of Bristol

Key topics

Learning objectives

- Be able to consult with teenagers and understand the guidelines regarding confidentiality and consent.
- Be able to describe the normal process of puberty and when to refer.
- Be able to understand the harms associated with risk-taking behaviour in adolescents.
- Be able to demonstrate awareness of how depression presents in young people and the risks associated with it.
- Be able to recognise presentations that suggest an underlying eating disorder.

For simplicity, in these child health chapters the term 'parent' encompasses any adult who has a parental role and is regularly caring for children; the term 'child' means any person from birth to the age of 18.

Essential Primary Care, First Edition. Edited by Andrew Blythe and Jessica Buchan.
© 2017 John Wiley & Sons, Ltd. Published 2017 by John Wiley & Sons, Ltd.
Companion website: www.wileyessential.com/primarycare

Consulting with teenagers

We may recall being an adolescent ourselves, but that doesn't always help us know how to consult with teenagers. Perhaps we are concerned that we won't know how to connect with young people when we no longer relate to their interests or views on the world, perhaps we fear that they won't open up or perhaps we are unsure whether to treat them as a child or as an adult. So much change happens in a few years that there is a big difference between consulting with a 13- or 14-year-old and consulting with the same person at 17 or 18. We need to adapt our consultation skills to the individual's stage of development.

At the start of adolescence, most children are wholly dependent on their parents. This can be seen in the GP surgery, where most young teens consult with their parents and defer to them for decisions about their care. Only a few years later, these same children are independent to varying degrees; a handful are even parents themselves. In reality, many older teenagers still need their parents for many aspects of their lives but take increasing responsibility for themselves and their health and may consult the GP on their own. This poses particular challenges, as adolescents may physically look adult (even towering over their parents), but not all will think or understand in an adult way.

Early teenagers think in a very concrete way; abstract thought develops later. This means that they can be quite 'black and white' about health issues. For instance, they may think that our health advice about smoking causing heart disease doesn't relate to them, as it doesn't affect their immediate experience. This can make teenage health promotion much more effective on a society basis (e.g. tackling advertising or the availability of cigarettes).[1] It doesn't mean we shouldn't try to give accurate information and promote healthy behaviours. Adolescence is a stage where new health behaviours are laid down, and the child moves away from family values and starts their own exploration. It is well documented that behaviour that starts in adolescence is carried into adulthood, so it is important that behaviours like safe sex, exercise and a healthy diet are tackled in adolescence. We need to make sure that the information that our teenage patients get from their peer group is accurate. It is especially important that our advice and information are tailored to the priorities of the patient, as we discussed in Chapter 7.

We risk alienating our patients if we lecture them or try too hard to be their friend. Instead, we need to be curious about teenagers' experiences and thinking, and ask what will best help them. We also need to speak to them with the empathy and respect we would give an adult patient. We must assess their cognitive abilities and tailor the way we present information accordingly. Forming a good relationship with teenagers makes it more likely that they will seek help for their problems. There are some excellent websites we can point teenagers to, which can help back up the information we provide (see Top tip box).

> **Top tip: sources of information for teenagers**
>
> - **www.talktofrank.com** This site gives expert and up-to-date advice about drugs and their effects, and where to get help.
> - **www.brook.org.uk** Brook Advisory Services is a sexual health charity that provides services, advice and education on all aspects of sex, including contraception, relationships and sexually transmitted infections, to young people. It also runs advisory centres and a helpline.
> - **www.b-eat.co.uk** Beat is a charity that provides information and support to patients with eating disorders. It is not specific to teenagers, but it does run a 'youthline' telephone service.

Confidentiality and consent

There are also issues with confidentiality and consent in a consultation with a child under 16. Children and adolescents have a right to see the doctor, and we should respect patient confidentiality as we do for adults, unless not disclosing information about the young person to another party would cause the child harm. The Royal College of General Practitioners (RCGP)'s adolescent health group has produced leaflets for parents and adolescents to promote the right of young people to seek advice from their GP or nurse about any problem.

Case study 16.1a

Cindy Jefferies is 15. She consults her GP and brings in a friend from school. Cindy says her parents don't know that she has come but she is thinking about having sex with her boyfriend and wants to go on the pill.

Can the GP keep Cindy's confidence?
GPs will see teenagers under 16 on their own, but we should encourage the young person to discuss the consultation with their parents. The GP should assess whether Cindy has sufficient intelligence and maturity to understand what

(treatment) is proposed and its implications, including risks and alternatives. This general test of competence for treatment in under-16s is known as 'Gillick competence', after a mother who campaigned against health service guidance that would mean her daughters under the age of 16 could receive confidential contraceptive advice from a doctor without her knowledge.[2] One of the judges who ruled on the case, Lord Fraser, set out the 'Fraser guidelines',[3] which relate specifically to contraception in the under-16s (see Box 16.1). If a child refuses to involve their parents but we don't think they are competent, we need to seek child protection advice, as outlined in the General Medical Council (GMC)'s 0–18 guidance.[4]

The GP consults with Cindy and finds that she has a mature outlook and has not yet had sex but is planning ahead. Cindy refuses to involve her parents. Cindy understands and retains the information the GP gives her and is able to ask sensible questions about taking the pill. The GP asks about Cindy's boyfriend. He is also 15 and a virgin.

Cindy is proposing having sex under the age of 16, which is illegal. What is the duty of the doctor with regard to the law?
The age of consent for intercourse, both heterosexual and homosexual, is 16 in England, Scotland and Wales, and 17 in Northern Ireland. It is illegal to have sex if either partner is under this age, even if they give consent. Surveys suggest that 1 in 3 people have had sex before the age of 16.[5] We also know that despite good access to contraception, teenage pregnancy rates are higher in the UK than in any other country in Europe, and our young people are disproportionately affected by sexually transmitted infections. The GP can advise Cindy of the legal position but cannot stop her having sex. Her health is at risk if she feels unable to seek health advice and contraception. If Cindy was under 13, she would not be able to consent to sex by law, and it would be child sexual abuse. It is also important that the GP finds out about Cindy's boyfriend. If he was older than Cindy or in a position of power, it would be harder for the relationship to be truly consensual and the GP would be concerned about sexual abuse.

Box 16.1   Giving contraceptive advice and/or treatment to the under-16s

The doctor should be satisfied that:
1. The patient understands the doctor's advice.
2. The patient cannot be persuaded to inform their parents or to allow the doctor to inform their parents that they are seeking contraceptive advice.
3. The patient is very likely to continue having sexual intercourse with or without contraceptive treatment.
4. Unless they receive contraceptive advice or treatment, the patient's physical or mental health, or both, are likely to suffer.
5. It is in the patient's best interests to receive contraceptive advice or treatment, or both, without parental consent.

Source: Adapted from Fraser guidelines.[3]

Puberty

Puberty is the process in which the human body goes through stages of development, called Tanner's stages (Table 16.1), to become capable of reproduction. The timing of these stages varies by individual, and is influenced by genetic and environmental factors. There is a trend to puberty starting earlier than in previous generations.[7] Puberty starts earlier in girls, beginning with breast development between 8 and 12. Next, androgen secretion promotes pubic hair growth and acne may start. Growth rate then accelerates. Menarche occurs 2–3 years after puberty begins. Puberty ends for girls around 16, with growth rate first slowing and then stopping altogether. For boys, the obvious external signs of puberty are slower, as the first change is a subtle increase in testicular size at between 12 and 13 years. Boys develop pubic hair 1 or 2 years later, with a growth in penile and scrotal size, and accelerated

Table 16.1 Stages of puberty (based on Tanner's stages).[6]		
Stage	**Males**	**Females**
Stage 1 (Prepubertal)	Testes <3 ml No sexual hair Basal rate of growth 5–6 cm/year	Elevation of papilla Growth 5–6 cm/year
Stage 2	Scrotum and testes enlarge, reddening of scrotal skin and change of texture Sparse hair at base of penis	Breast bud appears, aerola enlarges Sparse growth of hair on labia Growth accelerates 7–8 cm per year
Stage 3	Penile enlargement Coarser pubic hair Growth accelerates to 7–8 cm/year	Breast tissue grows beyond aerola Pubic hair coarser Peak rate of growth up to 8 cm/year
Stage 4	Scrotum enlarges further, penile length increases Pubic hair covers pubis region but not medial thigh Peak velocity of growth to 10 cm/year	Projection of areola and papilla form a secondary mound Growth decelerates
Stage 5 (Adult)	Adult genitalia and hair distribution Growth decelerates and stops around 17 years	Adult breast Growth stops around 16 years

Table 16.2 Causes of delayed puberty.

Underlying pathology	Causes	Comments
None	Constitutional delay	May be a similar history in parents or siblings
Hypothalamic suppression	Systemic illness Malnutrition, including anorexia or Crohn's disease	Consider if known chronic disease or underweight patient
Chromosome abnormalities	Klinefelter's syndrome (extra X chromosome in boys) Turner's syndrome (absent or incomplete X chromosome)	May be tall, slender, gynaecomastia. Associated with (minor) learning disabilities Short stature, primary amenorrhoea, may have dysmorphic features
Gonadotropin-releasing hormone deficiency	Hypothyroidism Gonadal failure Pituitary lesion/hypopituitarism Chemotherapy/radiotherapy	Kallmann's syndrome is hypogonadotrophic hypogonadism; sense of smell may be diminished or absent
Anatomical causes	Imperforate hymen, absence of uterus or vagina	Girls may have symptoms of a monthly cycle without bleeding

Case study 16.2

Sam Smith, age 14, is brought to see the GP by his parents. He is distressed that he is 'not developing' like his friends. He has grown in height but has always been shorter than his peers and hasn't started puberty.

How should the GP approach this?

1. History should cover previous growth and development, including cognitive development, review of previous growth charts, if available, and congenital anomalies – is there a general delay or are there delays in other areas? The GP should ask about his sense of smell (Kallmann's syndrome). If Sam is underweight, is there evidence of poor nutrition or a history of abnormal eating patterns? The GP should cover past medical history (chronic illness can delay puberty) and drug history (steroid use can delay growth). What was the parents' pattern of growth and puberty?

2. Physical examination should record weight, height and body mass index (BMI) on a growth chart. Estimate the Tanner stage (Table 16.1)[6] and other signs of puberty. Is there any sign of acne, voice changes and increased musculature? Do not be reassured by pubic hair, as this may reflect the activity of the adrenal glands rather than the hypothalamic–pituitary axis.[8] The midparental centile is an estimated height that the child should reach at 18. To calculate the mean parental centile, add the parents' heights and divide by 2, then add 7 cm for a boy or subtract 7 cm for a girl. Final height is still

normal for a boy within 10 cm of midparental centile and 8.5 cm for a girl, so it is not a very accurate prediction, but it can help parental and child expectations and estimate whether a child is following an appropriate centile. Check visual fields and fundoscopy, because a craniopharyngioma can cause visual loss and papilloedema.

3. In 95% of boys, puberty starts between 9.5 and 13.5 years. The first change is testicular size, and this can be measured by a string of beads of different volumes called a Prader's orchidometer. Puberty is said to start when the testes start enlarging (they are 1–3 ml in the prepubertal boy; 4 ml with reddening and thickening of the scrotal skin suggests puberty starting; >12 ml is adult size).[8]

4. Blood tests are usually done in secondary care, as hormone levels in this age group are difficult to interpret. Gonadotrophin levels will be low in a prepubertal child.

Sam is 153 cm and 40 kg, so is on the 10th centile for height and weight; previous records show this was always the case. His father is 176 cm and his mother 152 cm, so his expected height is 171 ± 10 cm. If he follows his centile, he will reach the lower end of this target. However, he has no signs of puberty on examination.

In this case, the GP needs to know when to refer; a boy with no signs of testicular enlargement by 14 will need investigating in secondary care. A specialist sees Sam and, after investigation, diagnoses 'constitutional delay'. In other words, Sam is expected to go through normal puberty but at the older end of the age range. Although 90% of delay is constitutional, it can be treated with low-dose sex steroids to develop skeletal and

muscle mass and avoid the psychological consequences of delayed puberty. In Sam's case, the specialist opts for watchful waiting, and Sam's puberty starts normally a few months later.

growth rate. The boys' growth spurt starts later, is faster (up to 10 cm a year) and ends later than in girls, at around 17 years old, when the epiphyseal growth plates fuse. Puberty is delayed if there are no signs of puberty by 13 for a girl and 14 for a boy (see Table 16.2); 2% of adolescents complain of delayed puberty, and the majority of these are boys.

Primary amenorrhoea

If a teenage girl has not had her first period by 14, she should be assessed for the development of secondary sexual characteristics and referred if these are not present. It can be worth waiting until age 16 if other features of puberty are apparent and she is otherwise developing normally. Genetic factors play a role, and a family history should be taken; if her mother was late with her menarche, constitutional delay is more likely. Turner's syndrome is a chromosomal abnormality with an absent or deficient X chromosome. We also need to consider rare but important anatomical causes, ranging from an imperforate hymen to the absence of a vagina or uterus. In the former case, she may get all the symptoms of a monthly cycle, including abdominal pain, but without bleeding. All secondary causes of amenorrhoea (see Chapter 26) can cause primary amenorrhoea, and pregnancy should always be considered.

Drugs and alcohol

Children tend to take the cue for their behaviour, values and beliefs from their families. This begins to change in adolescence, when young people become more aligned with their peer group than their families and develop their self-identity. For some, this may result in questioning family beliefs and values; for others, it includes exploring adult behaviours, including sexual behaviour. This experimentation can be healthy, but it can be harmful when the young person engages in smoking, drinking alcohol, drug misuse or getting involved in crime.

The continuity of these behaviours into adulthood is well documented.[1] Engaging in one risk-taking behaviour increases the likelihood of others. For instance, those who use alcohol are much more likely to have sex at a younger age.[9] Although young people report drinking less than they used to, the number of alcohol-related hospital admissions for males aged 15–24 rose by 57% from 2002 to 2010; the increase was even greater for females, where admissions rose by 76% in the same age group (from 15 233 to 26 908).[10]

GPs may become aware of alcohol or drug issues during a consultation, or it may be the parents who seek help because they have noticed a change in their teenager. Withdrawal and moodiness are general signs that alert parents. These may be caused by many factors. We should ask about specific markers, such as money going missing from the home or the teenager being drunk or smelling of alcohol, as well as specific warning signs of drug-taking, such as bloodshot eyes, dilated pupils or finding drug paraphernalia in the house. Parents can find useful information online (see Top tip box). Often, issues only come to light because the young person drops out of social activities, gets into trouble for the first time or is truant from school. GPs have a role in advising parents and young people about the negative effects of drinking and drugs, and can tell them how to reduce the risk of harm. There is some evidence that children who delay the time of their first drink may reduce their long-term risk of harmful drinking. Other factors that protect the young person include: a supportive relationship with their parents, having their first drink at home and learning about the effects of alcohol from parents rather than peers.[9] If we discover that a young person is using drugs and alcohol, we should signpost and refer them to specialist services. (See Chapter 8 for more on alcohol and drug misuse.)

Mood

There is a common perception that moodiness in teenagers is normal, even that sporadic psychological distress is to be expected. Therefore, parents and doctors may be reluctant to medicalise low mood, seeing it as a developmental stage. But we need to recognise that depression is easy to miss in a teenager, and the risks of doing so are significant. Anxiety disorders are also common, and often coexist with depression. Symptoms of anxiety in teenagers predict depression in adulthood. They are underdiagnosed and undertreated at all ages (see Chapter 24). Teenagers themselves may not recognise symptoms because they haven't got the life experience to give their current emotional state context. They may not know how to seek help, or they may be afraid that their concerns will be dismissed out of hand. Parents may think their teenager's withdrawal or moodiness is normal and not intervene. There is also some evidence that GPs spend less time consulting with teenagers, and that when they do pick up on psychological problems, they are less likely to put specific plans or follow-up in place.[11] The evidence that teenagers should expect to suffer psychologically through their teenage years is lacking; most do not.

Case study 16.1b

Cindy Jefferies attends with her mother 6 months after her GP prescribed the pill. Cindy is now 16. The GP notices from the medical record that she did not collect another pill prescription after the initial 3 months she was given. Cindy's mum says that she is worried about Cindy's mood. Cindy split up with her first boyfriend 3 months ago and became very withdrawn. She spent a lot of time in her room, became tearful and moody and stopped seeing her friends. Cindy's parents thought she would get over the break-up, but now they are concerned by Cindy's ongoing withdrawal and weight loss. Yesterday, her mother noticed some cuts on Cindy's arms. She tried to talk to Cindy about this but Cindy started yelling at her to leave her alone and said that she didn't want to live anymore. Cindy spends the consultation with her head bowed, avoiding eye contact and picking at the sleeve of her jumper. She does not speak.

As well taking a history of depression, what else should the GP screen for?
Depressed teenagers are more likely to engage in risk-taking behaviours; we should screen depressed teenagers for alcohol and drug use (and should screen teenagers taking drugs and alcohol for depression). We should also assess risk of self-harm and suicide: is Cindy harming herself in any other way (see Box 16.2)? Cindy told her mother that she doesn't want to live. Is this a recurrent thought? Has she acted on, or thought about acting on, such thoughts? We would want to assess for evidence of psychosis, which may present with withdrawal and is linked to drug use. We would also want to ask about anxiety and panic symptoms. Cindy has lost weight. Is this a somatic feature of depression or a presentation of associated eating disorder?

What are the risks of missing depression in teenagers?
There is the risk of immediate harm from self-harm and suicide. Linked risk-taking behaviours also increase morbidity and mortality. Depression in teenagers can be chronic and relapsing, which affects their psychological well-being, but also impacts on their education through time off school, truancy or school refusal and poor concentration. The long-term effects include poor mental health persisting into adulthood.

How does the management of depression in teenagers differ from that in adults in primary care?
Drug treatment is initiated by specialists, not GPs; in 2003, the Committee on Safety of Medicines (CSM) advised against using selective serotonin reuptake inhibitors (SSRIs) for depression in children and adolescents because of concerns about the possibility of increased suicidal thinking associated with these drugs in this age group. In mild or moderate depression, drug therapy is likely to be used only when other psychological therapies, such as cognitive behavioural therapy (CBT), have been tried and not had a good response.

After spending time with Cindy and her mum, and speaking to Cindy on her own, the GP is concerned that she is significantly depressed and at further risk of self-harm. She has very low self-esteem and body dysmorphia. She has been trying to control her food intake, as she thinks she is fat (despite having a BMI at the lower end of normal), and this has resulted in a cycle of bingeing and vomiting. The GP refers her to the child and adolescent mental health team by telephone and follows this up with a written referral letter. They see her later that week and diagnose depression and bulimia. (See Chapter 24 for more on depression.)

Box 16.2 Addressing self-harm in primary care

- Self-harm is not just attention-seeking (many patients do it in secret and try to hide the evidence).
- The patient causes intentional harm to themselves, including inflicting pain (such as cutting the skin or head-banging), ingesting poisons and engaging in reckless behaviour.
- Self-harm is not always done with suicidal intent, but patients should be assessed for suicidal ideation. Self-harmers are more at risk of serious harm and suicide.
- Self-harm is often used by patients as a way to relieve emotional distress: anxiety, self-loathing, sadness, anger or feelings of 'emotional numbness'.
- It can be very distressing for family and friends to witness self-harm behaviour, and it can be difficult for GPs to know how to address it.
- Patients self-harm for different reasons, and we should try and understand the emotions they experience that lead to the self-harm behaviour. Getting our patients to identify triggers will also help them recognise when they are at risk.
- We should be understanding, not judgemental. Patients who self-harm need to be listened to and risk-assessed.
- We should explain the risks, such as scarring and serious harm, and signpost support.
- We can suggest alternative behaviours, such as punching a cushion to vent angry feelings, using an ice cube on the skin instead of something sharp or drawing with red pen on the skin instead of drawing blood.
- Parents and patients need to know where to access emergency support in a crisis or if risks escalate.

Eating disorders

Eating disorders often emerge in adolescence. They are commoner in girls, but also happen in boys, and they affect all cultures and backgrounds. Anorexia is a low BMI (<17.5 kg/m^2) associated with excessive control of eating. Bulimia is associated with cycles of uncontrolled bingeing (overeating) and purging (behaviour to compensate for the overeating, such as vomiting or laxative abuse), with either a normal or a low weight. Parents or teachers may notice signs of weight loss or odd behaviour around food, such as skipping meals or being excessively picky about food, developing an obsession with exercise, going to the bathroom soon after eating and stashing food. Teenagers may present with mood changes or their periods becoming irregular or stopping. They may seek help directly for an eating disorder, but it is often a hidden problem, so GPs need to be aware of the presentations that should prompt questions about eating problems (see Table 16.3).

Table 16.3 Assessing eating disorders in primary care.

Presentations that may suggest an eating disorder

Depression, anxiety, low mood or self-harm, including overdose
Underweight patient, or parents or patient complaining of weight loss or not being able to gain weight
Scanty or irregular periods/short stature/delayed puberty
Complaints of nausea/vomiting/dizziness/faints
Unexplained hypokalaemia (from vomiting)

The SCOFF questionnaire – to detect eating disorders

- Do you ever make yourself **S**ick because you feel uncomfortably full?
- Do you worry you have lost **C**ontrol over how much you eat?
- Have you recently lost more than **O**ne stone in a 3-month period?
- Do you believe yourself to be **F**at when others say you are too thin?
- Would you say that **F**ood dominates your life?
Two or more positive answers should prompt further questioning.

Areas to ask about if a patient discloses food or eating issues

Associated symptoms:
- tiredness
- poor concentration
- low mood, anxiety, poor self-esteem
- self-harm and suicidal ideation
Associated behaviours:
- vomiting
- laxative abuse
- excessive exercise

Areas to assess on examination

Height and weight: BMI < 14 kg/m^2 needs urgent intervention
Pulse: May have slow pulse or arrhythmia
Blood pressure: Hypotension. Blood pressure <90/70 or postural drop >10 mmHg indicates need for urgent intervention
Muscle weakness: Test ability to stand from sitting without using hands, or ability to squat
In bulimia, we may see dental decay (if the patient is vomiting) or calluses on the back of the hand (if the patient is inducing vomiting). In anorexia, we may see lanugo hair and delayed puberty.

Investigations in primary care, initially and for monitoring (follow guidance from secondary care)

Full blood count (FBC), erythrocyte sedimentation rate (ESR), urea and electrolytes (U&Es), creatinine, glucose, liver function tests (LFTs) and thyroid function tests (TFTs)
Electrocardiogram (ECG)
Dual-energy X-ray absorptiometry (DEXA) scan

Case study 16.1c

Cindy is started on an SSRI; this is used for her depression, but is also used in bulimia, where it can help break the cycle of bingeing and purging. There is no evidence medication helps in anorexia. Cindy engages well with CBT, and her parents are prepared to learn how best to help her. They all realise that the treatment of eating disorders can take a long time, but Cindy has a better prognosis through early recognition and appropriate support. The GP is asked to monitor Cindy's serum potassium; patients who purge through vomiting risk dangerous hypokalaemia.

SUMMARY

The teenage years are a period of intense and rapid change. Children transition into adults through physical growth, sexual maturation and cognitive development. A challenge for doctors is to understand what constitutes 'normal' at each stage of development. Adolescents may be distressed when they are not growing and maturing like their peers, but puberty happens at different times and different rates for different individuals. Parents and doctors may miss depression if they believe that teenage angst and mood swings are normal. Misdiagnosis can cause immediate harm, and there is evidence that untreated mental health issues in adolescence persist into adulthood. Amidst all this change is the pressure teenagers feel to develop a 'self-identity'. For some, this self-awareness results in dislike of their bodies, and even in eating disorders; others engage in risk-taking behaviour and experiment with drugs, alcohol and sex. GPs need to develop rapport with their teenage patients and aim to support them in developing physical and mental health for life, while recognising and helping teenagers at risk.

Now visit **www.wileyessential.com/primarycare** to test yourself on this chapter.

REFERENCES

1. Viner R, Macfarlane A. ABC of adolescence: health promotion. *BMJ* 2005;**330**:527–9.

2. Wheeler R. Editorial: Gillick or Fraser? A plea for consistency over competence in children *BMJ* 2006;**332**:807.

3. Gillick v West Norfolk & Wisbech Area Health Authority [1985] UKHL 7. Available from: http://www.bailii.org/uk/cases/UKHL/1985/7.html (last accessed 6 October 2015).

4. General Medical Council. *Principles of Confidentiality. 0–18 Years: Guidance for all Doctors*. London: GMC; 2013.

5. Faculty of Sexual & Reproductive Health Care. Contraceptive Choices for Young People. March 2010. Available from: http://www.fsrh.org/pdfs/ceuGuidanceYoungPeople2010.pdf (last accessed 6 October 2015).

6. Blondell RD, Foster MB, Dave KC. Disorders of puberty. *Am Fam Physician* 1999 Jul;**60**(1):209–18, 223–4.

7. Pitteloud, N. Editorial: managing delayed or altered puberty in boys. *BMJ* 2012;**345**:e7913.

8. Palmert M, Dunkel L. Clinical practice: delayed puberty. *N Engl J Med* 2012;**336**:443–53.

9. Department for Children, Schools and Families. Impact of Alcohol Consumption on Young People – A Systematic Review of Published Preview. Available from: dera.ioe.ac.uk/11355/1/DCSF-RR067.pdf (last accessed 6 October 2015).

10. Alcohol Concern. Statistics on alcohol. Available from: http://www.alcoholconcern.org.uk/help-and-advice/statistics-on-alcohol/ (last accessed 6 October 2015).

11. Iliffe S, Williams G, Fernandez V, et al. Treading a fine line: is diagnosing depression in young people just medicalising moodiness? *Br J Gen Pract* 2009;**59**(560):156–7.

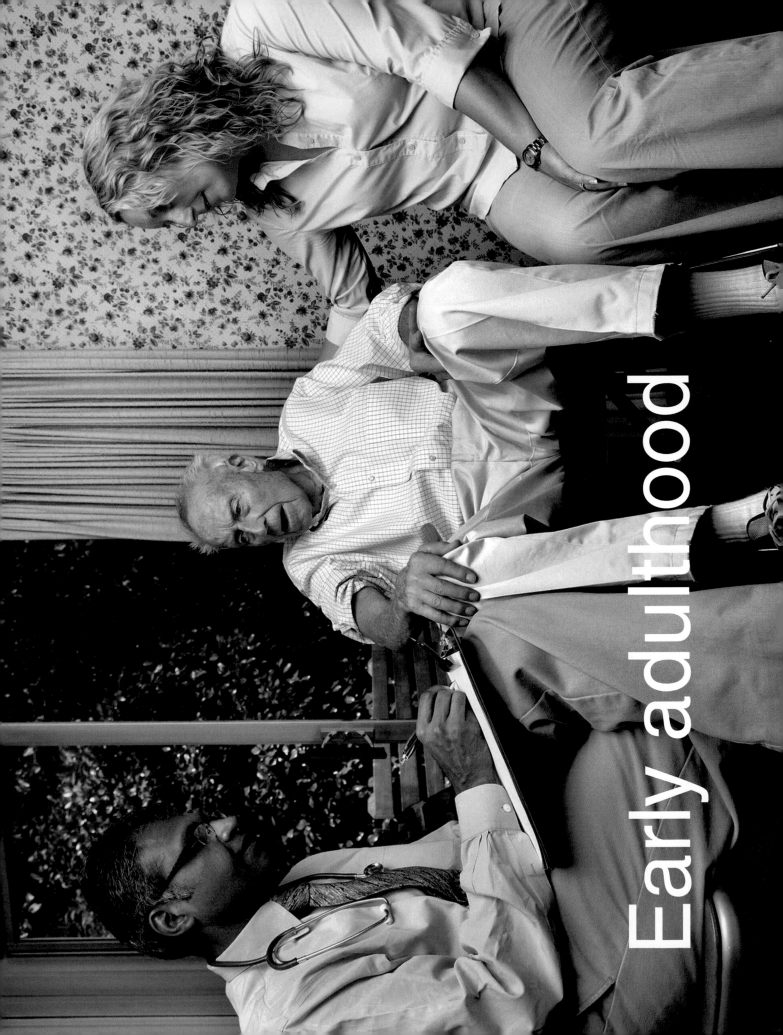

Early adulthood

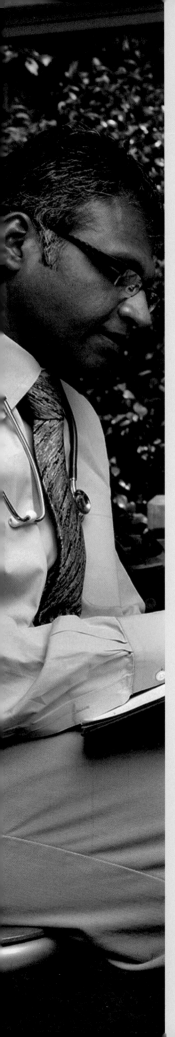

CHAPTER 17
Respiratory tract infections

Lucy Jenkins
Teaching Fellow in Primary Care, University of Bristol

Key topics

Learning objectives

- Be able to assess and manage patients with a cough, sore throat and nasal congestion.
- Be able to discuss the pros and cons of antibiotic use in respiratory infections.
- Be able to diagnose and give advice on glandular fever.

Essential Primary Care, First Edition. Edited by Andrew Blythe and Jessica Buchan.
© 2017 John Wiley & Sons, Ltd. Published 2017 by John Wiley & Sons, Ltd.
Companion website: www.wileyessential.com/primarycare

Coughs and colds

The case studies in this section illustrate the management of coughs and colds in adults in general practice. Chapter 13 outlined the assessment and management of children presenting with coughs and colds. It is December, and Dr Boyle's morning surgery is split into telephone triage followed by face-to-face appointments. The first two patients he is asked to phone have 'cold/cough' next to their names (Case studies 17.1 and 17.2).

Case study 17.1 Telephone call 1

Jeremy Jordan is a 48-year-old businessman who is concerned that he has a nasty cold which needs some treatment. He has been unwell for 3 days, with a blocked nose, sneezing, sore throat and an annoying cough.

What should the GP do next?
A full history is essential, especially if a problem is going to be managed over the phone. Examination and investigations are not needed to diagnose the common cold. Jeremy's history is typical; nasal discharge is also common, and some patients complain in addition of a hoarse voice due to laryngitis. General malaise often occurs, but fever is low-grade and less common than in children; if associated with headache and myalgia, it may point to influenza.

As always, it is important to ask about a patient's concerns and expectations and to rule out serious illness. The common cold is largely a self-limiting illness, but the vague symptoms can mimic other serious illnesses, and some groups are at higher risk of complications.

What are the red flags for the common cold?
Alarm signs needing face-to-face assessment are severe headache, upper airway distress, swallowing difficulties suggesting obstruction and lower respiratory distress

suggesting pneumonia. A review of a patient's past history is also necessary. Smoking, diabetes, pre-existing respiratory disease, immunosuppression and pregnancy all increase the risk of complications.[1]

Dr Boyle is happy that Jeremy is low-risk and does not require an appointment or prescription. He still wants treatment, though: what could the GP suggest?
The GP should educate Jeremy so that future similar illnesses can be self-managed. The GP should explain the natural history of colds and advise on symptom management, and should safety-net for complications of a cold (e.g. sinusitis or lower respiratory tract infections (RTIs); in younger children, otitis media is a more common complication).[2]

Jeremy's main concern is that he has an important meeting today and he may pass an infection on to a senior colleague, who is pregnant.

What should the GP advise?
There is no clear guidance about missing work or school with a cold. A common-sense approach should be taken, with the emphasis on careful hygiene, including hand-washing, to minimise spread.

Top tip: advice for patient with colds

A GP might say: 'Unfortunately, colds are very common: adults experience an average of two to four colds per year. Most symptoms resolve after 1 or 2 weeks, although a mild cough can last a bit longer. Antibiotics do not work for colds, so we do not use them, but there are lots of things that you can do to help yourself get better. We recommend rest if you are tired, eating well, drinking lots of fluids and taking paracetamol if you have a headache or muscle aches. Some people find that over-the-counter treatments such as lozenges and throat sprays help with a sore throat or congestion.'

Case study 17.2a Telephone call 2

Colin Carson is 52 years old and has had a cough with green sputum for 2 weeks. Dr Boyle's initial questions reveal that Colin has been feeling unwell and is worried, as he was previously admitted with a chest infection 2 years ago. He is a smoker.

What is the differential diagnosis?
It sounds like Colin has a chest infection, either acute bronchitis or pneumonia. He needs a face-to-face assessment. If he had asthma, chronic obstructive pulmonary disease (COPD) or other pre-existing lung conditions, he would be at risk of infective exacerbations (see Chapter 30).

Lower respiratory tract infections: bronchitis and pneumonia

Bronchitis and pneumonia both present with cough and sputum, and may also cause wheeze, breathlessness and systemic features. Bronchitis is inflammation of the bronchial tree. It is more common (44 per 1000 adult population[3]) than pneumonia (5–11 per 1000 adult population[4]). In patients who are otherwise well, bronchitis is usually self-limiting. Pneumonia is inflammation of the lung parenchyma and carries a significant risk of complications, so antibiotics are indicated. In primary care, the following clinical signs are useful for determining the risk of pneumonia:[5]

- absence of a runny nose;
- presence of breathlessness;
- crackles and reduced breath sounds;
- tachycardia >100 bpm;
- fever >37.8 °C.

Blood tests for the inflammatory marker C-reactive protein (CRP) can also help determine the risk of pneumonia, but they are less useful than the signs just listed and their results are not immediately available in primary care.[5] Chest X-ray results are not usually available quickly enough in primary care to help diagnose pneumonia, but they are useful if underlying pathology is suspected (see section on Follow-up and other possible diagnoses).

Pneumonia may be managed in the community if the patient is well enough. If the patient is unwell (including those with oxygen saturations of <92%) or has significant comorbidity, admission may be required. The CRB-65 is an adapted scoring system (based on the British Thoracic Society CURB-65 score) used to assess people with suspected pneumonia[4] and predict mortality (see Box 17.1). The score may overestimate the risk, so GPs should use clinical judgement to prevent inappropriate admissions.[6] Complications such as effusion, emphysema, abscess and septicaemia contribute to the mortality rate of 6–12% for those requiring admission.[4]

National Institute for Health and Care Excellence (NICE) guidance suggests treatment following local antibiotic guidelines in patients who are systemically ill or have a comorbidity or immunosuppression.[8] More specifically, it advises antibiotics for patients >65 years with at least two of the following, or >80 years with at least one of the following:

- hospitalised in the last 12 months;
- heart failure;
- diabetes;
- on steroids.

Follow-up and other possible diagnoses

Routine follow-up of bronchitis is not necessary. However, if the patient has repeated infections, the GP should consider spirometry to rule out COPD if there is a smoking history. Likewise, any persistent cough warrants further investigation, especially if there are any red-flag symptoms for lung cancer. Chronic cough has a number of causes; the GP should broaden the history to include reflux, allergic symptoms, cardiovascular systems review and medications. Those with pneumonic changes on a chest X-ray are often given a repeat X-ray 8 weeks later to check changes have resolved. People who have had pneumonia can feel very tired afterwards – even those who are normally fit and well.

Sinusitis

Sinusitis is unpleasant, and patients can feel unwell for 2.5 weeks (see Figure 17.1). This may be the reason that GPs often prescribe antibiotics despite guidance that they are not

---

Box 17.1 Adapted CURB-65 score for use in primary care

- Confusion (recent).
- Respiratory rate >30.
- Systolic blood pressure <90.
- Age >65.

Consider admission for patients with one or two of these criteria. Admit those with three.

Case study 17.2b

Colin has a temperature of 37.4 °C, pulse 80 bpm and respiratory rate 20 breaths/minute. He has a mild wheeze, but no other chest signs, and he seems reasonably well.

What is the diagnosis and how should the GP treat him?
Colin has acute bronchitis. This is usually self-limiting, so the GP should advise on self-care. This is an excellent opportunity for health promotion, and Dr Boyle should make the link between Colin's smoking and this illness. He should then offer him information and advice on smoking cessation, and help if Colin does want to stop smoking.

Colin wonders if there is anything he can have for the cough or if an inhaler would help
GPs tend not to prescribe cough-suppressant medication, as there is little evidence of benefit, although patients may report short-term symptomatic relief and generally it is safe. There is no evidence for β2 agonists in acute bronchitis in the absence of underlying obstructive lung disease.[7]

When are antibiotics indicated in acute bronchitis?
It is important not to prescribe antibiotics inappropriately, as this may medicalise a self-limiting illness, discourage self-management and promote further consultations with similar symptoms in future. In addition, it is an unnecessary cost to the patient and health service. (See Chapter 13 for tips on discussing the balance of benefit versus harm of antibiotic use.)

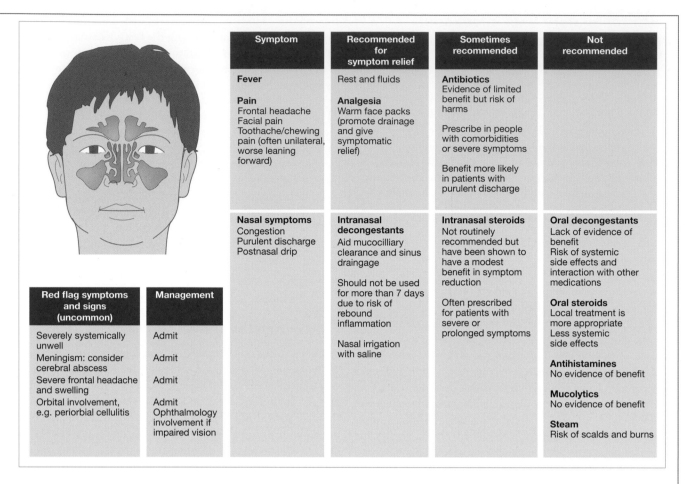

Symptom	Recommended for symptom relief	Sometimes recommended	Not recommended
Fever	Rest and fluids	**Antibiotics** Evidence of limited benefit but risk of harms	
Pain Frontal headache Facial pain Toothache/chewing pain (often unilateral, worse leaning forward)	**Analgesia** Warm face packs (promote drainage and give symptomatic relief)	Prescribe in people with comorbidities or severe symptoms Benefit more likely in patients with purulent discharge	
Nasal symptoms Congestion Purulent discharge Postnasal drip	**Intranasal decongestants** Aid mucocilliary clearance and sinus drainage Should not be used for more than 7 days due to risk of rebound inflammation Nasal irrigation with saline	**Intranasal steroids** Not routinely recommended but have been shown to have a modest benefit in symptom reduction Often prescribed for patients with severe or prolonged symptoms	**Oral decongestants** Lack of evidence of benefit Risk of systemic side effects and interaction with other medications **Oral steroids** Local treatment is more appropriate Less systemic side effects **Antihistamines** No evidence of benefit **Mucolytics** No evidence of benefit **Steam** Risk of scalds and burns

Red flag symptoms and signs (uncommon)	Management
Severely systemically unwell	Admit
Meningism: consider cerebral abscess	Admit
Severe frontal headache and swelling	Admit
Orbital involvement, e.g. periorbial cellulitis	Admit Ophthalmology involvement if impaired vision

Figure 17.1 Sinusitis.

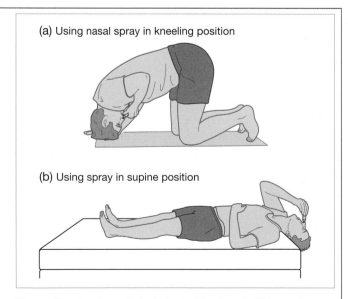

(a) Using nasal spray in kneeling position

(b) Using spray in supine position

Figure 17.2 How to apply topical nasal treatments. This can be done in two positions. Insert the nozzle into the nostril and angle at 30°.

indicated for acute sinusitis. A Cochrane review showed slight benefit of antibiotics in reducing secretions and time to cure, but there was no difference in terms of pain or activities of daily living.[9] There were relatively high levels of antibiotic side effects, low risk of serious complications from acute sinusitis and increasing problems with antibiotic resistance. In practice, many GPs prescribe antibiotics for patients with severe symptoms, or those lasting 7 days or more.

Chronic sinusitis

Sinusitis lasting more than 12 weeks is known as chronic sinusitis. It is common, especially in smokers and atopic individuals, including asthmatics.[10] It causes nasal congestion, rhinorrhoea, a sensation of facial pressure and a reduced sense of smell. Facial pain is less common than in acute sinusitis, and dental infections should always be excluded, especially if cheek swelling is present. Careful examination in primary care with an otoscope will show any underlying congestion, polyps, septal deviation or foreign body.

Nasal steroids in spray or drops form the mainstay of treatment. Compliance is important, as is correct use (Figure 17.2). Nasal douching with saline is also beneficial.[11] In some cases, a prolonged 12-week course of antibiotics or a 2-week course of

Top tip: red-flag symptoms in sinusitis

The following may indicate nasopharyngeal carcinoma:
- Unilateral symptoms.
- Persistent blockage.
- Blood-stained discharge.
- Proptosis or diplopia.
- Neurological signs.

Box 17.2 Centor criteria

- History of fever.
- Tonsillar exudates.
- No cough.
- Tender anterior cervical lymphadenopathy.

Three or four of these criteria make infection with group A β-haemolytic *Streptococci* (GABHS) more likely, and antibiotics should be considered. Zero or one makes GABHS unlikely.

Table 17.1 FeverPAIN scoring system for sore throat.

Score 1 for each of	
Fever	Fever in the last 24 hours
P	Purulence of tonsils
A	Rapid attendance (patient seen within the first 3 days of symptoms starting)
I	Inflamed tonsils
N	No cough or coryza

Score 0 or 1: Treat with simple measures
Score 2 or 3: Deferred antibiotics
Score 4 or 5: Immediate antibiotics (60% of these will have a streptococcal sore throat)

oral steroids may be beneficial. If patients are not responding to this, referral to ENT is indicated, as for red-flags symptoms (see Top tip box).

Sore throat: pharyngitis and tonsillitis

The principles of managing sore throats in adults are similar to those in children (see Chapter 13). The terms 'pharyngitis' and 'tonsillitis' describe which part of the oral cavity is predominantly affected. The challenge for a GP is to identify those who need antibiotics, and to manage expectations and symptoms in those who do not; 40% of acute throat infections will be better within 3 days regardless of treatment, and by day 7, 85% of patients with a throat infection will have recovered regardless of the causative organism.[12]

Management is largely with analgesia; in adults with tonsillitis, ibuprofen has been shown to be more effective than paracetamol or aspirin.[13] The Centor criteria (see Box 17.2)[13] are recommended by NICE and the Scottish Intercollegiate Guidelines Network (SIGN) for the identification of infections likely to be caused by the bacteria group A β-haemolytic *Streptococci* (GABHS). The PRISM study looked into this further, and developed the FeverPAIN scoring system, which is designed to be sensitive to all streptococcal sore throats and to guide treatment (see Table 17.1).[14] The scores suggest which infections may be caused by bacteria, but this is not necessarily a good predictor of symptom severity or complication rates. A UK study based in general practice looked at symptoms and signs to see if any were useful in predicting the commonest complications of quinsy, otitis media, sinusitis and cellulitis.[15] Severe tonsillar inflammation and severe earache were shown to be independent predictors of complications.

When antibiotics are given, local guidelines should be followed. Usual treatment is phenoxymethylpenicillin for 10 days; a macrolide is an alternative if the patient is penicillin-allergic.

In secondary care, adults with severe tonsillitis are often treated with oral steroids, and some GPs may do this for patients with severe symptoms. The GP should immediately refer patients who have stridor or respiratory difficulty. Other patients who need referral are those with severe dehydration, inability to take oral medications, severe systemic symptoms or severe complications like quinsy.[16]

Referral for tonsillectomy in adults with recurrent tonsillitis is advised if they have had five or more episodes per year of sore throat due to tonsillitis; the episodes should have been disabling and have prevented normal functioning.

Top tip: sore throat in immunosuppressed patients

Sore throat should be taken seriously in immunosuppressed patients such as those on disease-modifying antirheumatic drugs or those with a known haematological malignancy or human immunodeficiency virus (HIV).

- Consider admission if these patients are unwell. Have a low threshold to discuss with specialists.
- If admission is not needed, take a full blood count (FBC) and check the results the same day. Have urgent discussion with specialists if white cell count is low.
- Carbimazole (used to treat hyperthyroidism) can cause idiosyncratic neutropaenia, so these patients also need an urgent FBC. Withhold the drug until the result is available and seek specialist advice as necessary.

Glandular fever

Glandular fever, or infectious mononucleosis, is caused by the Epstein–Barr virus (EBV). Many people have mild forms of it in childhood, which are simply treated as nonspecific viruses. It is often called the 'kissing disease' as it is spread by droplet and direct contact. Young adults are more likely to be symptomatic, with prolonged fever and sore throat, swollen lymph nodes and aching joints. Often, these are initially treated as bacterial tonsillitis and the diagnosis is made on blood tests later on. As it is a virus, initial management is conservative, with rest, fluids and analgesia. Stress and alcohol are thought to prolong recovery times so are best avoided.

In young adults, the acute infection usually resolves in 3 weeks, but a persistent malaise and fatigue can occur, which can be quite debilitating. Similar symptoms can occur with a nonspecific postviral fatigue, and in a prolonged form in chronic fatigue syndrome. For postviral fatigue, the GP should take a sensitive and sensible approach. Patients should be advised that short-term rest and slowing the pace of life are necessary. General advice about healthy eating and gradually

increasing activity is important. It is essential to ask about mood and to watch for signs of depression. The good news is that the prognosis is excellent and, given adequate time, the vast majority of patients make a full recovery.

Mild initial complications include secondary bacterial infections and a rash with amoxicillin. Patients may initially present with right upper quadrant pain, which is caused by a self-limiting viral hepatitis or splenomegaly. Patients with glandular fever should therefore be advised to avoid contact sports, as there is a low risk of splenic rupture. Serious complications are rare, and infection usually gives lifelong immunity, so infection later in life is unusual.

SUMMARY

Textbook symptoms of RTIs are more common in adults than in children, and a thorough history and examination will usually give the diagnosis without the need for further investigations. These infections are usually self–limiting, and the GP's role includes patient education. Knowledge of the natural history of these conditions is essential, and by sharing this with the patient and advising on self-care and over-the-counter treatments, the GP can empower the patient to self-manage in the future. While uncommon, there are some serious complications of these infections, and it is important to be able to identify and manage these.

Now visit **www.wileyessential.com/primarycare** to test yourself on this chapter.

REFERENCES

1. NICE. Common cold. NICE Clinical Knowledge Summaries. November 2011. Available from: http://cks.nice.org.uk/common-cold (last accessed 6 October 2015).

2. Heikkinen T, Jarvinen A. The common cold. *Lancet* 2003;**361**(9351):51–9.

3. Wark, P. Bronchitis (acute). *BMJ Clin Evid* 2011;**1508**. Published online 20 June 2011: http://www.ncbi.nlm.nih.gov/pmc/articles/PMC3275297/ (last accessed 6 October 2015).

4. Lim WS, Baudouin SV, George RC, et al. BTS guidelines for the management of community acquired pneumonia in adults: update 2009. *Thorax* 2009;**64**(Suppl. 3):iii1–55.

5. Falk G, Fahey T. C-reactive protein and community-acquired pneumonia in ambulatory care: systematic review of diagnostic accuracy studies. *Fam Pract* 2009:**26**;10–21.

6. McNally M, Curtain J, O'Brien KK, et al. Validity of British Thoracic Society guidance (the CRB-65 rule) for predicting the severity of pneumonia in general practice: systematic review and meta-analysis. *Br J Gen Pract* 2010;**60**(579):e423–33.

7. Becker LA, Hom J, Villasis-Keever M, van der Wouden JC. Beta2-agonists for acute bronchitis. *Cochrane Database Syst Rev* 2011;**7**:10.1002/14651858.

8. NICE. Respiratory tract infections – antibiotic prescribing: prescribing of antibiotics for self-limiting respiratory tract infections in adults and children in primary care.

NICE Clinical Guideline 69. July 2008. Available from: https://www.nice.org.uk/guidance/cg69 (last accessed 6 October 2015).

9. Lemiengre MB, van Driel ML, Merenstein D, et al. Antibiotics for clinically diagnosed acute rhinosinusitis in adults (review). *Cochrane Database Syst Rev* 2012;**10**:10.1002/14651858.

10. Ah-See KL, MacKenzie J, Ah-See KW. Management of chronic rhinosinusitis. *BMJ* 2012;**345**:e7054.

11. Harvey R, Hannan SA, Badia L, Scadding G. Nasal saline irrigations for the symptoms of chronic rhinosinusitis (review). *Cochrane Database Syst Rev* 2007;**3**:10.1002/14651858.

12. National Prescribing Centre. Management of common infections in primary care. *MeReC Bulletin* 2006;**17**:3.

13. SIGN. Management of sore throat and indications for tonsillectomy. Scottish Intercollegiate Guideline 117. April 2010. Available from: http://www.sign.ac.uk/pdf/sign117.pdf (last accessed 6 October 2015).

14. Little P, Hobbs FDR, Moore M, et al. Clinical score and rapid antigen detection test to guide antibiotic use for sore throats: randomised controlled trial of PRISM (primary care streptococcal management). *BMJ* 2013;**347**:f5806.

15. Little P, Stuart B, Hobbs FDR, et al. Predictors of suppurative complications for acute sore throat in primary care: prospective clinical cohort study. *BMJ* 2013;**347**:f6867.

16. NICE. Sore throat – acute. NICE Clinical Knowledge Summaries. October 2012. Available from: http://cks.nice.org.uk/sore-throat-acute (last accessed 6 October 2015).

CHAPTER 18
Low back pain

Jessica Buchan
GP and Teaching Fellow in Primary Care, University of Bristol

Key topics

Learning objectives

- Be able to demonstrate how to assess someone who says, 'My back hurts'.
- Be able to identify when further investigation and referral are warranted in a patient presenting with back pain.
- Be able to describe the natural history of nonspecific low back pain and nerve root pain.
- Be able to advise on evidence-based management strategies for nonspecific low back pain and nerve root pain.
- Be able to identify patients at risk of developing chronic low back pain, and describe strategies to reduce the impact of chronic back pain.

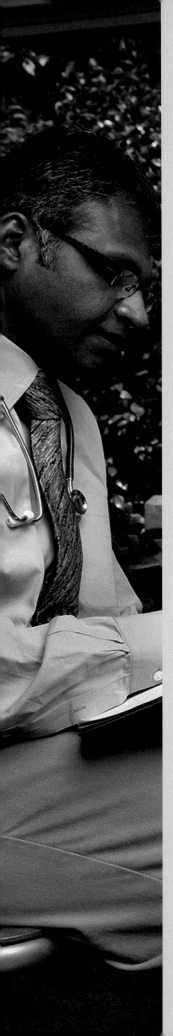

Essential Primary Care, First Edition. Edited by Andrew Blythe and Jessica Buchan.
© 2017 John Wiley & Sons, Ltd. Published 2017 by John Wiley & Sons, Ltd.
Companion website: www.wileyessential.com/primarycare

The burden of back pain

Low back pain is common. Most people will suffer at least one episode of low back pain in their lives; up to a third of the population suffer with back pain each year. Most people with back pain do not consult their GP, but at least a fifth do,[1] resulting in up to 2.6 million people seeking GP advice every year.[2] Patients may want:

- reassurance that there is no serious underlying cause for the pain;
- reassurance that their pain won't persist or cause permanent disability;
- advice on managing the pain;
- advice on managing daily activities including work; or
- advice on how to aid recovery or prevent recurrences.

The GP's task is to thoroughly assess the patient with back pain and know when to investigate or refer and when to reassure. Most episodes of acute nonspecific back pain are self-limiting and resolve in 1 week to 1 month (see Table 18.1), but they can recur, or result in residual symptoms.

Whatever the underlying cause, we need to acknowledge that back pain can result in considerable pain and disability.

Table 18.1 Definition of low back pain.

Pain, muscle tension or stiffness between the bottom of the ribs and the top of the legs, with or without leg pain (sciatica)	
Acute	<6 weeks
Subacute	6–12 weeks
Chronic	>12 weeks

As well as assessing symptoms, we need to assess the impact those symptoms have. For instance, patients with acute back pain may struggle to work, particularly if they have a manual job. It is estimated by the Office of National Statistics (ONS) that 30.6 million days of work were lost in the UK in 2013 due to musculoskeletal conditions (including back pain). This is more days than from any other cause, and results in a considerable burden for society.[3]

Assessing back pain in primary care

Acute back pain can be very painful, but severity of pain is not necessarily an indicator of underlying disease. Most cases (at least 90%) seen in primary care are 'nonspecific', meaning that there is no underlying cause that can be diagnosed. This is not easy for patients, or even doctors, to understand when they are used to the concept of the pathological diagnosis.

Several structures in the back can cause or contribute to pain, including the joints, discs, muscles and connective tissue. Examination and imaging cannot accurately tell us exactly which structure is causing the pain. We often call such pain 'mechanical back pain', because the pain is thought to arise from the way that the different structures work with one another. It is more important that the GP can differentiate patients who have nerve root pain, or possible spinal pathology such as malignancy, infection, fracture or inflammatory conditions such as ankylosing spondylitis, from those in whom a precise diagnosis is neither possible nor useful.

Case study 18.1 provides an example of the approach to adopt in assessing low back pain.

Case study 18.1a

Stuart Clarke, an IT manager, aged 43, slid and fell on the grass playing football last night. He tells his GP, Dr Edward Davies, that he had a mild dull pain in his lower back at the time, but since waking this morning the pain has been severe. He describes his back as feeling 'as if it is going to give way' when he walks. The pain is localised to the left side of his lumbar spine, radiating into the top of the left buttock.

How might Dr Davies assess Stuart?

- **Preparation:** Check the records. Is there an existing medical condition, medication or past history he should be aware of?
- **Watch the patient walk into the room:** Does Stuart look unwell? Is he in pain? What is his gait like?
- **Gather biomedical information:** Take a history of the presenting symptoms, including the mechanism of injury. Assess the pain: do symptoms suggest nerve root pain (see Box 18.1)?

- **Assess red-flag symptoms:** These make a serious cause more likely (see Box 18.2). Cauda equina syndrome should not be missed. Has Stuart noticed any change to or loss of control of his bowels or waterworks? Specifically, has he had difficulty passing urine? Has he noticed any numbness in or around his back passage?
- **Assess risk factors** for specific underlying causes of pain (see Box 18.3).
- **Medication:** What has Stuart already tried to relieve his pain? Are there any contraindications to medication Dr Davies might prescribe?
- **Gather social information:** Ask how the symptoms are impacting on Stuart's work and home commitments. He doesn't have a manual job, but he may have to do a lot of driving, or he could be a carer for someone at home.
- **Assess ideas, concerns and expectations:** What does Stuart think is going on? What is he concerned

about? What was he hoping for in coming to see the GP today? This helps Dr Davies tailor his explanation and management plan.

- **Examination:** This can be difficult in a patient with acute back pain. Reduced straight leg raising (SLR) is sensitive for disc herniation. The patient should lie supine, with the legs exposed, and be asked to raise first one leg, then the other. Normal is 80–90°. The nerve root is not stretched before 30°. A lower-limb neurological examination is essential if there are symptoms suggestive of nerve root pain. Saddle numbness and anal tone should be assessed with a rectal examination, if indicated.

After taking a history and examining Stuart, Dr Davies diagnoses a simple mechanical back injury. Stuart seems very concerned that he has sustained a serious injury to his back. Dr Davies delves a little deeper into his expectations for the consultation and discovers that

he wanted a 'scan' on his back to know what 'damage' he's done.

How can Dr Davies explain nonspecific back pain?
'Simple' or 'nonspecific' means there is no serious problem or disease of the back; it does not mean the pain is mild (it can be quite severe). However, the pain should improve quite quickly: usually within a week or so. Most patients initially off work with acute back pain return to work within the month.

What about the role of imaging?
There are no tests (including magnetic resonance imaging (MRI)) that can pinpoint a cause in nonspecific back pain. Lumbar X-ray and computed tomography (CT) scans give a high radiation dose and positive findings are rare. Unnecessary tests also have financial and workload costs for the health care service, can inconvenience patients and can cause undue concern. MRI should only be considered in nonspecific pain if spinal fusion is being considered.[4]

Box 18.1 Assessing pain

- **Site:** Where is the pain? Is it localised or radiating? Nerve root pain such as sciatica tends to be felt more in the back of the leg than the back itself and can radiate to the foot or toes.
- **Onset:** Ask the patient to describe the onset; a sudden onset of acute pain preceded by minor trauma (e.g. lifting or twisting) is reassuring for simple mechanical back pain, although patients with osteoporosis or spinal metastases may precipitate a spinal compression fracture with little to no trauma.
- **Character:** What is the pain like? How severe is it? What precipitates it? Pain on movement is more likely to be mechanical pain, whereas constant unremitting pain indicates possible serious spinal pathology, while pain that is worse after rest may indicate an inflammatory arthropathy. A sudden and severe pain in the central spine that is only relieved by lying down could indicate a fracture.

- **Radiation:** Radiation of pain, numbness or weakness in the lower limbs indicates nerve root pain. Bilateral lower-limb neurological symptoms may indicate cauda equina syndrome.
- **Associated features:** Back pain associated with abdominal pain may indicate an intraabdominal cause, such as a leaking abdominal aneurysm or pancreatitis, especially in a systemically unwell patient.
- **Timing:** What timescale is the patient describing? Persistent pain may need investigation, especially if the pain is constant or getting worse. A sudden and severe back pain, especially in an unwell patient, can indicate a serious cause, such as fracture or infection.
- **Exacerbating and relieving factors**
- **Severity**

Box 18.2 Red-flag symptoms

- Bowel or bladder dysfunction or saddle anaesthesia. These suggest cauda equina syndrome, which needs careful assessment and should not be missed.
- Bilateral, widespread or progressive neurological signs and symptoms.
- Night pain.

- Thoracic pain.
- Systemic feelings of being unwell, fever or weight loss. Red flags raise suspicion of a serious cause, but they are not diagnostic and the whole clinical picture should be taken into account.

Box 18.3 Risk factors for a serious underlying cause of back pain

- Presentation under 20 or over 55 years old.
- Current or past malignancy[5] known to metastasise to bone (e.g. prostate, breast, lung).
- Immunosuppression: patient is HIV positive or is on steroids or immunosuppressant medication.
- Fracture risk: older age, prolonged corticosteroid use, presence of contusion or abrasion.[5]

- History of significant trauma.
- Pain worse in the mornings, other joint involvement or family history of inflammatory arthropathy. These may indicate ankylosing spondylitis.
- Structural abnormalities.

Table 18.2 Management of serious causes of back pain.

Cause	Findings from history or examination	Management
Nerve root pain	Cauda equina syndrome suspected on examination	Immediate admission for neurosurgical assessment with a view to decompression
	Progressive or significant neurological deficit on examination	Urgent referral: neurosurgical investigation, e.g. MRI, and opinion on decompression
	History of nerve root pain not resolving after 6 weeks	MRI. Referral for orthopaedic spinal or neurosurgical opinion (depending on local referral pathways), ideally within 3 weeks
Fracture	Traumatic fracture: significant history of trauma; risk increases with age	Immediate admission for assessment if traumatic fracture is suspected
	Compression fracture: risk increases with age, steroid use, known osteoporosis and being female	Imaging. MRI recommended, but lumbar X-ray (AP and lateral) can show compression fractures; CT also used. May need referral for pain relief or for reduction of the fracture and immobilisation if the fracture is unstable. Isotope bone scans are useful to identify occult fractures including osteoporotic fractures, primary bone malignancies and metastases.
Malignancy, e.g. primary spinal tumour or spinal metastases	Known or previous history of malignancy	Urgent 2-week-rule referral (can also request MRI/other investigations, e.g. blood tests, to aid diagnosis, but do not delay referral)
	History of unremitting back pain/night pain or weight loss	
Infection/discitis	Severe pain, unrelenting pain at rest, fever, localised tenderness. May be insidious onset. Risks include male patient in late middle age, recent spinal surgery and spinal injection	Bloods: full blood count (FBC) shows leucocytosis, inflammatory markers raised. Blood cultures. Admit for imaging, isolation of organism and treatment (antibiotics)
Inflammatory arthropathy	Morning stiffness	Bloods: FBC may show leucocytosis, inflammatory markers can be raised and HLA-B27 is strongly associated with ankylosing spondylitis
	Pain worse after sleep or rest	Consider MRI spine, depending on local guidelines
	Family history of ankylosing spondylitis	Quick referral to rheumatology if inflammatory arthropathy is suspected
	Other joints may be involved	
Structural	Significant gait or spinal abnormality	Quick referral for orthopaedic opinion

---

Investigations and referral

If we suspect a specific underlying cause for back pain (see Table 18.2), investigation and treatment depend on the cause. Blood tests can show raised inflammatory markers in infection (e.g. discitis, malignancy or rheumatological conditions). Anaemia, raised alkaline phosphatase, raised calcium or raised prostate-specific antigen would make us suspicious of an underlying malignancy. HLA-B27 is strongly associated with ankylosing spondylitis.

Case study 18.1b

Dr Davies has explained to Stuart that nothing on the history or examination indicates that he has done any serious or lasting damage to his back and that the pain should settle over the next week or so, although it can sometimes last for a few weeks. He doesn't need a scan at this stage.

What advice can Dr Davies give?
- **Analgesia:** Initially take regular analgesia and reduce to as-required medication as the pain reduces. A benzodiazepine for a few days can be used if there is severe paraspinal muscle-spasm pain. Gabapentin or Pregabalin can be considered for nerve root pain.
- **Promote self-management:** Do usual activities as much as possible, keep active and take exercise. Heat or cold packs may help, as may sleeping on the side with a small firm cushion between the knees or lying on the back with knees bent and supported with several pillows.
- **Encourage return to work:** As soon as symptoms allow (Stuart does not need to wait to be pain free), return to work. Consider a Med3 'fit note' to suggest any adaptations the employer could make (e.g. regular breaks to stand and mobilise).
- **Explain natural history:** Back pain can recur, a bit like headaches can; usually, each episode clears up quickly, and with pain relief people can usually do all their normal activities.

Outcome
Stuart's initial back pain cleared up, but he had a further couple of minor episodes over the following 6 months. These prompted him to lose some weight, make some adjustments to his workstation and start an exercise programme.

Nerve root pain (radiculopathy) assessment and management

Sciatica (or lumbar radiculopathy) is caused when one or more of the lumbar nerve roots are compressed where they leave the lumbosacral spine (see Figure.18.1). This can occur in:
- disc herniation (90% of cases);
- spondylolithesis (when one vertebra slips forward on another);
- spinal stenosis (narrowing of the spinal canal);
- infection, tumour or bony injury (rare).

The patient experiences unilateral pain down the back of the leg to below the knee, which is usually worse than the back pain. The pain can reach, or only be felt in, the foot or toes. Nerve root compression causes symptoms of numbness, weakness or loss of tendon reflexes. Stretching the sciatic nerve exacerbates symptoms, so patients often report that the pain is worse when sitting or walking for long periods and is relieved by lying down. Reduced SLR was found by a Cochrane review group to be a very sensitive (but less specific) test for disc herniation.[4]

The prognosis for acute sciatica is not as good as for non-specific back pain, but most cases settle in 2–4 weeks,[6] although it can take a few months for a herniated portion of the disc to fully regress. Up to one-third of patients have pain that persists. In the absence of red flags or significant or progressive neurological deficit, we can initially advise conservative management similar to that used in simple mechanical back pain; physiotherapy can also be tried. Patients may benefit from epidural steroid injections in the acute phase.[7] We need to refer patients urgently with significant muscle wasting or weakness, loss of reflexes or a positive Babinski reflex, or if signs are progressive, as these indicate risk of permanent damage to the nerve.

If symptoms haven't settled in 6–8 weeks, a spinal surgeon or neurosurgeon should assess the patient and an MRI scan is

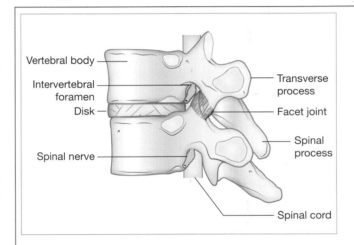

Figure 18.1 Sciatica caused by compression of the lumbar nerve roots.

Top tip: explaining slipped discs

Patients often use the term 'slipped disc', but this is not an accurate pathological description and may confuse patients, who can form an image of their discs being 'out of place'. In the younger age group, compression of a nerve root is most likely to occur from the soft inner material of the disc (the nucleus pulposus) bulging out through a tear in the outer covering (the annular ligament). Some GPs describe this to patients as the disc being like a jam donut with a tough skin, which sits between the bony vertebra and acts like a shock absorber. The disc itself doesn't move, but if the thick skin is torn, the jam bulges out, causing pain by pressing on the structures around it, such as nerves. Over time, the jam gets reabsorbed and the pain resolves.

indicated. Early surgery, such as microdisectomy, probably results in better short-term pain relief and perceived recovery rates compared to conservative therapy with eventual surgery if needed, even if there is no evidence of different outcomes at 1 year.[8] In an associated paper, the authors concluded that early surgery is likely to be cost-effective compared to conservative treatment.

Cauda equina syndrome

This is a rare neurological emergency requiring immediate admission and urgent surgical decompression to prevent permanent neurological damage. It is usually caused by a central disc herniation at L4/5 or L5/S1 pressing on the cauda equina (a mass of nerves so called because it looks like a horse's tail at the end of the spinal cord). Trauma, infection or malignancy can also compress this area and need to be treated accordingly.

Presentation

Onset can be insidious, and not all patients complain of back pain; 30–50% of patients have an incomplete syndrome. Look out for:
- Bilateral sensory loss or motor weakness in the legs.
- Urinary retention on presentation. Over 50% of patients have retention, and the syndrome can also cause overflow incontinence or loss of urethral sensation.
- Loss of perineal and perianal sensation ('saddle anaesthesia').
- Sexual dysfunction, constipation or faecal incontinence.

Other causes of back pain

Back pain can be the presenting symptom of other pathology in the pelvis, abdomen or even skin.
- **Urinary:** Patients with urinary tract infection (UTI) can present with low back pain; it is usually associated with other features of urine infection. Flank or renal angle pain can indicate pyelonephritis, or a renal calculus.
- **Gynaecological:** Dysmenorrhoea can be felt in the back. Back pain with menstrual irregularities, vaginal discharge or increased abdominal girth may indicate ovarian pathology. If the patient is pregnant, labour can present with acute back pain.
- **Abdominal:** Pain radiating from the abdomen through to the back can indicate pancreatitis, a duodenal ulcer or leaking abdominal aortic aneurysm.
- **Shingles**: Shingles causes a burning sensation over the skin of the back. Back pain, localised to a dermatome, can be the first symptom of shingles, and is soon followed by a vesicular rash.

Managing chronic nonspecific back pain

Most episodes of simple mechanical back pain will resolve spontaneously. However, once pain has persisted for 6 weeks, the number of patients who go on to develop chronic pain and

---

Case study 18.2

Karen Thorne, aged 36, had a very similar initial episode of back pain to Stuart (Case study 18.1). Karen's pain started after she twisted to lift her toddler out of her car 9 months ago. Karen now gets daily pain, which improves with rest. She has no nerve root pain, and examination and initial blood tests did not indicate any underlying pathology. An MRI was normal. Karen has now had to give up her job as a school cook. She did not tolerate a course of physiotherapy, as she felt it was aggravating her symptoms. She was recently referred to the pain clinic and now takes three different daily painkillers. She is struggling financially, and blames her depression on her pain. She feels angry with the doctors for 'not getting to the bottom' of her symptoms.

What aspects of Karen's situation make her more likely to be chronically disabled by back pain?
We don't know why some patients develop persistent pain. But there are elements of Karen's case that put her at higher risk of poor outcomes. Karen's attitude suggests passivity towards her symptoms, and she tends to avoid activity for fear of worsening the pain. These are known as 'yellow-flag' symptoms (see Box 18.4). GPs should be aware of yellow flags in patients who develop persistent pain. Manual workers are more at risk of losing their jobs

due to back pain than office workers; this reduces activity, which increases the risk of depression, as does chronic pain. As depression increases pain perception, patients can find themselves in a vicious cycle.

What is the role of exercise in chronic back pain?
Exercise, postural advice, manual therapy and acupuncture have all been shown to be of some benefit for pain that persists, is severe or doesn't resolve with initial self-help.[10] Guidelines are not specific about the type of exercise that is helpful,[11] but GPs often recommend keeping active using aerobic exercise (e.g. walking) or attending a supervised exercise class for muscle strengthening or postural control. There is no good evidence for specific back exercises. Depending on local pathways, GPs may be able to refer into structured exercise programmes. A randomised controlled study of patients with back pain across 64 practices in the southwest of England found that a prescription for exercise from a GP (along with behavioural counselling from a nurse) helped with back pain and functioning at 3 months. This effect was also found for massage and for lessons in the Alexander technique.[12] If pain is affecting work, patients may also benefit from an occupational assessment at work, with workplace adaptations and postural advice.[11]

Box 18.4 Yellow-flag symptoms

- Poor physical functioning.
- High levels of distress.
- Passive, negative or fearful attitude to pain (e.g. avoiding activity for fear of triggering symptoms).

It is worth bearing in mind that a patient does not have to have any of these symptoms to develop chronic back pain.

disability increases proportionally. Up to 7% of adults are chronically disabled by back pain,[9] which can result in loss of employment, depression and dependence on prescription medication.

It is helpful if GPs can recognise those at high risk of poorer outcomes in chronic back pain early on. This can result in less frustration for both patient and doctor, as they can adjust their expectations of recovery and suggest who may benefit from psychological treatments (such as cognitive behavioural therapy, CBT), as well as physical treatments. National Institute for Health and Care Excellence (NICE) guidance suggests that patients should be referred for a combined psychological and physical treatment programme when a less intensive treatment has failed and the patient has a high degree of psychological distress.[11]

Most people will suffer with low back pain at some point in their lives; commonly, this is 'nonspecific', meaning that no serious underlying cause can be found. GPs see a lot of patients presenting with low back pain, and we need to decide which of these patients needs further investigation or referral. Even when back pain is nonspecific, it can become chronic, resulting in ongoing pain and disability for the patient. This also puts pressure on health care services, and it impacts on society when people are unable to work. The challenge for primary care is to reduce the impact of back pain. We should assess the patient's attitudes and beliefs about back pain, manage physical symptoms, provide education about the nature of low back pain and offer evidence-based management strategies.

SUMMARY

 Now visit **www.wileyessential.com/primarycare** to test yourself on this chapter.

REFERENCES

1. Macfarlane GJ, Jones GT, Hannaford PC. Managing low back pain presenting to primary care: where do we go from here? *Pain* 2006;**122**:219–22.

2. Bevan S, Passmore E, Mahdon M. Fit for work? Musculoskeletal disorders and labour market participation. The Work Foundation 2007. Available from: http://www. theworkfoundation.com/assets/docs/publications/44_fit_for_ work_small.pdf (last accessed 6 October 2015).

3. ONS. Full report: sickness absence in the labour market, February 2014. Available from: http://www.ons.gov.uk/ons/ rel/lmac/sickness-absence-in-the-labour-market/2014/rpt--- sickness-absence-in-the-labour-market.html (last accessed 6 October 2015).

4. Van der Windt DA, Simons E, Riphagen II, et al. Physical examination for lumbar radiculopathy due to disc herniation in patients with low-back pain. *Cochrane Database Syst Rev* 2010:**17**(2);CD007431.pub2.

5. Downie A, Williams CM, Henschke N, et al. Red flags to screen for malignancy and fracture in patients with low back pain: systemic review. *BMJ* 2014;**347**:f7095.

6. Koes BW, van Tulder MW, Peul WC. Diagnosis and treatment of sciatica. *BMJ* 2007;**334**(7607):1313–17.

7. Stafford MA, Peng P, Hill DA. Sciatica: a review of history, epidemiology, pathogenesis and the role of epidural steroid injection in the management. *Br J Anaesth* 2007;**99**(4):461–73.

8. Peul WC, van Houwelingen HC, van den Hout WB, et al. Surgery versus prolonged conservative treatment for sciatica. *N Engl J Med* 2007;**356**(22):2245–56.

9. Campbell J, Colville L. ABC of pain: management of low back pain. *BMJ* 2013;**347**:f3148.

10. Savigny P, Watson P, Underwood M. Early management of persistent non-specific low back pain: summary of NICE guidance. *BMJ* 2009;**338**:b1805.

11. NICE. Low back pain: early management of non-specific low back pain. NICE Clinical Guideline 88. 2009. Available from: http://www.nice.org.uk/guidance/CG88 (last accessed 6 October 2015).

12. Little P, Lewith G, Webley F, et al. Randomised controlled trial of Alexander technique lessons, exercise, and massage (ATEAM) for chronic and recurrent back pain. *BMJ* 2008;**337**:a884.

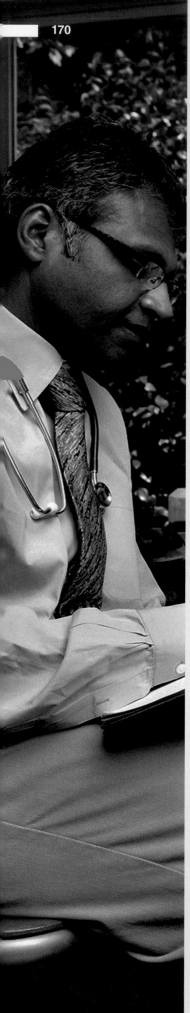

CHAPTER 19
Heartburn and dyspepsia

Jessica Buchan
GP and Teaching Fellow in Primary Care, University of Bristol

Key topics

Learning objectives

- Be able to conduct a consultation with an adult who presents with heartburn (reflux-like symptoms) or dyspepsia, and discuss treatment options.
- Know when to investigate heartburn or dyspepsia to exclude serious pathology.
- Know when to test for *Helicobacter pylori* and how to treat it.

Definition of heartburn and dyspepsia

Patients use lots of different terms to describe the sensations of heartburn and dyspepsia, so GPs need to clarify exactly what their patients are experiencing. This chapter uses the definition used by the ROME criteria, which differentiates heartburn from dyspepsia.[1] Heartburn is a burning sensation felt behind the sternum, rising towards the throat, and can be associated with an acid taste in the mouth. It is usually worse after eating or drinking, and when bending or lying down. In contrast, dyspepsia is a discomfort in the epigastric region of the stomach. It can be associated with a bloated feeling, fullness after eating or nausea.[2] Uncomplicated heartburn is usually caused by acid reflux, but dyspepsia has a higher chance of being caused by peptic ulcer disease. It's important to make sure that the patient is not describing symptoms that are more likely to be angina, gallstone disease or a cancer of the oesophagus, stomach, gallbladder or pancreas. Figure 19.1 shows the common causes of heartburn and dyspeptic-like symptoms.

Diagnosing and managing heartburn

Gastro-oesophageal reflux disease

With reflux, there is little correlation between the severity of symptoms and the pathological severity found on endoscopy. A degree of acid reflux is normal, and often doesn't cause symptoms. If the reflux is excessive or prolonged, the oesophagus can becomes inflamed: so-called 'oesophagitis'. Reflux can cause sore throat, hoarseness, cough and chest pains. These atypical symptoms need appropriate assessment before assigning them to reflux, but if no cause is found, patients are often tried on reflux medication. Smoking, alcohol, stress and anything that increases abdominal pressure, such as pregnancy, central obesity, an abdominal mass or even tight clothing, can increase the likelihood of acid refluxing. Acid reflux can also occur if the tone of the cardiac sphincter of the stomach is reduced, such as in hiatus hernia, causing acid to leak into the oesophagus, or if food doesn't move quickly down the oesophagus (poor peristalsis).

GPs ask about all medication that a patient takes, whether prescribed or not; some Chinese medicines and body-building supplements contain steroids that damage the oesophageal mucosa and can cause heartburn (see Table 19.1).

Endoscopy is not required if there are no alarm symptoms (see Table 19.2), but strictly speaking a diagnosis of gastro-oesophageal reflux disease (GORD) can only be made on endoscopy. If the mucosa has a normal appearance, it is called 'endoscopically negative reflux disease', which is found in up to half all patients who undergo an endoscopy for heartburn.[3]

Oesophageal cancer

Oesophageal cancer is on the increase, and is now the ninth most common cancer in the UK. Adenocarcinoma is associated with obesity and chronic acid reflux (although smoking

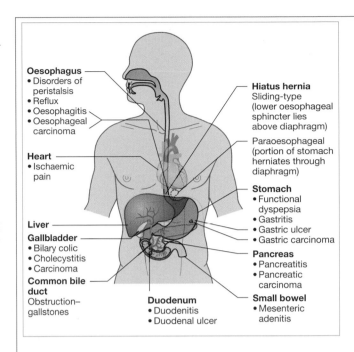

Figure 19.1 Causes of heartburn and dyspeptic-like symptoms.

Table 19.1 Medicines that can contribute to dyspepsia and reflux symptoms.

Can damage the mucosa	Nonsteroidal anti-inflammatory drugs (NSAIDs) – suspend use if referring patient[3]
	Corticosteroids
	Tetracycline antibiotics
	Bisphosphonates – should be taken with plenty of water, and the patient should stay upright for at least half an hour after ingestion
Can affect oesophageal motility	Calcium-channel blockers
	Nitrates
	Tricyclic antidepressants
	Anticholinergics

plays a part). Squamous cell carcinoma of the oesophagus is strongly correlated with smoking.[4] Unfortunately, the disease has to be quite advanced to cause alarm symptoms (see Table 19.2). GPs urgently refer anyone who presents with persistent or progressive dysphagia, and are alert to the earlier (but less easily defined) symptom of discomfort or pain on swallowing (odynophagia), which may warrant an endoscopy.[4] Chronic reflux causes premalignant cell change in the mucosa, termed 'Barrett's oesophagus'. The absolute risk of this progressing to overt carcinoma is low (5% in men and 3% in women),[5] but most patients undergo surveillance endoscopy and take long-term proton-pump inhibitors (PPIs).

Table 19.2 Alarm symptoms in dyspepsia and uninvestigated reflux.[3]

Urgent referral for endoscopy	Dysphagia: difficulty swallowing – needs urgent endoscopy at any age
	Progressive, unintentional weight loss
	Persistent vomiting
	Severe persistent pain, pain that radiates to back, pain that wakes the patient from sleep
	Symptoms or signs of gastrointestinal bleeding, including iron-deficiency anaemia
	Recent persistent onset in a patient over 55 (new-onset epigastric pain in an elderly person is a worrying symptom and suggests serious pathology)
	Epigastric mass on palpation
Other risk factors – consider endoscopy (urgent referral if worsening of symptoms)	Known Barrett's oesophagus or dysplasia
	Previous gastric ulcer
	Previous gastric surgery over 20 years ago
	Family history of gastric cancer
	Pernicious anaemia
	NSAID use
	Patients over 50 with longstanding (5 years) reflux symptoms with other risk factors, such as being white, male or obese

Case study 19.1

Richard Rider is 43 years old. He attends his GP, Dr Nick Pasad, with 'heartburn'. Dr Pasad notices that Richard looks anxious as he rubs his sternum. He says that he wouldn't have bothered, but his wife made the appointment. Dr Pasad finds out that Richard is experiencing a burning sensation behind the sternum, with an acidic taste in his mouth. He doesn't have any upper abdominal pain or discomfort. He's had similar symptoms following a 'big night out' for years. For the last 3 or 4 months, symptoms have occurred with other triggers, such as after eating a big meal. Symptoms settle with Gaviscon (an alginate) he's purchased from the local pharmacy.

What else should Dr Pasad ask Richard about his symptoms?

- **Exclude angina:** Richard does not get the symptoms when he exercises (e.g. climbing stairs or going for a walk).
- **Check alarm features:** Richard has not felt nauseated, vomited or had any difficulty swallowing. He has not had the sensation of food or drink sticking in his gullet. He has not lost weight, or ever noticed black or dark stools.
- **Contributing factors:** Dr Pasad asks about all the medication Richard takes – prescribed or not. Richard says he occasionally takes an ibuprofen (once every 2 weeks) for intermittent pains in his knees. He has never smoked. He enjoys four or five pints when he

goes to the pub twice a week. He knows his usual diet is not good: he is a fan of take-away curry and fried chicken.

Dr Pasad notices that Richard mentioned his wife persuaded him to come. Why is this important?
This is a cue. It's important to find out Richard and his wife's ideas, concerns and expectations. This may not only help Dr Pasad tailor his explanation and address the patient's fears, but also give him some important information he needs to be aware of. Dr Pasad asks, 'What would your wife say if she were here?' Richard explains that her father died from stomach cancer a few years ago and she wants him to have an endoscopy, but he is not keen.

Why is timing of symptoms important?
Richard mentions that his symptoms worsened 3–4 months ago. They haven't progressed since then. This may hold a clue as to the cause of Richard's symptoms and help guide management. For example, if Richard had regularly started using ibuprofen at this time, he may have developed an NSAID-related ulceration, and Dr Pasad would be more likely to refer for endoscopy. Dr Pasad discovers that Richard's job changed 4 months ago. He moved from an active job in a carpet warehouse to an administrative role, because of his knees. He has put

on a considerable amount of weight since then. Richard also misses the camaraderie of the shop floor and goes out for a drink with colleagues more frequently.

On examination, Richard's body mass index (BMI) is 28 (overweight). He is not pale or jaundiced. His blood pressure is 146/88. Abdominal examination is unremarkable, and he doesn't have any epigastric tenderness. Knee examination reveals some crepitus, but he has a full range of movement, with no localised tenderness.

Outcome

Dr Pasad advises lifestyle changes, including weight loss and alcohol reduction (this is also important for his knee pain and blood pressure). He advises paracetamol instead of ibuprofen, and that Richard book a further appointment to review his knees and recheck his blood pressure. Dr Pasad prescribes a month's course of a PPI, with follow-up at 4 weeks, and discusses alarm or persistent symptoms that would indicate the need for urgent review (see Table 19.2).

Lifestyle change in heartburn

Weight loss and refraining from heavy, fatty or spicy food (especially close to bedtime) may help symptoms, but they are also important for general health. Patients with dyspepsia should trial a reduction in caffeine intake, and reduce alcohol intake. If symptoms are prominent on lying flat, it can help to raise the head of the bed. These measures can reduce the frequency and severity of episodes, but are unlikely to fully resolve these unpleasant symptoms.[6] Many patients need medication, which should not be withheld on lifestyle grounds.

Top tip: heartburn and alcohol intake

Heartburn is often one of the first clues to the GP that their patient is drinking too much alcohol, and a sensitive and thorough assessment of alcohol intake is prudent.

Other treatment for heartburn

- Mild or very intermittent heartburn can respond to as-required alginates or antacids, bought over the counter. These can help mild symptoms, but there is no evidence that they heal inflammation.[3]
- Aim to stop drugs that may exacerbate symptoms. GPs often prescribe a 4-week course of a PPI. PPIs work by blocking the production of stomach acid, and can be bought over the counter.
- Although there is little evidence that treating *Helicobacter pylori* reduces reflux symptoms,[6] the National Institute for Health and Care Excellence (NICE) recommends that patients with reflux who have not had an endoscopy are treated as for uninvestigated dyspepsia[3] and tested for *H. pylori*, because of the association with peptic ulcer disease and gastric cancer. If *H. pylori* is found, it should be treated.
- If symptoms persist, some patients may benefit from 1 month's trial of H_2 receptor antagonists. Although in trials H_2 receptor antagonists have been found less beneficial overall than PPIs, individual patients may benefit.[3]
- Treatment should be stepped down if symptoms are controlled. Some patients use on-demand therapy: taking medication as required, or intermittent courses of regular medication. Some

patients can be controlled on low-dose PPIs. GPs aim for the patient to have reflux symptoms less than once a week. Refer those not responding to treatment.

- With proven oesophagitis on endoscopy, if symptoms aren't controlled after 1 month's course of a PPI, GPs may extend the course, double the dose or try alternative medications, such as an H_2 receptor antagonist which can be added to a PPI at night if nocturnal symptoms are prominent.
- Treatment may be long–term, but should be reviewed at least annually, and stepped down where possible.

Diagnosing and managing dyspepsia

As we have already stated, dyspepsia is a discomfort in the epigastric region of the stomach that can be associated with a bloated feeling, fullness after eating or nausea.[2] Most people with dyspepsia do not need an endoscopy, and if they do, a visible cause is often not seen. This is known as 'functional dyspepsia'. GPs need to be alert to other causes of similar dyspeptic-like symptoms or epigastric discomfort (see Table 19.3).

Functional dyspepsia is thought to be a combination of gastric dysmotility and sensitivity to stomach distension. It is more common in patients with depression and anxiety, but it's hard to untangle cause and effect, as symptoms often come and go over a long period of time. Symptoms may affect mood, as they have a negative impact on quality of life. Symptoms may respond to acid suppression, especially if there is acid reflux or epigastric pain, rather than 'postprandial dysmotility' (where the patient feels full after eating). There is a modest benefit from eradicating *H. pylori*, and antidepressants are sometimes used. There is currently no evidence that psychological therapies are effective.[2] There is less evidence for lifestyle change than in heartburn, but it makes sense that if patients can identify triggers, they can avoid them.

Peptic ulcer disease and gastritis

The problem with dyspepsia is that endoscopy is the only way to accurately diagnose an underlying gastric cause, but GPs don't want to subject all their patients to an expensive and invasive test when it is not necessary. Endoscopy is reserved for patients who present with alarm symptoms (see Table 19.2), and when treatment fails to control symptoms as for heartburn. For patients with dyspepsia without alarm symptoms,

Table 19.3 Differential diagnosis of chronic dyspeptic symptoms.

Cause	Symptoms/signs	Tests
Oesophagitis	Heartburn, acid taste in mouth, can be worse after eating	If the patient is well, with no alarm features of risk factors, review medication and stop culprits (see Table 19.1)
Hiatus hernia	Acid taste in mouth, heartburn, worse for bending/lying 10% of the population have one and may be asymptomatic	Consider full blood count (FBC), haematinics, liver function tests (LFTs), urea and electrolytes (U&Es), calcium to check for other causes. Consider upper abdominal ultrasound in dyspepsia
Gastritis	Epigastric pain, can be worse for eating, especially fatty spicy food or alcohol	If there are no alarm or risk factors, trial treatment with PPI or test for and treat *H. pylori*
Peptic ulcer disease	Epigastric pain and tenderness Gastric ulcer is classically worsened by eating, so weight loss is possible if the patient is afraid to eat Duodenal ulcer classically worse at night and helped by eating, but this is not diagnostic. Can radiate through to back if penetrating Anaemia, haematemesis, melena indicate bleeding ulcer Perforation causes severe constant pain, tacycardia and an acute abdomen	If alarm features are urgent, refer via 2-week rule for endoscopy, and consider endoscopy if other risk factors are present (see Table 19.2) Admit immediately if bleeding or perforation is suspected
Oesophageal carcinoma	As oesophagitis, but with difficulty swallowing, food regurgitation, pain on swallowing and weight loss	If suspected, refer urgently for endoscopy under 2-week rule
Gastric carcinoma	As gastric ulcer, but with loss of weight and poor appetite, constant, and with less relation to eating Vomiting and dysphagia, especially if near pylorus On examination, possible epigastric mass If metastases, jaundice/enlarged liver may be present	FBC – iron-deficiency anaemia, abnormal LFTs If suspected, refer urgently for endoscopy under 2-week rule for suspected upper gastrointestinal cancer
Gallstone disease	Classic biliary colic is constant right upper quadrant pain lasting half an hour or more Epigastric pain and intolerance of fatty foods also common Fever indicates acute cholecystitis or cholangitis Murphy's sign is tenderness in right hypocondrium on inspiration if gallbladder inflamed[a]	Check FBC, LFTs, U&Es, calcium, albumin, inflammatory markers LFTs: raised conjugated bilirubin and alkaline phosphatase (alanine transferase (ALT) and aspartate transaminase (AST) rise with obstruction) Upper abdominal ultrasound shows gallstones and biliary dilatation (magnetic resonance cholangiopancreatography, MRCP) Endoscopic retrograde cholangiopancreatography (ERCP) can diagnose and remove stones
Biliary carcinoma	As gallstone disease, but with weight loss Enlarged gallbladder may be palpable Jaundice	LFTs, FBC, inflammatory markers. If suspected, refer urgently under 2-week rule for suspected upper gastrointestinal cancer
Chronic pancreatitis	Epigastric pain (+/− left hypocondrium), may be worse for lying down and improved by sitting. Radiates to the back Diarrhoea/steatorrhoea caused by malabsorption Other signs of malabsorption, e.g. anaemia or vitamin B deficiency, causing sore mouth/tongue or peripheral neuropathy	FBC may show anaemia Haematinics may show low iron, vitamin B12 and folate in case of malabsorption Hypocalcaemia, if malabsorption Glucose: diabetes can develop LFTs can show biliary obstruction Amylase raised, in case of acute attack Initially, upper abdominal ultrasound. Abdominal X-ray can show pancreatic calcification Needs computed tomography (CT)/magnetic resonance imaging (MRI)/MRCP

Table 19.3 (*Continued*)

Cause	Symptoms/signs	Tests
Pancreatic carcinoma	Severe unremitting deep epigastric pain goes to back Jaundice Weight loss Anorexia Hepatomegaly	If suspected, refer urgently under 2-week rule for suspected upper gastrointestinal cancer
Superior mesenteric ischaemia	Older patients, known arteriosclerosis, central colicky abdominal pain after eating and diarrhoea Possible systolic murmur over abdominal aorta	If suspected, admit

[a] Courvoisier's law states that, in the presence of jaundice, an enlarged gallbladder is unlikely to be due to gallstones; pancreatic or biliary carcinoma is more likely.

GPs should stop any medication that could cause or worsen gastritis or peptic ulceration. GPs may start a PPI as a trial treatment (particularly if NSAIDs are implicated) and check a full blood count (FBC) to assess for anaemia.

Upper abdominal ultrasound is often used to investigate upper abdominal discomfort. Classic biliary colic tends to consist in episodes of constant pain (which is not colicky) in the right upper quadrant, lasting at least half an hour, rather than the more vague frequent epigastric discomfort of dyspepsia.

See Table 19.3 for the other causes of chronic dyspeptic symptoms.

Helicobacter pylori

Until the discovery of this spiral-shaped bacteria in 1982, it wasn't thought possible that a bacterium could survive in the hostile environment of the stomach. The Australian physicians Dr Barry Marshall and Dr Robin Warren were awarded the Nobel Laureate in Physiology or Medicine for 2005 for the discovery. Linking the bacteria to gastritis and peptic ulcer disease has revolutionised the management of dyspepsia. No one really knows if *H. pylori* causes duodenal ulcer or is just associated with it; for instance, it has been proposed that it may delay ulcer healing.[7,8] The puzzle is that *H. pylori* is commonly found in people with no symptoms and who never develop peptic ulcer disease. However, it is also rare to have peptic ulcer disease without the presence of *H. pylori*, and since eradication therapy was introduced, there has been a dramatic fall in ulcer recurrence.[3]

> **Top tip: testing for *H. pylori***
> - *H. pylori* is easy to test for and the stool antigen test is accurate at detecting current infection.
> - Advise patients to stop PPIs or H_2 blocker for at least 2 weeks prior to endoscopy, *H. pylori* stool antigen or breath-testing.
> - Antibiotics in the preceding 4 weeks can also result in a false-negative result for *H. pylori* testing.

> **Case study 19.2**
>
> Melanie Mowbury is 38. She sees her GP, Dr Sarah Reaves, complaining of daily epigastric pain and discomfort over the last few months. Melanie feels uncomfortably full after eating, but also has a gnawing pain if she is hungry. Her job as a primary school teacher is very busy, and she often skips meals. She sometimes gets reflux symptoms if she has a spicy or fatty meal. She has not had any weight loss, vomiting, haematemesis or melaena (alarm symptoms for urgent endoscopy with dyspepsia of any age). She is usually fit and well; she is very active and runs marathons. She has been taking daily antacids, but the relief doesn't last long. She does not smoke or drink. There is no family history of oesophageal or gastric cancer. On examination, she is of a slim build, with a BMI of 21. Abdominal examination reveals epigastric tenderness but no masses. She tells Dr Reaves that she really wants medication that is going to resolve her symptoms.
>
> *How should Dr Reaves investigate Melanie?*
> Dr Reaves should check FBC and ferritin (iron-deficiency anaemia would indicate the need for urgent endoscopy). She may also check inflammatory markers. Abnormal liver function tests (LFTs) might indicate gallstone disease. Dr Reaves also organises an upper abdominal ultrasound.
>
> Dr Reaves discusses testing for *H. pylori*. Guidelines advise either sending a stool antigen test to check for *H. pylori*, with eradication therapy if present, or starting a daily PPI for 4 weeks and testing for *H. pylori* if symptoms are not controlled or return on stopping acid suppression. Melanie opts for the former.

Her results are as follows:
- FBC and LFTs normal;
- upper abdominal ultrasound unremarkable;
- stool antigen test positive for *H. pylori*.

What treatment does Melanie need?
If a patient with dyspepsia tests positive for *H. pylori*, they are offered 'triple therapy'. This is a 7-day twice-daily regime of full-dose PPI with two antibiotics (commonly either metronidazole and clarithromycin or amoxicillin and clarithromycin, avoiding antibiotics that the patient is allergic to or has been exposed to in the past year.

Melanie asks her GP if she will need to stay on the PPI and if she should have a test to 'check the infection has cleared'. She does not: she can stop the PPI, and only needs retesting if symptoms recur.

Gastric cancer

Gastric cancer has a poor outlook and spreads early. Patients present with epigastric pain, which, as with peptic ulcers, can be relieved by food and antacids. Treatment with a PPI can result in some regression of the ulcer. However, pain is more likely to be persistent and severe; pain that wakes the patient from sleep indicates a serious underlying cause needing urgent investigation. Beware the older male smoker with upper abdominal pain and weight loss.

SUMMARY

The majority of patients with symptoms of indigestion are managed in primary care. Most patients with reflux and dyspepsia do not need endoscopy. The discovery of the bacterium *H. pylori* and the introduction of effective acid-blocking treatment have revolutionised the management of these conditions. Epigastric pain can also result from pathology in the pancreas or gallbladder. GPs need to remain alert for serious underlying causes of symptoms. Rates of oesophageal and gastro-oesophageal-junction cancer are on the increase, and gastric cancer is common, with a poor prognosis and no effective screening programme.

Now visit **www.wileyessential.com/primarycare** to test yourself on this chapter.

REFERENCES

1. Mostafa R. Rome III: the functional gastrointestinal disorders, third edition, 2006. *World J Gastroenterol* 2008;**14**(13):2124–5. Available from: http://www.wjgnet.com/1007-9327/14/2124.pdf (last accessed 6 October 2015).

2. Ford A, Moayyedi P. Clinical review: dyspepsia. *BMJ* 2013;**347**:f5059.

3. NICE. Dyspepsia: management of dyspepsia in adults in primary care. NICE Clinical Guideline 184. September 2014. Available from: http://www.nice.org.uk/cg184 (last accessed 6 October 2015).

4. Lagergren J, Lagergren P. Clinical review: oesophageal cancer. *BMJ* 2010;**341**:c6280. Available from: http://www.bmj.com/content/341/bmj.c6280 (last accessed 6 October 2015).

5. Jankowski J, Barr H, Ken Wang K, Delaney B. Clinical review: diagnosis and management of Barrett's oesophagus. *BMJ* 2010;**341**:c4551. Available from: http://www.bmj.com/content/341/bmj.c4551 (last accessed 6 October 2015).

6. Fox M, Forgacs I. Clinical review: gastro-oesophageal reflux disease. *BMJ* 2006;**332**:88–93.

7. Hobsley M, Tovey FI, Bardhan KD, et al. Does *Helicobacter pylori* really cause duodenal ulcers? No. *BMJ* 2009;**339**:b2788.

8. Ford AC, Talley NJ. Does *Helicobacter pylori* really cause duodenal ulcers? Yes. *BMJ*. 2009;**339**:b2784.

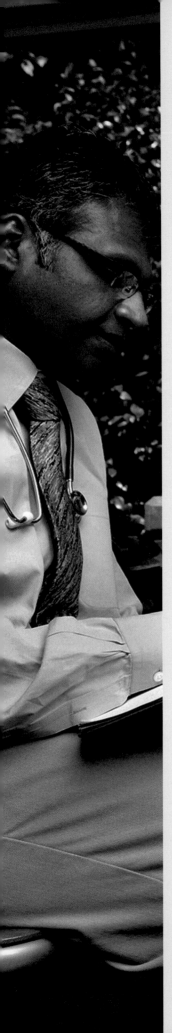

CHAPTER 20

Diarrhoea and rectal bleeding

Andrew Blythe
GP and Senior Teaching Fellow, University of Bristol

Key topics

Learning objectives

- Be able to conduct a consultation with an adult who presents with diarrhoea.
- Be able to explain how to exclude serious pathology that might be causing diarrhoea.
- Be able to give advice to someone suffering from irritable bowel syndrome.
- Be able to conduct a consultation with an adult who presents with rectal bleeding.

Essential Primary Care, First Edition. Edited by Andrew Blythe and Jessica Buchan.
© 2017 John Wiley & Sons, Ltd. Published 2017 by John Wiley & Sons, Ltd.
Companion website: www.wileyessential.com/primarycare

Causes of diarrhoea

The term 'diarrhoea' means different things to different people, so, while recognising that it's a slightly embarrassing thing to talk about, it is worthwhile asking the patient to explain exactly what they are experiencing. Is the stool watery or just loose? How often are they opening their bowels? For some people, opening their bowels several times a day is normal; for others, it is once every other day. This variation determines what frequency they perceive to be abnormal.

Gastroenteritis

If the diarrhoea started suddenly within the last few days, then gastroenteritis is the most likely cause. Gastroenteritis may be caused by food poisoning or by airborne noroviruses. Diarrhoea is usually the predominant symptom in food poisoning, whereas vomiting usually predominates with a norovirus.

Cases of food poisoning peak in the summer, when people leave food out of the fridge and get their barbeques out. *Campylobacter* is the commonest cause of food poisoning in the UK. Two-thirds of all chickens sold in the UK are contaminated with *Campylobacter*, so if chicken is not cooked thoroughly, campylobacter gastroenteritis can ensue.[1] This causes diarrhoea with crampy abdominal pain.[2] There is often blood in the stool, and other features such as fever, aching joints and headache are common. The illness is self-limiting and typically lasts about 2–4 weeks, but it can last for longer. *Salmonella*, *Shigella* and *Escherichia coli* cause a similar clinical picture.

Noroviruses tend to be most prevalent in the winter months. They are highly infectious, and if someone in hospital is identified as having norovirus, the ward has to be closed down. This puts even greater pressure on the hospital, because emergency hospital admission reaches its peak in the winter.

Causes of chronic diarrhoea

If the diarrhoea has lasted more than 2 weeks then infection becomes much less likely, although if the patient has been abroad, giardia is still a possibility. It can be tested for by asking the lab to look for it specifically in a stool sample. The older the patient, the more we need to take seriously the possibility of bowel cancer. Current National Institute for Health and Care Excellence (NICE) guidelines recommend that if a patient is

---

Case study 20.1

Samira Saunders, age 65, presents to her GP with a 6-day history of crampy abdominal pains that are eased by paracetamol. Over that time, she has been opening her bowels three times a day. The GP thinks gastroenteritis is a possibility and suggests that she submits a stool sample for microscopy and culture. The next day, before the stool test has been reported, she returns to see the GP because the pains are worse and her stool has become watery; there is no blood in it. She is worried that something more serious is wrong.

What other questions should the GP ask her?
- Has she been vomiting?
- Has she been feeling feverish?
- Has she lost weight?
- Does anyone else with whom she lives feel unwell?
- What did she eat before this episode of pain and diarrhoea started?
- Is she taking any new medication, such as antibiotics?
- Has she had any operations in the past?

She has continued to drink and is eating small amounts. She can't remember what she ate before this started. Her husband feels well. She has not been vomiting and does not feel feverish. She has not lost weight. She had two children delivered vaginally. She had a cholecystectomy 12 years ago. Her only regular medication is amlodipine for her high blood pressure.

On examination, she looks well. Her temperature is 37.0 °C. Her pulse is 90 bpm and regular. Her abdomen is not distended, but she is mildly tender on the right side on deep palpation. There is no guarding.

What diagnoses should be considered in addition to the possibility of gastroenteritis?

Bowel and ovarian cancer are possibilities. She has had an altered bowel habit, but not long enough to warrant urgent investigation of her lower gastrointestinal tract. However, if it is found that she has an iron-deficiency anaemia then the possibility of bowel cancer will be increased. Ovarian cancer can present with abdominal pain, and sometimes diarrhoea. The tenderness in her right iliac fossa could be due to ovarian pathology, so if her symptoms persist, the GP should check her serum CA125, do a pelvic examination and consider requesting a pelvic ultrasound scan.

The GP requests a few blood tests: full blood count (FBC), C-reactive protein (CRP), urea and electrolytes (U&Es) and liver function tests (LFTs). The next day, he receives the report of these tests and the stool sample.

FBC:
- Haemoglobin 121 g/l (normal range 120–155 g/l).
- Total white cell count 9.0×10^9/l (normal range $4.0–10.0 \times 10^9$/l).
- Platelet count normal.

CRP:
- 56 (normal <5).

Stool:
- No *Cryptosporidium* seen on microscopy.
- *Campylobacter* isolated on culture. Sensitivities are available; please discuss if treatment contemplated. Do not send repeat clearance specimens unless new symptoms occur.
- No *Salmonella* isolated.
- No *Shigella* isolated.
- No *E. coli O157* isolated.

Outcome

Ms Saunders has campylobacter gastroenteritis. Abdominal pain, rather than diarrhoea, can be the dominant symptom with campylobacter. The GP does not prescribe antibiotics (these can make the diarrhoea worse). Ms Saunders is relieved to know what has been causing her symptoms, and 2 days later she is feeling better, but is still opening her bowels a bit more often than normal.

Case study 20.2

Darren Doyle, age 23, presents to his GP because he has been feeling generally unwell for about 3 months. He has lost his appetite, feels nauseated and has lost weight. He has been opening his bowels up to 10 times a day. He describes his stool as being 'like porridge', and sometimes it contains fresh blood. His abdomen is painful at times. He no longer has the energy to play football. The GP suspects that he may have inflammatory bowel disease.

What other questions should the GP ask him?
- Has anyone in his family suffered from bowel problems? Both ulcerative colitis and Crohn's disease have a genetic component.
- Has he travelled abroad in the last 6 months?
- Does he smoke? The symptoms of Crohn's disease are made worse by smoking.

When the GP examines him, what should she look for?
She should examine his pulse, look for pallor of his conjunctivae, palpate his abdomen and perform a rectal examination.

She finds that his pulse is 100 bpm and regular. He does not look pale. He is tender on both sides of his abdomen, but there is no guarding or rigidity. His anus shows fissures and he is tender on digital rectal examination. These findings support a diagnosis of Crohn's disease.

What tests should the GP do?
The most important tests that the GP should do are FBC and plasma viscosity or CRP.

She finds Mr Doyle's plasma viscosity is 1.92 (normal range 1.5–1.72 mPa/s) and his haemoglobin is 124 g/l (normal range 130–170 g/l).

Outcome
The GP refers Mr Doyle to a gastroenterologist, who takes rectal biopsies which confirm the diagnosis of Crohn's disease. He is started on Asacol, and over the next few months he regains his energy and starts playing football again.

---

over 60 and has had a change in their bowel habit, they should be referred urgently in order to rule out bowel cancer.[3] Weight loss and rectal bleeding increase the probability that the patient has bowel cancer.[4]

If the patient has had repeated episodes of diarrhoea with or without rectal bleeding then we should consider the possibility of inflammatory bowel disease.

Other causes of chronic diarrhoea include coeliac disease, hyperthyroidism and alcohol misuse. Table 20.1 gives a more comprehensive list of the causes of diarrhoea and the tests that can be done to diagnose them.

Conducting a consultation about diarrhoea

History

Table 20.2 lists the issues that we should ask about in someone who presents with diarrhoea. Two principle aims underpin these issues: we are looking for clues that might suggest serious

pathology and considering the effects of the diarrhoea. Is the person dehydrated? Does the diarrhoea mean that they can no longer rely on their contraceptive pill, because they are not absorbing it properly? Can they continue to work, or do they present a risk to others?

Examination

Examining the patient will help us to assess their degree of dehydration and may give clues about the underlying cause. Drowsiness indicates severe dehydration. A rapid pulse may indicate dehydration, and in cases of inflammatory bowel disease, may indicate a severe flare-up. Patients with hepatitis A may be jaundiced and might be tender in the right hypochondrium. Patients with gastroenteritis may be mildly tender throughout the abdomen, but will not demonstrate guarding or rigidity. Patients with inflammatory bowel disease may be more tender throughout the abdomen. If we are concerned about the possibility of bowel cancer then we must do a digital rectal examination.

Table 20.1 Causes of diarrhoea.

Cause	Type	Subtype	Investigation
Very common			
Gastroenteritis	Food poisoning	Viral: hepatitis A	Serology: IgM
		Bacterial: *Campylobacter, Salmonella, Shigella, E. coli*	Stool for microscopy, culture and sensitivity (MC&S)
		Protozoa : *Giardia*	
	Norovirus		
Medication	Antibiotics		
	Metformin		
IBS			Diagnosis of exclusion Faecal calprotectin < 50 ng/ml
Coeliac disease			Serum IgA tissue transglutaminanse (tTG), FBC and serum ferritin
Reasonably common			
Inflammatory bowel disease	Ulcerative colitis		CRP, plasma viscosity, FBC, faecal calprotectin and colonoscopy
	Crohn's disease		
Bowel cancer			Colonoscopy or barium enema
Hyperthyroidism			Thyroid function tests (TFTs)
Alcohol misuse			LFTs, mean cell volume (MCV) and AUDIT questionnaire

Table 20.2 Issues to ask about in someone who presents with diarrhoea.

Subject	Issue
Stool	Onset and duration
	Consistency
	Blood in/on stool
	Frequency of opening bowels
Associated symptoms	Abdominal pain/cramps/discomfort
	Nausea/vomiting
	Fever
	Aching joints
Signs of dehydration	Headache
	Tiredness
	Urinary frequency
Food	In cases of acute onset, what did they eat in the 24 hours before the diarrhoea started?
Foreign travel	Risk of unusual infectious diseases
Red flags	Weight loss
	Previous or existing malignancy
Medication	Medicines that might be causing the diarrhoea
	Over-the-counter preparations that they might have tried to stop the diarrhoea
	Medication that they might not be able to rely on because of the diarrhoea (e.g. contraceptive pill)
Home and work	Does anyone else that they live with have similar symptoms?
	Does their job involve handling food?

Management

If the patient has had diarrhoea for 3 days or more, it is worthwhile sending a stool sample for microscopy, culture and sensitivity (MC&S). Most laboratories will test routinely for *Campylobacter*, *Shigella*, *Salmonella* and *E. coli*, as well as looking for ova and parasites. If the patient has travelled abroad then it is worthwhile testing for *Giardia*.

If food poisoning is suspected:

- The patient should be reminded about the importance of hygiene and hand-washing.
- If the patient is on a contraceptive pill, they cannot rely on it and need to take extra contraceptive precautions for the duration of the diarrhoea, and for 2 days afterwards.
- The patient should be encouraged to drink clear, still fluids. They should drink an extra 200 ml each time they pass a loose stool. For older people, oral rehydration salts dissolved in a glass of water may be a better option.
- Loperamide stops diarrhoea and is available over the counter to stop diarrhoea. It may be worth taking if the patient is about to go on a long journey.
- If the laboratory confirms food poisoning, the local public health team should be notified. It may then investigate the origin of the food poisoning.
- There is usually no need to prescribe antibiotics, because most cases of food poisoning are self-limiting and one of the commonest side effects of antibiotics is diarrhoea.
- If their job involves handling food, the patient should not return to work until they have been free of diarrhoea for 48 hours.

Top tip

Whenever we review someone who is on an angiotensin-converting enzyme (ACE) inhibitor, diuretic or metformin, we must remind them that if they develop diarrhoea or vomiting, they should stop these medicines temporarily. If they do not stop these medicines, they are at risk of developing acute renal failure as the result of dehydration.

Irritable bowel syndrome

'Irritable bowel syndrome' (IBS) is a term used to describe a common cluster of symptoms, which often includes diarrhoea. The other symptoms include bloating, abdominal discomfort relieved by defecation and an erratic bowel habit. In some sufferers, the main problem is constipation, not diarrhoea. The pathophysiology is not well understood, but it seems that there are a variety of disease processes at play, including a disturbance of the $5HT_3$ and $5HT_4$ pathways that mediate the sensation of bowel evacuation.[5] Social and environmental factors play a role, too. Although it doesn't lead to more serious physical problems, IBS can have a major effect on the sufferer's quality of life, and it is often accompanied by symptoms of anxiety and depression. As many as 1 in 10 people may suffer from IBS. It develops in adults in their 20s and 30s and can continue into middle age. It is twice as common in women as it is in men.

Diagnosing IBS

There is no test for IBS, so it can only be diagnosed once more serious causes have been excluded by taking a careful history, followed by an examination and appropriate investigation. IBS usually starts in early adulthood; it does not start in middle or old age. If someone in their 40s or 50s complains of abdominal discomfort, bloating or an irregular bowel habit and has not had these symptoms before, we should start by considering the possibility of cancer.[6] Bloating can be a presentation of ovarian cancer. In IBS, the bloating gets worse during the course of the day; when the patient wakes in the morning, their tummy is flat again; in patients with ovarian cancer, the bloating persists. Abdominal pain can be a presentation of many types of cancer (stomach, pancreas colon and kidney), so all of these diagnoses should be considered, especially if the patient is not young. In IBS, the pain is relieved by defecation; if this isn't the case, we should question the diagnosis of IBS.

It is often difficult for GPs to rule out the possibility of inflammatory bowel disease and so they end up referring the patient to a gastroenterologist for a colonoscopy. The availability of a test for faecal calprotectin may help GPs to be more confident about excluding inflammatory bowel disease.[7] Calprotectin is produced by inflammatory processes in the bowel and is secreted into the lumen. A low level of faecal calprotectin (<50 ng/ml) makes inflammatory bowel disease very unlikely.

Coeliac disease also needs be excluded before we can make a diagnosis of IBS. Measuring the serum level of tissue transglutaminase is a good way of doing this.

Guidelines exist to help diagnose IBS.[8] The most widely used diagnostic criteria are those devised by the Rome committee. In order to diagnose IBS, the patient must have had recurrent abdominal pain or discomfort for at least 3 days a month in the last 3 months, in association with at least two of the following features:

- improvement on defecation;
- onset associated with change in frequency of stool;
- onset associated with a change in appearance of stool.

Managing IBS

Managing IBS involves a combination of lifestyle advice and medication.

We should tell the patient that there are two types of fibre: soluble (such as oats and linseed) and insoluble (such as bran). Insoluble fibre usually makes the symptoms of IBS worse. Eating more soluble fibre normally helps, particularly if bloating is a dominant symptom. Patients with IBS often have stressful lives and eat 'on the go'. We should recommend that they set aside time to eat at regular intervals and drink at least eight

Table 20.3 Medication used for managing IBS.

Medication	Example	Indication
Antispasmodic	Mebeverine	Bloating and abdominal discomfort
Antidiarrhoeal agents	Loperamide	Diarrhoea
Laxatives	Ispaghula, senna (not lactulose)	Constipation
Tricyclic antidepressants	Amitriptyline	Pain, diarrhoea and anxiety and depression associated with IBS
Selective serotonin reuptake inhibitors	Citalopram	Quality-of-life issues

cupfuls of fluid a day, but they should avoid drinking too much caffeine. If diarrhoea is a problem, we should suggest that they avoid sorbitol.

Table 20.3 lists the medication that can be used to manage IBS.

Rectal bleeding

Rectal bleeding can be the first symptom of bowel cancer, but more frequently it has a benign cause such as haemorrhoids or an anal fissure. It's not feasible or desirable to perform a sigmoidoscopy or colonoscopy on everyone presenting with rectal bleeding, so GPs have to make a judgement about the risk of cancer. The risk increases with age. Amongst men over the age of 80, the positive predictive value (PPV) of rectal bleeding is 4.5%, but amongst men under 60 the PPV is less than 1%[9] (see Chapter 38 for further discussion of the risk of cancer).

Patients can normally feel haemorrhoids, and sometimes they are itchy. An anal fissure makes defecation painful. Therefore, if a patient does not complain of pain, a lump or itching around their anus, the risk of bowel cancer is thought to be greater. When the bleeding is from a haemorrhoid or fissure, the patient normally sees bright red blood on the toilet paper or on the surface of the stool. If the blood is mixed in with the stool, the risk of cancer or inflammatory bowel disease is higher. However, there is some evidence that placing too much store in the pattern of bleeding and anal symptoms could be unwise. One study[10] asked a group of GPs to refer all patients over the age of 40 for colonoscopy if they presented with new rectal bleeding. Of 99 patients, 8 were found to have a bowel cancer, and these patients could not be predicted by the nature of the rectal bleeding.

Current NICE guidance states that GPs should refer a person urgently to exclude bowel cancer if they are 50 or over and have unexplained rectal bleeding. Weight loss, change in bowel habit, abdominal pain and iron deficiency anaemia each increase the risk of bowel cancer when added to rectal bleeding. Therefore GPs should consider making an urgent referral if a person under the age of 50 has rectal bleeding alongside any of these features.

Haemorrhoids

Haemorrhoids tend to develop as the result of constipation. They are common in pregnancy and in people with hepatic portal hypertension. Treatment is aimed at making defecation easier – eating more fruit and vegetables and drinking more water. Faecal softeners like lactulose can help too. Local anaesthetic ointments and suppositories, sometimes in combination with a corticosteroid, can soothe the pain. If haemorrhoids bleed frequently, the GP can make a referral for banding or sclerotherapy.

Anal fissures

Anal fissures may coexist with haemorrhoids and are also the result of constipation. They can be exquisitely painful. If faecal softeners are not helpful, topical glyceryl trinitrate (GTN) or diltiazem can help by relaxing the anal sphincter. It this is ineffective, anal dilatation under anaesthetic may be needed.

SUMMARY

Campylobacter gastroenteritis is the commonest cause of acute-onset diarrhoea. This is a self-limiting illness, but it can cause dehydration and interfere with the absorption of medicines. Diarrhoea that continues for several weeks may be the result of inflammatory bowel disease, coeliac disease or bowel cancer. IBS is common and often causes episodic loose stools with bloating. There is no specific test for IBS, and the diagnosis can only be made once other causes of the symptoms have been excluded. IBS does not start in later life. Rectal bleeding is most commonly the result of haemorrhoids and/or an anal fissure, but in a new presentation it is always important to consider the possibility of bowel cancer, particularly in elderly men. NICE has published guidelines on which patients with diarrhoea and/or rectal bleeding should be referred urgently to look for bowel cancer.

Now visit **www.wileyessential.com/primarycare** to test yourself on this chapter.

REFERENCES

1. Food Standards Agency. Food Survey Information Sheet 04/09. A UK survey of campylobacter and salmonella contamination of fresh chicken at retail. 2009. Available from: http://webarchive.nationalarchives.gov.uk/20120206100416/ http://food.gov.uk/science/surveillance/fsisbranch2009/ fsis0409 (last accessed 6 October 2015).

2. Skirrow MB. Campylobacter enteritis: a 'new disease'. *BMJ* 1977;**2**:9.

3. NICE. Suspected cancer: recognition and referral. NICE guideline NG12. Available from http://www.nice.org.uk/ guidance/NG12/chapter/1-recommendations#lower-gastrointestinal-tract-cancers. (last accessed 1 January 2016)

4. Hamilton W, Coleman MG, Rubin G. Easily missed? Colorectal cancer. *BMJ* 2013;**346**:f3172.

5. Jones R. Irritable bowel syndrome: management of expectations and disease. *Br J Gen Pract* 2004;**54**:490–1.

6. NICE. Irritable bowel syndrome in adults: diagnosis and management of irritable bowel syndrome in primary care. NICE Clinical Guideline 61. February 2015. Available from: http://www.nice.org.uk/guidance/cg61/resources (last accessed 6 October 2015).

7. NICE. Faecal calprotectin diagnostic tests for inflammatory diseases of the bowel. October 2013. NICE Diagnostic Guidance 11. Available from: http://www.nice.org.uk/ guidance/dg11/resources/faecal-calprotectin-diagnostic-tests-for-inflammatory-diseases-of-the-bowel-1053624751045 (last accessed 6 October 2015).

8. Spiller R, Aziz Q, Creed F, et al. Guidelines on the irritable bowel syndrome: mechanisms and practical management. *Gut* 2007:**56**(12):1770–98.

9. Hamilton W, Lancashire R, Sharp D, et al. The risk of colorectal cancer with symptoms at different ages and between the sexes; a case-control study. *BMC Med* 2009;**7**:17.

10. Metcalf JV, Smith J, Jones R, Record CO. Incidence and causes of rectal bleeding in general practice as detected by colonoscopy. *Br J Gen Pract* 1996;**46**(404):161–4.

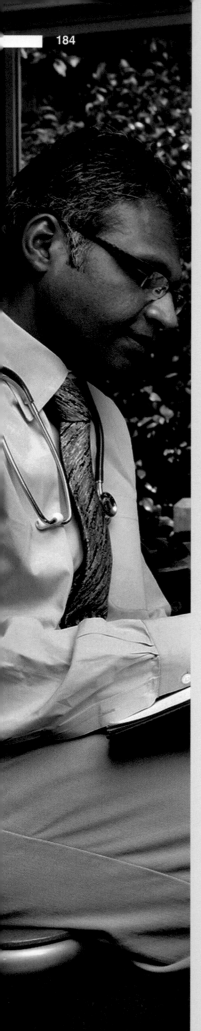

CHAPTER 21
Common skin conditions

Matthew Ridd
Consultant Senior Lecturer in Primary Care, University of Bristol

Key topics

Learning objectives

- Be able to diagnose and manage someone with psoriasis, acne or eczema.
- Be able to diagnosis and give advice on treatment to someone with one of the other common inflammatory skin disorders.
- Be able to identify pigmented lesions that require referral.
- Be able to diagnose and advise on treatment of common skin infections.

Essential Primary Care, First Edition. Edited by Andrew Blythe and Jessica Buchan.
© 2017 John Wiley & Sons, Ltd. Published 2017 by John Wiley & Sons, Ltd.
Companion website: www.wileyessential.com/primarycare

Introduction

Dermatoses (diseases of the skin) are common. Up to 55% of the overall population in the UK has had some form of skin disease, and around a quarter of people visit their GP with a skin problem every year.[1] The most commonly seen problems are covered in this chapter; they have been divided into the inflammatory dermatoses, pigmented lesions and infections. The majority of patients with these conditions are diagnosed and managed exclusively in primary care.

To be able to approach skin problems with confidence, we first need to learn how to describe them (see Table 21.1). Not only will this help us diagnose the problem, but it will also help when discussing or making referrals to dermatology specialists.

Inflammatory dermatoses

The term 'inflammatory dermatoses' encompasses a range of conditions in which there is acute inflammation of the skin. The most common long-term diseases in this group are eczema, psoriasis, acne, rosacea, lichen planus and hidradenitis suppurativa.[1]

People with these conditions experience changes in the appearance and comfort of their skin to varying degrees of severity and bodily involvement, which can be distressing for both patients and their carers. Assessment of severity should be based both on the appearance of the skin and on the impact on the individual's quality of life. Impairments can be functional (e.g. where the conditions affects the hands or feet), social (e.g. avoidance of swimming, bullying for school-age children, low levels of employment and income for adults) and psychological (depression and anxiety).

While doctors and nurses can provide advice and support, current treatments seek only control, not cure, so patients and carers have to learn to self-manage their conditions. Combined with the unpredictable nature of disease, this can place a considerable burden on patients and their carers. In addition, there are significant costs to patients and the health service for therapy and repeat consultations.

Psoriasis

Psoriasis is common (prevalence 1.0–2.5%), with predominantly skin and joint manifestations. It is characterised by scaly skin lesions, which can be in the form of patches, papules or plaques. Psoriatic arthritis affects approximately 1 in 5 people with psoriasis. Patients should be advised to promptly report any joint pain, swelling or stiffness so that it can be referred early for investigation and treatment.

The most common form of psoriasis (80–90%) is chronic plaque, which usually presents between 15 and 30 years of age, or after 40 years of age. It is usually a long-term condition, but spontaneous remission may occur in about a third of people. Figure 21.1 shows psoriatic plaques on the trunk.

Guttate psoriasis is a variant that usually presents in children and young adults. It may be triggered by an acute

Table 21.1 Common dermatology terminology.	
Term	**Description**
Papule	A palpable lesion, usually less than 5 mm in diameter
Nodule	A palpable lesion greater than 5 mm in diameter
Plaque	A flat lesion greater than 5 mm in diameter
Cyst	A papule or nodule that contains fluid, so is fluctuant
Vesicles	Fluid-filled blisters less than 5 mm in diameter
Pustules	White or yellow vesicles
Bulla	A large, fluid-filled blister
Macule	A smooth area of colour change less than 15 mm in diameter
Abscess	A localised collection of pus

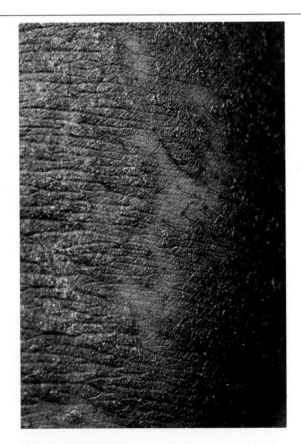

Figure 21.1 Psoriatic plaques on the trunk. *Source*: Morris-Jones, R (ed.) (2014) *ABC of Dermatology*, 6th edn. Reproduced with permission of John Wiley & Sons, Ltd.

streptococcal infection (usually of the throat). Small, round or oval (2 mm to 1 cm in diameter) scaly pink or red papules are usually seen in large numbers all over the body, but particularly the trunk and proximal limbs. It is usually self-limiting, resolving within 3–4 months of onset, but around a third of people with guttate psoriasis go on to develop classic plaque disease.

Other, less common types of psoriasis are pustular psoriasis (localised and general) and erythrodermic psoriasis. Nail psoriasis can occur with all types of psoriasis and is particularly common in people with psoriatic arthritis. Psoriatic nail changes include pitting, discolouration and onycholysis.

Box 21.1 Drugs associated with onset or worsening of psoriasis

- Antibacterials, such as tetracycline and penicillin.
- Antimalarials.
- Beta blockers.
- Gemfibrozil.
- Lithium.
- Nonsteroidal anti-inflammatory drugs (NSAIDs).
- Angiotensin-converting enzyme (ACE) inhibitors.
- Trazodone.
- Terfenadine.

Case study 21.1

Mark is a 20-year-old trainee chef with no significant past medical history. He attends the surgery because he's worried about a pink scaly rash that has recently developed on his elbows and knees. While not very self-conscious about his looks, his boss has noticed and quipped 'That better not be catching', and he's recently started dating a waitress he's met through work.

What should the GP do?
Ask whether there are any rashes elsewhere on his body. While psoriasis classically affects the extensor surfaces of the elbows and knees, it also commonly affects the trunk, scalp, gluteal cleft and genitals; Mark may be reluctant to disclose the latter unless directly asked.

Ask if he has been unwell recently with a sore throat or started any new tablets. Streptococcal infections are strongly associated with guttate psoriasis, and certain drugs have been associated with the onset or worsening of psoriasis (see Box 21.1).

Ask about smoking, alcohol and cardiovascular disease (CVD) risk factors. Smoking and excess alcohol consumption are more common in people with psoriasis, and people with psoriasis are at increased risk of a diabetes mellitus, hypertension and coronary heart disease. Cardiovascular risk should be assessed using appropriate tools, and possible treatments should be discussed (see Chapter 9).

Ask if he has been under any stress recently, and how the rash has affected him. Although patients commonly report a link, there is no good quality evidence that stress is associated with onset or worsening of psoriasis. The psychological and social impact of psoriasis, however, can be significant, and the effect on the individual is not necessarily related to the severity of skin involvement.

Ask about any joints pains and bowel symptoms. Inflammatory bowel disease is more common in people with psoriasis

Examine the areas he's already identified, but also get him to undress and check the rest of his body, offering a chaperone if this includes buttocks/genitals.

What should the GP tell him?
Tell him that he has psoriasis, which is a common skin condition that isn't infectious and comes in various forms. He probably has the plaque type, in which case it is something which he will probably have to live with long-term.

What treatment can the GP offer him?
Treatment with topical preparations: a potent topical corticosteroid (applied once a day) plus a topical vitamin D preparation (applied once a day). The GP should advise him that these should be applied at different times of the day (e.g. one in the morning and the other at night). Emollients can help with itch and reduce scale, but if scale is a particular problem, preparations containing salicylic acid may help. They should advise him not to apply potent corticosteroids for more than 8 weeks at any one site; after 8 weeks, he should take a 4-week 'treatment break', during which vitamin D preparations may be continued. Alternative treatments include coal tar preparations and short contact dithranol.

The GP should invite him to come back if he's having problems or his symptoms are worsening; otherwise, they should arrange a follow-up appointment 4–6 weeks from now to assess treatment efficacy and acceptability.

They should offer referral for second- and third-line treatments (e.g. phototherapy or systemic therapy) if topical treatments alone are expected not to be effective, which is more likely if there is extensive disease or nail involvement.

Acne

Acne (also known as acne vulgaris) affects 9 out of every 10 adolescents between 14 and 19 years of age. However, it also commonly persists or develops outside of these ages. Only 14% of people will see their GP about it, and an even smaller proportion (0.3%) will see a dermatologist.

Clinical features include open (blackheads) and closed (whiteheads) comedones, and inflammatory lesions (papules, pustules, nodules and cysts). These are illustrated in Figures 21.2 and 21.3. With time, scarring can also develop. Lesions may be present on the face, neck, chest or back.

Important differential diagnoses include rosacea and perioral dermatitis. Acne is also a clinical feature of polycystic ovarian syndrome, which can affect up to 10% of women to some degree.

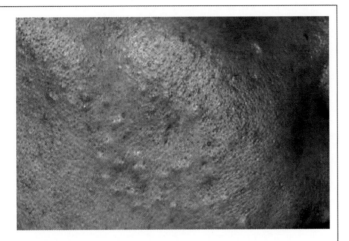

Figure 21.2 Closed comedones. *Source*: Morris-Jones, R (ed.) (2014) *ABC of Dermatology*, 6th edn. Reproduced with permission of John Wiley & Sons, Ltd.

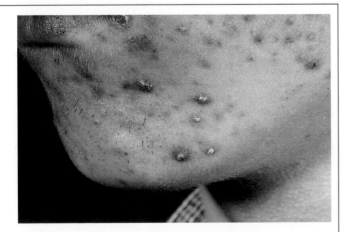

Figure 21.3 Inflammatory papules and pustules in acne. *Source*: Morris-Jones, R (ed.) (2014) *ABC of Dermatology*, 6th edn. Reproduced with permission of John Wiley & Sons, Ltd.

Treatment

The aims of treatment are to improve appearance, relieve psychological distress and prevent scarring. The means by which the different treatments work are summarised in Table 21.2. It is important that patients know to allow 6–8 weeks (3–6 months in the case of combined oral contraceptives (COCs)) before stopping or changing a new treatment. Most treatments are long-term, with the exception of topical and oral antibiotics, where the recommendation is 12 weeks.

Topical treatments

Topical retinoids come in various formulations and strengths, and are recommended for all types of acne. When inflammatory lesions are present, they should be combined with antimicrobial therapy or benzoyl peroxide (BPO). Skin irritation, which is common, may be minimised by using lower-concentration or cream-based formulations, and some patients may find their acne worsens before it improves. Adapalene appears to be the best tolerated, whereas tazarotene may be more efficacious. Topical retinoids should be avoided during pregnancy because of concerns about teratogenicity.

Topical antibiotics, usually clindamycin or erythromycin, are recommended for mild to moderate acne when inflammatory lesions are present. Because of the risk of antibacterial resistance, they should be prescribed in combination with retinoids or BPO.

BPO similarly comes in different formulations and strengths (from 2.5 to 10.0%). It produces rapid improvement in inflammatory lesions and is commonly prescribed in combination with other agents. It has bactericidal properties, thereby minimising bacterial resistance. Skin irritation is common – more so with higher concentrations – but usually resolves with continue use. Patients should be warned that BPO may bleach clothing, bedding and hair, and that it fluoresces in ultraviolet light, which can be a problem in night clubs. Since all retinoids except adapalene are unstable with BPO, these agents should be applied separately.

Other topical treatments include azelaic acid and salicylic acid. Azelaic acid is an alternative to topical retinoids that is well tolerated but can cause hypopigmentation in darker-skinned

Table 21.2 Mechanism of actions of different acne treatments.

Acne treatment	Mechanism of action
Topical retinoids	Comedolytic and sometimes anti-inflammatory
Antibiotics	Antimicrobial and anti-inflammatory
Benzoyl peroxide (BPO)	Antimicrobial, plus weakly anti-inflammatory and comedolytic
Salicyclic acid	Desquamating and comedolytic
Hormonal agents	Sebosuppressive
Oral retinoids	Comedolytic, sebosuppressive, antimicrobial and anti-inflammatory

patients. Salicylic acid is less potent than retinoids and may be used when patients cannot tolerate standard agents.

Systemic treatment

Systemic treatments are reserved for people with more severe or extensive disease, such as when the application of creams to the back may be difficult. Options in primary care are oral antibiotics and, for women, hormonal therapies. Isotretinion (Roaccutane) is a specialist-initiated treatment only, so requires referral.

No one oral antibiotic has been shown to be more effective than others, but not all will work equally well for individual patients. Commonly prescribed antibiotics are doxycycline, lymecycline, tetracycline and erythromycin. Resistance is becoming an increasing problem, so it is prudent to refer to local antimicrobial guidelines. Antibiotics should be prescribed with a topical retinoid or BPO to minimise the development of bacterial resistance and improve treatment efficacy.

For women with acne, hormonal treatments in the form of a combined (oestrogen and progesterone) oral contraceptive may be a particularly good choice if they also need contraception. While some COCs are purported to be more 'skin-friendly', clinical practice is to avoid norethisterone-containing COCs. There is little evidence of difference between the different types available, including cyproterone acetate.[2] Cocyprindiol (Dianette) is licensed for the treatment of antibiotic-refractory acne, but carries a higher risk of venous thromboembolism (VTE) (see Chapter 26). Progestogen-only pills (POPs) may worsen acne. Androgen-receptor blockers, such as cyproterone acetate and spironolactone, provide an alternative, hormonal, noncontraceptive treatment option.

Isotretinoin is the best treatment for severe inflammatory acne. It is prescribed in secondary care and requires monitoring and supervision. Any risks in relation to mental health, self-harm and even suicide are very small. Adequate contraceptive precautions must be taken by females to avoid pregnancy.

Case study 21.2

Kirsty is a 16-year-old student who has come to see the GP about her acne, which started about 2 years ago. She's tried various over-the-counter treatments (which contain BPO), but nothing seems to have made much difference. As a result, she's started using make-up to cover it up. It's started to get her down: she's in the final year of her GCSEs and really wants to have better-looking skin by the end-of-year ball in a month's time.

What should the GP do?
Identify and address ideas or concerns about lifestyle and diet. Acne is not linked with poor facial hygiene – the central discolouration in blackheads is oxidised melanin, not dirt! Diet is not related to acne, but smoking is associated with increased severity.

Ask if she is taking any regular medication. Acne can also be caused or exacerbated by drugs, such as corticosteroids, lithium and phenytoin.

Enquire sensitively about how has it is affected her (socially and emotionally). People with acne commonly lack confidence and have a poor self-image.

Ask if she is in/about to start a sexual relationship. If so, is she using or does she need contraception?

Some hormonal contraceptives may worsen or help improve acne.

Examine all acne-prone areas, including her back, and document the physical severity in her medical records (see Table 21.3). The GP may need to ask her to remove her make-up in order to examine her face.

What should the GP advise?
The GP should reassure her that while there is no 'cure', it takes time for treatments to work and sometimes a trial of several different treatments may be required. There are effective treatments for all grades of acne.

She should be realistic about the timescales required for treatments to work – it may not be possible to improve her skin as much as she would like before her forthcoming social event, for example.

The GP should involve her in the decision-making, if appropriate by referring her to an online decision aid (see Further Reading/Resources box at end of chapter). For mild–moderate acne, her options include topical and oral treatments (see Table 21.4). The GP should arrange follow-up in 6–8 weeks.

Table 21.3 Assessment of acne severity.

Severity	Features
Mild	Predominantly noninflammatory lesions (comedones), with few inflammatory (papules and pustules) lesions, typically limited to the face
Moderate	More inflammatory lesions on the face, and often mild truncal disease
Severe	Widespread inflammatory lesions, nodules, cysts and scarring. Facial lesions are often accompanied by widespread truncal disease

Table 21.4 Treatment options for people with acne, according to severity.

	Comedonal acne	Mild–moderate papulopustular acne	Moderate–severe papulopustular/ moderate nodular acne	Severe nodular/ conglobate acne
First-line	Topical retinoid	Topical retinoid + BPO BPO + clindamycin	Isotretinoin	Isotretinoin
Second-line	Azelaic acid or BPO	Systemic antibiotics[a]	Systemic antibiotics + topical retinoid Systemic antibiotics + azelaic acid Systemic antibiotics + topical retinoid + BPO	
Female-only options		Hormonal antiandrogens + topical treatment Hormonal antiandrogens + systemic antibiotics		

[a] In case of more widespread disease/moderate severity, initiation of a systemic treatment can be recommended.
Source: Adapted from European Dermatology Forum (2011) *Guideline on the Treatment of Acne*. Available from: http://www.euroderm.org/edf/index.php/ edf-guidelines/category/4-guidelines-acne (last accessed 6 October 2015).

Other inflammatory dermatoses

Atopic eczema is most common among infants and young children (see Chapter 15). However, the condition will persist in a significant proportion of patients into adulthood, where individuals will commonly have the other 'atopic' conditions of asthma and hayfever. The principles of treatment are the same in adults as in children: avoidance of irritants, regular moisturisation and use of topical corticosteroids and/or calcineurin inhibitors for prevention or treatment of 'flares'.

Rosacea (also known as acne rosacea) is characterised by facial flushing with erythema, telangiectasia, papules and pustules affecting the forehead, cheeks, nose and chin (see Figure 21.4). It is distinguished from acne by the absence of comedones and seborrhea. It can also affect the eyes (blepharitis), and over time rhinophyma can develop (where, due to sebaceous-gland hyperplasia, the nose becomes lumpy and disfigured). Treatments include topical metronidazole gel or azelaic acid for mild to moderate rosacea and oral antibiotics (e.g. oxytetracycline, tetracycline) for more severe disease.

Hidradenitis suppurativa is characterised by recurrent painful nodules, most commonly in the axillary and inguinal areas. These lesions often recur at the same sites over years. It is associated with smoking and obesity, so lifestyle advice is important. Treatment is guided by disease severity, the mainstay being topical or oral antibiotics (which are thought to act through their anti-inflammatory properties, as bacterial swabs are frequently sterile) and surgery. Simple excision and drainage of boils, however, has a high rate of recurrence and should be avoided.

Lichen planus affects 1–2% of the population and is characterised by itchy, shiny, flat-topped, purple papules, often crossed by fine white lines (Wickham's striae). The lesions are most commonly found on the front of the wrists, lower back, ankles, mouth and genitals. Treatment is usually with potent topical or oral corticosteroids.

Seborrheic dermatitis (or seborrheic eczema) comes in infant and adult forms – but the two are probably unrelated conditions. Infantile seborrhoeic eczema affects babies under

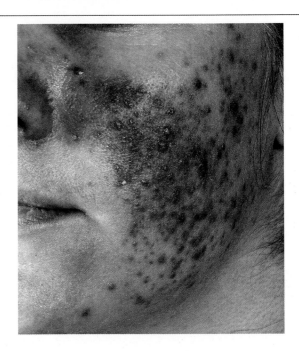

Figure 21.4 Rosacea. *Source*: Morris-Jones, R (ed.) (2014) *ABC of Dermatology*, 6th edn. Reproduced with permission of John Wiley & Sons, Ltd.

the age of 3 months, who present with 'cradle cap' or erythematous scaling of the nappy area, face, chest, back and limb flexures. The adult version affects scalp, face (creases around the nose, behind ears, within eyebrows) and upper trunk. Treatment is usually with a topical antifungal, sometimes in combination with a mild corticosteroid.

Pigmented lesions

Patients will commonly ask their GP to check spots or moles, sometimes prompted by a partner or a news article, and often as an aside to the main reason for their visit. The majority of people will be worried about possible skin cancer. What should be considered and done when this happens?

Start by asking about the lesion itself: Has the patient noticed any change in size, shape or colour? Irregularity in the margins of the lesion or the colour within it are particularly relevant. Has the lesion become symptomatic: itching, painful, bleeding, crusting or inflamed? It is then worth asking about risk factors for skin cancer: sun exposure (in particular, sunburn) and a personal or family history of skin cancer.

Melanomas

A melanoma of the skin is a malignant tumour arising from melanocytes in the skin. Figure 21.5 shows an example of the most common sort of melanoma: superficial spreading melanoma. Factors that increase the risk of melanoma include: a high density of freckles or a tendency to freckle in the sun; a large number of normal moles; five or more atypical moles; pale skin that does not tan easily and burns; sun exposure, particularly blistering sunburn; and increasing age.

To assess the possibility of melanoma, take a history and examine the lesion in good light. The appearance of melanomas can vary depending on the type (superficial spreading melanoma, nodular melanoma and lentigo maligna melanoma make up 90% of all diagnosed malignant melanomas) and site. Use the 'ABCDE' checklist to guide the assessment (see Table 21.5). Pigmented lesions that 'stand out from the crowd' because they are different (the 'Ugly Duckling sign') are a cause for concern, especially if they are changing.

Lesions which are suspicious for melanoma should not be removed in primary care. Instead, patients should be referred, urgently (within 2 weeks), if there is:

- A new mole appearing after the onset of puberty that is changing in shape, colour or size.
- A long-standing mole that is changing in shape, colour or size.
- A mole that has three or more colours or has lost its symmetry.
- A mole that is itching or bleeding.
- Any new persistent skin lesion, especially if it is growing, pigmented or vascular in appearance, or if the diagnosis is not clear.
- Nail changes, such as a new pigmented line in the nail or something growing under the nail.

Surgery is the only curative treatment for melanoma. Prognosis is dependent on the thickness of the primary melanoma and the number of mitoses present.

Other pigmented lesions

Melanoma can sometimes be difficult to distinguish from benign lesions, which include:

- **Moles (or melanocytic naevi)**: Benign localised collections of melanocytes, which are usually oval or round, flat or protruding, from a few millimetres to several centimetres in diameter and from pink or flesh tones to dark brown or black in colour.

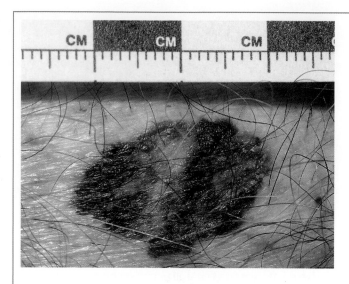

Figure 21.5 Superficial spreading melanoma. *Source*: Morris-Jones, R (ed.) (2014) *ABC of Dermatology*, 6th edn. Reproduced with permission of John Wiley & Sons, Ltd.

Table 21.5 ABCDE checklist for melanomas.

	Feature of pigmented lesion that should raise suspicion of melanoma
A	Asymmetry
B	Border irregularity
C	Colour variegation or changes
D	Diameter greater than 6 mm
E	Evolutionary changes in colour, size, symmetry, surface characteristics and symptoms

- **Seborrhoeic keratosis (or basal cell papillomas/senile warts)**: Benign flat, raised or pedunculated lesions, which vary in colour from yellow to dark brown. They appear to be stuck on to the skin like barnacles.
- **Dermatofibromas (or fibrous histiocytoma)**: Firm nodules, often yellow-brown in colour, which most often occur on the legs and arms. They may arise from trauma, such as an insect bite.
- **Freckles (or ephilides)**: Small, flat, brown marks arising on the face and other sun-exposed areas.
- **Lentigines (or sun spots)**: Larger and more defined than freckles. Arise in middle age and are most often found on the face and hands.
- **Pigmented basal cell carcinoma (or rodent ulcer)**: Brown, blue or greyish lesions that arise in otherwise normal-appearing skin, growing slowly over months or years.

Some GPs use a dermatoscope, a hand-held light magnifier, to visualise subsurface structures and distinguish between these different lesions.

Common skin infections

Shingles

Shingles is characterised by a painful blistering rash which follows a unilateral, dermatomal distribution, most commonly seen in older adults. It is caused by reactivation of the varicella virus, so anyone who has previously had chickenpox (varicella) may subsequently develop shingles. Before the rash appears, patients often complain of pain and general malaise. The diagnosis is made clinically, and treatment with an oral antiviral, ideally within 72 hours of the onset of the rash, reduces the severity and duration of symptoms.

A common complication is post-herpetic neuralgia, which is pain persisting after the rash has healed. The risk increases with age, and in 2014 a varicella vaccination programme was introduced in the UK for people aged 70 years and older. If non-immune pregnant women come into contact with someone with chickenpox or varicella, they are at risk of developing chickenpox, and their baby foetal varicella syndrome.

Herpes simplex

The *Herpes simplex* virus commonly causes blisters and sores. Lesions can occur almost anywhere, but type 1 is associated with lesions around the mouth (cold sores) and face, whereas type 2 causes genital infection (genital herpes). Infections may reappear periodically. The diagnosis is usually clinical for cold sores, but sexual health screening is recommended for genital lesions. Topical or oral antivirals (e.g. aciclovir) are commonly prescribed for oral and genital lesions, respectively, although symptoms usually resolve in 7–10 days even without treatment. Pregnant women with active lesions near time of delivery need specialist advice to avoid passing infection on to their newborn.

Fungal nail infections

People are often bothered by the appearance of abnormal-looking toenails. It is important to distinguish between discolouration and deformity that has been caused by systemic diseases such as psoriasis, subungual malignant melanomas and fungal nail infections (onychomycosis).

Fungal nail infections affect toenails more frequently than fingernails. Typically, the nails feature white or yellow spots or streaks, with scaling and thickening (see Figure 21.6). The diagnosis should be confirmed before starting antifungal treatment, by sending nail clippings for microscopy and culture. Mild superficial infection may be treated with amorolfine 5% nail lacquer. More severe infections require oral antifungals, usually terbinafine. Treatment is prolonged: up to 12 months for toenail infections treated with amorolfine. So, the question is, for a condition that does not pose a risk of serious harm, does the patient want to take a tablet every day for several months?

Warts and verrucae

Common warts are usually easily diagnosed and are caused by the human papilloma virus (HPV). They can appear anywhere, but are most commonly seen on the hands and feet. Plantar warts – warts on the soles of the feet – are also called 'verrucae' (see Figure 21.7). Although warts can be cosmetically unsightly, they are not harmful. In children, without treatment, 50% of warts disappear within 1 year, and two-thirds are gone in 2 years. They are more persistent in adults, but they clear up eventually. They are usually spread by direct skin-to-skin contact, or indirectly via contact with contaminated floors or surfaces.

Patients often seek treatment from their GP, but none of the treatments are very effective. A randomised study of the treatment of verrucae, comparing 12 weeks of treatment by topical salicyclic acid 50% with cryotherapy (freezing the verrucae with liquid nitrogen), showed that the cure rate for both treatments was only 14%.[3] The preparations of salicylic acid that are available over the counter are usually less than 50%.

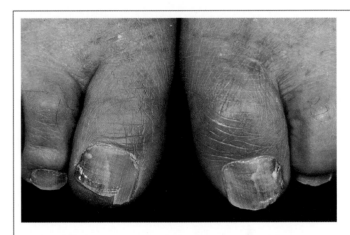

Figure 21.6 Oncychomycosis. *Source*: Morris-Jones, R (ed.) (2014) *ABC of Dermatology*, 6th edn. Reproduced with permission of John Wiley & Sons, Ltd.

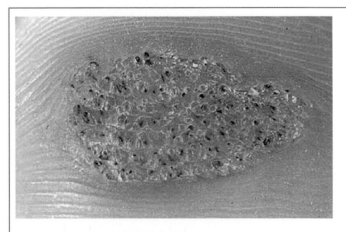

Figure 21.7 Verruca. *Source*: Morris-Jones, R (ed.) (2014) *ABC of Dermatology*, 6th edn. Reproduced with permission of John Wiley & Sons, Ltd.

Molluscum contagiosum

Molluscum contagiosum is a very common viral skin infection caused by the molluscum contagiosum virus (MCV). The majority of cases occur in preschool children. Lesions appear in clusters anywhere on the body (except the palms of the hands and the soles of the feet) and have a characteristic pinkish or pearly white popular appearance, with a central umbilicus. Molluscum contagiosum is a self-limiting condition that will typically resolve spontaneously within 18 months. Treatment (squeezing, piercing or cryotherapy) is not usually recommended.

Cellulitis

Cellulitis is a bacterial infection of the skin and subcutaneous tissue, characterised by a hot, raised, tender area of skin. Always consider underlying predisposing factors (diabetes, obesity, venous disease, pregnancy) when making the diagnosis. It may be accompanied by lymphangitis (infection within the lymph vessels), which is seen as a red line running from the cellulitis to the lymph glands that drain the affected area. It is usually caused by *Streptococcus pyogenes* and *Staphylococcus aureus* and is treated with systemic antibiotics (flucloxacillin or erythromycin). Previously, when cellulitis was severe or extensive, GPs would have to admit patients for intravenous antibiotics. Nowadays, in most parts of the country, it's possible for nurses to give this treatment in the patient's home.

Impetigo

Impetigo is a common superficial bacterial infection of the skin, often caused by *Streptococcus* and/or *Staphylococcus* species, and predominantly seen in children. It may occur by itself (most commonly around the nose and mouth) or as a complication of other skin diseases, such as eczema. It is characterised by multiple vesicles or pustules, which evolve into golden crusted plaques (see Figure 21.8). Localised infections can be treated with topical antibiotics (fusidic acid), but more extensive or severe infection may require oral antibiotics (flucloxacillin or erythromycin). It is highly infectious, and children should stay away from school until the lesions are dry and scabbed over, or, if the lesions are still crusted or weeping, for 48 hours after antibiotic treatment has started.

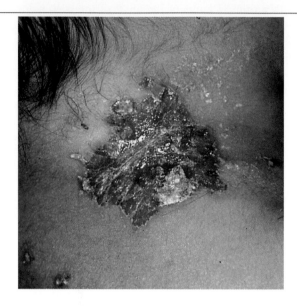

Figure 21.8 Impetigo. *Source*: Morris-Jones, R (ed.) (2014) *ABC of Dermatology*, 6th edn. Reproduced with permission of John Wiley & Sons, Ltd.

Further reading/resources

General
- Ashton R, Leppard B, Cooper H. *Differential Diagnosis in Dermatology*, 4th edn. Abingdon: Radcliffe Publishing; 2014.
- **www.bad.org.uk** The British Association of Dermatologists (BAD). Provides a range of patient information leaflets and guidelines for health care professionals.
- **www.britishskinfoundation.org.uk** The British Skin Foundation, the UK's only charity dedicated to skin research.
- **www.dermnetnz.org** DermNet NZ, an authoritative and free website based in New Zealand, written and reviewed by dermatologists, other health professionals and medical writers.

Acne
- **sdm.rightcare.nhs.uk/pda/acne/** Acne treatment decision aid.

Eczema
- **www.eczema.org** National Eczema Society.
- **www.nottinghameczema.org.uk** Nottingham Support Group for Carers of Children with Eczema.

Psoriasis
- **www.psoriasis-association.org.uk** Psoriasis Association.
- **www.papaa.org** Psoriasis and Psoriatic Arthritis Alliance.

Skin problems are one of the most common reasons for patients to see their GP. They can be broadly divided into inflammatory conditions (which include eczema, psoriasis and acne), pigmented lesions and infections of the skin. When assessing patients, it is important to identify any concerns about the origin or nature of the problem; to consider the psychosocial impact as well as the physical appearance of the problem; and, for many conditions, to establish realistic expectations about treatment. The burden of treatment for some problems can be as significant as the underlying disease itself. In addition to providing information and prescriptions, primary care clinicians can help support patients through ongoing review and, where needed, referral for specialist advice or treatment.

SUMMARY

Now visit **www.wileyessential.com/primarycare** to test yourself on this chapter.

REFERENCES

1. Schofield J, Grindlay D, Williams H. *Skin Conditions in the UK: A Health Care Needs Assessment*. Nottingham, UK: Centre of Evidence Based Dermatology, University of Nottingham, 2009.

2. Arowojolu AO, Gallo MF, Lopez LM, Grimes DA. Combined oral contraceptive pills for treatment of acne. *Cochrane Database Syst Rev* 2012(**7**):CD004425.

3. Cockayne S, Hewitt C, Hicks K, et al. Cryotherapy versus salicyclic acid for the treatment of plantar warts (verrucae): a randomised controlled trial. *BMJ* 2011;**342**;d3271.

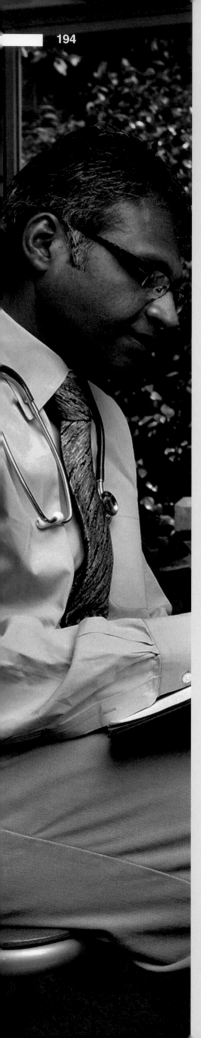

CHAPTER 22

Headache

Andrew Blythe
GP and Senior Teaching Fellow, University of Bristol

Key topics

Learning objectives

- Be able to diagnose someone with migraine.
- Be able to advise a sufferer of migraine on the treatment options available to them.
- Be able to identify a patient who may have a space-occupying lesion causing their headache.
- Be able to identify a patient who has a subarachnoid haemorrhage or meningitis.
- Be able to describe the other serious causes of headache.

Essential Primary Care, First Edition. Edited by Andrew Blythe and Jessica Buchan.
© 2017 John Wiley & Sons, Ltd. Published 2017 by John Wiley & Sons, Ltd.
Companion website: www.wileyessential.com/primarycare

Types of headache

For a significant proportion of the population, headaches are a regular and disabling feature of life. Two-thirds of the respondents in a postal survey conducted in Staffordshire said they had suffered a headache within the last 3 months and 14% reported a moderate degree of headache-related disability.[1]

Migraine and tension-type headache are responsible for the vast majority of headaches. Between them, they carry a huge burden of disability and result in time off work. Migraine and tension-type headache are classified as primary headaches, because they are not caused by another condition. Secondary headaches are headaches caused by another disorder, such as trauma, vascular disease, tumours, noxious substances and infection.

Migraine affects about one in eight of the adult population,[2] but it is probably underdiagnosed in primary care and is often mistaken for the less severe tension-type headache. Both conditions, migraine and tension-type headache, can result in patients taking large quantities of pain killers, which in turn can become the cause of the headache; this is referred to as 'medication-overuse headache'.

It is usually possible to identify primary headaches on the basis of the history alone. Asking the patient to keep a diary of their headaches is often helpful; doing this saves time in the consultation and can be very useful in establishing the pattern to the person's headaches.

Migraine

Migraine is a condition which causes recurring, throbbing headaches that usually last 4–72 hours. The headaches are often unilateral and are accompanied by nausea and sometimes vomiting and/or photophobia. Before the onset of each headache, the sufferer can experience a number of neurological symptoms, referred to as an 'aura'. Visual disturbance is the commonest form of aura; patients can be aware of a hole in their visual field (a scotoma), and sometimes they can see flashes of light or bright jagged edges (fortification spectra). All of these symptoms are illustrated in Figure 22.1.

Less frequently, an aura can take the form of tingling, numbness or weakness. By definition, an aura lasts for less than an hour; if the symptoms last longer than this, an alternative diagnosis should be considered. Some sufferers experience an aura without going on to develop a headache.

Migraine without aura is the commonest type of migraine. Table 22.1 contains the diagnostic criteria for migraine without aura recommended by the International Headache Society.[3]

Migraines are about three times more common in women than in men. They often run in families, and can affect the sufferer for decades. Many things can trigger a migraine, including a change in the environment (altitude, light and temperature) and stress. Changes in oestrogen levels can be a trigger too, so migraines can be linked to the menstrual cycle

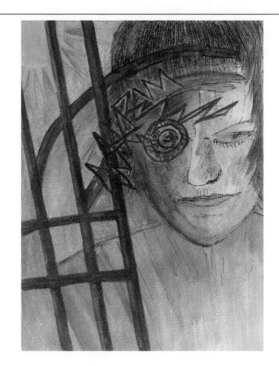

Figure 22.1 'Another Wasted Day'. *Source*: Reproduced with permission from Migraine Action.

Table 22.1 International Headache Society's diagnostic criteria for migraine without aura.
At least five attacks with these three criteria:
1 Headache lasts 4–72 hours
2 Headache has at least two of the following characteristics
a Unilateral
b Pulsating
c Moderate or severe in intensity
d Aggravated by or causing avoidance of routine activity
3 During the headache, there is at least one of the following:
a Nausea and/or vomiting
b Photophobia and phonophobia
And headache is not attributable to another disorder

and can be worse for those on the combined oral contraceptive (COC) pill. Certain foods, like cheese and chocolate, are said to trigger migraines, but the evidence for this is lacking.

If migraines start occurring two or more times a month, the patient may want to consider prophylaxis.[5] Table 22.2 lists the different medications that can be used as prophylaxis. Of these, propanolol is the first one to try.

Case study 22.1a

Charlotte Campbell is 31. She has suffered from migraines since the age of 16. Over the last year, they have become more frequent, such that now she gets an attack about once a month. She knows that an attack is coming on because she sees a shimmering spot in the centre of whatever she is looking at, which makes it impossible for her to read. This spot disappears after about 15 minutes, and then she gets a throbbing pain on the side of her head (the side varies) and starts to feel nauseated. Once or twice, she has vomited. She often has to go to a darkened room and lie down, but this isn't always possible. Up until now she has taken ibuprofen and paracetamol to ease the headache, but these are no longer proving effective. She works part time in an office and is worried about getting behind with various deadlines. She has two young children, aged 5 and 3.

What can her GP do to help?

The account of her headaches is typical of migraine with aura. The GP should conduct a brief examination: check her pulse, blood pressure, fundi and visual fields. Assuming that this examination is normal, they can be positive about the diagnosis and reassure her that she does not need further tests.

The GP should ask about contraception. If she is on the COC pill, she should stop this, because it is contraindicated in migraine with aura. Taking the COC pill

in the presence of migraine with aura increases the risk of ischaemic stroke. The progestogen-only pill (POP), implant, coil and depo progestogen are all safe alternatives.

Charlotte can be offered a triptan;[4] this is a 5HT receptor agonist which mediates vasoconstriction. There are several different types of triptans, and they come in different preparations (tablets, nasal sprays, subcutaneous injections and dissolvable wafers), which have different speeds of onset. The subcutaneous injections and nasal sprays are the quickest to take effect. Taking a triptan at the start of a headache can abort the migraine, and if the headache returns, another dose can be taken. Triptans work best alongside a nonsteroidal anti-inflammatory drug (NSAID) or paracetamol. Because of the risk of causing constriction, triptans are contraindicated in patients with coronary heart disease.

If Charlotte would like something to stop the nausea, she could be prescribed an antiemetic.

Her stress at work seems to be a contributory factor. The GP could discuss this with her in more detail and explore ways of minimising or managing this stress.

Charlotte may also want more information about migraine. She can be directed to the websites of Migraine Action (www.migraine.org.uk) and the British Association for the Study of Headache (BASH) (www.bash.org.uk).

Table 22.2 Medication for preventing migraine.

Medication	Advantages	Contraindications	Side effects/problems
Propranolol	Effective first-line treatment Once-a-day, cheap, safe	Asthma, peripheral artery disease	Cold peripheries, tiredness
Topiramate	Effective first-line treatment	Pregnancy (teratogenic)	Can interfere with effectiveness of contraception Have to titrate up the dose
Amitriptyline	Useful if patient is also suffering from depression	Cardiac arrhythmia	Dry mouth, blurred vision, constipation Widely used, but evidence of effectiveness is lacking

Ultimately, a patient cannot be cured of their migraine, but treatment can reduce the severity and frequency of attacks such that the patient's quality of life is preserved.

Tension-type headache

Although there is a blurred boundary between tension-type headache and migraine without aura, tension-type headache differs from migraine in several respects:[6]
- Patients tend to describe tension-type headache as a band or feeling of pressure across their forehead; it is usually bilateral.

In contrast, patients with migraine describe the headache as throbbing or pulsating and the pain is usually unilateral.
- Tension-type headache is not as severe as migraine, although patients can describe any sort of headache as severe.
- Mild nausea can be a feature of tension-type headache, but vomiting and photophobia are not consistent with the diagnosis.
- Tension-type headaches tend to be briefer than migraines. Sufferers of migraine have a continuous headache that lasts for up to 3 days, whereas tension-type headaches come and go.

Tension-type headaches are best managed with simple analgesia, such as paracetamol, aspirin or ibuprofen.[6,7] Opiates should be avoided. It is important to treat any underlying depression and provide reassurance. That reassurance comes from taking a detailed history, listening to the patient's worries and examining them carefully. Amitriptyline can be used for prophylaxis, and people who suffer from chronic tension-type headaches may benefit from a course of acupuncture.

Cluster headache

Cluster headache is a relatively rare but underdiagnosed cause of headache. It is a type of trigeminal autonomic cephalalgia and is very different from migraine and tension-type headache. Unlike migraine, it is commoner in men. It causes a very severe headache that recurs day after day for up to 2 months, then goes away for several months. The headache starts in the morning and makes the sufferer feel agitated. The pain may be so severe that the patient bangs their head against a wall. In association with the headache, the patient has watery eyes, a blocked nose, swelling of the eyelid and sweating. Cluster headaches are difficult to treat, but they do respond to triptans, given by subcutaneous injection or nasal spray, and high-flow oxygen. If we suspect someone has cluster headache, we should refer them to a neurologist. Often, because the headache is so severe, the patient presents to A&E and is referred from there.

Causes of headache that should not be missed

When a patient presents with a headache, the patient and their GP often worry about the possibility of a brain tumour. The headache caused by brain tumours is nonspecific; it tends to be episodic and responds initially to simple analgesia. It is not possible to spot someone who has a brain tumour simply from a description of their headache.[8] However, the chance of a patient who presents with a headache having a brain tumour is very low (less than 1 in 1000), providing there are no other worrying symptoms or concerning features in the history. Most brain tumours present with other symptoms, such as seizures, numbness, weakness or personality change. Table 22.3 lists the features that should raise the suspicion of a tumour or something else requiring urgent attention.

In cases of acute-onset headache, there are other serious causes to consider. Any type of meningitis can cause a headache.

Case study 22.1b

When Charlotte first came to her GP for help, she was on the POP. Ibuprofen and paracetamol were not helping her headaches, so she accepted the GP's offer of taking a triptan when needed. That was 3 years ago. She has just submitted a request for another 24 sumatriptan tablets. The GP scrutinises her medical records and notes that over the last year, she has been requesting sumatriptan more and more frequently. Now it looks as if 24 tablets are lasting her just 3–4 weeks. She has also had prescriptions for co-codamol (paracetamol and codeine) at various times over the last year.

What should the GP do?
The frequency with which she is requesting sumatriptan and co-codamol raises the possibility that she has developed **medication-overuse headache**. Patients can easily fall into the trap of taking too much analgesia. Sometimes, they start taking tablets before they do anything that they think might bring on a headache. Doctors fuel the problem by prescribing more analgesia and relenting to the request for stronger analgesia.

The GP signs the prescription for sumatriptan but attaches a note asking her to make an appointment to see them for a review of her headaches. She appears in surgery a week later and the GP asks what her headaches are like.

'I seem to get a headache every day now', she says. 'They are making my life really difficult. I'm constantly worried when the next one is going to start—it's always at a really awkward time, like when Tom, my youngest, is having a bad time with his asthma, or when I've got to stay late at work. Perhaps I need a scan or something. It can't be right, getting them this often.'

The GP reviews the history and nature of her headaches and does not identify any new features. In particular, she doesn't vomit with the headaches. The headaches do not wake her at night. She has not experienced any weakness and has not had any fits. When the GP probes more about what she is doing to control these headaches, she says that she takes a sumatriptan tablet as soon as she feels a headache coming on; this is about 4 days a week. Often this doesn't work, so she takes two co-codamol tablets. When things are really bad, she can take up to six co-codamol tablets over the course of the day.

What should the GP advise?
Her account is consistent with medication-overuse headache. The GP should explain this to her. The only solution is to stop all her analgesia. This will not be easy; she should stop the triptan abruptly, but she will need to be weaned off the co-codamol, because it contains codeine. It may be prudent to seek the advice of a neurologist in this situation. When she stops her medication, it's likely that Charlotte will experience rebound headaches, but after a month or so her headaches should start to settle. The GP could consider starting some prophylaxis for migraines.

Table 22.3 Features indicative of a serious diagnosis.

Feature	Possible diagnosis
Onset over 50 years	Giant-cell arteritis
Previous cancer (especially breast, lung and melanoma which metastasise to the brain)	Brain secondaries
Human immunodeficiency virus (HIV) infection	Cryptococcal meningitis, cerebral toxoplasmosis and neurosphyllis (all less likely if the patient is on antiretroviral medication)
Headache getting progressively worse over several days	Brain tumour/abscess
Headache on waking	Brain tumour /abscess
'Worst headache ever'/thunderclap headache	Subarachnoid haemorrhage
Headache triggered by valsalva-type manoeuvre (coughing, sneezing)	Anything that causes raised intracranial pressure
Seizures	Brain tumour
Altered consciousness	Encephalitis, meningitis
Early-morning vomiting	Raised intracranial pressure due to space-occupying lesion
Fever	Encephalitis, meningitis
Weight loss	Brain tumour or cerebral tuberculosis (TB)
Loss of power	Transient ischaemic attack (TIA) or stroke

Table 22.4 Examination of someone with a headache.

Examination	Interpretation
Conscious level	Decreased in encephalitis, meningitis and severe CO poisoning
Temperature	Raised in encephalitis, meningitis
Blood pressure	Increases as intracranial pressure rises
Neck stiffness	Present in meningitis and subarachnoid haemorrhage
Palpations of temples	Tender in giant-cell arteritis
Fundoscopy	Papilloedema indicative of raised intracranial pressure
Cranial nerves	Cranial nerve palsies may be indicative of space-occupying lesion
Gait and coordination	May be abnormal with space-occupying lesion or CO poisoning
Range of movement in cervical spine	May be reduced in tension-type headache and patients with degenerative disease of the cervical spine
Mini mental-state exam	Impaired with CO poisoning

In the UK, meningitis is usually viral or bacterial. In patients who come to the UK from tropical areas, cerebral tuberculosis and cerebral malaria have to be considered.

Case studies 22.2 and 22.3 illustrate two of the most serious causes of acute-onset headache: meningitis and subarachnoid haemorrhage. They also demonstrate the importance of a physical examination in someone with a new headache. Table 22.4 lists the aspects of physical examination that should be undertaken in order to exclude serious pathology.

When should we request a CT of head?

A computed tomography (CT) scan of the head will show up most space-occupying lesions, so having access to CT scans makes the work of the GP a bit easier. When GPs have access to CT of the head, their referral rate to neurology clinics falls dramatically. GPs request a CT scan in cases where the headache has slightly unusual features or is associated with persistent vomiting. If a patient has seizures, worsening headache or signs of increased intracranial pressure, GPs will arrange urgent admission. A CT of the head is not a particularly expensive test

Case study 22.2

On a Monday afternoon, the flatmate of Callum Cooper, age 19, phones the GP surgery. The flatmate is worried because Callum has been unwell for 3 days and started vomiting today. Over the weekend, it appeared that Callum had flu; he was tired, hot and had a headache. Callum has been in bed for most of the time since then. The vomiting is new and his headache seems to be getting worse. The GP sees from Callum's notes that apart from childhood asthma and an episode of knee pain a few years ago, Callum has previously been well. He is not on any regular medication.

The GP decides to visit Callum immediately and tells the receptionists that she will be a bit late starting her afternoon surgery. On arrival, the flatmate takes her to Callum, who is lying in a darkened bedroom (the curtains are shut). Callum is alert and says his head and neck hurt.

His pulse is 82 bpm and his temperature is 38.0 °C. The GP lifts his head off the pillow and detects definite neck

stiffness. His blood pressure is 132/76 mmHg. Suspecting meningitis, she inspects him carefully for a rash; there is none. His chest sounds clear and abdominal examination is normal. He is able to sit up and walk.

What should the GP do now?
The fever, photophobia, headache and neck stiffness suggest meningitis until proven otherwise. She should phone for an urgent ambulance and give him a dose of an antibiotic that is effective against meningococcus. Most GPs carry benzyl penicillin for this purpose. She gives 1.2 mg by intramuscular injection.

Outcome
On arrival in hospital, Callum has a lumbar puncture. This gives a diagnosis of viral meningitis. He is sent home later that day and improves slowly over the coming week.

Case study 22.3

Will Wareham is 35. He is the first patient on the GP's list on Monday morning. She has not met him before. She sees from his notes that he injured his knee playing rugby a few years ago and had an episode of back pain 2 years ago. He is not on any regular medication. He tells her that he has a bad migraine that began yesterday afternoon. He has been taking some co-codamol that he had left over from the time that he had a bad back, but it is not helping.

What questions should the GP ask him?
- Where is the headache? Is it changing in intensity? Has he had anything like it before?
- Does he feel nauseated or has he vomited?
- Does he mind the bright light?
- Has he had a head injury recently?
- Has he experienced any tingling, numbness or weakness in his limbs?
- Has he felt hot or shivery?

He says he hasn't had anything like this before and hasn't had a migraine attack in the past. He assumed it was a migraine because his mother used to have bad

migraines. He says that the headache is getting worse. Immediately, these things make the GP suspicious. He admits feeling mildly nauseated and he has mild photophobia. There are no other positive findings in his history. His temperature is 36.7 °C and his pulse is 72 bpm. His blood pressure is 144/84 mHg. He has definite neck stiffness. His optic discs are normal, as is the rest of the cranial nerve examination.

What is the likely diagnosis?
This is not migraine. The worsening headache and neck stiffness point to a subarachnoid haemorrhage. The textbook description of a subarachnoid haemorrhage is that of 'the worst headache ever, like being struck on the back of the head', but sometimes the history is a little more insidious.

Outcome
The GP arranges an urgent hospital admission. On arrival at hospital, Will has a computed tomography (CT) scan of his head, which reveals a subarachnoid haemorrhage.

and exposes the patient to less ionising radiation than a plain X-ray of the lumbar spine.[9]

Giant-cell arteritis (temporal arteritis)

In anyone over the age of 50 who presents with a headache, we need to consider the possibility of giant-cell arteritis. This causes inflammation of the temporal arteries. The patient often complains of pain on combing their hair or when chewing (jaw

claudication). In fact, amongst the elderly, a headache brought on by chewing is almost pathognomonic of giant-cell arteritis. If we suspect that a patient has giant-cell arteritis, we should request an urgent erythrocyte sedimentation rate (ESR) or plasma viscosity and start treatment with high-dose steroids. This is essential because, if left untreated, giant-cell arteritis can cause blindness. A high ESR makes the diagnosis more likely and should prompt us to refer the patient to an ophthalmologist, who will consider performing the definitive diagnostic test:

a temporal artery biopsy. Giant-cell arteritis is associated with polymyalgia rheumatica, so the patient may also complain of pain, weakness or stiffness in their shoulders and hips.

Carbon monoxide poisoning

If cookers or heating appliances are not maintained properly or do not have the correct flue, they may slowly poison the occupants of a home by raising the concentration of carbon monoxide. Carbon monoxide binds to haemoglobin more competitively than oxygen, so it deprives the body of its oxygen supply. Headache is the commonest symptom of carbon monoxide poisoning; it is present in 90% of cases. The other symptoms include nausea and vomiting, dizziness, impaired consciousness and subjective weakness. As a result, carbon monoxide poisoning can be mistaken for migraine, tension-type headache, gastroenteritis or depression. To raise awareness of carbon monoxide poisoning, the Department of Health recommends that GPs make use of the mnemonic 'COMA' when they see a patient who complains of a headache:[10]

- **C** = Do any **C**ohabitees or **C**ooccupants have similar symptoms?
- **O** = Do the symptoms get better when you go **O**utside?
- **M** = Do you **M**aintain your heating appliances and cookers properly?
- **A** = Do you have a carbon monoxide **A**larm?

Most GPs have breath analysers for the detection of carbon monoxide that they use in smoking-cessation clinics. GPs can use these if they suspect a person has carbon monoxide poisoning. If the patient has been in an affected area within the last 6 hours, carbon monoxide should be detectable. However, if the patient smokes then it is difficult to interpret the result. When a meter is not available to them, GPs can take a sample of venous blood to check the level of carboxyhaemoglobin. The key to treatment is high-flow oxygen (to displace the carbon monoxide). GPs can start treatment in their surgery and arrange transfer to A&E. It's also important to tell the patient that they should not return to their home until the appliances have been checked.

> ### Top tip
>
> Be wary about attributing a chronic headache to sinusitis or an error of refraction. Consider other causes first.

SUMMARY

Headache is an extremely common symptom, experienced by most people at some time in their life, and is usually managed by the patient. For some sufferers, headaches can cause significant disability for many years. Migraine and tension-type headache account for the vast majority of headaches. Cluster headache is much less common and causes a very severe headache that recurs over the course of several weeks. Triptans are useful medicines for managing both migraine and cluster headache, but, when prescribing pain-relieving medication for headache sufferers, GPs need to be alert to the possibility of medication-overuse headache. GPs must also be able to identify the rare and serious causes of headache, which include meningitis, subarachnoid haemorrhage, temporal arteritis and carbon monoxide poisoning. Brain tumours are a rare cause of headaches and usually present with additional symptoms.

 Now visit **www.wileyessential.com/primarycare** to test yourself on this chapter.

REFERENCES

1. Boardman H, Thomas E, Croft PR, Millson DS. Epidemiology of headache in an English district. *Cephalalgia* 2003;**23**:129–37.

2. Steiner T, Scher AI, Stewart WF, et al. The prevalence and disability burden of adult migraine in England and their relationships to age, gender and ethnicity. *Cephalalgia* 2003;**23**:519–27.

3. Headache Classification Committee of the International Headache Society. The international classification of headache disorders: 2nd edition. *Cephalalgia* 2004;**24**(Suppl. 1):1–60.

4. Pringsheim T, Becker WJ. Triptans for symptomatic treatment of migraine headache. *BMJ* 2014;**348**:g2285.

5. Fenstermacher N, Levin M, Ward T. Clinical review: pharmacological prevention of migraine. *BMJ* 2011;**342**:d583.

6. NICE. Headaches: diagnosis and management of headaches in young people and adults. NICE Clinical Guideline 150.

September 2012. Available from: http://www.nice.org.uk/guidance/CG150 (last accessed 6 October 2015).

7. Duncan CW, Watson DPB, Stein A. Diagnosis and management of headache in adults: summary of SIGN guidance. *BMJ* 2008;**337**:a2329.

8. Kirby S. Headache and brain tumours. *Cephalalgia* 2010;**30**(4):387–8.

9. Kernick D, Williams S. Should GPs have direct access to neuroradiological investigation when adults present with headache? *Br J Gen Pract* 2011;**61**:409–11.

10. Department of Health and Public Health England. Carbon monoxide poisoning: recognise the symptoms and tackle the cause. 21 November 2013. Available from: http://www.gov.uk/government/publications/carbon-monoxide-poisoning (last accessed 6 October 2015).

CHAPTER 23

Fits, faints and funny turns

Andrew Blythe
GP and Senior Teaching Fellow, University of Bristol

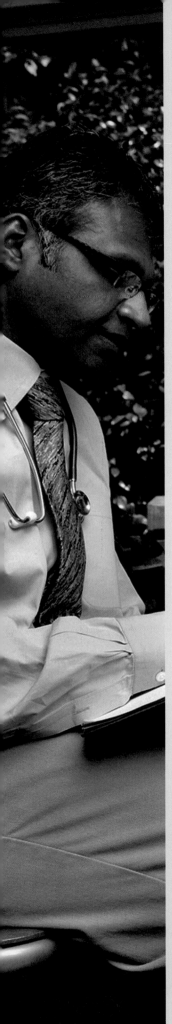

Key topics

Learning objectives

- Be able to conduct a consultation with someone who has experienced transient loss of consciousness.
- Be able to conduct an annual review for someone who has epilepsy.
- Be able to assess someone who has experienced episodes of vertigo.

Essential Primary Care, First Edition. Edited by Andrew Blythe and Jessica Buchan.
© 2017 John Wiley & Sons, Ltd. Published 2017 by John Wiley & Sons, Ltd.
Companion website: www.wileyessential.com/primarycare

Transient loss of consciousness

Transient loss of consciousness, such as that described in Case 23.1, is a common scenario in patients of all ages. There are many causes, but the four broad headings we should consider are:

- *neurogenic* causes of syncope – this includes simple faints (vasovagal attacks);
- *orthostatic* (postural) hypotension;
- *cardiac* causes of syncope;
- *epilepsy*.

Neurogenic syncope

Neurogenic syncope most often occurs because stimulation of the vagal nerve results in simultaneous slowing of the pulse and a sudden drop in blood pressure, which together cause a decrease in cerebral perfusion. This can be triggered by fear, such as that caused by the thought of having blood taken, micturition or defecation. Carotid sinus syndrome is another cause of neurogenic syncope; a tight collar or turning of the head results in pressure on the carotid artery, causing slowing of the pulse. The main risk of harm from neurogenic syncope is that of an injury, such as a fracture, as a result of falling.

Orthostatic hypotension

Orthostatic hypotension can be the result of autonomic dysfunction, volume loss (such as that caused by a gastrointestinal bleed or profuse diarrhoea) or medication – diuretics, in particular.

Cardiac syncope

Cardiac syncope carries a substantial risk of death. Cardiac output stops or is compromised by an arrhythmia or structural abnormality of the heart, such as severe aortic stenosis.

Epilepsy

Epilepsy covers a range of conditions in which abnormal electrical activity of the brain causes a seizure. Not all types result in loss of consciousness.

Taking a history

The key to working out which of these pathologies is responsible for the transient loss of consciousness is taking a detailed history from the patient and an eye witness.

Preceding events, provocation and posture

We begin by asking the patient about what they remember in the run up to the loss of consciousness. What were they doing? Had they being standing for a long time, or had they been exercising? Vasovagal attacks tend to occur when someone has been standing for a while; orthostatic syncope occurs soon after getting up; and cardiac syncope and epileptic seizures can occur at any time, in any posture. If the loss of consciousness occurs during exercise, this should alert us to a possible cardiac cause. Epileptic seizures can be triggered by sleep deprivation and alcohol or substance misuse.

Case study 23.1a

It's Friday morning and Dr Emma Evershed is the duty GP in an inner-city practice. The receptionist asks if Dr Evershed will phone Mr Walters urgently, because his wife, Pam, has had 'a peculiar turn'.

How should Dr Evershed approach the phone call to Mr Walters?
As the GP, Dr Evershed has rapid access to all Mrs Walter's notes on the computer. She checks her age, medical history and medication and quickly reads the notes from her most recent consultations. This information helps direct her list of possible diagnoses. She phones Mr Walters and assesses the level of urgency. She doesn't assume that Pam has made a full recovery – it may be necessary to summon an ambulance. She asks Mr Walters some basic triage questions: Is she conscious? Is she breathing normally? What colour is she? Can she speak normally? Does she have any weakness of her face or limbs? Does she appear to be in any pain? Does she have a fever? The possibilities that she wants to exclude at this stage are stroke, myocardial infarction, pulmonary embolus, hypovolaemic shock and sepsis. These are emergencies.

Outcome
Pam Walters is 53. Her only medical history of note is hypertension, for which she is on an angiotensin-converting enzyme (ACE) inhibitor. Her husband says that she seems ok now (the answers to all Dr Evershed's questions are 'no'), but he is very worried because this morning, while they were doing some shopping, she suddenly went pale and said she felt peculiar. Then she collapsed and lost consciousness for a few seconds. He says she isn't prone to faints. They are meant to be flying to Spain tomorrow morning for a holiday.

Dr Evershed asks Mr Walters if he can pass the phone to Pam. 'My husband is a bit of a worrier', says Pam. 'I feel fine now. I don't think I blacked out for very long. I was able to get myself up and felt better when I got outside the shop and had some fresh air. I don't think I really need to see you. I've got a lot of packing to do.' After a bit of negotiation, it's agreed that Mr Walters will bring Pam to the surgery in about an hour.

Prodromal symptoms

We next ask the patient if they had any symptoms that preceded the loss of consciousness. Before neurogenic syncope, people often feel nauseated, sweaty, warm or lightheaded; sometimes, their vision goes blurry or dark. People with cardiac syncope may feel breathless or sweaty or have palpitations, or they may not have any warning. People with epilepsy may experience a feeling of déjà vu.

Description of the event

We then ask the eye witness what they saw. Did the patient change colour? People often go pale during neurogenic or cardiac syncope; during an epileptic seizure, they may appear blue. During an epileptic seizure, patients may go rigid, jerk all or some of their limbs and clench their teeth. Jerking the limbs is not pathognomonic of epilepsy – it can happen during neurogenic syncope too, although usually the person's limbs will be floppy in that case. If the patient bit their tongue or was incontinent of urine, that would make epilepsy more likely, but incontinence can occur during neurogenic syncope too.

Recovery period

We ask how long the patient was unconscious for. In neurogenic or cardiac syncope, it is rarely more than 20 seconds. Finally, we ask about the recovery period. People who have experienced neurogenic or cardiac syncope usually feel back to normal within a few minutes, whereas people who have had a seizure can take hours or sometimes even a couple of days to feel back to normal, and their memory of events may be vague.

Table 23.1 summarises the key features of the history that help to differentiate the causes of transient loss of consciousness.

Investigation and management

For someone who has experienced a transient loss of consciousness, our examination should be focussed on the cardiovascular system. In particular, we should check the rate and rhythm of their pulse, listen to their heart and measure their blood pressure lying and standing (see Top tip box). We should also ask the patient to walk; this is a quick way of checking that they have no gross neurological deficit.

> **Top tip: checking for orthostatic hypotension**
> - Lay patient down for 10 minutes. Check blood pressure.
> - Help them stand. Check blood pressure 3 minutes later.
> - Blood pressure and pulse should rise on standing.
> - Orthostatic hypotension is confirmed if systolic blood pressure falls by >20 mmHg, or if diastolic blood pressure falls by >10 mmHg.

Table 23.1 Differentiating neurogenic syncope, cardiac syncope and epilepsy.

	Neurogenic syncope	Cardiac syncope	Epilepsy
Age		More likely in elderly	Any age. Onset more common in childhood
Relevant history		On cardiac medication Dementia, Parkinson's	More common in people with learning disability
Posture	After prolonged standing	Any position	Any position
Precipitant	A shock, opening bowels, cough, tight collar	None/exercise	Sleep deprivation, flashing lights, alcohol, drugs
Prodrome	Feeling lightheaded Vision blurry/darkened Nausea	Palpitations, chest pain, short of breath	Feeling of déjà-vu/jamais vu
Period of unconsciousness	Brief: 20–30 seconds	Brief	Minutes
Colour	Looks pale	May be pale	May be cyanosed
Abnormal movements while unconscious	Body floppy		Body rigid All limbs jerk rhythmically Tongue-biting
Recovery	Quick Sometimes, nausea and feeling tired	Quick	Prolonged Aching muscles Feeling tired

The only essential test is a 12-lead electrocardiogram (ECG), to look for abnormalities that might suggest cardiac syncope (Table 23.2). We might also consider checking their full blood count (FBC) to look for anaemia. If the ECG does reveal telltale abnormalities, we should make an urgent referral to a cardiologist (within 24 hours).

Other things that should prompt urgent referral to a cardiologist are:[1]

- syncope during exercise;
- family history of sudden cardiac death;
- new breathlessness;
- heart failure;
- heart murmur.

Requesting a 24-hour ECG is unlikely to be helpful unless the patient has daily symptoms.[1]

If there was a clear provoking factor for the loss of consciousness, it occurred while standing and the patient experienced prodromal symptoms, neurogenic syncope is likely. If, in addition to this, there is no drop in blood pressure and a 12-lead ECG is normal, then there is no need for further investigation. We can reassure the patient, explain why they lost consciousness and give them some advice on what to do if this happens again. If they feel that they are about to faint, they should lie down and put their legs up to promote blood flow to the brain. If there isn't room to lie down, they should sit down with their knees up and put their head between their knees. Unless the syncopal episode was caused by coughing, they can still drive.

Epilepsy

The classification of epilepsy can be confusing. The current system of classification (see Table 23.3) is a descriptive one. The word 'complex' is used to denote impairment of

Table 23.2 Abnormalities on 12-lead ECG that suggest cardiac syncope.

Rate < 50 bpm
Heart block
Right or left bundle branch block
Ventricular arrhythmia
Sustained atrial arrhythmia (e.g. atrial fibrillation)
QT interval too short (<350 ms) or too long (>450 ms)
ST-segment or T-wave abnormalities

Case study 23.1b

When Dr Evershed calls Mrs Walters, she notes that Mrs Walters looks well and walks normally into the consulting room. Dr Evershed asks her to go through the morning's events again. Mrs Walters and her husband had got up early and had walked into town. They had been shopping for about an hour, and Mrs Walters was standing in a queue, when she suddenly felt lightheaded and then fell to the ground. Her husband says she looked pale. He wasn't able to check her pulse at the time, but she came round within a few seconds. She did not bite her tongue and was not incontinent. Mr Walters is sure that he did not see her twitch or jerk any of her limbs. One of the assistants had asked if she should call for an ambulance, but Mrs Walters had insisted this was not necessary. She left the shop and sat on a bench for a minute or two, then they got a taxi home and phoned the doctor's surgery.

What other questions should Dr Evershed ask Mrs Walters?
She should ask if she felt sweaty or nauseated. Did she feel short of breath or experience any palpitations? Has she had any similar episodes in the past? Has anyone in her family had any heart problems?

Outcome
Mrs Walters says 'no' to these things, but says there was one occasion earlier in the morning when she was aware of her heart racing briefly.

Examining her, Dr Evershed is surprised to find that her pulse is 92 bpm and is irregularly irregular. Her apex rate is the same. Her blood pressure is 124/76 mmHg and her heart sounds are normal; there are no murmurs.

Dr Evershed asks the practice nurse to do an ECG. This confirms atrial fibrillation, with a rate of around 90–100. This is a new diagnosis and suggests that the syncopal episode this morning was due to an arrhythmia. Dr Evershed explains this to Mrs Walters, makes an urgent referral to a cardiologist and breaks the bad news to Mr and Mrs Walters that they need to think about cancelling their holiday.

What were the clues that this was cardiac syncope?
Mrs Walters' history of hypertension and her palpitations were the main clues. However, the fact that she lost consciousness after walking and when she had been standing for a while seemed to point towards a diagnosis of neurogenic syncope. This case illustrates the importance of keeping an open mind, carefully considering possible differential diagnoses and carrying out a cardiovascular examination and ECG in someone who has had a transient loss of consciousness. For more information on the management of atrial fibrillation, see Chapter 29.

Table 23.3 Classification of epilepsy.

Focal	Simple focal
	Complex focal
	Focal evolving into secondarily generalised seizures
Generalised	Absence
	Atypical absence
	Myoclonic
	Clonic
	Tonic-clonic
	Atonic

consciousness, while a 'partial seizure' is one in which consciousness is preserved. The words 'focal' and 'generalised' are used to describe the extent to which the seizure affects the body; 'generalised' implies that the whole body is involved.

For a long time, epilepsy has been a somewhat neglected chronic disease in the UK, despite the fact that it affects around 1 in 100 to 1 in 200 people[2] and carries a risk of premature death.[3] Much of the excess mortality results from accidents that occur when someone has a fit: drowning, burns and falls. The highest mortality is observed in young men. People are also at greater risk of dying from epilepsy if they drink too much alcohol, if they fail to collect their prescriptions for antiepileptic drugs or if they are depressed. All these things are linked: alcohol makes depression worse, and people who are depressed may be less likely to take medication as instructed.

A diagnosis of epilepsy can have a very negative effect on all aspects of the sufferer's life. There is still some social stigma attached to the diagnosis. The word 'seizure' stems from the belief that the sufferer was 'seized by a spirit'. The unpredictability and frequency of fits for many people is extremely difficult to live with and can cause depression. If epilepsy is not well controlled, it is a bar to driving and to doing many jobs. As a result, the patient's socioeconomic status is affected. On top of this, a lot of the medication that is used to control epilepsy has unpleasant side effects.

There is also evidence to suggest that some people may have been incorrectly diagnosed with epilepsy and may be on inappropriate medication.

The situation is improving, though. GPs (steered by a new contract in 2004) have focussed more of their attention on people with epilepsy. The main roles of the GP are:

- Identifying and referring people who might have epilepsy.
- Prescribing and monitoring antiepileptic medication.
- Conducting annual reviews to check that the epilepsy is well controlled and its impact is minimised.

Meanwhile, as the result of National Institute for Health and Care Excellence (NICE) guidance,[4] hospital neurology services have begun offering appointments more quickly to someone suspected of having epilepsy. Many hospitals employ epilepsy specialist nurses who can support and advise patients and their GPs. All of these improvements should result in more people being diagnosed correctly and in those who do have epilepsy remaining seizure-free or having fewer fits. The aim is to improve sufferers' quality of life and reduce their risk of death.

Assessing and referring someone who might have had an epileptic fit

In the section on Transient Loss of Consciousness, we reviewed the features of the history that support a diagnosis of epilepsy – the features before, during and after the loss of consciousness (Table 23.1). Remember, it is essential to get a history from an eye witness.

Spotting someone who might have partial epilepsy is more tricky. The seizures may take the form of relatively innocuous movements, such as lip-smacking, or they may be confused with panic attacks.

Seizures can be caused by brain tumours or structural abnormalities. It is important to ask about other neurological symptoms, in particular weakness, numbness and visual changes, before going on to perform a neurological examination.

If a GP suspects epilepsy, the current NICE guidelines recommend an urgent referral, with the intention that the patient is seen by a neurologist within 2 weeks. This urgency stems from the fact that if it is epilepsy, the patient is at risk of having another seizure. The National General Practice Study of Epilepsy showed that within a year of having their first seizure, two-thirds of people suffered a recurrence (i.e. a second fit).[5] The risk of recurrence is highest amongst children, those over 59 and those who've had a partial seizure. But even for adults who have had a single complex, generalised, tonic-clonic seizure, there is a roughly 70% chance that they will have another fit within 3 years.

At the time of referral, the GP needs to make clear to the patient the potential risks of epilepsy and advise them to:

- Inform the Driver and Vehicle Licensing Agency (DVLA): until instructed otherwise, they should not drive.
- Avoid going near water or machinery, unless supervised.
- Inform their employer.

The neurologist usually makes the diagnosis based on the history and examination, but will do some investigations. A magnetic resonance imaging (MRI) scan is required to rule out structural abnormalities of the brain. This is particularly important if there are any focal features to the seizure. The neurologist may also request an electroencephalogram (EEG). A normal EEG doesn't rule out the possibility of an epileptic seizure, but an abnormal EEG supports a diagnosis of epilepsy and is associated with an increased risk of having a second seizure.

A crucial decision that the neurologist has to make with the patient is whether or not to start antiepileptic medication immediately. NICE recommends that it is started after a second fit, but gives the neurologist discretion whether or not to start it after the first.

There are a growing number of antiepileptic drugs. Monotherapy is preferable, but many people end up on a combination of drugs. The choice of drug is dictated by the type of seizure, the age and gender of the patient and any other medication the patient may be on. Sodium valproate and lamotrigine are the first-line drugs for preventing generalised tonic-clonic seizures. Sodium valproate has a greater teratogenic risk, so for women of child-bearing age, lamotrigine is best.

Conducting an annual review of someone with epilepsy

Although most GPs do not have expertise in selecting the most appropriate antiepileptic drugs, they are well placed to take a holistic review of the patient who has epilepsy.

Addressing the patient's concerns

As in the review of any chronic disease, it's important to identify at the outset what, if any, concerns the patient has; this might be a potential side effect of their medicine, or it might be difficulty finding a job.

Assessing control

Assessing the current control of the epilepsy involves asking the patient when they last had a fit and finding out how often they have a seizure. If they have had a seizure within the last year, the GP should explore, in a sensitive manner, their adherence with the medication. If they are not taking it regularly, it may be because they are concerned about side effects. If they are taking the medication as instructed, the GP might consider increasing the dose of one of the antiepileptic drugs or contacting the neurologist for advice.

Despite being on a combination of several antiepileptic drugs, some patients' epilepsy may be very difficult to control and they may have prolonged fits: status epilepticus. For this eventuality, the GP can prescribe buccal midazolam or rectal diazepam, which the patient's carer can administer to stop the seizure.

Contraception issues

As well as being teratogenic, some antiepileptic drugs, such as phenytoin, have an enzyme-inducing effect and increase the metabolism of the combined oral contraceptive (COC) pill and progestogen-only pill (POP). If a woman uses one of these forms of contraception, it is advisable for her to switch to an alternative method. NICE recommends that a woman on enzyme-inducing antiepileptic medication takes an oral contraceptive containing at least 50 µg of ethinyl oestradiol. If she wants to get pregnant then the GP should ask the neurologist to review her, explain the risks and give advice about switching to the safest antiepileptic drug.

Assessing mood

Depression is very common amongst people with epilepsy, so it's worthwhile exploring this possibility during an annual review. Many antiepileptic drugs affect mood, so if someone does appear depressed, the first option to consider is switching to another drug. GPs have to be very cautious about starting antidepressant medication, because some antidepressants increase the risk of seizure and interact with antiepileptic medication. Psychological therapy is preferable and safer.

Work and home

People with poorly controlled epilepsy may struggle to find work and may be in receipt of benefits. Often, they need their GP to write letters to explain their diagnosis and treatment. Sometimes, they just need someone who will listen to them and understand the difficulties they face.

Warnings

An annual review is also an opportunity to reiterate advice that the patient should never go near water or machinery by themselves. If the patient has been fit-free for 5 years, they may be able to ask for their ordinary driving licence again. The rules on this change, but they are readily accessible in the DVLA document 'At a Glance Guide to Current Medical Standards of Fitness to Drive'.[6] People cannot drive a lorry or bus until they have been fit-free and off all antiepileptic medication for 10 years.

The outcome of an annual review might be a referral to the neurologist or the epilepsy specialist nurse, or simply renewal of the existing prescription.

Dizziness

'Dizziness' can be used by patients to describe all sorts of things. Some people use the term to convey a general sense of unease. If they feel like this a lot of the time, it might be that they are suffering from anxiety. Some use it to describe feeling lightheaded, others to describe presyncope or an illusion of movement (vertigo).

Vertigo is not a diagnosis, it is a symptom. People describe it as feeling like they are on a boat or have just come off a merry-go-round. The existence of vertigo implies that there is a vestibular problem. Despite the fact that it is a common reason for people consulting their GP, a recent systematic review[7] concluded that no good studies have been done on the epidemiology of vertigo in primary care; most studies of the causes of vertigo have been done in secondary care. Here we will consider what are thought to be the three commonest causes of vertigo: benign paroxysmal positional vertigo (BPPV), acute vestibular neuronitis (often referred to as 'labyrinthitis') and Meniere's disease.

Benign paroxysmal positional vertigo

BPPV is probably the commonest cause of vertigo. It is characterised by recurrent brief episodes of vertigo that come on a second or two after the patient moves their head in a certain direction, such as when they turn their head on their pillow or get out of bed. It may be accompanied by nausea or vomiting.

It is commonest in people over the age of 50. Although the episodes only last a few seconds, sufferers can have numerous episodes in a day.

We think that BPPV is caused by free-floating debris in the posterior semicircular canal. This debris acts like a plunger, causing persistent movement of the endolymph after the sufferer has stopped moving their head. It is this movement of the endolymph that gives the illusion of movement.

BPPV is diagnosed using the Hallpike manoeuvre,[8] which can be done in the GP surgery (Figure 23.1). If the manoeuvre produces horizontal nystagmus, the diagnosis is confirmed and we can reassure the patient. BPPV does not progress to something worse.

Because the episodes are so brief, there is no role for medication. However, it is possible to dislodge the debris that causes the vertigo using the Epley manoeuvre (see Figure 23.2). A Cochrane review[9] concluded that the Epley manoeuvre is better than sham manoeuvre or control at producing resolution of vertigo. It is a safe treatment, but some patients experience a recurrence. For those who do not experience benefit, vestibular rehabilitation can be helpful. Vestibular rehabilitation consists of exercises that help patients to use other sensory inputs – sight and proprioception – to overcome their vertigo.

Acute vestibular neuronitis (labyrinithitis)

Acute vestibular neuronitis tends to occur in younger adults and has a sudden onset. It can follow respiratory tract symptoms and so it is thought to have an infective cause. The bout of vertigo can last for several days before subsiding and is often accompanied by nausea or vomiting. Repeated bouts of vertigo can occur over the next few weeks, but each bout is less severe and is followed by complete resolution. It's very unlikely that someone will get acute vestibular neuronitis for a second time, so if they experience a bout of vertigo months later, it's worthwhile reviewing the diagnosis; it may be Meniere's disease or BPPV.

Someone with acute vestibular neuronitis may have unprovoked nystagmus on looking forward. In this scenario, it is important to exclude the possibility of a cerebellar stroke. To do this, the GP should examine all the cranial nerves, check finger-to-nose coordination, look for dysdiadochokinesia and ask the patient to stand without holding on to anything. Someone who has had a cerebellar stroke will have poor coordination and will not be capable of standing.

Sufferers of acute vestibular neuronitis normally need treatment with an antiemetic such as prochlorperazine. If necessary, this can be given in buccal form or as an intramuscular injection.

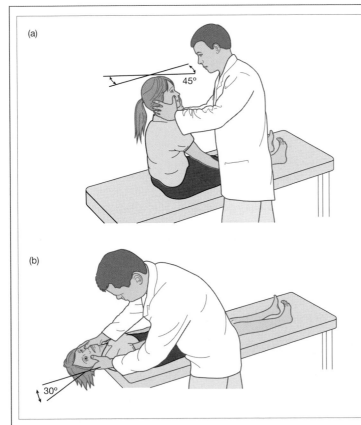

- Ask the patient to sit on the couch and tell them that in order to make an assessment of their dizziness you will tip them backwards while looking at their eyes.

- Warn them that this may feel unpleasant for a little while and may reproduce their symptoms, but you will support their head at all times and ensure that they are safe.

- They must be seated on the couch in such a way that when you tip them backwards, their head can hang over the edge of the couch.

- With the patient sat upright on the couch, turn their head towards yours and ask them to fix their eyes on your forehead.

- Hold their head by placing one hand on each side of it, then tip it backwards until it is 30° below horizontal.

- Keep them in this position for 30 seconds. Ask them to keep their eyes fixed on the same position on your forehead.

- You are looking for nystagmus. A horizontal nystagmus in which the fast movements are directed towards the lowermost ear suggests that they have BPPV.

- Sit the patient upright and repeat the procedure with the patient's head turned to the other side. You will need to get on the other side of the couch to do this.

Figure 23.1 Hallpike manoeuvre.

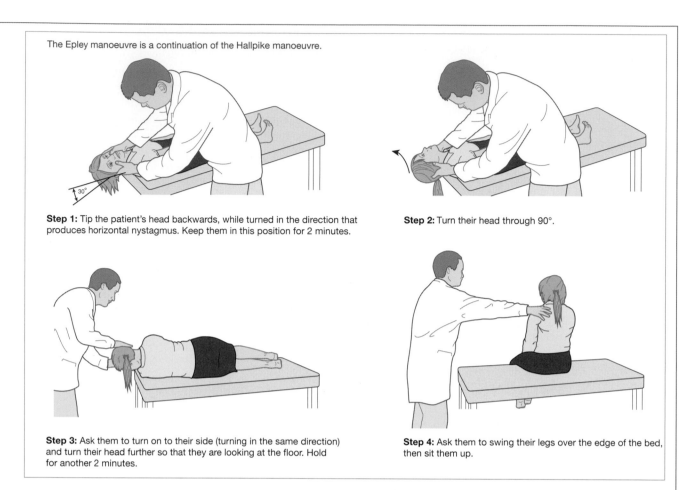

The Epley manoeuvre is a continuation of the Hallpike manoeuvre.

Step 1: Tip the patient's head backwards, while turned in the direction that produces horizontal nystagmus. Keep them in this position for 2 minutes.

Step 2: Turn their head through 90°.

Step 3: Ask them to turn on to their side (turning in the same direction) and turn their head further so that they are looking at the floor. Hold for another 2 minutes.

Step 4: Ask them to swing their legs over the edge of the bed, then sit them up.

Figure 23.2 Epley manoeuvre.

Meniere's disease

In Meniere's disease, the vertigo is combined with audiological symptoms: tinnitus, hearing loss and a feeling of fullness in the ear. It is the presence of these audiological symptoms that differentiates Meniere's disease from BPPV and acute vestibular neuronitis. The bouts of vertigo last for longer than those in BPPV; they can last anything from 10 minutes to 12 hours.

The underlying problem in Meniere's disease seems to be an increase in volume of the endolymph and dilatation of the endolymphatic spaces.

Meneriere's disease is a progressive disease. After each bout of vertigo, there is a further deterioration in the patient's hearing. GPs can treat Meniere's disease with antiemetics and betahistine, but often a referral to an ear, nose and throat (ENT) specialist is needed. Second-line treatment consists of diuretics and sometimes surgery.

Other causes of dizziness

A cholesteatoma is a rare cause of vertigo. This is one reason why it is important to examine the ear with the auroscope. If there is a crust or suspicious lesion arising from the attic, a referral to ENT is prudent.

Remember, having a good sense of balance is not just down to having normal vestibular function. Vision and proprioception make an important contribution to our sense of balance. If someone complains of feeling unsteady, we should check these sensory functions, too.

SUMMARY

People use the term 'having a funny turn' to describe many different symptoms. It's important to obtain a first-hand account from a witness and establish early on whether the patient lost consciousness. Someone who has had an unprovoked transient loss of consciousness may have an underlying cardiac problem, so we should take a cardiovascular history and perform a 12-lead ECG. Neurogenic syncope can be identified by the relationship to posture and the presence of a provoking factor and prodrome. Epilepsy is common and is a cause of sudden death. Making an early diagnosis and starting antiepileptic medication can reduce the risk of recurrent fits. GPs should offer people with epilepsy an annual review. Vertigo is an abnormal sensation of movement. If the cause is BPPV, it may be helpful to perform the Epley manoeuvre.

Now visit **www.wileyessential.com/primarycare** to test yourself on this chapter.

REFERENCES

1. NICE. Transient loss of consciousness ('blackouts') management in adults and young people. NICE Clinical Guideline 109. August 2010. Available from: http://www.nice.org.uk/guidance/cg109 (last accessed 6 October 2015).

2. Bell GS, Sander JW. The epidemiology of epilepsy: the size of the problem. *Seizure* 2001;**10**(4):306–14.

3. Risdale L. Avoiding premature death in epilepsy. *BMJ* 2015;**350**:10.

4. NICE. The epilepsies: the diagnosis of the epilepsies in adults and children in primary and secondary care (update) NICE Clinical Guideline 137. January 2012. Available from: http://www.nice.org.uk/guidance/cg137 (last accessed 6 October 2015).

5. Hart YM, Sander JW, Johnson AL, Shorvon SD. National General Practice Study of Epilepsy; recurrence after a first seizure. *Lancet* 1990;**336**:1271–4.

6. Drivers Medical Group. For medical practitioners: at a glance guide to the current medical standards of fitness to drive. DVLA, Swansea. November 2014. Available from: http://www.gov.uk/government/uploads/system/uploads/attachment_data/file/418165/aagv1.pdf (last accessed 6 October 2015).

7. Hanley K, O'Dowd T, Considine N. A systematic review of vertigo in primary care. *Br J Gen Pract* 2001;**51**: 666–71.

8. Dix MR, Hallpike CS. The pathology, symptomatology and diagnosis of certain disorders of the vestibular system. *Proc Roy Soc Med* 1952;**45**;341–54.

9. Hilton M, Pinder D. The Epley (canalith repositioning) manoeuvre for benign paroxysmal positional vertigo. *Cochrane Database Syst Rev* 2002;**1**:CD003162.

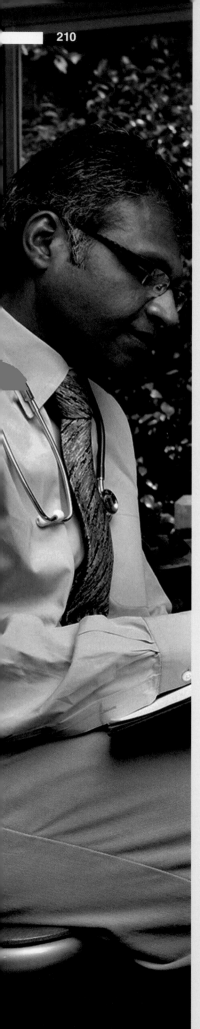

CHAPTER 24

Depression, anxiety and self-harm

David Kessler
Reader in Primary Care Mental Health, University of Bristol

Key topics

Learning objectives

- Feel confident in making an assessment of someone you think might have depression or anxiety.
- Be able to describe to someone the treatment options for depression and anxiety.
- Feel confident reviewing someone who is on antidepressant medication.

Essential Primary Care, First Edition. Edited by Andrew Blythe and Jessica Buchan.
© 2017 John Wiley & Sons, Ltd. Published 2017 by John Wiley & Sons, Ltd.
Companion website: www.wileyessential.com/primarycare

Introduction

GPs are often the first point of contact for people in distress or crisis. As well as providing support and advice at these difficult times, it is an important part of our role to assess whether the distress is likely to pass quickly, or whether it is part of a more pervasive pattern of unhappiness. We are ideally placed to do this; we provide continuity of care and often know something of the person's history and family background. We can assess the impact of their social context and medical history on their present state.

At some point, this pervasive pattern of worry and unhappiness becomes a clinical disorder called 'depression' or 'anxiety'. There is no absolute rule to tell us when this is the case; psychological distress is one of the most contested areas of medical diagnosis. Social attitudes to depression have become more open and tolerant over the last 20–30 years, and there are a number of factors that have contributed to this change. There has been a change in the public perception of depression; it is not a complete reversal, but there is no doubt that the illness is less hidden than it was. In 1992, the Royal Colleges of Psychiatry and General Practice launched the Defeat Depression Campaign, which had three broad aims: to educate health professionals (particularly GPs) to improve recognition and management; to educate the general public to encourage them to seek help earlier; and to reduce stigma. A few years earlier, in 1989, Prozac, the first of a new class of antidepressants, the selective serotonin reuptake inhibitors (SSRIs), was introduced.

One consequence of changing social attitudes and the widespread perception of the beneficial effects of the SSRIs has been a massive growth in the diagnosis of depression and the prescribing of antidepressants. In fact, the evidence suggests a steady rise in the prescribing of antidepressants since the 1970s; with year-on-year growth, there are now more than 40 million prescription items per annum. For some, this has gone too far, and has led to concern that ordinary distress has been medicalised. Whether or not this is the case, GPs manage more cases of depression than any other group of health professionals, and our knowledge and attitudes have a formative effect.

Definition

Low mood and anxiety are universal human experiences, and depression and anxiety disorders exist on a continuum with persistent low mood and worry. Defining the point at which these normal experiences become pathological is important; an example of widely used criteria is those of the American Psychiatric Association (APA), as set down in the Diagnostic and Statistical Manual of Mental Disorders 5 (DSM5) for 'major depressive episode'.

DSM5 definition of a major depressive episode

All three of the following features must be present:
  A. Depressed mood or a loss of interest or pleasure in daily activities for more than 2 weeks.
  B. Mood represents a change from the person's baseline.
  C. Impaired function: social, occupational, educational.

In addition, at least five out of these nine specific symptoms should be present nearly every day:
1. Depressed mood or irritable most of the day, nearly every day, as indicated by either subjective report (e.g. feels sad or empty) or observation made by others (e.g. appears tearful).
2. Decreased interest or pleasure in most activities, most of each day.
3. Significant weight change (5%) or change in appetite.
4. Change in sleep: insomnia or hypersomnia.
5. Change in activity: psychomotor agitation or retardation.
6. Fatigue or loss of energy.
7. Guilt/worthlessness: feelings of worthlessness or excessive or inappropriate guilt.
8. Concentration: diminished ability to think or concentrate, or more indecisiveness.
9. Suicidality: thoughts of death or suicide, or has suicide plan.

Anxiety is more complicated. There are a number of anxiety disorders, including panic disorder, social phobia and agoraphobia, but the most prevalent is generalised anxiety disorder (GAD), which may occur with or without episodes of panic.

DSM5 definition of generalised anxiety disorder

A. Excessive anxiety and worry occurring more days than not for at least 6 months, about a number of events or activities (such as work or school performance).
B. The person finds it difficult to control the worry.
C. The anxiety and worry are associated with three (or more) of the following six symptoms (with at least some symptoms present for more days than not for the past 6 months):
  (a) restlessness or feeling keyed up or on edge;
  (b) being easily fatigued;
  (c) difficulty concentrating or mind going blank;
  (d) irritability;
  (e) muscle tension;
  (f) sleep disturbance (difficulty falling or staying asleep, or restless unsatisfying sleep).
D. The anxiety, worry, or physical symptoms cause clinically significant distress or impairment in social, occupational or other important areas of functioning.
E. The disturbance is not due to the direct physiological effects of a substance (e.g. a drug of abuse, a medication) or a general medical condition (e.g. hyperthyroidism).

Epidemiology

Depression and anxiety are known as the 'common mental disorders'. Between 8 and 12% of the population experiences depression in any one year, and mixed anxiety and depression is even more common. Women are twice as likely as men to be diagnosed with one of these disorders. Common mental disorders peak in middle age (45–54), with rates between 1 : 5 and

1 : 4 of the population, and the lowest rates are in those aged 70–74. However, it is important to remember that the rate of depression in the elderly who are in care in homes is much higher: up to 20%. Poorer people, the long-term sick and the unemployed are more likely to remain unwell for longer. In fact, people with long-term physical conditions have higher than expected rates of depression. This applies to a range of very common conditions, such as neurological disorders (including stroke), rheumatological disorders, cardiovascular disease (CVD), diabetes and chronic obstructive pulmonary disease (COPD). Depression and anxiety tend to be recurrent relapsing conditions, and a substantial proportion of those who receive appropriate treatment remain depressed for long periods of time.

In this chapter, we will focus mainly on depression or mixed depression and anxiety; the treatments are similar or the same, and most of the research evidence from primary care concerns depression.

Diagnosis

Depression and anxiety are 'primary care disorders'; most people with these common mental disorders are diagnosed and treated in general practice. Despite increasing openness about psychological distress, there is still a concern that many patients with depression go undiagnosed in primary care. There are a number of reasons for this. Depression and anxiety are often associated with other chronic illnesses, and physical needs may seem more pressing to both doctor and patient in the context of relatively brief consultations. Many patients are reluctant to talk to their GP about their emotional distress; they may be

ashamed or fear that they will be stigmatised by being labelled as mentally ill; they may doubt their GP's capacity to respond in an appropriate or useful way.

Many patients who present with medically unexplained symptoms are suffering from depression and anxiety. This includes a greater than expected likelihood of depression or anxiety in those with the main four functional somatic syndromes: irritable bowel syndrome (IBS), non-ulcer dyspepsia, chronic fatigue syndrome and fibromyalgia. But it also includes a much larger group of patients with single symptoms, rather

Table 24.1 Management of somatic symptoms associated with psychological distress.

Strategy	Acknowledge the reality of the somatic distress, as well as the importance of the underlying psychological symptoms
	Identify serious somatic symptoms and exclude underlying physical disorder
	Don't overinvestigate; it can reinforce somatic anxiety in the long term by encouraging a pattern of presentations of somatic worry relieved by tests
	Explore patients' perspectives, their health beliefs and how they explain or attribute their symptoms
	Introduce the idea that the symptoms are associated with and indeed may be caused by psychological distress
	Begin to address the psychological distress

Case study 24.1

Helen Hodgson, age 37, is talking to her GP:

I've always been a worrier, I know that. My mother was the same. My husband says I'm always needing someone to tell me everything is going to be Ok. He gets annoyed with me sometimes, but he is so forgetful and I worry about him. I do worry about everything, especially my family. Sometimes I sit here in the armchair and it just feels as though something else awful is going to happen and I've no idea what it is. I just feel sweaty and shaky and my heart starts beating really fast. Then, the other day in the supermarket, I just suddenly felt really dreadful, I suddenly started shaking and sweating, and I felt faint and I thought I was going to pass out. It was really scary. I'm finding it more and more difficult to get things done, even normal things like making dinner; I've just lost interest. I feel sad and I don't know what's happening to me. It's all really getting me down.

Helen's story illustrates how depression, anxiety and somatic symptoms occur together. She suffers from both trait and state anxiety; she has a background of

vulnerability to anxiety in her personality, and this has developed into an acute illness. She gives a clear description of a panic attack. She refers at the end to her low mood. In this sense, the recognition of psychological distress is not difficult. However, it is possible that agreeing such a diagnosis with Helen will be more challenging. Bodily symptoms are as prominent as psychological symptoms throughout her account. They are interwoven with each other and with thoughts about her family history and social situation. Her penultimate statement, 'I don't know what's happening to me', captures her bewilderment in the face of this mix of psychological and somatic distress and environmental hardship, and gives us an idea of the GP's task. For example, it is possible that Helen might present to her GP with concerns about whether she has a serious disease: perhaps something wrong with her heart. Listed in Table 24.1 are some of the strategies which may be useful in this situation.

Remember: a diagnosis of depression or anxiety may not be helpful if the patient whose diagnosis it is does not agree with you.

than syndromes. Patients often present physical symptoms when they are depressed and anxious, and psychological disorders often find a somatic expression. Presenting a physical symptom to the GP provides a legitimate reason for the consultation for many patients, as well as being a way of addressing concerns about possible underlying physical illness. Depression and anxiety both amplify and distort patients' fears and thoughts about their bodily symptoms.

Variations in presentation

Depression and anxiety can present to the GP in different ways; we have already mentioned the effect of comorbid physical illness and somatisation. Age and culture can also have an influence. Once again, there are no hard and fast rules, but it is important to be sensitive to some of the possible variations in presentation.

Culture

It has been said that non-Western cultures may not view depressive symptoms in the same way as the dominant UK culture. We have already argued that depression and anxiety are human universals, but local sociocultural factors shape the way the experience of persistent worry and low mood are viewed, and thus how they present to GPs. This has been a topic of study in transcultural psychiatry, and research tends to indicate that although terminology may vary from culture to culture, the underlying experience is very similar. For example, in Zimbabwe, the Shona have a concept of 'Kufungisisa' or 'thinking too much'; an apt descriptive term for nonspecific stress-related misery.[1] The idea that 'overthinking' can be unhealthy is not entirely strange to us, and on closer study there is considerable overlap with our notion of depression and anxiety, and recognition that the state described is one of pathological misery.

What is important is not the exact meaning of different cultural terms, but the GP's sensitivity to the needs of the individual patient, and their ability to understand the distress and its meaning in the patient's cultural context.

Age

The key symptoms of depression and anxiety are similar at different ages, but there are often different emphases. Although the moody withdrawn adolescent is a cliché, the strongest evidence of variation comes from comparing older adults to young adults. Older adults are more likely to present to their doctors with agitation and somatic symptoms, even hypochondriasis, while younger adults are more likely to experience guilt and complain of loss of libido.[2] 'Lifecourse epidemiology' aims to understand how determinants of health and illness act and interact through a person's life. There is increasing evidence that the 'trajectory of risk for major depression' can be established early in life, often as a result of childhood trauma.[3]

The biopsychosocial assessment

In recent years, assessment of depression in primary care for the Quality and Outcomes Framework (QOF) has involved the use of questionnaires such as the Patient Health Questionnaire-9 (PHQ-9) (see Figure 24.1), HAD-D or Beck Depression Inventory to count symptoms. Although symptom counts can be useful, depression and anxiety are both disorders that exist in the biological, social and psychological domains; it does not make sense to focus on symptoms alone, and a broader assessment is essential. There are a number of factors that contribute to the onset of depression and that can maintain and prolong an episode. A formal biopsychosocial assessment (see Table 24.2) encourages GPs to ask about those areas in which recovery can take place.

Patient Health Questionnaire – 9 (PHQ–9)

Over the **last 2 weeks**, how often have you been bothered by any of the following problems? (Use '√' to indicate your answer)	Not at all	Several days	More than half the days	Nearly every day
1. Little interest or pleasure in doing things	0	1	2	3
2. Feeling down, depressed, or hopeless	0	1	2	3
3. Trouble falling or staying asleep, or sleeping too much	0	1	2	3
4. Feeling tired or having little energy	0	1	2	3
5. Poor appetite or overeating	0	1	2	3
6. Feeling bad about yourself – or that you are a failure or have let yourself or your family down	0	1	2	3
7. Trouble concentrating on things, such as reading the newspaper or watching television	0	1	2	3
8. Moving or speaking so slowly that other people could have noticed? Or the opposite – being so fidgety or restless that you have been moving around a lot more than usual	0	1	2	3
9. Thoughts that you would be better off dead or of hurting yourself in some way	0	1	2	3

FOR OFFICE CODING   0   +   ____   +____ +____

= Total Score: ____

If you checked off **any** problems, how **difficult** have these problems made it for you to do your work, take care of things at home, or get along with other people?

Not difficult at all	Somewhat difficult	Very difficult	Extremely difficult
☐	☐	☐	☐

Figure 24.1 Patient Health Questionnaire-9 (PHQ-9). A score of >10 has 88% sensitivity and specificity for identifying a major depressive disorder. The score increases with severity of depression. Developed by Drs. Robert L. Spitzer, Janet B.W. Williams, Kurt Kroenke and colleagues, with an educational grant from Pfizer Inc.

Table 24.2 Biopsychosocial assessment.

Area of questioning	Current symptoms, including duration and severity
	Personal history of depression
	Family history of mental illness
	The quality of interpersonal relationships with partner, children and/or parents
	Living conditions
	Social support
	Employment and/or financial worries
	Current or previous alcohol and substance use
	Suicidal ideation
	Discussion of treatment options
	Any past experience of, and response to, treatments

Top tips: approaching a consultation in which the patient may have depression

If we suspect depression, we should ask the patient what they think.

Ask about drugs and alcohol.

Don't be frightened to ask about suicidal thoughts: they are common in depression and patients usually feel relieved to talk about them. We can say, 'Have you had any thoughts about harming yourself or wanting to take your life?, or, 'Sometimes when people feel very low, they have thoughts of ending their life. Have you had any thoughts like that?'

Assess suicidal risk: this is difficult, but the following are associated with greater risk:

- male sex;
- drug and alcohol abuse;
- history of previous self-harm;
- severe depression;
- comorbid personality disorder.

In addition, it makes sense to be aware of clear and detailed plans, final acts (such as writing a note) and social isolation.

Conversely, good social support and being responsible for the care of young children can be protective factors.

Management

The management of depression and anxiety in UK primary care is based on the idea of the stepped-care model. The underlying principle of this model is that the intervention offered should be the least intrusive possible and appropriate to the severity of the illness. Table 24.3 outlines the stepped-care model for depression, while Table 24.4 shows the model for GAD.

Table 24.3 Stepped care for depression.

Focus of the intervention	Nature of the intervention
Step 1: All known and suspected presentations of depression	Assessment, support, psychoeducation, active monitoring and referral for further assessment and interventions
Step 2: Persistent subthreshold depressive symptoms; mild to moderate depression	Low-intensity psychological and psychosocial interventions, medication and referral for further assessment and interventions
Step 3: Persistent subthreshold depressive symptoms or mild to moderate depression with inadequate response to initial interventions; moderate and severe depression	Medication, high-intensity psychological interventions, combined treatments, collaborative care and referral for further assessment and interventions
Step 4: Severe and complex depression; risk to life; severe self-neglect	Medication, high-intensity psychological interventions, electroconvulsive therapy, crisis service, combined treatments, multiprofessional and in-patient care

Table 24.4 Stepped care for generalised anxiety disorder (GAD).

Focus of the intervention	Nature of the intervention
Step 1: All known and suspected presentations of GAD	Assessment, support, psychoeducation, active monitoring and referral for further assessment and interventions
Step 2: Diagnosed GAD that has not improved after education and active monitoring in primary care	Low-intensity psychological interventions: individual non-facilitated self-help, individual guided self-help and psychoeducational groups
Step 3: GAD with an inadequate response to step 2 interventions or marked functional impairment	Choice of a high-intensity psychological intervention (cognitive behavioural therapy (CBT)/applied relaxation) or a drug treatment
Step 4: Complex treatment-refractory GAD and very marked functional impairment, such as self-neglect or a high risk of self-harm	Highly specialist treatment, such as complex drug and/or psychological treatment regimens; input from multiagency teams, crisis services, day hospitals or in-patient care

Table 24.5 Thought distortions.

Thought distortion	Example
Exaggeration/catastrophising	Everything seems extreme: difficulties turn into disaster. You exaggerate problems and the harm they can cause. You underestimate your ability to deal with problems: 'Now I have upset her, our friendship is over and I'll end up with no friends.'
Overgeneralisation	You make broad statements that emphasise the negative. For example, if someone criticises you, you think, 'I am a failure', and, 'Nobody likes me'.
Ignoring the positive	You only seem to remember and dwell on negative events. You dismiss good experiences as 'unimportant': 'So what if I finished my work? It's what I'm supposed to do.'
All-or-nothing thinking	You see things in black and white. If something falls short of perfection, it is a failure.
Jumping to conclusions	You interpret what happens in a negative way, without any facts to support your view. For example, you indulge in **mind-reading**: you assume someone feels or thinks badly of you without checking it out: 'He thinks I'm a bore' or 'She's really laughing at me.' Or you may do some **fortune-telling** (or even better, **misfortune-telling**): you are sure that things will turn out badly, without any evidence: 'This is never going to work'.
Labelling	You deal with your mistakes (and other people's) by using general labels: 'I'm a bad mother.' This is very demoralising when you keep doing it.
Personalisation	You assume responsibility for things that aren't really under your control: 'It's my fault he started drinking again.'
'Should' or 'shouldn't' thoughts	You tell yourself how you ought to act, feel or think: 'I should please everyone' or 'I shouldn't have to put up with this.'

The stepped-care model is based on the idea that many who come in at step 1 with relatively mild symptoms will improve with minimal intervention and not progress to steps 3 or 4. The model should be applied flexibly, so that people who are seriously unwell should not be held back in one of the lower steps when they need urgent treatment. For the model to work, there must be wide access to a range of low-intensity psychological interventions. These include psychoeducation, facilitated self-help and some forms of group therapy. Until the last few years, this has been an aspiration, but the roll-out of the initiative to Improve Access to Psychological Therapies (IAPT) has made it increasingly possible to respond appropriately to the needs of patients in primary care. In addition, IAPT includes resources for the provision of 'high-intensity' one-to-one psychotherapy for those who are more unwell.

Psychological therapies

The psychological therapy with the most extensive evidence base is cognitive behavioural therapy (CBT). This grew out of psychodynamic psychotherapy, the type of psychological treatment pioneered by Sigmund Freud, but has incorporated learning from cognitive science and behaviourism. One of the insights of CBT is that negative thoughts about oneself or one's experiences are associated with low mood; CBT teaches people to address these thoughts by asking questions about them, and asserts that learning how to address these negative thoughts can lead to improvements in mood.

Negative thoughts seem to come 'automatically', and often take the form of thought distortions or error. Table 24.5 outlines

Table 24.6 Questioning negative thoughts: a process and a technique that can be learned.

Questions that patients find useful	'What is the evidence that my thought is true?'
	'Is there an alternative explanation for what happened?'
	'What's the worst that could happen, and could I live through it?'
	'What would I tell a friend in my position?'
	'What is the effect of my believing this negative thought? How would I feel if I thought about it more realistically?'
	'What should I do now?'

some typical thought distortions that occur in depression, while Table 24.6 gives some suggestions for questioning the validity of those thoughts (known as 'Socratic questioning').

As well as exploring thoughts, CBT also encourages patients to invest in behaviour change. Other psychotherapies are effective for depression and anxiety, and the evidence base for treatments such as interpersonal therapy (IPT) and brief psychodynamic psychotherapy is increasing.

Patient surveys suggest that two out of three prefer psychological treatments to antidepressants. However, many find psychotherapy challenging, and the drop out rate is high; it is the responsibility of referring clinicians to explain something about psychotherapy so that their patients can begin to make an informed decision about whether it is right for them.[4]

Antidepressants

In spite of the increasing availability of psychological treatments, the most widely used treatment for depression and anxiety is antidepressant drugs. The SSRIs have replaced the older tricyclic antidepressants (TCAs) and the monoamine oxidase inhibitors (MAOIs) as the first-line drugs, in part because they are much safer in overdose. In addition to more severe depression, antidepressants are also recommended for those with mild to moderate depression who have not responded to initial interventions, including low-intensity psychological therapies. They may be chosen as a first preference by some patients, although a brief period of 'active monitoring' with a planned review is often advised. In addition, the National Institute for Health and Care Excellence (NICE) recommends that antidepressants are considered for those with persistent 'subthreshold' symptoms of depression when they have lasted for at least 2 years, there is past history of moderate to severe depression or other treatments have failed. 'Subthreshold depression' is a way of describing an illness where low mood is accompanied by some of the associated symptoms listed in the DSM5 definition of major depression, but fewer than five.

Top tips: prescribing antidepressants

- SSRIs are the first choice among the antidepressants.
- Patients should always be advised that it is likely to be a few weeks before they feel any benefit from the drugs.
- Patients should be advised that they may experience adverse effects: gastrointestinal upset, temporary increase in anxiety and sexual dysfunction are all common.
- The patient should be reviewed after 2 weeks. If there is improvement, this interval can be increased, although ongoing support is an important part of GP care.
- It is recommended that drug treatment is continued for at least 6 months, if effective.
- These drugs should not be stopped suddenly, but over a period of about 4 weeks; otherwise, a discontinuation syndrome (commonly, dizziness, headache, nausea and lethargy) can occur.

Benzodiazepines

This class of drugs was probably overprescribed in general practice in the past; they have the potential to give rise to dependence, and are commonly sold on the street. Because of these risks, they should be prescribed with caution, and clear instructions should be given to the patient that the prescription is unlikely to be long-term. Nonetheless, they remain an effective adjunct in the short-term management of acute anxiety[5] and are often used during the initial treatment phase of mixed anxiety and depression, when SSRIs can exacerbate anxiety symptoms and restlessness.

When treatment fails

A surprisingly large proportion of patients treated for depression do not significantly improve. In one primary care survey,[6] half of those who had taken antidepressants for at least 6 weeks were not better. For those who have not responded to antidepressants, CBT should be considered, and vice versa; there is no reason why psychotherapy and drug treatment should not be combined. In addition, various pharmacological strategies have been suggested, including swapping between antidepressants (evidence is weak) and adding an additional psychotropic drug, such as a second antidepressant of a different class or an antipsychotic drug. It is generally advised that advice be sought from a psychiatrist if drug therapy is to be augmented in this way.

Even for those that do recover from an episode of depression, we need to acknowledge that this can be a recurring and relapsing illness. When depressed people are recovering, GPs still have an important role. We should review the episode with them and make a plan for future action based on the following:

- What has been the pattern of depressive episodes in their life? Are there any obvious triggers or warning signals? It is worthwhile asking patients to list these, and to seek help if they occur.
- What treatments have been effective? Do they need to have a lower threshold for seeking help?
- What activities and life changes have helped them recover, and how can these be maintained?
- The need for continuing antidepressants should be reviewed regularly; current advice is to continue treatment for 6 months after remission of symptoms. In cases where depression is recurrent, it is advised to treat for 2 years.[7]

Controversies in depression and anxiety

Voices within and outside of the medical profession have expressed alarm at the 'medicalisation of unhappiness'. A recent example is the change in the new version of the DSM. In the previous version, DSM IV, a recent bereavement excluded a diagnosis of major depression. In DSM5, this exclusion has been removed. While some argue that this medicalises normal grief, others maintain that it means that depressed patients who have experienced loss get the care they need.

Linked to this is concern about the high volume of antidepressant prescribing. In 2012, in the UK, there were more than 40 million prescription items for these drugs, and most of them were written in primary care. It is true that many of these are short prescriptions or repeats for those on long-term treatment, but the rise in prescribing shows no signs of abating, and the indications for the use of these drugs continue to be extended beyond depression. For example, many commentators deplore the growing use of medication to treat 'social anxiety'.

Personality disorder, depressed mood and recurrent self-harm

It is important to think about other possible causes of disturbed mood. Depression is more common in psychotic disorders, and where there is evidence of prolonged episodes of overactivity and disinhibited behaviour, bipolar disorder must be considered. GPs will also encounter patients whose mood is disturbed and who self-harm, but whom psychiatrists do not categorise as having a mental illness; they are often described as having a 'personality disorder'. People with personality disorders have persistent problems in social relations and social functioning. They seem to have a more limited range of feelings, behaviours and coping skills. These adverse patterns of behaviour are established fairly early on in adult life. ***Borderline personality disorder (BPD)*** is one of the more common, and is characterised by unstable and intense interpersonal relationships, self-perception and moods. These feelings can lead to both self-harm and impulsive behaviour. Such disorders and behaviours should not be dismissed as 'untreatable'; there is a growing body of evidence for effective interventions.

Patients with BPD tend to seek help, while those with, for example, antisocial personality disorders tend to avoid engagement with services. There are no specific drug treatments; the studies that suggest that second-generation antipsychotics or mood stabilisers are helpful tend to be small and thus underpowered. Treatment is behavioural and psychotherapeutic, and much of it is best delivered in a specialist setting. Nonetheless, there are important general principles of care which link directly into the GP's long-term commitment to their patients' welfare. These include working in partnership with the patient, encouraging autonomy and offering consistency and reliability. People who have BPD have often suffered trauma or abuse; they can experience changes in care as rejection or even abandonment, and it is important for their GP to be aware of this. It is not uncommon for this group of patients to develop very high expectations of their doctor and to be angry and upset when these expectations are not fulfilled.

It is not always possible to avoid crises with this group of patients. It is best to try and anticipate them and to make contingency plans to limit their impact on the patient and those around them. One way of doing this is to produce a written plan with the patient based on a discussion of a previous event. It is essential to involve families and carers in these plans.

Case study 24.2

Emma first presented to child and adolescent mental health services with low mood and repeated attempts at self-harm. These ranged from frequent self-cutting to more dangerous behaviours, including driving a car into a wall. Although she stayed in school and later found employment, her behaviour became more disordered and challenging as she started to abuse drugs, especially alcohol and cocaine. Her mood appeared labile and unpredictable, and for a while psychiatrists considered a diagnosis of bipolar affective disorder. Various drug treatments, including mood stabilisers, antipsychotics and benzodiazepines, proved of little benefit, although she actively sought repeated benzodiazepine prescriptions. She was eventually diagnosed with BPD.

As Emma grew into adulthood, her acts of self-harm became more frequent and more serious. She discloses that she was sexually abused as a child.

She has engaged with long-term dialectical behavioural therapy (DBT). This has had some effect in helping her feel safe and contained, and has let her start to make sense of her difficult history. She still has crises; these are often triggered by what appear to be relatively minor stresses and are associated with drug or alcohol abuse and self-harm. Her treatment is ongoing. Emma, her family, her GP and the psychiatric team accept that this is a long-term process, but that progress is possible.

Depression and anxiety are the common mental disorders, and are most often managed in primary care; they form a core part of the GP's workload. Depression and anxiety are often associated with other chronic illnesses, and physical needs often seem more pressing. Mental disorders still carry stigma, and this too can lead to delayed diagnosis. Antidepressants are often prescribed in primary care, and these drugs can be effective for both anxiety and depression. There is a commitment to make psychological therapies more accessible in primary care, and an emphasis on the 'stepped-care model', in which the intervention offered is the least intrusive and most appropriate to the severity of the illness. GPs have an important role in managing depression: in diagnosis, in setting the illness in the context of their patient's life and other illnesses, in helping their patient make informed decisions about treatment and in providing continuity.

SUMMARY

Now visit **www.wileyessential.com/primarycare** to test yourself on this chapter.

REFERENCES

1. Patel V, Gwanzura F, Simunyu E, et al. The phenomenology and explanatory models of common mental disorder: a study in primary care in Harare, Zimbabwe. *Psychol Med* 1995;**25**(6):1191–9.

2. Hegeman JM, Kok RM, van der Mast RC, Giltay EJ. Phenomenology of depression in older adults compared with younger adults: meta-analysis. *Br J Psych* 2012;**200**(4):275–81.

3. Gilman S. The life course epidemiology of depression. *Am J Epidemiol* 2007;**166**(10):1134–7.

4. Barnes M, Sherlock S, Thomas L, et al. No pain, no gain: depressed clients experiences of cognitive behavioural therapy. *Br J Clin Psychol* 2013;**52**:347–64.

5. Baldwin DS, Anderson IM, Nutt DJ, et al. Evidence-based guidelines for the pharmacological treatment of anxiety disorders: recommendations from the British Association for Psychopharmacology. *J Psychopharmacol* 2005;**19**(6):567–96.

6. Thomas L, Kessler D, Campbell J, et al. Prevalence of treatment resistant depression in primary care: cross-sectional data. *Br J Gen Pract* 2013;**63**:852–8.

7. NICE. Depression in adults: the treatment and management of depression in adults. NICE Clinical Guideline 90. October 2009. Available from: http://www.nice.org.uk/guidance/cg90 (last accessed 6 October 2015).

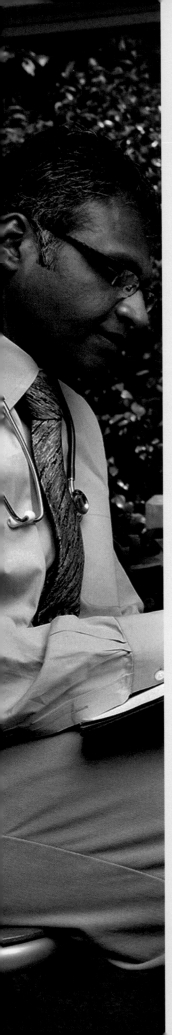

CHAPTER 25
Sexual health and dysuria

Lucy Jenkins
Teaching Fellow in Primary Care, University of Bristol

Key topics

Learning objectives

- Be able to assess and manage patients presenting with dysuria and vaginal discharge.
- Be able to manage recurrent urinary tract infections and candidiasis.
- Be able to carry out a sexual history and examination.
- Be able to identify those at high risk of sexually transmitted infections.
- Be able to investigate and manage sexually transmitted infections in general practice.
- Be able to understand the role of the GP in chlamydia screening, identification of high-risk patients and the interface with sexual health clinics.

Essential Primary Care, First Edition. Edited by Andrew Blythe and Jessica Buchan.
© 2017 John Wiley & Sons, Ltd. Published 2017 by John Wiley & Sons, Ltd.
Companion website: www.wileyessential.com/primarycare

Sexually transmitted infections: a historical perspective

Dysuria and discharge commonly occur in sexually transmitted infections (STIs). STIs are infections spread primarily through sexual contact; they were previously known as venereal diseases and have been documented throughout history. Laws passed in 1161 were targeted at reducing the spread of 'the perilous infirmity of burning'. Later, the surgeon to Richard II and Henry IV described this burning to be a 'certain inward heat and excoriation of the urethra', which supports the idea that this condition was gonorrhoea.[1] Further writings on the 'impure embrace of infected persons' that degenerated into 'ulceration and putrefaction of the genital organs and terminated in death' likely describe syphilis, which was common in the 1500s and onwards. Shakespeare refers to the illness in many of his plays as 'pox'. Venereal disease is discussed in *Measure for Measure*: commenting on a brothel madam, Lucio, a citizen of Vienna, says, 'I have purchased…many diseases under her roof'.[2]

Medicine has developed rapidly in the last 500 years, but dysuria is still a common symptom, and STIs remain a problem today.

Dysuria and urinary tract infections

Dysuria is painful or difficult urination. It may seem trivial, but can be very distressing.

Dysuria in women

If a woman presents to her GP with dysuria, she is most likely to have a urinary tract infection (UTI). This is the commonest bacterial infection managed in primary care, and analysis of midstream sample by microscopy, culture and sensitivity (MC&S) is one of the tests most frequently requested by GPs. UTIs are much more common in women than in men, as the female urethra is shorter and opens nearer the anus. By the age of 24 years, one in three women will have had a UTI. Annual incidence increases with age.

Case study 25.1

Dr Kirsty Dyer conducts a telephone consultation with Cara Cooper, age 24. For the last 48 hours, Cara has been passing small amounts of urine quite frequently, with some burning and mild suprapubic pain. She has no fever, loin pain or vaginal discharge. She takes the combined oral contraceptive (COC) pill, and her last period was 1 week ago. She has tried over-the-counter alkalinising sachets, but these have not helped much.

What is the most likely diagnosis?
This history fits with an uncomplicated lower UTI. 'Lower' describes symptoms affecting the bladder, causing cystitis, and the urethra, causing urethritis. An uncomplicated UTI is one caused by a typical pathogen in a person with a normal urinary tract and normal renal function.

What investigation should Dr Dyer do to confirm the diagnosis?
A urine dip is a useful, quick and easy near-patient test. The presence of nitrites alone has a positive predictive value (PPV) of about 80%, while nitrites with leucocytes/ blood (see Figure 25.1) have a PPV >90%.[3] However, the absence of nitrites does not rule out the possibility of a UTI in a symptomatic patient.

Dr Dyer offers Cara an appointment in the surgery, but she is too busy with work to attend. What are the other options?
Dr Dyer offers Cara empirical treatment. This means treating a presumed clinical diagnosis without it being confirmed. Dr Dyer combines the clinical information from

the history with her knowledge about likely organisms and their local antibiotic sensitivities. The usual organisms causing UTIs are *Escherichia coli* (the most common), *Staphylococcus saprophyticus* and *Proteus mirabilis*. In terms of treatment, often trimethoprim or nitrofurantoin are given; a 3-day course is adequate for an uncomplicated UTI. Trimethoprim is effective because it is concentrated in the renal tract and is effective against Gram-negative organisms, but it is important to check local microbiological guidelines, as resistance patterns can vary.

Cara visits Dr Dyer again 2 days later, complaining of ongoing dysuria with pinkish-coloured urine and new loin pain. She is feeling hot and unwell, and has vomited twice. Examination reveals a temperature of 38°C, a regular pulse of 92 bpm and a soft abdomen with left loin tenderness.

What is the diagnosis?
This picture fits with acute pyelonephritis, an upper UTI. Dr Dyer needs to decide whether or not Cara needs hospital admission. This would be necessary if she were unable to take oral fluids or medications, or was systemically unwell. Assuming she is well enough for home treatment, a broad-spectrum antibiotic such as ciprofloxacin or co-amoxiclav is appropriate, depending on local guidelines. These are usually given for 7–14 days. A midstream specimen of urine (MSU) is essential at this stage. Cara must be advised to seek review if her symptoms are worsening.

Should Dr Dyer have sent an MSU initially? What are the advantages of this?

In this case, the management was reasonable; with typical symptoms and a suggestive urine dip, it is reasonable to start empirical treatment without sending or waiting for an MSU.

Urine microscopy looks for red blood cells, white blood cells and epithelial cells. A pyuria is the presence of elevated numbers of white cells (>10 white cells/mm³). If a bacterium is present, the total number of organisms is counted (colony count); in the UK, the cut-off is 10^5 CFU/ml to diagnose a UTI.

The advantages of sending an MSU are that it confirms the diagnosis, guides treatment and enables microbiological monitoring of infection rates and resistance. Also, a sterile pyuria (white cells but no growth) can be a sign of another infection, such as chlamydia. A possible disadvantage is the cost of an investigation that might not affect management. In addition, it may delay treatment. Contamination can result in inconclusive results and the need to repeat the test.

Cara attends Dr Dyer again 3 years later. She has been away at university but has had three or four UTIs each year. She is fed up and worried that something may be wrong.

Does she need further investigations or referral for treatment?

Recurrent UTIs can be diagnosed in non-pregnant women who have two or more UTIs in 6 months or three or more in 1 year.[4] Many GPs would do a urinary tract ultrasound at this stage, and if this was normal, they would consider treatment options. These include self-initiated antibiotics, postcoital antibiotics for women whose symptoms occur after intercourse and prophylaxis with a daily low-dose antibiotic. There is good evidence that prophylaxis reduces recurrences. It is important to check local guidelines and balance treatment with the risk of resistance and side effects, and to review treatment at 6 months. Further investigation or referral for UTI is needed for those with persistent haematuria after treatment (see Chapter 32), renal problems, past urological surgery, stones, possible fistula or multidrug-resistant infections.

Women may try postcoital voiding, wearing cotton underwear and douching to prevent UTIs, but there is little evidence for the efficacy of any of these. There is mixed evidence for cranberry products and evidence of some benefit from local oestrogen treatment in postmenopausal women where atrophic vaginitis is felt to be contributing.[4]

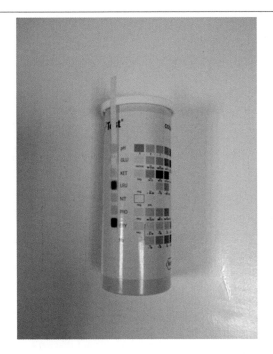

Figure 25.1 Urine testing strip, showing positive for nitrites (pink) and leucocytes (purple).

Top tip: advice to adult patients on collecting an MSU

- Advise the patient to wash their hands first, and ideally the genital region (with nonbactericidal soap).
- Women should hold open their labia and men retract the foreskin.
- Pass some urine into the toilet first before collecting the sample directly into the laboratory container.

Top tip: dysuria in pregnancy

Always ask a woman with dysuria whether or not she might be pregnant.

UTI is more common in pregnancy, due to urinary stasis caused by progesterone reducing muscle tone in the ureters. There is a higher risk of cystitis progressing to pyelonephritis, and an association with preterm labour. Therefore, in pregnant women, an MSU should always be sent and antibiotic treatment should be for 7 days. It is important to check gestation and antibiotic safety guidelines before prescribing.

Dysuria in men

If a young man presents to his GP with dysuria, chlamydia is the most likely diagnosis. UTIs are rare in men under 50 years and uncommon in men over 50. UTI symptoms are similar to those in women. A detailed history is essential to look for an underlying cause, such as prostate disease, renal stones or immunosuppression. It is appropriate to start empirical treatment, but, in men, an MSU must be sent and follow-up

Table 25.1 Noninfective causes of dysuria in men and women.

Cause	Symptoms	Diagnosis	Treatment
Detrusor instability 'irritable bladder'	Dysuria, frequency, urgency and incontinence	Often clinical Urodynamics may confirm	Fluid modification Bladder drill and pelvic floor exercises Anticholinergic medication
Inflammatory skin conditions, e.g. dermatitis and lichen sclerosis	Dryness, soreness, itch, fissures	Clinical diagnosis Biopsy for lichen sclerosis or planus	Emollient Potent steroid for lichenoid conditions, with monitoring, as there is a risk of malignant change
Postmenopausal atrophic vaginitis (women only)	Dysuria, vulval or vaginal dryness	Relevant history Dryness, dysuria and superficial dyspareunia	Topical oestrogen Consider systemic hormone replacement therapy (HRT) (see Chapter 33)

Table 25.2 Infective causes of dysuria in men and women.

Cause[a]	Diagnosis	Treatment
Urethritis (in men, most commonly due to gonorrhoea)	Swabs for nucleic acid amplification test (NAAT)	Ceftriaxone and azithromycin Full STI screen Contact-tracing
Nongonococcal urethritis (also known as nonspecific urethritis) Most commonly due to chlamydia, but can be caused by other organisms; in 20–30%, no organism is identified	Swabs for NAAT	Azithromycin
Genital *Herpes simplex*	Clinical, virology swabs	Aciclovir

[a] Full details in section on Sexual Health Epidemiology and Sexual Health Services.

Top tip: atypical UTIs

A UTI may present atypically with confusion, fever or nonspecific illness, especially in older patients.

Top tip: what is abnormal vaginal discharge?

- Discharge is abnormal is if it smells, is itchy, is associated with soreness or has blood in it.
- Any change from normal for an individual woman needs review.
- Change in volume may warrant investigation; excess discharge can occur with genital malignancy.

---

arranged. Referral for urological assessment should be made for men who fail to respond to antibiotic treatment or who have complicated or recurrent infections or persistent haematuria. Obstructive lower urinary tract symptoms in men that are commonly caused by benign prostatic hyperplasia and prostate cancer are covered in Chapter 32.

Tables 25.1 and 25.2 describe other causes of dysuria in men and women.

Vaginal and penile discharge

Vaginal discharge

A normal (physiological) discharge in women of reproductive age is clear or white, mucoid and odourless. It varies with the menstrual cycle and hormonal changes, and thus it tends to be increased during pregnancy, around the time of ovulation and

in women taking the COC pill. Abnormal discharge has various causes, as listed in Tables 25.3 and 25.4.

The most common cause for abnormal discharge is infection, usually due to bacterial vaginosis (BV) and candidiasis (thrush). A sexual history and swabs are essential if the diagnosis is not clear from the clinical history. Vaginal and speculum examination are essential if pelvic inflammatory disease (PID) is a possibility.

A charcoal swab for MC&S will identify candidiasis, BV and trichomonas. An endocervical swab for nucleic acid amplification test (NAAT) is the gold standard for identifying

Table 25.3 Noninfective causes of abnormal vaginal discharge.

Cause	Nature of discharge	Associated symptoms	Treatment
Cervical ectropion	Clear and watery	May be on COC pill	Cryotherapy
Atrophic vaginitis due to oestrogen deficiency, or in prepubertal, breastfeeding and menopausal patients	Clear and watery May be bloodstained, but remember postmenopausal bleeding is endometrial cancer until proven otherwise	Relevant history Dryness, dysuria and superficial dyspareunia	Topical oestrogen
Foreign body: retained tampon, retained products of conception/surgery	Grey or bloodstained purulent with extreme odour	Relevant history May develop pain Risk of systemic infection	Removal antibiotics also usually given
Cancer	Excessive discharge can be an early sign; later, it is often bloody with an offensive odour	Ask about pain, menstrual and other bleeding, smears and weight loss	Depending on diagnosis, may include surgery, chemotherapy or radiotherapy

Table 25.4 Infective causes of abnormal vaginal discharge.

Cause	Nature of discharge	Associated symptoms	Treatment
Candidiasis (thrush)	Thick white, curdlike	Vulval itch, dysuria and dyspareunia Erythema and oedema on examination	Antifungal: pessary/cream ± oral stat fluconazole
Bacterial vaginosis (BV)	White/grey watery, fishy odour	Usually none	Metronidazole or clindamycin
Trichomonas	Profuse yellow/green, frothy discharge with offensive odour	Itch	Metronidazole
Chlamydia and gonorrhoea	May cause discharge if associated with cervicitis, but often asymptomatic	Abnormal bleeding, dysuria and pain	Antibiotics, depending on local guidelines

Case study 25.2

Rachel Roberts, age 32, visits Dr Rufus Samson. Rachel has no major past medical history, although she did have two recent courses of antibiotics for sinusitis. She has a creamy white thick discharge with vulval itch. She has mild dysuria and intercourse was sore last night. She has had similar symptoms before, but they only lasted a few days. She is sure this can't be sexually transmitted as she has been married for 10 years.

Examination reveals thick, white, creamy discharge with vulval erythema and oedema.

What is the most likely diagnosis and what will Dr Samson do next?
The history and examination findings support a thrush (candida) infection. In this case, culture is not required: empirical treatment is appropriate. Topical or vaginal antifungal treatments with imidazoles (e.g. clotrimazole cream or pessaries) can be bought over the counter or prescribed. Oral treatment with a one-off dose of oral fluconazole is equally effective.

It is important that Dr Samson checks that Rachel is not pregnant; a week-long course of topical treatment is indicated in pregnancy. The oral treatments are not licensed for use in pregnancy or breastfeeding, although they are at times used for resistant candidiasis in women who are breastfeeding.

Rachel is really worried as she has 'never had an infection down there before'. What can Dr Samson say to reassure her?
Dr Samson explains that candidiasis is common (it affects 75% of women of reproductive age[5]). It does not cause lasting harm, and it is *not* an STI (although candida may be passed on during intercourse, and the physical trauma of intercourse may trigger it in predisposed individuals). It is caused by a yeast which commonly lives in and around the vagina and on the skin. It multiplies when the conditions are right, causing symptoms. This can also happen in specific

circumstances when the usual vaginal bacterial flora is altered, such as in pregnancy, diabetes, or immunosuppression.

What can Rachel do to treat her thrush and prevent it from recurring?
General advice is to ensure good hygiene, wear loose cotton clothing and avoid perfumed products. There is no evidence for the effectiveness of natural therapies, such as diet modification, live yoghurt and tea tree oil.

Less commonly, men can get symptoms on their penis with a candidal balanitis. If this is the case, her partner will also need treatment.

Rachel has two further episodes in the next 6 months, which resolve with over-the-counter treatment. When her symptoms return, she visits Dr Samson again.

What can Dr Samson do next?
He performs swabs to rule out any other coexisting infections. A charcoal high vaginal swab shows Candidia++

and group B *Streptococcus* (GBS)+. A vaginal NAAT swab is negative for chlamydia and gonorrhoea.

The swab results confirm the clinical diagnosis of thrush. Treatment is only indicated if there are symptoms, as asymptomatic carriage rates of candida are high, at 10%.[6]

Often reported in swabs, GBS is a harmless commensal and does not cause a discharge. It therefore does not require treatment unless the woman is pregnant, as the infection can be dangerous for newborn babies. Pregnant women carrying GBS are given antibiotics in labour.

Dr Samson wants to rule out diabetes and immunosuppression, which are risk factors for recurrent candidiasis. The usual treatment for recurrent symptoms would be a longer course of oral and topical treatment (at least 1 week) and then maintenance treatment. This consists of 6 months of once-weekly oral or topical treatment, which usually has good effect. Infection during this period would suggest resistance and specialist advice should be sought.

Top tip: a presentation of diabetes

- Candidiasis is a common presentation of diabetes.
- Candidiasis is oestrogen-dependent and is therefore rarely seen in prepubertal or postmenopausal women, so consider and look for other diagnoses in these cases.

chlamydia and gonorrhoea. The patient can carry out a low vaginal self-swab for these last two infections; this is the method used in the UK screening programme.

Penile discharge

Penile discharge is associated with urethritis and is a sign of infection. Patients should therefore be referred to a sexual health clinic for investigations and treatment.

Candidiasis in men rarely causes discharge. It presents with balanitis, which is inflammation of the glans and foreskin. Balanitis can also be bacterial, due to Staphylococci, Streptococci or coliforms. It is common in young men with nonretractile foreskins and older men with diabetes. Treatment is topical antifungals or oral antibiotics.

Sexual health epidemiology and sexual health services

Historic events go some way to explaining the changing epidemiology of STIs over the last 100 years. Peaks during both world wars were followed by another peak with the 'Free Love' movement in the 1960s, when there was also easy access

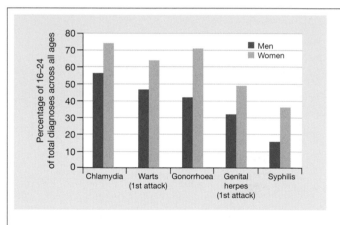

Figure 25.2 Percentage of STIs diagnosed in young people (16–24 years), United Kingdom, 2008. *Source*: Rogstad, KE (ed.) (2011) *ABC of Sexually Transmitted Infections*, 6th edn. Reproduced with permission of John Wiley & Sons, Ltd.

to the contraceptive pill and antibiotic treatments. A temporary fall followed the advent of acquired immunodeficiency syndrome (AIDS) in the 1980s and 90s, but this is now seen as a more treatable disease, and in recent years the incidence of STIs has been increasing. This is seen especially in young people, with those in the 16–24 age group accounting for around half of all newly diagnosed STIs in the UK[7] (see Figures 25.2 and 25.3). This is thought to be due to unsafe sexual practice and a comparatively high rate of partner change. In addition, teenage girls are more susceptible to chlamydia than adults, due to a more immature cervix and increased use of the COC pill.

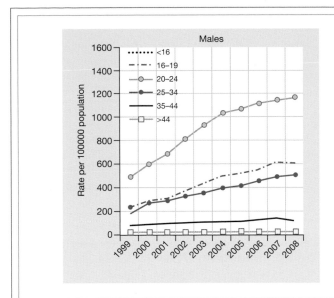
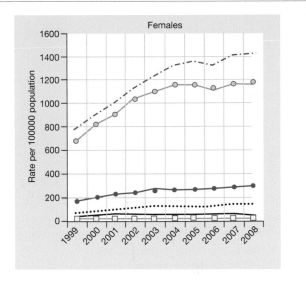

Figure 25.3 Diagnoses of uncomplicated chlamydia infection in genitourinary clinic by sex and age group in the United Kingdom, 1999–2008. *Source*: Rogstad, KE (ed.) (2011) *ABC of Sexually Transmitted Infections*, 6th edn. Reproduced with permission of John Wiley & Sons, Ltd.

Chlamydia diagnoses are increasing in young people. In part, this is due to increased screening, more sensitive tests and easier access to services. Because many patients are asymptomatic, the true prevalence of infection is higher than the recorded prevalence. While symptoms may be minimal or absent, the long-term complications of untreated chlamydia can be serious; they include infertility, chronic pelvic pain and ectopic pregnancy. Bloodborne infections are a significant worldwide cause of morbidity and mortality.

Sexual health services

While improved sex education and political will are essential to addressing the issue, health professionals are central not only in managing STIs but also in education and in preventing spread and future infection. At the inception of the NHS, patients were only given direct access to two services without first going to their GP: accident and emergency departments and sexual health clinics. Now, sexual health care is provided by a mix of primary and secondary care in a variety of settings.

The current public health strategy is to improve sexual health outcomes by providing accurate, high-quality and timely information, preventative interventions and early, accurate and effective diagnosis and treatment of STIs, including human immunodeficiency virus (HIV).[8] Patients should have rapid access to confidential, open-access, integrated sexual health services in a range of settings, accessible at convenient times and working with other specialities when appropriate. The aim is 'joined-up provision that enables seamless patient journeys across a range of sexual health and other services, to include community gynaecology, antenatal and HIV treatment and care services in primary, secondary and community settings'.[8]

UK services have been stratified to three levels:

- All GPs offer level 1 services: testing women for STIs and assessing and referring symptomatic men.
- Level 2 services involve primary care teams with a specialist interest: sexual health screening, treating and managing partner notifications.
- Level 3 refers to specialist services: sexual health clinics, abortion and community family planning.[9]

The structure and organisation of health services is always changing, and the reality is that while some patients prefer specialist clinics, these services do not have the capacity to manage all STIs. Many are thus treated in primary care. GPs often provide level 2 services and offer guidance and referral for level 3 services. GPs also have an essential role in promoting sexual health and educating patients about safe sex, contraception and relationships.

Specialist services can provide full screening, microscopy with immediate results and contact-tracing. They are particularly important for more complex and high-risk patients, some of whom might struggle to access primary care. They also provide advice and support to GPs. Contact-tracing is done by sexual health clinics. As a minimum, an attempt should be made to contact all of a patient's sexual partners from the 3 months prior to their diagnosis of a STI.

Who is at risk?

STIs are more common in women, men who have sex with men and young adults. They are also seen more frequently in black Africans, commercial sex workers and returned travellers who had sexual contacts abroad.

In addition, the following can increase risk:

- unsafe sex: not using barrier contraception;
- concurrent partners, multiple partners, recent partner change;
- STI in partner;
- another STI;
- mental health problems;
- using drugs or drinking excess alcohol.

Taking a sexual history in primary care

In 2013, the British Association for Sexual Health and HIV (BASHH) produced an international guideline accredited by the National Institute for Health and Care Excellence (NICE) for consultations requiring sexual history-taking. This covers communication, components of the history and documentation. It emphasises the importance of ensuring confidentiality; a patient's attendance at a sexual health clinic is not routinely disclosed to the GP without the patient's explicit consent.[10]

As detailed earlier in this chapter, a comprehensive full sexual history is needed in specialist clinics but may be felt to be time-consuming, unnecessary and intrusive in the primary care setting. Indeed, it has been shown that in low-risk asymptomatic patients, too many detailed questions may reduce the truthfulness of responses and uptake for screening.[11]

So, a history in primary care may be shorter. A good approach is to start with nonintrusive, open questions to decide if the patient is low or high risk, and then to direct further questioning from there.

Regardless of the level of detail, these consultations require sensitive questioning, skilled consulting and reassurance regarding confidentiality. In particular, a nonjudgemental approach is essential; as a doctor, one needs to recognise one's own feelings and to ensure that the patient's age, gender, ethnic, cultural and religious beliefs do not influence one's interaction with them.

For patients under 16, their competency should be assessed using the Fraser guidelines (see Chapter 16). The history should include questions to assess any safeguarding concerns. Table 25.5 describes history, examination and investigations of STIs in primary care.

Top tip: managing STIs

- Stat doses increase adherence.
- Contact-trace; partners should be treated.
- The patient must avoid unprotected intercourse until treatment is complete.
- Screen for other STIs, as they often coexist.
- Educate patients to reduce risk of recurrence.
- Discuss contraceptive needs.

Case study 25.3 Pelvic inflammatory disease and chlamydia

Jasmine Jameson, age 24, books a telephone consultation with Dr Sam Rodgers as she has had some intermenstrual bleeding. Dr Rodgers establishes that Jasmine normally uses condoms, but not always. She has not missed a period and has no symptoms of postcoital bleeding, dysuria, vaginal discharge or abdominal pain. Jasmine has recently split up with her boyfriend.

What are the possible causes of Jasmine's bleeding, and does she need any investigations?
Intermenstrual bleeding may be physiological, but it always needs assessment. It has many possible causes, including the COC pill, endometrial polyps, uterine fibroids, endometrial hyperplasia or cancer, cervicitis and cervical, vulval or vaginal cancer. Dr Rodgers therefore suggests that Jasmine attends for a pelvic examination and swabs to rule out an STI and find the cause of her abnormal bleeding.

Jasmine asks to see Dr Rodgers again 2 months later, as she now has pelvic pain. He learns that she didn't book the appointment he previously suggested. Jasmine is feeling unwell with fever and bilateral pelvic pain. Further history reveals she is experiencing dyspareunia and ongoing intermenstrual bleeding.

On examination, Jasmine is febrile with lower abdominal tenderness, adnexal tenderness and cervical excitation

What should Dr Rodgers do next?
Guidance from BASSH is that in any sexually active woman under 25 with recent-onset pain and localised tenderness, we should think about PID, rule out pregnancy and send swabs, but these should not delay treatment, which should be started empirically.[12]

PID is infection of the upper genital tract; it is usually an ascending infection from the endocervix, although it can be descending. One-quarter is caused by chlamydia and gonorrhoea. It is more common in patients under 25 years and in those with a history of previous STIs, new or multiple partners and recent uterine instrumentation. Multiple antibiotics are needed to cover all possible causative organisms. Complications include tubo-ovarian abscess, recurrent pelvic infection, ectopic pregnancy and infertility. Patients who are unwell should be referred to hospital, where they may be treated with intravenous antibiotics, and laparoscopy may be performed if the diagnosis if uncertain. If managed in primary care, local antibiotic guidelines should be followed, early review should be arranged and the patient should be advised to seek further help if they deteriorate. It is essential to offer a full STI screen, to advise on barrier contraception and to organise contact-tracing.

Table 25.5 Assessment of sexual health problems.

History (if symptomatic)	Examination (usually reserved for symptomatic patients)
Presenting complaint Specific symptoms: • discharge • itch • soreness • urinary symptoms • dyspareunia • abdominal pain • lumps • rashes or ulcers • fever In women: • menstrual history • abnormal bleeding • smears Contraceptive use Sexual history: • number of partners in last 6 months • gender of partners • type of intercourse • risk in partners PMH, including: • previous STIs • medications • allergies • social history • vaccinations Risk factors for blood borne STIs: • injecting drug use • tattoos/body piercing • medical procedures • blood transfusions	Appearance of genitalia: • discharge • ulcers • warts Vaginal examination in women Consider proctoscopy if anal symptoms or history of anal intercourse
	Investigations (should be done at time of presentation)
	NAAT is the gold standard for identifying chlamydia and gonorrhoea Females: • Charcoal swab for MC&S if vaginal discharge is present. Can self test • Endocervical swabs • First catch urine (less sensitive) Males: • First catch urine (best) • Urethral swab Consider: • Urethral, pharyngeal and rectal swabs if contact with gonorrhoea • Testing vesicular fluid for herpes simplex Offer screening for blood borne infections especially to high risk patients

---

Top tip: screen for asymptomatic chlamydia

Chlamydia is mostly asymptomatic, especially in men, so remember to ask about risk factors in consultations and have a low threshold for offering screening tests.

The National Chlamydia Screening Programme

The English National Chlamydia Screening Programme targets people aged under 25 years. Tests are available from general practice, sexual and reproductive health services and a range of other venues, such as pharmacies.

Screening for chlamydia mostly meets the Wilson and Jungner criteria for a good screening test.[13] It is an important condition. It is asymptomatic in 50–88% of men and women and has a known natural history.[10] The test is acceptable and validated, and there are facilities and clear policies for the evidence-based treatment. The cost of case-finding is economically feasible.

In terms of the screening programme, it has been shown that entirely opportunistic screening does not reach those most at risk. The Scottish Intercollegiate Guidelines Network (SIGN) has produced guidance on who to screen, focussing on those with symptoms and those asymptomatic individuals who are in the highest-risk groups.[14] This includes men and women under 25 years, and screening is therefore targeted at this group.

Focus groups with young people suggest that those offering screening should use the word 'test', not 'screen', and normalise the process. 'All young people should have a Chlamydia test once a year and with every new partner.'[15] It should be explained that no examination is necessary and that individuals can self-test if they wish. For young men, it is important to explain clearly that the test is painless, free, easy to do and easy to treat.

Other sexually transmitted infections

Genital warts

After chlamydia, genital warts (see Figure 25.4) are the second most common STI in the UK. They are often recurrent. They are usually painless, but can cause some itching or discharge in women. The warts are caused by human papilloma virus (HPV) strains 6 and 11. These are not the types which are associated with cervical cancer, but they are targeted alongside the cervical cancer-associated strains 16 and 18 in the HPV vaccination programme for girls in secondary school. The diagnosis is clinical. GPs may prescribe topical treatment for warts, but sexual health clinics can treat them more effectively with treatments such as cryotherapy, so referral is advisable.

Gonorrhoea

Gonorrhoea is asymptomatic in 50% of women and 10% of men. Men with gonorrhoea are commonly symptomatic, with urethritis and dysuria, and can develop prostatitis. In women, gonorrhoea can present with vaginal discharge, dysuria and abnormal bleeding, and it can cause PID. It can also cause rectal and pharyngeal infections, which are usually asymptomatic in women and mostly asymptomatic in men, or which may present with pain or anal discharge.

Gonorrhoea can cause the same complications as chlamydia, and disseminated infection can cause fever, rash and joint symptoms. Swab for NAAT can provide diagnosis, but urethral, pharyngeal and rectal swabs are also advised if someone has had contact with gonorrhoea. Culture to assess antibiotic sensitivities is important, as resistance is common. Referral to sexual health services is essential.

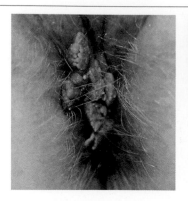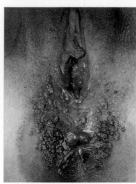

Figure 25.4 Genital warts. *Source*: Rogstad, KE (ed.) (2011) *ABC of Sexually Transmitted Infections*, 6th edn. Reproduced with permission of John Wiley & Sons, Ltd.

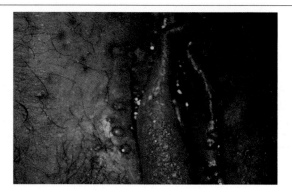

Figure 25.5 Genital herpes. *Source*: Beigi, RH (ed.) (2012) *Sexually Transmitted Diseases*. Reproduced with permission of John Wiley & Sons, Ltd.

Genital *Herpes simplex*

Genital *Herpes simplex* (see Figure 25.5) is usually diagnosed clinically with painful blisters, but can be confirmed by taking a swab for polymerase chain reaction (PCR) testing. It is usually a recurrent condition, although recurrences tend to be milder than the initial episode and can be self-limiting. Oral antiviral treatment with aciclovir may be prescribed by the GP, but sexual health assessment is advised to screen for other STIs and to counsel the patient regarding the diagnosis.

Other causes of genital lumps and ulcers

An examination is essential for all patients presenting with lumps or ulcers. These are often benign, and include pearly penile papules, fordyce spots and common skin problems such as molluscum contagiosum, skin tags, lichen planus and sebaceous cysts. Less common causes include syphilis, vulval cancers and Behcet's and Crohn's disease, all of which should be managed by specialists.

Bloodborne sexually transmitted infections

These infections are commonly sexually transmitted, but can also be transmitted from mother to child during pregnancy and childbirth, and through blood products and tissue transfer. Hepatitis, HIV and syphilis are diagnosed by serology. GPs can offer blood tests to high-risk patients, but must be aware of incubation periods. Confirmed cases must be referred for specialist care.

Human immunodeficiency virus and acquired immunodeficiency syndrome

While there is no cure for HIV, developments in prophylaxis and treatment in developed countries mean that prognosis in the UK is much improved, although worldwide the epidemic continues. Like many STIs, HIV infection can be asymptomatic.

The natural history of HIV is that a glandular fever-type seroconversion illness occurs 1–6 weeks after initial infection. This is self-limiting and may be asymptomatic. An asymptomatic period of many years follows, before constitutional symptoms and opportunistic infections develop. These are referred to as the 'AIDS-related complex', a prodrome to AIDS. AIDS consists of severe immunodeficiency with life-threatening infections and unusual tumours.

Universal HIV testing is offered to everyone attending sexual health clinics, women attending for antenatal care or termination of pregnancy and people diagnosed with tuberculosis (TB) and hepatitis. In high-prevalence areas (>2 per 1000), it should be offered to all new patients registering with a GP and all patients being admitted to hospital.

In primary care, our role is to identify and offer testing to high-risk patients and to offer usual GP care to patients who are HIV positive. High-risk patients are those with another STI or conditions associated with HIV (certain infections and malignancies), and those who originate from high-prevalence regions (e.g. sub-Saharan Africa and India). The risk is also higher in men who have sex with men and those with a history of or current injecting drug misuse.

After initial infection, there is a latent period of up to 3 months, so a negative test should be repeated 3 months after the initial exposure. Men who have sex with men and injecting drug users should be offered annual tests.

Ideally, patients with HIV are under specialist care and monitoring. Patients are encouraged to consent to their GP being notified as to their diagnosis, but this does not always occur. This has potential to cause many problems, not least with prescribing and the risk of interactions with antiretroviral treatments. There have been suggestions that some HIV care could be transferred to primary care.[16] The rationale behind this is that because treatments have improved and regimes have been simplified, the disease now follows a stable and predictable course. HIV patients are living longer, and in some ways it has become a chronic disease like many others we manage in general practice. Patients with HIV are also developing the other diseases we manage every day that are covered in this book. Taking an integrated approach may reduce the risk of prescribing problems and possibly improve overall care.

Hepatitis B

Hepatitis B is transmitted via bodily fluids. Risk factors are similar to those for HIV. The incubation period is 6–23 weeks. Patients may be asymptomatic or may present with an acute hepatitis. Diagnosis is via serology, and treatment is conservative for the acute illness. The majority of patients clear the infection, but 10% become carriers; these are managed by specialist care and may be treated with antivirals and interferon. It is essential to advise these patients about 'safer sex', and close or high-risk contacts may be vaccinated.

Syphilis

Syphilis is caused by the bacterium *Treponema pallidum*. It is uncommon, but is increasing in incidence. The incubation period is 9–90 days, and GPs should investigate and refer any patients who may be at risk. Primary infection presents with a painless sore (chancre) in the genital region, and all patients with such lesions should be referred to a sexual health clinic for treatment with intramuscular penicillin. The sore lasts 2–6 weeks and then disappears, but secondary symptoms such as sore throat and rash may follow. The infection is usually latent for many years, but untreated people may develop tertiary or quaternary infection, which can cause granulomas in connective tissue and severe neurological and cardiovascular problems.

Dysuria is common, and UTIs are the commonest bacterial infections managed in primary care. They are much more common in women, and the incidence increases with age. The symptoms of a UTI can also be caused by chlamydia, an STI. Patients who suspect they have an STI can attend sexual health clinics without a referral, but many patients consult their GP first. Sensitive consulting skills are essential so that people feel comfortable and confident discussing potentially embarrassing symptoms.

SUMMARY

Now visit **www.wileyessential.com/primarycare** to test yourself on this chapter.

REFERENCES

1. Thomas Thomson. *History of the Royal Society: From its Institution to the End of the Eighteenth Century.* Cambridge: Cambridge University Press; 2011.

2. William Shakespeare. *Measure for Measure.* Hertfordshire: Wordsworth Editions; 2005.

3. Little P, Turner S, Rumsby K, et al. Developing clinical rules to predict urinary tract infection in primary care settings: sensitivity and specificity of near patient tests (dipsticks) and clinical scores. *Br J Gen Pract* 2006;**56**(529):606–61.

4. Gupta K, Trautner BW. Diagnosis and management of recurrent urinary tract infections in non-pregnant women. *BMJ* 2013;**346**:3140.

5. Mitchell H. Vaginal discharge – causes, diagnosis and treatment. *BMJ* 2004;**328**:1306–8.

6. Spence D, Melville C. Clinical review: vaginal discharge. *BMJ* 2007;**335**:1147–51.

7. Public Health England. Young people carry disproportionate burden of sexually transmitted infections in the UK. HPA.

2008. Available from: http://webarchive.nationalarchives.gov.uk/20140714084352/http://www.hpa.org.uk/NewsCentre/NationalPressReleases/2008PressReleases/080715annrep/ (last accessed 6 October 2015).

8. Department of Health. A framework for sexual health improvement in England. DOH. March 2013. Available from: http://www.gov.uk/government/publications/a-framework-for-sexual-health-improvement-in-england (last accessed 6 October 2015).

9. Department of Health. *The National Strategy for Sexual Health and HIV.* London: DOH; 2001.

10. Brook G, Bacon L, Evans C, et al. 2013 UK national guideline for consultations requiring sexual history taking. BASHH. 2013. Available from: http://www.bashh.org/documents/Sexual%20History%20Taking%20guideline%202013.pdf (last accessed 6 October 2015).

11. Pavlin NL, Parker R, Fairley CK, et al. Take the sex out of STI screening. Views of young women in implementing

Chlamydia screening in general practice. *BMC Infect Dis* 2008;**8**:62.

12. British Association for Sexual Health and HIV. UK national guideline for the management of pelvic inflammatory disease 2011. BASHH. June 2011 Available from: http://www.bashh.org/documents/3572.pdf (last accessed 6 October 2015).

13. Wilson MG, Jungner G. *Principles and Practice of Screening for Disease*. Geneva: WHO; 1968.

14. SIGN. Management of genital *Chlamydia trachomatis* infection. Scottish Intercollegiate Guideline 109. March 2009. Available from: http://sign.ac.uk/pdf/sign109.pdf (last accessed 6 October 2015).

15. Kalwij S, Macintosh M, Baraitser P. Screening and treatment of *Chlamydia trachomatis* infections. *BMJ* 2010;**340**:c1915.

16. Drugs and Therapeutics Bulletin. HIV services – what role for primary care? *DTB* 2011;**49**:85.

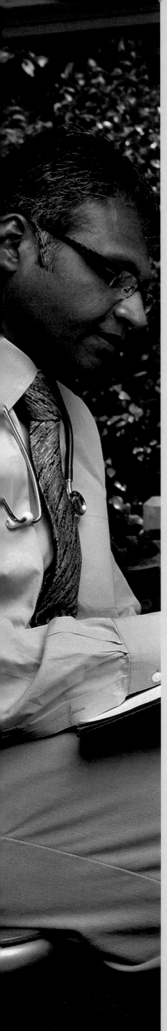

CHAPTER 26

Menstrual problems, contraception and termination of pregnancy

Jessica Buchan
GP and Teaching Fellow in Primary Care, University of Bristol

Key topics

Learning objectives

- Be able to assess, investigate and manage common menstrual disorders presenting in primary care.
- Be able to assess a woman's contraceptive needs and advise her on suitable methods, including postcoital contraception.
- Be able to safely prescribe the contraceptive pill.
- Be able to understand the role of the GP in termination of pregnancy.

Essential Primary Care, First Edition. Edited by Andrew Blythe and Jessica Buchan.
© 2017 John Wiley & Sons, Ltd. Published 2017 by John Wiley & Sons, Ltd.
Companion website: www.wileyessential.com/primarycare

Introduction

Menstruation is part of a woman's experience for nearly 4 decades of her life. Even though menstruation is a normal biological process, periods that are too heavy, frequent or painful can be very disruptive to normal activities. A regular monthly bleed is also seen by many women as indicative of normal health and fertility; when periods don't follow this pattern, or there is a change from a woman's usual cycle, it can cause anxiety. The Internet and media have also increased awareness of the symptoms of gynaecological cancer. A change in bleeding pattern does not necessarily mean that there is serious underlying pathology. Because the menstrual cycle is under the physiological control of a series of hormones, it can be easily and temporarily disrupted, so GPs must strike the balance between careful and thorough assessment and not overinvestigating. There are effective treatments for many of the common menstrual disorders, including many of the methods that are also used for birth control. Assessing a woman's contraceptive needs and being able to advise her on suitable methods should be part of any gynaecological assessment in primary care.

Top tip: be alert to social issues

Consultations for contraception, especially for emergency contraception, may hide many other issues that women are dealing with in their personal lives. Are they experiencing, or at risk of domestic abuse (see Chapter 28)? Are they working as a sex worker? Are they at risk of sexually transmitted disease? Patients with anorexia or other eating disorders may present for the contraceptive pill as a means to regulate infrequent periods (or may appear overly anxious about weight-gain side effects).

The menstrual cycle

Normal menstruation occurs every month from menarche (the first menstrual period) until menopause, unless interrupted by pregnancy. A menstrual cycle is measured from the first day a woman bleeds until the day before her next period and ranges between 21 and 35 days. The bleeding can last from 3 to 8 days, but is usually of 4–5 days' duration.

Women complain of four main problems about their periods:

- timing;
- pain;
- duration;
- quantity of blood loss.

The menstrual cycle is under the control of three sets of hormones, from the hypothalamus, the anterior pituitary gland and the ovaries. The first part of the menstrual cycle is the follicular phase. This phase can vary in length, which is why some women have longer menstrual cycles than others.

Follicle-stimulating hormone (FSH) from the anterior pituitary gland stimulates the development of a dominant follicle on the surface of the ovary. In the middle of the cycle, there is a surge in luteinising hormone (LH) that triggers the follicle to release an egg (ovum). Ovulation occurs 14 days prior to menstruation if the ovum egg is not fertilised. This second part of the cycle is the luteal phase. The ruptured follicle on the ovary forms the corpus luteum; this produces progesterone to prepare the endometrium for implantation. If the ovum is not fertilised, the corpus luteum degenerates, oestrogen and progesterone levels fall and the blood vessels of the endometrium constrict and shed as menstrual blood.

Taking a menstrual history

If a woman presents with problems with her periods, it's helpful to cover the following:

- Age of menarche.
- Clarification of the cycle: length of cycle, regularity, duration of bleeding, relationship of pain or other symptoms to bleeding and whether any aspect of menstruation has changed from the women's usual pattern.
- Is the patient currently sexually active? Has she ever been sexually active? Is there any chance of pregnancy? Has she ever been pregnant?
- Symptoms of pelvic pathology: vaginal discharge, pain on intercourse (especially deep pelvic pain), abnormal bleeding (e.g. spotting or bleeding between periods or bleeding after intercourse).
- Medication: hormones, steroids or drugs that increase prolactin. Past and current contraception, including impact on cycle.
- General health: weight, symptoms of bleeding disorders and other endocrine abnormalities.
- Is the patient up to date with smear tests? Has she ever had an abnormal smear or previous gynaecological problems or investigations?
- Psychological health, including eating disorders, depression and anxiety.
- Social factors, including impact of problem on work, social life and activity. Excessive exercise and stress can cause menstrual irregularities.
- Smoking history (smoking is known to worsen period pain).

Common menstrual problems

Timing

Women complain when their cycle differs from normal or if it is unpredictable. Their periods may not come when expected (delayed), be irregular (called 'oligomenorrhoea' when they are less frequent than expected) or stop altogether (secondary amenorrhoea). Primary amenorrhoea describes the situation where periods do not start by the expected age of menarche (see Chapter 16). Secondary amenorrhoea is when periods have stopped for 6 months or more, but in practice GPs often start investigations earlier than this, as women are often anxious when their periods alter or stop. Pregnancy is the commonest cause of amenorrhoea and should always be suspected and excluded first. Perimenopausal women are at risk of pregnancy if they stop contraception too early (see Chapter 33).

An occasional delayed or missed period is something many women experience, and this is because stress or a change in weight acts at the level of the hypothalamic–pituitary axis

(HPA). Extreme stress to the body, such as in anorexia, may cause persistent amenorrhoea. Pregnancy and menopause are common reasons for amenorrhoea. Investigations include taking a pregnancy test and checking hormone levels at particular points in the cycle. If indicated, thyroid and prolactin levels may also be helpful; there are a number of causes of raised prolactin.[1] Table 26.1 outlines some of the causes of amenorrhoea.

Table 26.1 Causes of amenorrhoea.

Level of problem	Cause	Areas to assess
Hypothalmic–pituitary axis (HPA): functional	Extremes of weight or rapid weight loss, e.g. anorexia Excessive exercise Chronic illness	Stress Exercise habits Changes in weight Food issues Body mass index (BMI)
Anterior pituitary gland: hyperprolactinaemia (suppresses follicle-stimulating hormone, FSH)	Can be: • Physiological – stress, pregnancy, puerperium, breast feeding • Pituitary tumour (90% are benign microadenomas) • Drugs, including antipsychotics, selective serotonin reuptake inhibitors (SSRIs) • Hypothyroidism	Galactorrhoea, infertility, hirsuitism, loss of libido (may indicate hyperprolactinaemia) Symptoms or family history of hypothryoidism Drug history, e.g. SSRIs Prolactinomas: usually small, but if large can cause pressure symptoms, e.g. headaches and visual-field defects
Pituitary gland: hypopituitarism	Surgery, trauma, irradiation Infiltration, e.g. sarcoidosis, tumour Sheehan's syndrome (pituitary infarct following postpartum haemorrhage)	Specific causes suggested by history, with varying degrees of endocrine dysfunction
Rise in gonadal hormones: exogenous	Taking oestrogen or progesterone May persist for up to 1 year after stopping the combined pill	Recent or current contraceptive
Ovarian	Polycystic ovarian syndrome (PCOS): excess androgen production (30% of amenorrhoea) Ovarian carcinoma Ovarian failure (commonly menopause; see Chapter 33)	Acne, weight gain, hirsuitism (may suggest polycystic ovaries) Bloating, pelvic pain
Anatomical	Usually cause primary amenorrhoea Ashermann's syndrome, where the endometrium is scarred following surgery	Whether periods are scanty or have stopped following surgery (e.g. dilatation and curettage for missed miscarriage or retained products of conception)

Case study 26.1

Catherine Bailey is 26. She is a postgraduate student. She presents to her GP, Dr Sofia Martin, with a 4-month history of amenorrhoea since stopping the combined contraceptive pill. She started her periods aged 13 and had an irregular cycle until she started the contraceptive pill. She split up with her boyfriend 6 months ago. Her last pill check records a body mass index (BMI) of 24 kg/m².

What questions should Dr Martin ask Catherine?
• Dr Martin needs to exclude pregnancy. She should ask Catherine if she thinks she might be pregnant. If Catherine is unsure or even if she thinks it is unlikely, Dr Martin should ask questions to assess the possibility (e.g. asking about recent sexual partners, what contraception she has used, adherence to contraception, pregnancy symptoms such as breast

tenderness and nausea) and offer Catherine pregnancy testing.

- She should ask Catherine about current stresses and changes in her weight or exercise pattern.
- What were Catherine's periods like at times when she was not on the pill?
- Has Catherine got any symptoms suggestive of hypothyroidism or a family history of this?
- Has Catherine got any symptoms or signs suggestive of polycystic ovarian syndrome (PCOS) (e.g. excess facial or body hair and acne)?
- Has Catherine ever been pregnant before? Has she got any known gynaecological problems?
- Does Catherine take any medication, whether prescribed or not? Think especially of drugs that raise prolactin.

Catherine says she had two periods when she first stopped the pill, so this isn't a post-pill amenorrhoea, and she doesn't think she is pregnant. She recalls having an irregular cycle before she started the pill, varying from 3 weeks to 8 weeks in length. She is handing in her dissertation, so is quite stressed, and she has gained a bit of weight (her BMI is now 26 kg/m²). Since her ex-boyfriend, she has had two casual partners, with whom she's used condoms for contraception. She is embarrassed about hair on her upper lip and acne and would like something to help these.

What should Dr Martin do next?
- Check and record BMI and blood pressure. PCOS increases the risk of hypertension and a raised blood pressure increases the risks of using the combined oral contraceptive (COC) pill.

- Undertake abdominal examination for masses, concealed pregnancy, and abdominal striae.
- Perform pelvic examination if sexually active, and offer sexually transmitted infection (STI) screening if indicated.
- Take serum blood for a hormone profile in the first week of the cycle (days 1–5). Testosterone or free androgen index can be raised in polycystic ovarian syndrome.
- Conduct a urine pregnancy test.
- Consider testing thyroid function, glucose levels and prolactin, depending on the symptoms and family history.
- Perform a pelvic scan, looking for polycystic ovaries and other ovarian pathology.

Outcome
Catherine has typical symptoms of PCOS and her free androgen index is slightly elevated at 5.1 (the Rotterdam diagnostic criteria are two out of three of: polycystic ovaries on ultrasound, oligomenorrhoea or anovulation and clinical or biochemical signs of hyperandrogenism).[2] Her symptoms could improve with weight loss. Catherine opts to go back on the pill, as this previously helped with her acne and facial hair and she wants contraceptive cover.

What else should Dr Martin cover when discussing PCOS?
She should give Catherine information on this common condition and advise on a healthy lifestyle (weight loss and increased physical activity), as she is more at risk of hypertension, type 2 diabetes and dyslipidaemias in later life.[2] Fertility can be reduced, but if she ovulates, pregnancy can occur naturally.

Intermenstrual or postcoital bleeding

It is important to clarify what women mean by 'irregular periods'; they may actually be describing abnormal bleeding that occurs between their periods (intermenstrual bleeding) or after intercourse (postcoital bleeding). Spotting between periods can be the result of a sexually transmitted infection (STI) such as chlamdyia or pelvic inflammatory disease (PID) (see Chapter 25).

A cervical ectropion occurs when the transition between the columnar cells that line the cervical canal and the squamous epithelium that covers the outside of cervix is visible (Figure 26.1). An ectropion is not harmful, but can bleed more easily, and is a cause of postcoital bleeding. It is more common with higher levels of oestrogen during pregnancy or when women are on the contraceptive pill.

Bleeding between periods or bleeding after intercourse can be a presentation of gynaecological cancer, and pelvic examination and speculum examination is required as part of assessment. Women with a suspicious-looking cervix need urgent

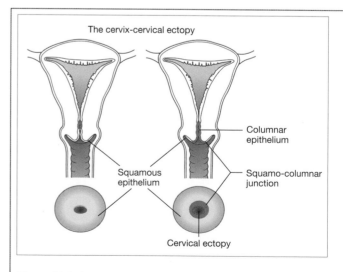

Figure 26.1 A cervical ectropion.

referral. Women with a normal-looking cervix should have pregnancy and STI excluded, but should still be referred urgently for specialist examination if there is persistent post-coital bleeding (especially if over 40), intermenstrual bleeding and vaginal discharge.[3] A smear is a screening test and does not exclude cancer or abnormal cells, so doctors should be wary of being reassured by a normal smear if they are suspicious. Colposcopy is the investigation of choice if cervical cancer is suspected.

Painful periods

It is common for women to experience some mild low abdominal or pelvic pain just before and for the first couple of days of their period. Self-help measures include warmth to the abdomen, such as a warm bath (avoid direct heat, due to burn risk), lying supine, massage and simple analgesia. Dysmenorrhoea is severe or persistent pain. Primary dysmenorrhoea has no underlying pathology; it is common in young women once they start ovulatory cycles and in smokers. If the patient is not sexually active and gives a classic history of pain that resolves within a few days, pelvic examination is unnecessary and a trial of treatment can be given. Most women have tried self-help measures before seeing their GP. GPs recommend regular non-steroidal anti-inflammatory drugs (NSAIDs). The contraceptive pill is often used to reduce pain and bleeding. Pill packets can be run together to reduce the number of bleeds.

Secondary dysmenorrhoea is pain that is caused by pelvic pathology. Women who are sexually active, have more severe or persistent pain or who develop new or different pain to usual should be investigated for underlying causes, such as:

- fibroids;
- PID;
- endometriosis;
- adenomyosis;
- adhesions;
- anatomical abnormalities.

Endometriosis

Endometrial tissue can deposit in sites outside the lining of the uterus, particularly in the pelvic cavity, such as on the ovaries, bowel or bladder, or in the pouch of Douglas. This can cause chronic pelvic pain and pain on intercourse, and is implicated in infertility. Other symptoms, such as urinary tract symptoms, painful defecation, backache or bleeding at extrapelvic sites, can also occur at the time of menstruation. Examination may be normal. Laparoscopy is the gold-standard investigation, but unless symptoms are severe or unusual, patients in primary care are often offered a trial of the contraceptive pill or an NSAID first.

Problems with excess or persistent bleeding

Menstrual loss is very subjective. It is more important to assess whether bleeding is limiting physical activity and social situations. Often, no underlying cause is found. Dysfunctional uterine bleeding is commonest at the extremes of a woman's fertile years, as it is associated with the anovulatory cycles that occur in the first few years after menarche or in the perimenopause (see Chapter 33).[4]

Secondary causes of excessive bleeding include anything that increases the surface area of the endometrium, such as fibroids. Systemic causes include hypothyroidism, bleeding disorders and cirrhosis of the liver. Menorrhagia is the commonest cause of anaemia in fertile women. If a woman presents with heavy periods, it is worthwhile checking her full blood count (FBC) and serum ferritin.

Treatment for menorrhagia

The Mirena intrauterine system (IUS) (see section on Intrauterine Contraceptives: the IUD and IUS) is now a first-line treatment for menorrhagia,[4] and has revolutionised its treatment. Many women were previously referred for hysterectomy. It is reported to result in better control and improved quality of life compared to other methods,[5] but the discontinuation rate may be higher. Other treatments include tranexamic acid, mefenamic acid and the combined oral contraceptive (COC) pill.

Postponing menstruation

Some women wish to delay their period; they may be going on holiday, getting married or sitting an exam. Women on the COC pill can try running two packets together, but the GP needs to warn them that breakthrough bleeding can occur. Alternatively, the GP can prescribe norethisterone (a progesterone), which the patient should start 3 days before her period is due. When she stops the medication, she will have a bleed 2–3 days later. Women should be warned that norethisterone taken in this way is not a contraceptive.

Assessing contraception needs

There is no perfect method of contraception. Women have different contraceptive needs at different times in their lives. One woman's priority may be reliability and not having to remember to take a pill every day, another woman may want a method that doesn't use hormones. GPs need to continue to review the suitability of a method for individual patients and to assess side effects (see Table 26.2).

The reliability (or success rate) of some contraceptives is dependent on the patient's using them correctly. The most reliable forms of contraception do not rely on the patient. Intrauterine devices (IUDs) are reliable because once they have been correctly fitted, they do not require the patient to do anything to make them work, as long as they are replaced on time. IUDs have a failure rate of less than 1%, meaning that out of 100 women, fewer than 1 will get pregnant in a year of use (it is actually closer to 1 or 2 women getting pregnant on the IUD over 5 years of use), compared to more than 80 who would get pregnant in a year if they didn't use any contraception.

Table 26.2 Comparing methods for contraception.

Patient priorities for contraception	Options
Reliability	Intrauterine device (IUD), implant or contraceptive injections are all less user-dependant than condoms or daily pills
Cycle control	COC pill tends to give more reliable cycle control Pill packets can be run together to 'skip' withdrawal bleeds. Although evidence is lacking, it is commonly recommended that women have a break to allow at least four bleeds per year
Nonhormonal	Copper IUD Some women opt for condoms, or use natural methods to assess the most fertile time in their cycle and avoid intercourse at that time, but the risk of pregnancy makes these options unsuitable for many women
No oestrogen (migraine with aura or oestrogen-dependant tumours)	The progesterone-only options include: • Progestogen-only pill (POP) • Injectable contraceptives • Implantable contraceptives • The Mirena IUS or nonhormonal copper IUD
Reversibility	POP, implantable contraceptives and IUD/IUS. Although the COC pill is reversible for most women, they should be warned that a few women do experience a delay in return to normal menstrual cycles

The contraceptive pill is quoted as having a failure rate anywhere between 0.3 and 9%, depending on how reliably a patient takes it.[6]

The combined oral contraceptive pill

The COC pill, often called 'the pill', has a long history of use and a number of positive benefits:
- doesn't interfere with intercourse;
- reversible (although, as discussed, cycles can take time to return to normal);
- regulates cycles and reduces pain and amount of bleeding;
- improves premenstrual tension;
- can improve acne (depending on the type of progesterone in the pill);
- reduces symptomatic fibroids and benign breast disease;
- reduces risk of ovarian, colorectal and endometrial cancer.

Risks of taking the pill

Women worry about the risks of taking oestrogen: there is an increased risk of venous thromboembolism (VTE). However, the clot risk in an otherwise healthy, non-pregnant woman is 5–10 in every 100 000 women. This rises to 20 on the pill, and 60 if a woman is pregnant. There are some important individual risk factors that must be assessed when prescribing the pill, as they may make the risks of taking the pill outweigh the benefits (see Table 26.3). It is the

individual risk that is important in cancers. Studies suggest that being on the pill may decrease a woman's overall risk of cancer, but there is a small increased risk of breast cancer (which returns to normal 10 years after stopping the pill), and an increased risk of cervical cancer linked to duration of use. If a woman has a strong family history of breast cancer, any increased risk could be unacceptable. The Faculty of Sexual and Reproductive Healthcare (FSRH) publishes guidance on the risks of the pill with underlying medical conditions.[7]

Side effects of the pill

Women may develop nausea, headaches and breast tenderness on the pill. Some women complain of mood changes or a change in libido. Side effects can improve on a different preparation. All COC pills contain the same oestrogen: ethinyloestradiol. What differentiates the different types of pill is the dose of oestrogen and the type of progesterone.

Oestrogen can cause the blood pressure to rise, so it is important to check the patient's blood pressure at least once a year when she is on the pill.

Breakthrough bleeding can occur on the pill, and tends to settle in the first few months. It is important to check that women do not have an underlying gynaecological cause for their bleeding. A pelvic and speculum examination should be performed, and a smear test if due, as well as sexual health testing, if indicated.

Table 26.3 Contraindications to the COC pill.

Contraindication	Risk factors for venous thromboembolism (VTE) (avoid if two present)	Risk factors for arterial disease (avoid if two present)
History of VTE or known condition that increases risk, e.g. systemic lupus erythematosus (SLE)/phospholipid syndrome	Family history of VTE in first-degree relative under 45	Family history of arterial disease in first-degree relative under 45
History of arterial thrombosis and transient ischaemic attacks. Heart disease associated with pulmonary hypertension or embolus risk	Obesity: avoid if BMI > 35 kg/m^2 (caution if BMI > 30kg/m^2)	Diabetes (avoid if complications present)
Focal migraine with aura	Long-term immobilisation	Blood pressure >140/90 mmHg Avoid if blood pressure >160/90 mmHg
History of cholestatic jaundice or liver disease	History of superficial thrombophlebitis	Obesity: avoid if BMI > 35 kg/m^2
Hormone-dependant cancer, including breast cancer (consider use if no recurrence after 5 years and no other suitable method)	Age over 35 (avoid over 50)	Age over 35 (avoid over 50)
Undiagnosed vaginal bleeding	Smoker (class as ex-smoker only when stopped for 1 year)	Smoker (class as ex-smoker only when stopped for 1 year)
Known pregnancy		Migraine without aura

Case study 26.2

Kelly is 19 and training to be a children's nurse. She visits Dr Rufus West as she wants to go 'on the pill'. She is asthmatic and takes a regular corticosteroid inhaler, which controls her symptoms. Her periods are regular but heavy and painful; she bleeds every 26 days.

What is it important for Dr West to assess?
- Is the pill the right method? Is Kelly looking for control of her periods and/or contraception? Is she planning a family soon?
- Does Kelly have any contraindications to taking the pill? What risk factors does she have? Has she ever had a migraine with aura? Is there a personal or family history of clots in the lungs or legs? Is there any chance of current pregnancy?
- Is Kelly on medication that could interfere with the pill, including nonprescribed medicines like the herbal preparation St John's wort?
- Does Kelly smoke?
- Have Kelly and her partner had up-to-date sexual health screening tests?
- Examination: BMI and blood pressure should always be checked and recorded.

Kelly has no contraindications to taking the pill. She wants a reliable method that can delay bleeding if she's on a night shift. Dr West discusses the Mirena IUS; this should lessen her bleeding (in many women, periods stop altogether) and is a reliable long-term form of contraception; she wouldn't have to remember to take it, which could help with a shift-work pattern. Kelly decides to read about this, but would like to start the pill today.

What information should Kelly be given about the COC pill?
Dr West doesn't assume that because Kelly is a trainee nurse, she knows anything about the pill. All women should have the opportunity to go through all the details of taking the pill. Women often stop the pill without seeking advice, so it's important to address misconceptions early (see Box 26.1). Kelly should also know what to do if she misses a pill; she should keep the information provided by the manufacturers in the pill packet handy.

Box 26.1 How to take the COC pill

- Start the pill on days 1–5 of your next period. If you are sure you are not pregnant, you can start the pill at a different time, but you will need to use condoms or abstain from sexual contact for 7 days after starting.
- Take the pill every day for 21 days, followed by a break from taking it for 7 days.
- During the 7-day break, you will have a bleed due to the withdrawal of the hormones; this bleed may be lighter than your usual period.
- During the 7-day break, you do not need any other form of contraception: you cannot get pregnant as long as the break is not longer than 7 days.
- It is very important that you do not miss any of the first seven pills in a packet: these pills stop ovulation (release of an egg) from occurring.
- If you do miss a pill, follow the 'missed pill' guidelines on the leaflet in your pill packet.
- Some women take two or even three packets 'back to back' to reduce the numbers of bleeds they have in a year. This is not harmful, but it is recommended that you have four periods a year.

- If you vomit within 2–3 hours of taking the pill, you should take another one.
- Continued vomiting or severe diarrhoea can affect absorption of the pill; follow the 'missed pill' guidelines.
- Most antibiotics do not affect the absorption of the pill, unless they are enzyme-inducing antibiotics, like rifampicin. You do *not* need to use additional contraception on most antibiotics: take your pill as usual.
- Other medicines, such as antiepileptics and the herbal preparation St John's wort, can also interfere with the pill working properly.
- To help make taking your pill a habit, it can be useful to link it to an activity like brushing your teeth. Some women find it helpful to set a reminder on their mobile phone.
- Discuss side effects with your GP, especially if you are thinking of stopping the pill. You can get pregnant if you stop the pill at the wrong time.
- There are some situations where the pill needs to be stopped immediately, so if you develop a severe headache, leg swelling, chest pain or breathlessness, you should seek urgent medical advice.

Progesterone-only methods of contraception

The progestogen-only pill

The progestogen-only pill (POP or mini-pill) does not contain oestrogen. It is a suitable alternative for women who are breast-feeding, have migraine with aura or are a smoker over the age of 35. Mini-pills usually need to be taken within 3 hours of the same time every day and are taken daily without a break. Cerazette can be taken within 12 hours of the time it is due. This development has made the mini-pill useful as a first-line contraceptive. Side effects include irregular or infrequent bleeding, and Cerazette especially may cause amenorrhoea.

Progesterone-only injectable and implantable contraception

Injectable progesterones are a reliable form of progesterone-only contraception. They are given every 12 weeks (for Depot Provera) or every 8 weeks (for Noristerat). They can be effective at reducing heavy or painful menstrual bleeding, but can cause amenorrhoea or irregular bleeding. There are concerns that they may cause reduced bone mineral density. Other methods are usually preferred in adolescents or those with other risk factors for osteoporosis. Women who've used injectable progesterones continuously for more than 2 years should be reviewed and offered other methods of contraception, especially if they are amenorrhoeic. Women should be advised that as the injectable contraception is long-acting, it is not immediately reversible; side effects such as unscheduled bleeding may persist for several months on stopping.

Progesterone-only implants are fitted under the skin with a small operation using local anaesthetic. They release a very small daily dose of hormone: less than in other hormonal methods. They are very reliable, and are also fully reversible on removal. Implants can cause irregular bleeding, but often make periods lighter, and one in five women stop bleeding. Although it's difficult for observers to see it when fitted, the implant can be felt; women should also be warned that it is visible under ultraviolet light.

Intrauterine contraceptives: the IUD and IUS

An IUD, 'the coil', is a small piece of plastic coated with either copper (copper IUD) or progesterone hormone (Mirena IUS). Both types are fitted by insertion through the cervical canal. Once fitted, the copper coil can stay in place for up to 10 years, and the Mirena coil for 5 years. Both types are reliable methods. The copper coil makes periods heavier, but women choose it because it is nonhormonal and doesn't interfere with their normal cycle. The Mirena coil is used as a treatment for heavy, painful periods. With both types, there is a risk of expulsion, and rarely (fewer than 2 women in 1000), the coil can perforate the muscle of the uterus. After fitting, the threads of the coil protrude through the cervical canal. The threads should be monitored to check the coil is in the right place: if they are not visible or are shortened, a pelvic ultrasound is needed to assess the position of the coil. If a woman becomes pregnant with a coil in situ, the risk of an ectopic pregnancy is increased.

Case study 26.3

Alice O'Connell, age 28, wants a prescription for the 'morning-after pill', after the condom her partner used came off at about 10 pm last night. She has only been with her current sexual partner for a few weeks and she is starting a business. She tells her GP, Dr Sofia Martin, that it is very important to her that she doesn't get pregnant at the moment.

What are Alice's options?
There are two types of pill that can be taken after intercourse to prevent pregnancy, or she can have a copper coil (IUD) fitted as long as she is not already pregnant. Dr Martin should check when Alice's last period was and if there have been other episodes of unprotected intercourse in this cycle. The IUD is the most reliable form of postcoital contraception and can be used 5 days after intercourse or within 5 days of the earliest calculated date of ovulation (14 days prior to the next expected period, which would be day 14 of a 28-day cycle).

Alice wants to know more about the morning after pill
Levonelle is a progesterone pill that can be used up to 72 hours after intercourse. Ulipristal acetate (EllaOne) is a selective progesterone receptor modulator that acts by inhibiting ovulation. It may also act on the endometrium and prevent implantation. It is at least as effective as Levonelle, and can be used up to 5 days after intercourse.

What are the contraindications to the hormonal methods of emergency contraception?
There are no absolute contraindications to Levonelle, except acute porphyria. If a woman is on enzyme-inducing medication then an increased dose of Levonelle is advised, or a copper coil should be fitted. The safety of ulipristal acetate has not been established in breastfeeding, so it is advised that breastfeeding is avoided for a week after use. Ulipristal should also not be used repeatedly in the same cycle.

Alice decides to opt for the coil, but would like to take Levonelle now in case there is any delay or problem getting the coil fitted. Dr Martin gives Alice a prescription and the number for her local family-planning clinic so she can arrange for the coil to be fitted. This will give her ongoing contraception – or the coil can be removed during her next period.

What should Dr Martin advise Alice about taking Levonelle?
- Levonelle may not be effective if Alice vomits within 2 hours of taking the pill, so she should return for a replacement dose.
- Alice can expect her next period to occur within 3 days of the expected date, but some women bleed sooner than this. If the bleed is delayed by 7 days or is unusually light, she should perform a pregnancy test.
- If Alice does not get the coil fitted, she should use barrier methods or abstain from intercourse until she has bled.

Postcoital contraception

Women who take Levonelle as a precaution when they have missed contraceptive pills should be advised to restart their usual method of contraception within 12 hours of taking it. They should also use a barrier methods for 7 days if they are on the COC pill, and for 2 days if they are on the POP. Due to concerns that Ulipristal may reduce the effectiveness of hormonal contraception, barrier methods are currently recommended up to 14 days after use depending on the method. New guidelines also suggest hormonal contraception may interfere with the efficacy of Ulipristal so shouldn't be restarted for 5 days after use.[8]

Termination of pregnancy

Women need good education about family planning and access to contraception if the current high rates of unwanted pregnancies are to be reduced. In 2012, the total number of abortions in England and Wales was 185 122. For women aged between 15 and 44, the abortion rate was 16.5 per 1000 women. The rate was highest in women in their early 20s (31 per 1000 women aged 21).[9]

Termination is legal in the UK under the Abortion Act 1967, if it fulfils certain criteria. The pregnancy must be less than 24 weeks' gestation and terminating the pregnancy must:
1. reduce the risk to a woman's life; or
2. reduce the risk to her physical or mental health; or
3. reduce the risk to the physical or mental health of her existing children; or
4. prevent the baby's being born with a serious mental or physical handicap.

Most terminations are performed under clause 2. If there is a serious risk to the mother's health or life or a risk of serious handicap to the child, there is no upper gestational age limit.

Some doctors argue for the reduction of the legal gestational age, as with advances in care it is increasingly possible for neonates of 23 or 24 weeks to survive outside the womb. GPs may disagree with termination on moral or religious grounds, and there is no obligation on them to refer for a termination. The General Medical Council (GMC) advises that doctors should be clear about their stance with the patient, make it clear the patient has the right to see another doctor and provide information about alternative services.[10]

The options for women include medical termination using mifepristone plus a prostaglandin, or surgical suction termination after 7 weeks. Medical termination is usually used if the pregnancy is over 12 weeks. The role of the GP is to discuss the options with the woman and/or her partner (although note that the woman's partner cannot consent to or refuse abortion on a woman's behalf) and provide counsel to help them reach the best decision for them. Often, this takes more than one consultation. In some areas of the UK, women can self-refer to organisations that are contracted to the NHS to provide assessment and carry out terminations. GPs should provide women with information about these organisations to allow them to self-refer.

SUMMARY

Menstruation is a normal biological process, but can cause problems for women. Excess bleeding can cause anaemia, and heavy bleeding or painful periods negatively impact quality of life. Women may see their GP for advice on controlling their cycle. Hormonal treatment can make periods lighter, more regular or less frequent, or can be used to postpone bleeding. In the younger woman, hormonal treatment can also offer contraceptive cover. However, GPs need to be alert to when abnormal bleeding needs further investigation.

 Now visit **www.wileyessential.com/primarycare** to test yourself on this chapter.

REFERENCESS

1. Levy A. Interpreting raised prolactin levels. *BMJ* 2014;**348**:g3207.

2. Royal College of Obstetricians and Gynaecologists. Long-term consequences of polycystic ovarian syndrome. Green Top Guideline 33. 2007. (Revised November 2014.) Available from: https://www.rcog.org.uk/globalassets/documents/guidelines/gtg_33.pdf (last accessed 6 October 2015).

3. NICE. Referral guidelines for suspected cancer. NICE Clinical Guideline 27. June 2005. (Modified April 2011.) Available from: https://www.nice.org.uk/guidance/cg27 (last accessed 6 October 2015).

4. NICE. Heavy menstrual bleeding: investigation and treatment. NICE Clinical Guideline 44. January 2007. Available from: https://www.nice.org.uk/guidance/cg44 (last accessed 6 October 2015).

5. Gupta J, Kai J, Middleton L, et al. Levonorgestrel intrauterine system versus medical therapy for menorrhagia. *N Engl J Med.* 2013;**368**(2):128–37.

6. Trussell J. Contraceptive failure in the United States. *Contraception* 2011;**83**:397–404.

7. Faculty of Sexual and Reproductive Health Care. UK medical eligibility criteria for contraceptive use. November 2009. (Revised May 2010.) Available from: http://www.fsrh.org/pdfs/UKMEC2009.pdf (last accessed 6 October 2015).

8. Faculty of Sexual and Reproductive Health Care. Available from: http://www.fsrh.org/pdfs/CEUStatementQuickStartingAfterUPA.pdf (last accessed 6 October 2015).

9. Department of Health. Abortion statistics, England and Wales: 2012. April 2014. Available from: http://www.gov.uk/government/uploads/system/uploads/attachment_data/file/307650/Abortion_statistics__England_and_Wales.pdf (last accessed 6 October 2015).

10. General Medical Council. Good Medical Practice: personal beliefs and medical practice – guidance for doctors. 2013. Available from: http://www.gmc-uk.org/guidance/ethical_guidance/21171.asp (last accessed 6 October 2015).

CHAPTER 27
Pregnancy

Jessica Buchan
GP and Teaching Fellow in Primary Care, University of Bristol

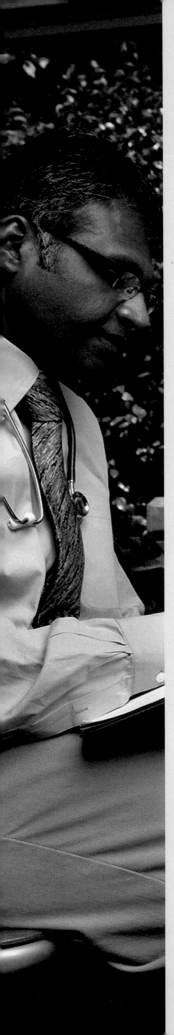

Key topics

Learning objectives

- Be able to give preconceptual advice and advice in early pregnancy.
- Be able to take a history, initiate investigations and know when to refer couples who have difficulty conceiving.
- Be able to describe the antenatal screening programme in the UK.
- Be able to manage common problems presenting to primary care in pregnancy and the purpureum.

Essential Primary Care, First Edition. Edited by Andrew Blythe and Jessica Buchan.
© 2017 John Wiley & Sons, Ltd. Published 2017 by John Wiley & Sons, Ltd.
Companion website: www.wileyessential.com/primarycare

Preconceptual advice

All women benefit from maximising their health prior to pregnancy, so it is important for the GP to offer preconceptual advice. For instance, folic acid reduces the risk of foetal malformation but is most beneficial if taken prior to conception, so women have to be aware of its use before they get pregnant. Some consultations lend themselves naturally to preconceptual advice. During a contraception consultation, the GP can enquire about the patient's plans for future pregnancies. The review of women who are taking potentially foetotoxic medication such as Isoretinion (for acne) or antiepileptic drugs should include preconceptual advice. It is also helpful to ascertain pregnancy plans in women with coexisting health problems such as diabetes, for whom pregnancy would be higher-risk and who would benefit from specialist input prior to conception to maximise the control of the condition. Table 27.1 outlines pre-pregnancy counselling advice. When women present to the GP with difficulty getting pregnant, it is an ideal opportunity for the GP to give preconceptual advice at a time when the patient is often motivated to make changes to take care of their health.

Subfertility in primary care

Most women under 40 years old who don't use contraception and have regular intercourse will get pregnant within a year, and half of those that don't will do so naturally within 2 years of trying. When women don't conceive in this timeframe, the GP can start initial investigations, although if there is a predisposing factor, known cause of infertility or the woman is aged 36 or more, couples should be referred earlier for secondary-care investigations.[2] A cause for infertility is not always identified (in up to 25% of couples[2]), but investigations are important to guide management. Table 27.2 describes the history and examination that should be undertaken when a woman presents with difficulty conceiving. Table 27.3 outlines investigations in subfertility.

Table 27.1 Giving preconceptual advice.

Category	Action
• Lifestyle: • Diet and exercise • Weight • Smoking • Alcohol • Drugs (including risk of hepatitis or human immunodeficiency virus, HIV) • Occupation	Aim for a healthy body mass index (BMI) to improve chances of conception and reduce risks in pregnancy Stop smoking Stop alcohol in the first trimester to reduce the risk of miscarriage Does the patient require occupational health advice? Does her job put her at risk of radiation or other hazards?
Supplements	Take folic acid 400 µg daily (5 mg if high-risk), ideally a month prior to conception, to prevent neural-tube defects
Investigations: • Check immunity • Cervical screening programme • Sexual health testing	Check rubella immunity status Check whether there is a history of chickenpox or shingles – if there is not, check immunity If a smear is due, do it before conception, or it will need to be delayed until after birth
Specific risks	
Age	Most women over the age of 35 have normal pregnancies, but the risk of chromosome abnormalities and complications of pregnancy are increased
Preexisting conditions, e.g. diabetes	Preexisting conditions increase risk for mother and foetus Pregnancy may exacerbate chronic conditions Risks are reduced by good control
Foetotoxic medication	May need specialist input and alternative medication prior to conception
Past medical, obstetric or puerperal history	Assess risk of recurrence; may need a specialist opinion
Ethnicity	Screen for thalassaemia and sickle-cell anaemia if in a high-prevalence area Check family-of-origin questionnaire[1]
Family history/risk of genetic abnormalities	Consider specialist genetic counselling

Table 27.2 Initial history-taking to assess infertility in primary care.

Common cause of infertility in primary care	History
General	Previous pregnancies/abortions/miscarriages/ectopics Pre-existing children impact on eligibility for funding
Problems with intercourse	Frequency of coitus (two or three times a week is optimum) Painful or difficult intercourse Male erectile or ejaculation dysfunction
Age	Female fertility naturally declines with age (males to a lesser degree)
BMI	BMI <19 or >30 reduces fertility Men with a BMI >30 also have reduced fertility
Lifestyle	Smoking cigarettes or cannabis reduce fertility in both partners
Coexisting medical conditions	Poorly controlled diabetes affects fertility
Ovulation disorders (25%)[3]	Menstrual cycle in women Ask about galactorrhoea Acne or hirsutism may indicate androgen excess
Uterine or peritoneal disorders (10%)[3]	Significant fibroids can prevent implantation Endometriosis can cause pelvic adhesions
Tubal or cervical problem (20%)[3]	History of pelvic inflammatory disease or pelvic surgery
Male factors (30%)[3]	Testicular or inguinal surgery Previous infections causing orchitis, e.g. mumps Medication: sulphasalazine impairs spermatogenesis Ask about secondary sexual characteristics Gynaecomastia may indicate hyperprolactinaemia

Table 27.3 Investigations and causes of infertility.

Female	Test ovulation is occurring: day-21 progesterone (if low, repeat). Can do weekly if cycle is irregular
	Hormone profile: lutenising hormone (LH), follicle-stimulating hormone (FSH), testosterone, sex hormone-binding globulin, free androgen index
	Prolactin and thyroid function, if suggested by the history
Male	Semen analysis (if mildly abnormal, repeat at 3 months after lifestyle advice)
	If grossly abnormal (e.g. azoospermia), repeat as soon as possible. Refer if confirmed
	Target other investigations: HbA1c if erectile dysfunction
	Chromosome analysis if hypogonadism
	Before infertility treatment, check rubella status in woman
	Offer both partners testing for HIV and hepatitis C and B

Case study 27.1a

Shruti Gupta is a 28. She consults her GP, Dr Isobel Watson, because she is not getting pregnant. She came off the contraceptive pill 14 months ago.

What are the areas in the history and examination that Dr Watson should assess?
Dr Watson asks about Shruti's menstrual and contraceptive history (see Table 27.2).

Since stopping the pill, Shruti's periods have been regular, with a 28-day cycle, but heavy and painful. She was initially prescribed the pill to manage dysmenorrhoea.

Dr Watson sensitively enquires how often Shruti and her partner have intercourse, as infrequent intercourse lessens the chance of conception. She also asks about problems with intercourse. Shruti admits to intermittent deep dyspareunia since stopping the pill. She had blamed being tense; the couple are feeling the strain of trying to conceive.

Shruti has no other medical problems, has never been pregnant, had surgery or had any gynaecological investigations or procedures, and she doesn't take any medication. To her knowledge she has never had a pelvic infection. She doesn't smoke, and has reduced her alcohol intake to 1–2 units per week for the last year. She is taking folic acid.

On examination, Shruti's BMI is 22. A pelvic examination reveals tenderness in the posterior fornix.

What investigations should Dr Watson organise at this stage?
The most basic investigation Dr Watson is likely to organise is a day 1–5 hormone profile (FSH and LH) and a midluteal progesterone level on day 21 of Shruti's cycle (in a 28-day cycle), where day 1 is the first day of her next period. A pelvic scan is arranged in view of the dyspareunia and heavy, painful periods.

Shruti's partner sees his own GP, who organises semen analysis (see Top tip box and Table 27.4 for reference ranges for semen analysis).

Other tests will depend on the clinical situation. Dr Watson would only test thyroid or prolactin levels if Shruti was symptomatic or there was a strong family history of thyroid disorders. Sexually transmitted infection (STI) testing may be required, especially in view of the dyspareunia. Dr Watson discusses this with Shruti.

Shruti's pelvic scan is normal. She reports her husband had a low sperm count. Dr Watson refers her to secondary care, as her symptoms are suggestive of endometriosis.

What further tests can Shruti expect?
It is not uncommon for causes of subfertility to coexist. Laparoscopy is the gold-standard test to diagnose endometriosis. This is likely to be combined with a dye test to check the patency of Shruti's fallopian tubes.

Further investigations include assessing for ovulation disorders, which may benefit from medical treatment to stimulate the ovaries or from ovarian drilling.

Outcome
Shruti is diagnosed with mild endometriosis on laparoscopy, which is treated with ablation therapy. Shruti's partner makes lifestyle changes, including stopping smoking, and his sperm count returns to normal levels. Shruti finds out that she is pregnant 4 months later.

Table 27.4 Reference ranges for semen analysis.

Semen analysis	Normal values (minimum World Health Organization (WHO) reference values)[2]
Volume	Sample needs to be at least 1.5 ml to analyse
pH	7.2
Concentration (number of sperm per ml)	>15 million sperm/ml
Motility	>40% mobile, or 32% with progressive motility
Normal forms	>4% normal morphology

Top tip: instructions to men on how to perform a semen analysis

- Semen samples need to be assessed promptly. Men are usually advised to take their own sample directly to the laboratory or to do the sample there.
- The sample should be transported to the lab within the hour (ideally, within 30 minutes).
- An appointment needs to be made with the laboratory prior to arrival.
- Men should not ejaculate for 3 days before the test.
- The semen should be collected by masturbation directly into the provided container. The semen must not be collected from a condom, as these often contain spermicides.

Funding for in vitro fertilisation (IVF) on the NHS varies according to local guidelines, but is based on likelihood of success (body mass index (BMI) and age) and other access criteria, such as whether the couple already has children and whether they have previously had infertility treatment.

Case study 27.1b

Shruti consults Dr Isobel Watson as soon as she finds out she is pregnant. It is 5 weeks since her last period. She asks Dr Watson what she should do next.

What should Dr Watson discuss with Shruti?
Dr Watson calculates gestation from the date of the first day of the last menstrual period and estimates a delivery date 40 weeks later.

Gestation is now calculated more accurately by measuring the crown-to-rump length of the foetus on ultrasound at around 10 weeks' gestation.

Shruti is already taking folic acid (see Box 27.1), and should continue for the first 3 months of the pregnancy. She should also be offered vitamin D 10 μg daily. This is offered to all pregnant women in the UK, but it is especially important for women with a BMI >30 kg/m², women with little direct sun exposure to the skin and women whose families originate from South East Asia, Africa, the Caribbean or the Middle East.[3]

Dr Watson advises Shruti to use as few medicines as possible, and only if the benefit outweighs the harm; this means she should tell the pharmacist she is pregnant before purchasing any over-the-counter medications. Just because a medicine is herbal or is labelled as 'natural' does not mean it is safe for use in pregnancy.

Dr Watson advises a flu vaccination, which is free to all pregnant women in the UK and is offered by most surgeries between September and January. Shruti's midwife will offer her a whooping cough vaccine in later pregnancy.

Regarding diet, Dr Watson advises avoiding 'deli counter' produce, due to the risk of listeria and toxoplasmosis. This includes all uncooked meat, fish, soft cheeses and unpasteurised milk. She also advises avoiding food that has been sitting around and washing salads and vegetables thoroughly, even if they are labelled as 'washed and ready to eat'.

Shruti says she runs regularly and asks if it safe to continue to do so. Dr Watson explains that if Shruti already does moderate exercise, she can continue to do so (she would advise inactive pregnant women to start a gentle programme of exercise). She warns that she might not be able to exercise her usual amount, because it's common to feel very tired or lightheaded in the first trimester. Later in pregnancy, girth size and pressure symptoms can make some activities difficult or uncomfortable. Dr Watson checks that Shruti doesn't do excessive exercise or contact sports, which risk damage to the abdomen. She also advises avoiding saunas and hot tubs, which can cause overheating, and that she doesn't scuba dive. Sexual intercourse is safe throughout pregnancy, as long as there is no history of preterm rupture of membranes.

Dr Watson ends the consultation by asking Shruti to make a booking appointment with the midwife and gives her a pregnancy pack, which includes dietary advice and pregnancy information.

Box 27.1 Who should take additional folic acid in pregnancy

5 mg/day should be prescribed to women with:
- BMI >30 kg/m²;
- coeliac disease;
- diabetes;
- antiepileptic medication;
- family history of neural-tube defects;
- sickle-cell anaemia.

The antenatal screening programme

Pregnant women should have a booking visit with the midwife before 10 weeks so that a dating scan can be organised.[3] This is the longest of the antenatal visits. Its purpose is to give the patient information, form a plan for the pregnancy and birth, undertake screening and identify women who need additional care. The aim of antenatal care is to monitor the mother's psychological, social and physical well-being, with regular blood pressure checks and urinalysis, and maternal biochemical tests. Foetal health and well-being are also monitored. Foetal growth is checked by measuring the symphysis–fundal height, the foetal heartbeat is checked and, in the final stages of the pregnancy, foetal position is assessed. Ultrasound scans also check foetal growth and development. Nulliparous women are seen more frequently than women who have given birth before (see Table 27.5).

Screening for Down's syndrome

The dating scan at 10–13 weeks can be combined with a test for Down's syndrome, called the 'nuchal translucency scan'. This scan measures the thickness of a fluid collection at the back of the baby's neck. Women can also have a blood test to assess the risk of Down's at 11–14 weeks.[3] The most accurate calculation of risk can be made when these two tests are combined. Women who miss these tests can have a blood test between 15 and 20 weeks.[3] These are screening and not diagnostic tests. If the risk of Down's syndrome is estimated to be 1 in 150 or greater (in other words, in 150 pregnancies there is a chance that one baby will have Down's syndrome), this is considered high-risk and the woman is offered invasive diagnostic tests. Both aminocentesis and chrononic villus sampling gather foetal cells for chromosome analysis for a range of genetic conditions. Aminocentesis can be performed after 15 weeks; it takes a small amount of the amniotic fluid that surrounds the baby. Choronic villus sampling can be done earlier (between 11 and 14 weeks); it analyses a small amount of placental tissue. Both tests carry a small risk of miscarriage (around 1–2%).[4]

Problems in the first trimester

Most women first realise they are pregnant when they miss a period, but some present with pregnancy symptoms such as unexplained vomiting. Some women have few early symptoms, while others suffer fatigue (which can be extreme: see Chapter 11), frequent urination (due to the effects of BHCG) or breast tenderness. A few weeks into the pregnancy, nausea can start, with or without vomiting. The increased progesterone levels can cause

Table 27.5 UK antenatal screening.	
First visit to midwife	BMI Baseline blood pressure Urinalysis – for baseline protein, to detect diabetes and asymptomatic bacteruria Blood tests include: • Full blood count (FBC) – to detect anaemia • Haemoglobin analysis by electrophoresis for haemoglobinopathies, e.g. sickle cell/ Thalassaemia for those at risk[1] • Blood group, rhesus D status and red cell antibodies Rubella immunity status HIV Syphilis Hepatitis B
10–13 weeks	Dating scan. Gestational age calculated using crown–rump length
11–14 weeks	Down's screening via nuchal translucency scan
16–18 weeks	Glucose tolerance test for women with previous gestational diabetes
18–20 weeks	Foetal anomaly scan
25 weeks (for nulliparous women)	Blood pressure, urinalysis for proteinuria and symphysis fundal height measured from now on
24–28 weeks	Glucose tolerance test for women at risk of gestational diabetes
28 weeks	FBC and red cell antibody status Pertussis vaccination offered (to prevent whooping cough in newborns)
31 weeks (nulliparous women)	Review appointment with midwife
36 weeks	Assess position of baby
36 weeks	Repeat scan if 20-week scan showed a low placenta
38, 40 and 41 weeks	Review appointments with midwife for all pregnant women At 41 weeks, women are offered membrane sweep and induction of labour is considered

Case study 27.1c

Shruti Gupta returns to her GP when she is 13 weeks pregnant. She felt nauseated in the first trimester, but in the last 2 days she has started vomiting three or four times a day. She is keeping down regular sips of fluid but her urine is darker than usual and has a 'funny smell' to it. She has also noticed lower abdominal pain. She is worried she is having a miscarriage.

What should Dr Watson assess?
Nausea and vomiting are common in early pregnancy, and usually start about week 7. It is unusual for the symptoms to start or worsen after the first trimester, so in Shruti's case Dr Watson is looking for underlying causes. The GP should also assess for dehydration and perform a urinalysis for ketones. Women who are not keeping fluid or oral antiemetics down, and who show signs of significant dehydration or ketosis, should be admitted for fluid replacement.

Severe lower abdominal pain in early pregnancy is an ectopic until proven otherwise and needs urgent admission. Shruti says her pain is very mild, dull and suprapubic; it only occurs when she wants to pass urine. Dr Watson asks her about vaginal bleeding, which with or without abdominal pain can indicate a miscarriage. Most hospitals have an early pregnancy assessment unit where women who have possible signs of miscarriage can be booked for a scan. Multiple pregnancies can cause hyperemesis, but Shruti's dating scan 2 weeks ago showed a singleton viable intrauterine pregnancy.

On examination, Shruti is apyrexial; her blood pressure is 110/60 mmHg and there is no renal angle or abdominal tenderness. Urinalysis shows leucocytes+++, a trace of protein and blood, and is positive for nitrates. There are no ketones or glucose in the urine.

With Shruti's symptoms, examination findings and scan results, Dr Watson suspects a urinary tract infection (UTI). In view of her symptoms, she sends a sample for microscopy and culture and starts a 7-day course of empirical antibiotics (that are appropriate for use in pregnancy). Dr Watson also prescribes oral rehydration solution. Shruti declines antiemetics. Dr Watson makes Shruti aware that she should be seen as a matter of urgency if she develops more severe abdominal pain, loin pain, fever or vaginal bleeding, or if she is not keeping fluids down or passing a good amount of urine every 2 or 3 hours.

Outcome
Shruti is reviewed 48 hours later with urine microscopy and culture results. She has a proven urine infection, which is sensitive to the antibiotics she is taking. She feels much better. If Shruti was not improving at this point, she might need alternative or intravenous antibiotics, and admission should be considered.

constipation, and some women experience food cravings or aversions. Women may also experience mood changes. Signs of pregnancy include breast enlargement with visible veins under the skin of the breast, or darkening of the areola.

Urine infections in pregnancy may be asymptomatic, or have fewer of the usual signs. A proven simple urinary tract infection (UTI) or asymptomatic bacteriuria should be treated with antibiotics as per local guidelines.

Vomiting in pregnancy

This is often called 'morning sickness', as some women feel worse in the morning, but other women get nausea or vomiting at all times of day. Symptoms are different for different women in different pregnancies. Vomiting is unpleasant, but women can be reassured that it tends to resolve by the middle of the second trimester. There is no evidence of harm to the developing foetus. Rest, fluids, regular small carbohydrate-based snacks and meals and avoidance of fatty foods can all help. The use of antiemetic medication is generally restricted to women in whom the symptoms are daily and are preventing their normal activities.[5] Nausea in later pregnancy can be due to reflux, which usually responds to antacids.

Hyperemesis gravidarum is where severe vomiting leads to dehydration and electrolyte imbalance. Nausea and vomiting can indicate thyrotoxicosis, so thyroid function tests (TFTs) can be useful, as can checking electrolytes and liver function tests (LFTs). An ultrasound scan can diagnose a multiple or molar pregnancy.

Miscarriage and molar and ectopic pregnancy

Vaginal bleeding in pregnancy always needs assessment, although light bleeding can occur without miscarriage. GPs can refer to an early pregnancy assessment unit, which aim to see and assess women within a day of referral. From 6 weeks, an ultrasound scan can check the foetus is intrauterine and the pregnancy is viable. Another cause of vaginal bleeding is a molar pregnancy. This is the result of abnormal conception, where a mass of trophoblast cells grows in the uterus instead of an embryo. It can be indicated by a much higher than expected level of BHCG for the gestation and can be identified on an ultrasound. The molar pregnancy needs removal. It is closely followed up via the National Trophoblastic Screening Centre's surveillance programme to make sure women don't develop persistent or invasive trophoblastic disease requiring chemotherapy.

An ectopic is a pregnancy that implants outside the uterus, usually in the fallopian tubes. Early diagnosis does not save the pregnancy, but if the embryo grows big enough to rupture the tube, the internal bleeding can be sudden and life-threatening. Symptoms tend to start at 6 weeks with abdominal pain (usually on one side) and vaginal bleeding, and sometimes the patient feels faint or dizzy or complains of shoulder-tip pain. Women may be asymptomatic until sudden collapse. A scan may see the ectopic pregnancy in the fallopian tubes, or it can be picked up when the BHCG is high but there is no intrauterine pregnancy. It is possible for an ectopic to coexist with an intrauterine pregnancy in a multiple pregnancy.

Case study 27.2a

Jayda Jackson, aged 24, sees her GP, Dr Chris Pope, after a 'missed miscarriage' at 11 weeks. There was no foetal heartbeat visible on her dating scan. Jayda initially opted 'for nature to take its course', but eventually needed a surgical evacuation for retained products of conception (ERPC). Now Jayda is tearful and has a number of questions for her GP.

Jayda wants to know why she miscarried. She feels she is to blame, and recalls having a hot bath a few days prior to the scan

A miscarriage can be very upsetting. Women often feel guilty and blame themselves. Dr Pope explains that it is

more likely that a one-off isolated genetic fault meant that the baby was never going to survive. There is nothing Jayda or her partner could have done differently. Up to 20% of recognised pregnancies end in miscarriage, but many more pregnancies probably end before the woman even realises she is pregnant.

Jayda tells Dr Pope that she has a friend who is taking medication to prevent her miscarrying and wonders if she can be prescribed something. Dr Pope suspects Jayda's friend had recurrent miscarriages. Where a woman has had three or more miscarriages (or a second- or third-trimester miscarriage), the chances of another one occurring are much higher, because there is greater likelihood of an underlying cause. A common reason for recurrent early foetal loss is the presence of antiphospholipid antibodies. If this is diagnosed, heparin and low-dose aspirin improve the live birth rate. Otherwise, healthy pregnant women should avoid taking any unnecessary medication and follow healthy lifestyle advice. Most of these women go on to have a successful pregnancy.

Jayda feels reassured and asks how soon she should wait before she tries for another baby. Dr Pope explains that there is no clear medical evidence about this. Some women like to let their bodies 'get back to normal'. A miscarriage results in a period of grief, and some women find another pregnancy easier to cope with when they have had time to come to terms with it. Others want to try again as soon as possible. Dr Pope advises it may be sensible to at least wait until she has had one normal period. The advice would be different for an ectopic or molar pregnancy.

Common problems in the second and third trimesters

Many women feel better in the second trimester, when the symptoms of nausea and fatigue recede, and before the pressure symptoms of late pregnancy develop. The rise in intra-abdominal pressure can cause issues such as indigestion, haemorrhoids, varicose veins, urinary frequency and, in the later stages of pregnancy, shortness of breath. Posture changes, stretching of skin and muscle and the softening of ligaments due to the pregnancy hormones also make back and pelvic pain common. Fluid retention can cause pedal oedema and carpal tunnel syndrome, and can contribute to leg cramps. In late pregnancy, itch is common, and some women develop a pregnancy-related urticarial rash. Most of these complaints are troublesome and are managed with common-sense advice and support.

Top tip: examining the pregnant woman

- Check blood pressure and urinalysis, if not done in the last 1–2 weeks.
- From 20 weeks, a woman should be examined tipped slightly over to the left to reduce pressure on the inferior vena cava.
- Palpate the uterus gently, feeling for contractions, tenderness and foetal movements. Tenderness or a hard woody-feeling uterus may mean infection or a bleed.

- To check for extrauterine causes of abdominal pain in pregnancy (e.g. appendicitis), examine the woman on her side to displace the uterus.
- Vaginal examination in pregnant women is rarely indicated in primary care. If placenta praevia is suspected, examination can precipitate haemorrhage. If there are concerns about premature rupture of the membranes, examination needs to be done under sterile conditions, due to the risk of introducing infection.

Case study 27.2b

Jayda Jackson next sees Dr Pope when she is 15 weeks pregnant. She is concerned about her contact with her 18-month-old niece, who has developed chickenpox.

What should Dr Pope discuss with Jayda?
Chickenpox is infectious for 2 days prior to the rash developing. It is droplet-spread, and is highly infectious to people who are not immune. Most adults have had chickenpox as a child and are thus immune. If there is uncertainty, a blood test can check for antibodies to the varicella zoster virus. If Jayda is not immune, Dr Pope can arrange for her to be given varicella zoster immunoglobulin. Ideally, this is given within 4 days of exposure to the virus, but there is benefit up to 10 days.[6]

What are the risks of contracting chicken pox in pregnancy?
Pregnant women tend to get a more severe episode of chickenpox than children, and the risk of complications such as pneumonia or encephalitis is higher. The developing foetus is at risk of foetal varicella syndrome, especially in the first part of the second trimester. This results in foetal abnormalities. If the mother develops chickenpox in the 7 days before birth, the baby may develop a severe form of chickenpox. If pregnant women do develop chickenpox, specialist advice is needed to treat the mother and monitor the foetus[7] (see Table 27.6).

Jayda tells the GP that she clearly remembers having chickenpox one Christmas as a child, and there are photographs of her opening her presents covered in spots. This is reassuring.

However, Dr Pope notices Jayda hasn't collected her regular prescription for asthma inhalers recently. Jayda says she's been trying not to use inhalers as she didn't want to take steroids in pregnancy.

> *What should the GP discuss?*
> The risk of uncontrolled asthma in pregnancy far outweighs the risk from inhalers, and women should be encouraged to continue their usual asthma medications. Regular monitoring in primary care is crucial in pregnancy, as poorly controlled asthma has implications for foetal and maternal health, so there is a low threshold for specialist input. Asthma and migraine can improve or worsen during pregnancy.

Table 27.6 Infectious diseases in pregnancy.[6]

Infection	Presentation in pregnancy	Risk in pregnancy	Investigation and/or management
Rubella	Light pink rash Starts on face, spreads to trunk Joint pain/swelling Lymph nodes enlarged	*High* risk **First trimester:** 90% risk of congenital rubella syndrome, with mental impairment, heart defects, cataracts and deafness	Rubella and parovirus antibodies Seek specialist opinion if not immune Rising serial IgG and IgM titres suggest recent infection
Parovirus B19	Viral prodrome Erythema of the cheeks (look 'slapped')	Can cause intrauterine death and hydrops fetalis in the *first 20 weeks* if not immune	Parovirus IgG and IgM if exposed or infection is suspected
Chickenpox	Fever and malaise Then crops of vesicular spots that crust over	**First 20 weeks:** risk of foetal varicella syndrome **Near delivery:** risk of chickenpox in neonate	Test for varicella zoster IgG antibodies if no definite history of chickenpox/shingles
Measles	Widespread maculopapular rash, coryza and conjunctivitis	Intrauterine death, prematurity and risk of neonatal subacute sclerosing panencephalitis	If no vaccination or history of infection, test for measles IgG If not immune, give immunoglobulin
Cytomegalovirus (CMV)	Mononucleosis-like infection	Can affect foetal hearing and intellect Risk of malformations if congenital CMV	Test for CMV in pregnant women who appear to have glandular fever Refer if suspected
Toxoplasmosis	Lymphadenopathy, fatigue, headaches, myalgia History of handling cat faeces or eating undercooked meat	**First trimester:** foetal infection causing brain and eye damage, cognitive defects and intrauterine death **Late pregnancy:** risk of transmission	IgG antibodies to check immunity Intrauterine infection diagnosed by aminocentesis

Antenatal depression

The signs and symptoms of depression in the pregnant woman are the same as for depression in the general population (see Chapter 24). Antenatal depression may be missed, as the somatic symptoms of fatigue, insomnia, mood and appetite changes may be put down to pregnancy. GPs should assess psychological symptoms such as low mood and anhedonia with screening questions. Pregnant women with pre-existing depression risk abruptly stopping medication, as they may believe it will harm the foetus. Some selective serotonin reuptake inhibitors (SSRIs) used in the first trimester have been linked with cardiovascular abnormalities, but the evidence is conflicting.[8] There is a link between SSRI use and pulmonary hypertension in the neonate in the third trimester, and there is risk of withdrawal or toxicity in the newborn.[8] GPs should

Top tip: prescribing in pregnancy

- Medication should only be given if the benefits to the mother outweigh the risks to the developing foetus.
- Medication used in the first trimester carries the highest risk of causing congenital malformations; some medication used in the third trimester can cause withdrawal symptoms in the newborn.
- Always check the British National Formulary (BNF), which identifies the risks of various drugs in pregnancy and the trimester in which they should be avoided.
- Aim to use older drugs with a more established risk profile, use the smallest effective dose and discuss the pros and cons of use with the patient.

use an SSRI with the best safety data in pregnancy, so will usually seek secondary-care advice. Initiating medication for depression in pregnancy should be reserved for moderate to severe depression, where woman want to take it. Access to effective adjunct or alternative therapy, such as cognitive behavioural therapy (CBT), is important for maternal and foetal health.

Gestational diabetes

In pregnancy, any degree of glucose intolerance that appears is known as 'gestational diabetes'. It usually resolves after delivery, but can persist, and is a risk factor for the development of diabetes in later life. It is diagnosed using a glucose-tolerance test. Maternal diabetes increases the risk of large-for-dates babies, shoulder dystocia, preterm labour and pre-eclampsia. National Institute for Health and Care Excellence (NICE) guidelines recommend that women who have had previous stillbirths or large babies (over 4.5 kg), women with a high BMI (>30 kg/m^2), previous gestational diabetes or a first-degree relative with diabetes and women from an ethnic background with high diabetic risk (Middle Eastern, Black Caribbean or South Asian) should be screened.[3,9] Some argue that all pregnant women should be screened, as gestational diabetes can occur in women with no risk factors.

Women diagnosed with gestational diabetes are usually taught to self-monitor glucose, keeping fasting levels between 3.5 and 5.9 mmol/l and postprandial levels under 7.8 mmol/l. Foetal growth is monitored on monthly scans. If dietary measures don't control glucose or there is evidence of foetal macrosomia, insulin is usually started.

High blood pressure and pre-eclampsia

Pregnant women can have pre-existing hypertension; this is usually known about, or it can be picked up for the first time at the booking appointment. When high blood pressure > 140/90 mmHg occurs after 20 weeks, it is known as 'gestational hypertension', or as 'pre-eclampsia' if it is associated with proteinuria.[10] Mild disease is relatively common (1 in 100 pregnancies), but it can progress rapidly; severe pre-eclampsia is life-threatening. Hypertension and pre-eclampsia can result in intrauterine growth restriction, preterm labour and stillbirth. 'Eclampsia' is when the condition results in maternal convulsions.

Pre-eclampsia is more common in first pregnancies, women over 40, women with a previous or family history of pre-eclampsia, pre-existing diabetes, hypertension or chronic kidney disease, women with a BMI > 35 kg/m^2 and women with antiphospholipid syndrome.[10] Women at risk are offered low-dose aspirin from week 12.

Case study 27.1d

The practice nurse sees Shruti Gupta for her flu vaccination. Shruti is now 32 weeks pregnant. The nurse checks Shruti's blood pressure, and it is 146/94, which persists on repeat readings. She contacts Dr Isobel Watson, Shruti's GP.

What should Dr Watson do?
Dr Watson requests urinalysis and reviews Shruti straight away.

She checks Shruti's handheld maternal records; her booking blood pressure was 116/66 mmHg. She asks about symptoms; a frontal headache, epigastric pain, visual changes such as blurred vision, sudden swelling of the ankles or face and decreased foetal movements are concerning and indicate the need for urgent admission and assessment.

Shruti has proteinuria++. She has noticed some new ankle swelling and has a mild frontal headache. Dr Watson admits Shruti to the antenatal day assessment unit for blood pressure and foetal monitoring. She will also have blood tests to look for raised liver transaminases, thrombocytopenia and clotting abnormalities.

Outcome
Dr Watson later learns that Shruti's blood pressure continued to rise and she was started on Labetalol (a beta blocker used as an antihypertensive in pregnancy). She was discharged to community home monitoring but induced at 37 weeks due to reduced foetal growth.

Both mother and baby do well after delivery, and Shruti's blood pressure returns to normal 2 weeks later, so her medication is gradually reduced and stopped.

Case study 27.2c

Dr Chris Pope gets a message to telephone Jayda Jackson, who is now 37 weeks pregnant and complaining of itchy skin.

What diagnoses should the Dr Pope consider?
It is quite common in late pregnancy to develop dry itchy skin, especially over the abdomen, where the

skin is stretched. Emollients can help. Prurigo of pregnancy causes itchy bumps; steroid creams applied to the lesions can reduce itch and inflammation.
Dr Pope should also consider conditions unrelated to pregnancy, such as scabies. Obstetric cholestasis presents with intense pruritis without a rash, and abnormal LFTs where no other cause (e.g. gallstones)

can be found. The risk of intrauterine death and premature labour is increased in cholestasis, so the patient should be assessed by secondary care and give birth in hospital.

When Dr Pope telephones Jayda, she says she does have a rash. It started as itchy pink spots on her lower abdomen, and she thought it was due to a new fabric softener she'd use on her underwear. She does not have generalised itchiness: only the rash is irritating. This morning, the rash is red and angry-looking, with patches over her lower abdomen and on the outer thighs (Figure 27.1).

What is going on?
This is a typical history and appearance of pruritic urticarial papules and plaques of pregnancy (PUPPP), also known as 'polymorphous eruption of pregnancy'. The only cure is delivery. Most cases develop in the last few weeks, when the skin over the abdomen is most stretched. It is commoner in first pregnancies, heavy babies or multiple pregnancies. Emollients, steroid creams and antihistamines may help. Some antihistamines can be taken in late pregnancy, but they risk making the baby drowsy on delivery.

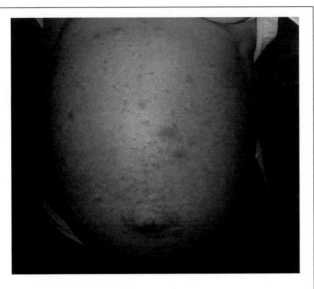

Figure 27.1 Pruritic urticarial papules and plaques of pregnancy (PUPPP) on abdomen. *Source*: via Wikimedia Commons.

The onset of labour

Many women experience Braxton Hicks 'practice contractions' for some weeks before the onset of labour. These are usually felt as a tightening sensation across the lower abdomen. Typically, labour starts with regular and increasingly intense contractions or back pains that become more frequent. Many women get a 'show' (a bloodstained thick plug of mucous from the cervix) before labour starts, or their waters break. Premature labour is labour before 37 weeks. After 42 weeks, the risk of intrauterine death increases, and induction is usually advised.

The membranes surrounding the baby and amniotic fluid may rupture prior to 37 weeks. Women may feel a 'pop' or a gush of fluid, but it may simply present with watery vaginal discharge. If a woman complains of increased vaginal discharge later in pregnancy, the GP should ask if it is watery. If premature rupture of the membranes is suspected, GPs refer the patient to the antenatal assessment unit. The woman may or may not go into spontaneous labour following rupture of the membranes, but there is a risk of ascending infection or too little fluid surrounding the baby (oligohydramnios), so it is vital that mother and baby are monitored for pyrexia and foetal distress.

Vaginal bleeding in late pregnancy can be from placenta previa, where the placenta covers or is close to the os; this is usually picked up on the 20-week scan and monitored during pregnancy. Abruption is where the placenta separates prior to delivery of the baby; the bleeding can be concealed. Abdominal pain, uterine tenderness and a woody-feeling hard uterus suggest the diagnosis. It is a cause of maternal shock and foetal distress.

Problems in the puerperium

The 6-week period after birth is known as the puerperium. The physiological changes of pregnancy return to the non-pregnant state. After delivery, the uterus contracts to approximately the size of a 20-week pregnancy, and then gradually contracts further; by 2 weeks, the GP should not be able to palpate the uterus abdominally. The bleeding after birth (lochia) reduces from bright red bleeding to a brownish discharge over a couple of weeks. A significant increase in bleeding or passing clots can indicate a secondary postpartum haemorrhage; combined with a bulky tender uterus, this may indicate retained products of conception.

Case study 27.2d

Jayda Jackson presents to Dr Pope at 8 days postpartum. She had an emergency caesarean section for failure to progress in labour. She is feeling hot and cold and shivery, as if she has flu.

What should Dr Pope consider?
Dr Pope considers all the usual sources of infection, including a urinary or chest infection, and even appendicitis. Sources of infection specific

to the puerperium include endometritis, retained products of conception and mastitis. Stitches can also become infected, so Dr Pope assesses these.

Jayda says that she thought her bleeding was settling, but for the last few days it has increased and become a bit smelly. She also has lower abdominal pain. On examination, she has a temperature of 38.2 °C and there is uterine tenderness.

In the absence of a UTI, it is likely that Jayda has a postpartum endometritis. This occurs in about 1–3% of births. Sepsis is still a leading cause of maternal death (10%) each year.[11,12] Vaginal swabs are usually taken; endometrial biopsy and ultrasound are rarely helpful. Jayda will need broad-spectrum antibiotics, based on local guidelines. She is treated in the community with oral antibiotics and reviewed within 48 hours. If she does not respond or there are signs of severe sepsis, she will need admission and intravenous antibiotics.

Dr Pope sees Jayda for review 2 days later, and she is much improved. She hasn't had a temperature for 24 hours, and the bleeding is beginning to settle. She asks when she can restart her contraception pill, as her husband is keen for their sex life to resume.

How should Dr Pope address this?
Women may ovulate after 21 days postpartum, so will need contraception. Women who are exclusively (or almost exclusively) breastfeeding and not having their period (so-called 'lactational amenorrhoea') may opt to use breastfeeding as a method of contraception for up to 6 months. Up to 2 in 100 women get pregnant using this method, so it is fairly reliable, but not as reliable as the contraceptive pill. For breastfeeding women, the progestogen-only pill (POP) or implant can be given from 21 days, and the progesterone-only injection from 6 weeks.

Dr Pope needs to check if Jayda is breastfeeding, as she should avoid oestrogen until the baby is 6 months old if so, as it may affect milk supply. He should perform the usual checks for starting contraception (Chapter 26).

Dr Pope also wants to check that Jayda is not describing pressure from her husband to resume intercourse (see Chapter 28). Jayda says her husband is very supportive, it's just that she feels guilty that she is spending all her time on the baby.

The GP notices Jayda seems flat in affect. She admits to having 'terrible baby blues'. She can't seem to stop crying and she is so anxious about the baby that she can't sleep.

How are baby blues different from postnatal depression and puerperal psychosis?
Baby blues occur around days 3–5 and are characterised by a transient low mood. Jayda may be developing postnatal depression. Dr Pope assesses Jayda's mood, suicidal ideation and feelings of attachment towards the baby. The Edinburgh Postnatal Depression Score (EPDS) is used as a screening tool.

Puerperal psychosis is a rare but serious condition that often has an acute onset a few days after birth, with psychotic delusions and hallucinations that may cause the mother either to harm her baby or to be unable to provide adequate care. Women suffering puerperal psychosis need admission to a specialist mother-and-baby unit.

Jayda is bonding well to her baby and has no suicidal ideation. She declines antidepressants and does well with increased family and community support.

SUMMARY

Community midwives now undertake much of the community care of pregnant women in the UK, but GPs still play a key role. Some women attend the GP specifically for health advice before they get pregnant, but one in six pregnancies remains unplanned.[13] Therefore, it is good practice for GPs to offer opportunistic pre-pregnancy counselling to all women of childbearing age. GPs also see couples who are finding it difficult to conceive, and must be able to give advice, know how and when to investigate and understand who is eligible for funding for infertility treatment. Pregnancy is the first time for many women that they have regular contact with the health service. Women are often told to contact their midwife or designated birth centre if problems arise in the pregnancy, but the GP may be the first to see them and needs to know how to assess and when and where to refer. Pregnant women present with any number of conditions that may be unrelated to the pregnancy, and the GP needs to consider the pregnancy in their advice and when proposing treatment.

 Now visit **www.wileyessential.com/primarycare** to test yourself on this chapter.

REFERENCES

1. Royal College of Obstetricians and Gynaecologists. Amniocentesis and chorionic villus sampling. Green Top Guideline 8. June 2010. Available from: https://www.rcog.org.uk/globalassets/documents/guidelines/gtg_8.pdf (last accessed 6 October 2015).

2. NICE. Fertility: assessment and treatment for people with fertility problems. NICE Clinical Guideline 156. February 2013. Available from: https://www.nice.org.uk/guidance/cg156 (last accessed 6 October 2015).

3. NICE. Antenatal care. NICE Clinical Guideline 62. March 2008. Available from: https://www.nice.org.uk/guidance/cg62 (last accessed 6 October 2015).

4. Public Health England. NHS Sickle Cell and Thalassaemia Screening Programme. 2013. Available from:http://www.sct.screening.nhs.uk (last accessed 6 October 2015).

5. Matthews A, Dowswell T, Haas DM, et al. Interventions for nausea and vomiting in early pregnancy. *Cochrane Database Syst Rev* 2010;**9**:CD007575.

6. Health Protection Agency. Investigation, diagnosis and management of viral rash illness, or exposure to viral rash illness, in pregnancy. January 2011. Available from: http://www.gov.uk/government/uploads/system/uploads/attachment_data/file/322688/Viral_rash_in_pregnancy_guidance.pdf (last accessed 6 October 2015)

7. Royal College of Obstetricians and Gynaecologists. Chickenpox in pregnancy. Green Top Guideline 13. September 2007. Available from: https://www.rcog.org.uk/globalassets/documents/guidelines/gtg_13.pdf (last accessed 6 October 2015).

8. SIGN. Management of perinatal mood disorders. Scottish Intercollegiate Guideline 127. March 2012. Available from: http://www.sign.ac.uk/pdf/sign127.pdf (last accessed 6 October 2015).

9. NICE. Diabetes in pregnancy: management of diabetes and its complications from pre-conception to the postnatal period. NICE Clinical Guideline 63. March 2008. Available from: https://www.nice.org.uk/guidance/cg63 (last accessed 6 October 2015).

10. NICE Hypertension in pregnancy: the management of hypertensive disorders in pregnancy. NICE Clinical Guideline 107. August 2010. Available from: https://www.nice.org.uk/guidance/cg107 (last accessed 6 October 2015).

11. French LM, Smaill FM. Antibiotic regimens for endometritis after delivery. *Cochrane Database Syst Rev* 2004;**4**:CD001067.

12. Royal College of Obstetricians and Gynaecologists. Bacterial sepsis following pregnancy. Green Top Guideline 64b. April 2012. Available from: https://www.rcog.org.uk/globalassets/documents/guidelines/gtg_64b.pdf (last accessed 6 October 2015).

13. Wellings K, Jones KG, Mercer CH, et al. The prevalence of unplanned pregnancy and associated factors in Britain. *Lancet* 2013;**382**:1807–16.

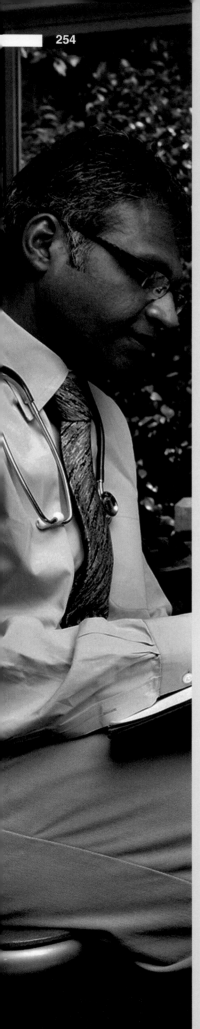

CHAPTER 28
Domestic violence and abuse

Gene Feder

Professor of Primary Care, University of Bristol

Key topics

Learning objectives

- Be able to recognise the different ways in which a victim of domestic violence or abuse might present to their GP.
- Be able to suggest sensitive ways of asking if someone is experiencing domestic violence and abuse.
- Be able to describe appropriate ways of responding to someone who discloses that they are the victim of domestic violence or abuse.

Essential Primary Care, First Edition. Edited by Andrew Blythe and Jessica Buchan.
© 2017 John Wiley & Sons, Ltd. Published 2017 by John Wiley & Sons, Ltd.
Companion website: www.wileyessential.com/primarycare

What is domestic violence and abuse?

Domestic violence and abuse (DVA) can be physical, sexual, emotional or financial and is perpetrated by adults who are, or who have been, intimate partners or family members, regardless of gender or sexuality. It forms a pattern of coercive and controlling behaviour. Adults can be from the extended family (e.g. a parent-in-law). In some cases, it may be teenagers or young adults who are violent or abusive towards family members, including their parents. It is not necessary for the perpetrators to live in the family home. Although DVA has a wide scope, most of the epidemiological and clinical research we discuss in this chapter focusses on intimate-partner violence. The perpetrator may be a partner or ex-partner; risk of serious injury to the victim (and their children) actually increases in the immediate aftermath of separation from an abusive partner, and harassment or stalking may persist for years after separation.

DVA consists of behaviours that potentially impact on health. Most, but not all, are illegal in most countries. The focus has traditionally been on criminal incidents of physical and sexual violence, such as physical or sexual assault. However, emotional abuse alone is also associated with long-term adverse physical and mental health effects. Aspects of emotional abuse may also constitute a criminal offence, including threats to kill, harassment, stalking and putting people in fear of violence. The central feature of the different types of DVA is the power and control that a perpetrator exerts over an intimate partner or ex-partner or other family member. This recurs, often gets worse with time and is potentially life-threatening.

Case study 28.1

Naomi Nightingale is 28. She has just registered with a new practice and comes to see the GP for the first time. She says she is having difficulty sleeping and wants something to calm her. It is a hot summer's day and the GP notices that she is wearing a long-sleeved top and looks anxious. She has completed a new-patient questionnaire and says that she drinks about 30 units of alcohol a week.

What questions might the GP ask her to find out if she is experiencing DVA?

- 'Sometimes people have problems sleeping because they are troubled by something going on in their lives. Are you troubled by anything at the moment? Are you afraid of anyone at home?'
- 'How are things at home? Is anyone upsetting or hurting you?'
- 'Do you feel safe at home?'

The scale of the problem

DVA occurs in all societies, regardless of ethnicity, age, class, religion, sexuality or disability. Internationally, DVA has no consistent demographic associations, other than relative poverty. Although it is prevalent across the socioeconomic spectrum, it is more common in families and communities that are relatively deprived, and there is a higher prevalence in countries with higher inequality. In the UK and north America, DVA, particularly intimate-partner violence, is more commonly perpetrated against younger women, and there is some evidence that women with disabilities are at increased risk. Coercive control, supported by patriarchal social structures, is a major cause of intimate-partner violence, although a full understanding of the causes of DVA requires analysis of factors at societal, community, relationship/family and individual levels (see Figure 28.1).

Domestic violence is a global public health problem, affecting millions who have to live with its consequences. The World Health Organization (WHO's) multinational violence against women study found that the prevalence of lifetime physical violence and sexual violence by an intimate partner, among ever-partnered women, varied from 15 to 71% in urban and rural settings in 10 countries. In the United Kingdom, as in the rest of the world, DVA is highly prevalent, and is more commonly perpetrated against women (see Figure 28.2), with more severe mental and physical health consequences than for DVA perpetrated against men. DVA also occurs in lesbian, gay, bisexual and transgender relationships.

Women experiencing DVA are more likely to need medical attention or hospitalisation and are more likely to fear for their lives. In this chapter, we mostly refer to women experiencing DVA, while acknowledging that it can also affect men. We hope that future research will help articulate the needs of male victims and inform effective interventions for men.

In women attending UK general practice, 41% have ever experienced physical violence from a partner or ex-partner, with 17% experiencing it in the past year. The prevalence of intimate-partner violence is higher in clinical populations than the general population, particularly in primary care, gynaecological, orthopaedic and gastroenterological services. This is not surprising in light of the associated health problems of survivors of domestic violence (see next section) and a consistent research finding that health care utilisation is higher among women who have a current or past history of abuse than among women with no history of abuse. Women with a current or past experience of DVA use primary care and specialist outpatient services more frequently, are issued with more prescriptions and are admitted to hospital more often than non-abused women.

Health impact

DVA damages health.[1] In the UK, two women are killed by their current or former male partner each week. In the USA, intimate-partner violence causes over 2 million injuries annually, with 550 000 people requiring medical treatment as a result. In women attending UK general practice, 21% have suffered a physical injury (bruising or worse) from assault by a partner. However, most patients' experience of DVA will be hidden from the doctor when presenting in primary care, without an obvious

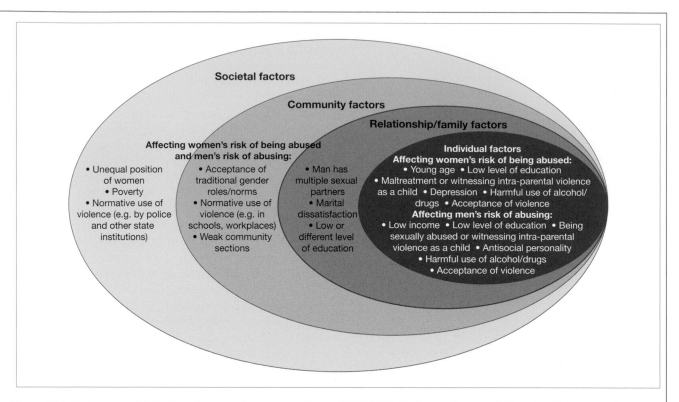

Figure 28.1 Factors associated with violence against women. *Source*: WHO 2012, *Understanding and Addressing Violence against Women: Overview*. Reproduced by permission of the World Health Organization.

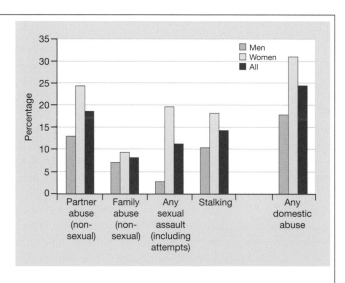

Figure 28.2 Crime Survey for England and Wales 2011/12. *Source*: Office for National Statistics licensed under the Open Government Licence v.3.0.

injury, as in Case study 28.1. DVA is more likely to present with short- and long-term health problems, which can persist after the abuse has ended.[2] These include chronic pain (e.g. headaches, back pain), increased minor infectious illnesses, neurological symptoms (e.g. fainting and fits), gastrointestinal

disorders (e.g. irritable bowel syndrome (IBS)) and gynaecological problems (e.g. sexually transmitted infections (STIs), vaginal bleeding, recurrent urinary tract infection (UTI)).[3] Women may present with these symptoms and conditions over many years, and are often referred to specialists for further investigation, without spontaneously disclosing their experience of abuse. In Australia, intimate-partner violence (a large subset of DVA) is the top contributor to death, disability and illness for women of reproductive age (15–44 years).[4] In these women, intimate-partner violence is the most important risk factor out of eight major risk factors for ill health, including raised blood pressure, adverse lipid profile and obesity. It accounts for 8% of the disease burden in this age group, while high blood pressure accounts for just 1%. Antenatal exposure to intimate-partner violence is associated with an increased risk of low birth weight and pregnancy complications.

The physical health associations of DVA are surpassed by the four- to fivefold increased risk of mental health problems, which can persist long after the violence has ceased (see Table 28.1). This is the case for depression, anxiety, post-traumatic stress disorder (PTSD), suicidal thoughts, suicide and substance misuse. Most of the epidemiological studies of DVA and mental health are cross-sectional, making conclusions about direction of causality uncertain, although recent longitudinal studies suggest that the effect is bidirectional: DVA precedes mental health problems, but mental health problems also increase vulnerability to abuse.[5]

Table 28.1 Potential presentations of DVA.

	Presentations
Psychological	Insomnia
	Depression and suicidal ideation
	Anxiety and panic disorder
	Somatoform disorder
	Post-traumatic stress disorder (PTSD)
	Eating disorders
	Drug and alcohol misuse
Physical	Obvious injuries, especially to the head and neck or multiple areas
	Bruises in various stages of healing
	Injuries from sexual assault
	Sexually transmitted infections (STIs)
	Chronic pelvic/abdominal pain
	Chronic headache
	Chronic back pain
	Numbness and tingling from injuries
	Lethargy
Pregnancy-related indicators	Miscarriages
	Unwanted pregnancy
	Antepartum haemorrhage
	Lack of prenatal care
	Low birth weight
General indicators/risk factors	Delay in seeking treatment of injuries
	Multiple presentations to general practice
	Recent separation or divorce
	History of child-maltreatment abuse
	Current maltreatment of child in family
	Age less than 40

Why should there be a specific role for health care in general, and primary care in particular?

The world is full of problems that have substantial health impact. For example, poor housing is associated with respiratory problems, from asthma to tuberculosis (TB). Doctors can advocate for better housing as active citizens and write letters for individual patients supporting their requests for rehousing, but treating the respiratory condition is their core business. Why should this be different for DVA?[6,7] First, because survivors of abuse identify doctors as the professionals they would most trust with a disclosure and want us to respond appropriately and safely (see Table 28.2).[8] Second, because there is

evidence from qualitative and quantitative studies for interventions that can improve outcomes for women experiencing recent or past DVA, for which doctors, and particularly GPs, can facilitate access.[9]

As with other conditions, the GP's expertise lies in recognition (diagnosis) of the problem, an appropriate response, consideration of the management options with the patient and – when appropriate – referral to effective specialist services. The key steps in the primary care response to DVA are asking patients about it, listening supportively, enquiring about immediate safety, offering referral to specialist services and providing ongoing support to the victim and her children.

Table 28.2 What women who have experienced DVA say they want from clinicians.[8]

Before disclosure or questioning	Understanding of the problem, including knowledge of community services and appropriate referral systems
	A supportive, welcoming and nonthreatening clinical environment
	Brochures and posters in the clinical setting
	Continuity of care
	Assurance about matters of privacy, safety and confidentiality
	Alertness to the signs of abuse and willingness to raise the matter
	Verbal and nonverbal communication skills that develop trust
	Compassionate, supportive and respectful attitude towards abused women
When the topic of domestic violence is raised	Nonjudgemental, compassionate and caring attitude when questioning about abuse
	Confidence and comfort in asking about domestic violence
	No pressure to disclose abuse; simply raising the topic can help women
	Raising of the issue of abuse on several occasions; a woman may disclose abuse at a later date
	A private and confidential environment, with sufficient time for the appointment
Immediate response to disclosure	Nonjudgemental attitude, with compassion, support and belief of experiences
	Acknowledgement of the complexity of the problem, and respect for the woman's unique concerns and decisions
	Putting the needs identified by the woman first, and help to ensure that social and psychological needs are met
	Taking time to listen, provide information and offer referrals to specialist help
	Validation of the woman's experiences, challenging of assumptions and provision of encouragement
	Response to any concerns about safety
Response in subsequent consultations	Patient and supportive attitude, giving the woman time to progress at her own therapeutic pace
	Understanding of the chronicity of the problem and provision of follow-up and continued support
	Respect for the woman's wishes, with no pressure to make any decisions
	Nonjudgemental attitude if the woman does not follow up referrals immediately
	Opportunity to disclose abuse at a later date

Asking about domestic violence and abuse

There is insufficient evidence for screening all female patients for experience of DVA, although this is a national health care policy in some countries, notably the USA. Yet, we know from interviews with survivors that it is difficult to spontaneously disclose to a doctor,[8] even one you trust and with whom you have a good relationship. That is because abuse is a highly stigmatised condition, and survivors often blame themselves for the abuse they have experienced, not least because of the perpetrator's insistence that it is their own fault.

So, when should a GP ask about current or past abuse? When a patient presents with one or more of a range of physical and psychological symptoms and illnesses that are associated with DVA (see Table 28.1), or if the GP has an intuition that there may be abuse in a family. Asking about abuse is a skill

that doctors need to learn. To facilitate disclosure, GPs can use a 'funnelling' technique, first asking a general question, such as, 'How are things at home?', and then asking more specific questions about abuse, depending on the initial response of the patient. These should cover different aspects of abuse: emotional abuse, fear, sexual abuse, physical abuse and safety. The mnemonic 'HARKS' is useful here (see Box 28.1). There is strong evidence from patient surveys and interviews that patients are not offended if doctors ask whether they are experiencing DVA.[10] If they are in a happy, safe relationship, they will say so.

Disclosure is only likely to occur if a woman feels that she can trust the doctor and practice. Having information about DVA in the practice, including telephone numbers for national helplines and local services (e.g. posters in waiting rooms, leaflets at reception and small, discreet, easily hidden credit cards in the toilets) may help women feel more able to

---

Box 28.1 HARKS questions for suspected DVA

- 'Have you felt **H**umiliated or emotionally abused by your partner or ex-partner, or anyone else in your family?'
- 'Are you now or have you ever been **A**fraid of your partner or ex-partner, or anyone else in your family?'
- 'In the past year, have you been forced to have any kind of sexual activity by your partner or ex-partner?' (Using the term '**R**ape' is usually not appropriate when asking about sexual violence, because patients may find it difficult to acknowledge that they have been raped.)
- 'Has your partner ever physically threatened or hurt you? Or have you been **K**icked, hit, slapped or otherwise physically hurt by your partner, ex-partner or another family member?'
- 'Are you **S**afe to go home?'

Box 28.2 Possible validation statements if a woman discloses DVA

- 'Everybody deserves to feel safe at home.'
- 'You don't deserve to be hit or hurt. It is not your fault.'
- 'I am concerned about your safety and well-being.'
- 'You are not alone. I will be with you through this, whatever you decide. Help is available.'
- 'You are not to blame. Abuse is common and happens in all kinds of relationships. It tends to continue.'
- 'Abuse can affect your health and that of your children.'

---

trust a practice. Posters stating that the practice is 'domestic violence-aware' and that the staff has received training about DVA can increase a woman's confidence that their GP or practice nurse will respond effectively and compassionately to disclosure. Alternatively, they may choose to contact a DVA specialist agency directly, without disclosing to a clinician.

Responding appropriately to disclosure

The immediate response of the GP must be validating of the woman's experience, asserting that the abusive behaviour is unacceptable and that the doctor will support her. The GP should express their empathy and state that no one deserves to be treated like that. We know from interviews with survivors of DVA that how a doctor (or other professional) responds to disclosure strongly influences whether a woman will trust them in further consultations or seek help in the future.[8] See Box 28.2 for appropriate validation statements.

GPs should always assess the risk of immediate harm by asking, 'Are you safe to go home?' Other useful questions can be, 'Are either you or your children in danger?', 'Has violence become more frequent or severe recently?', and, 'Are there weapons in the home?' If the answer to any of these questions suggests risk of immediate harm, then the woman should be helped to urgently contact either a specialist DVA service, the police (by dialling 999) or the local police domestic abuse reaction team (DART). This is an unusual situation in general practice, where the majority of cases of DVA are more akin to a chronic condition and the situation will not be urgent that day.

We have already emphasised how difficult it is for a patient to disclose abuse to a doctor. One of the reasons for this is fear that the perpetrator will discover the disclosure, endangering the patient further. This is a real risk if the perpetrator or someone known to the perpetrator gains access to the survivor's medical records or the records of children. General practices need robust policies to prevent this happening, including a disguised term or code for DVA on the front screen or problem list, in case the perpetrator attends a consultation with his partner. On one hand, a patient's exposure to DVA needs to be at the front of the patient's record, so that any doctor or nurse who sees the patient is aware of the problem; on the other, clear visibility of the problem on the screen might endanger the patient if she attends the GP consultation with the partner or another adult who is abusing her.

Offering referral

Referral to local specialist DVA advocacy services (e.g. local Women's Aid) should be offered to all women who disclose DVA, regardless of the nature of the abuse or the timeframe over which it happened. There is some evidence that domestic violence advocacy reduces the risk of further violence and may improve mental health and quality-of-life outcomes for survivors of DVA.[11] Even if a woman declines the referral, she will know that her GP is not ambivalent about discussing what is happening to her, and she may choose to be referred at another time. In this respect, DVA is different from other chronic conditions, such as diabetes, depression and atrial fibrillation, when specialist referral is often not necessary. Provision of specialist DVA services is patchy in the UK, particularly in the face of reduced public funding. It is essential that practices establish a link to a local service to which clinicians can refer patients, preferably in the context of integrated training, support and referral pathways, such as the Identification & Referral to Improve Safety (IRIS) programme.[12,13] These services can help assess risk to women and their children, provide advocacy and broker access to housing, criminal justice and social care support. The contact details for local and national DVA services and how best to access them should be documented in the practice handbook and the practice intranet, with easy accessibility for all locum doctors and other temporary staff. Each member of the primary health care team should at least be aware of the freephone 24-hour national domestic violence helpline run in partnership between Women's Aid and Refuge

(0808 2000247). This can give confidential support, help and information to women experiencing DVA, as well as their family, friends, colleagues and others calling on their behalf, including health professionals.

Children exposed to domestic violence and abuse

The damaging health and psychosocial effects of DVA cascade though the generations. Exposure to domestic violence during childhood and adolescence damages health across the lifespan. There is a moderate to strong association between children's exposure to interpersonal violence and internalising symptoms (e.g. anxiety, depression), externalising behaviours (e.g. aggression) and trauma symptoms. Children exposed to DVA are two to four times more likely than children from nonviolent homes to exhibit clinically significant problems. Children's exposure to DVA also damages social development and academic attainment. There is considerable variation in children's reactions and adaptation. This is partly explained by the presence or absence of other adversities in their lives (see Chapter 12). The overlap with direct maltreatment ranges from 40 to 60% of children exposed to DVA, who may also experience a range of other adversities, such as poverty, parental mental ill health, substance misuse and antisocial behaviour. The more adversities a child is exposed to, the greater the risk of negative outcomes.

Spontaneous disclosure by a child of exposure to DVA is rare. When should a GP suspect that there is DVA in a family? Some of the presentations that should bring the question to mind are the same as those that should raise the suspicion of direct child maltreatment: anxiety over fear-related behaviour or unexplained illness, running away from home, constant worry about possible danger or the safety of family members and evidence of injuries (see Table 12.4).

A central feature of good practice is speaking to the child or young person on their own in a way that is safe for them and for the parent who is experiencing domestic violence, seeking that parent's permission to do so. Other features of good practice for primary care professionals include: being realistic and honest about the limits of confidentiality (but promising to keep the child informed of what is happening); helping the child or young person to understand that they are not to blame for the DVA and that they are not alone; letting the child know that domestic violence is never acceptable; and being careful to acknowledge the child's experiences and helping them understand that it is not their responsibility to protect the nonabusive parent, while validating their concern and any action they may have taken to protect that parent. Children and young people can find it hard to talk for many reasons, including shame, guilt, torn loyalties, having received threats as to what will happen if they tell anyone, not wanting to leave home or split up the family and simply not having the language to express what is going on. Police and social services are trained to interview children. If a child discloses to the GP, it may be tempting to ask a lot of questions, but this is *not our role*. We need to find out enough to determine whether a referral is necessary, but we should try to use open-ended questions.

If a child is at risk of harm, the local safeguarding children procedures should be followed immediately. The decision to refer to children's social services is a fine judgement in relation to DVA exposure in the absence of direct maltreatment, hinging around the concept of significant harm: 'any impairment of the child's health or development as a result of witnessing the ill-treatment of another person, such as domestic violence'. Domestic violence advocacy services, which will be able to support the parent experiencing abuse, also have the expertise to assess children's needs and the need for referral. These services also undertake risk assessment for the parent and their children, a task beyond the capacity of most general practices. Supporting the parent experiencing DVA is crucial to protecting children exposed to that violence.

SUMMARY

DVA can be physical, sexual, emotional or financial, and is perpetrated by adults who are, or who have been, intimate partners or family members, regardless of gender or sexuality. It forms a pattern of coercive and controlling behaviour and is a violation of human rights, a major public health issue and a clinical problem that is increasingly recognised as a major challenge for health care services.

It is a global problem, present in all social classes and ethnic groups, with a higher prevalence and health impact among women – particularly mental health problems and chronic physical symptoms. GPs need to ask women about abuse, respond appropriately to a disclosure, check on safety and offer referral to a domestic violence advocacy organisation. Long-term support and follow-up may be necessary.[14]

 Now visit **www.wileyessential.com/primarycare** to test yourself on this chapter.

REFERENCES

1. Bewley S, Welch C. *ABC of Domestic and Sexual Violence.* London: Wiley Blackwell/BMJ Books; 2014.

2. Hegarty KL, O'Doherty LJ, Chondros P, et al. Effect of type and severity of intimate partner violence on women's health and service use: findings from a primary care trial of women afraid of their partners. *J Interpers Violence* 2013;**28**(2):273–94.

3. Howarth E, Feder G. *Prevalence and physical health impact of domestic violence.* In Howard LM, Feder G, Agnew-Davies (editors). Domestic Violence and Mental Health. London: RCPsych Publications; 2013.

4. Vos T, Astbury J, Piers LS, Magnus A, Heenan M, Stanley L, Walker L, Webster K. Measuring the impact of intimate partner violence on the health of women in Victoria, *Australia. Bull World Health Organ.* 2006 Sep;**84**(9):739–44.

5. Trevillion K, Oram S, Feder G, Howard LM. Experiences of Domestic Violence and Mental Disorders: A Systematic Review and Meta-Analysis. *PLoS ONE* 2012; **7**(12):e51740.

6. World Health Organization. *Responding to Intimate Partner Violence and Sexual Violence Against Women: WHO Clinical and Policy Guidelines.* Geneva: WHO; 2013.

7. Hegarty K, Taft A, Feder G. Working with the whole family when domestic violence is present: what do generalists need to know? *BMJ* 2008;**337**:a839.

8. Feder GS, Hutson M, Ramsay J, Taket AR. Expectations and experiences of women experiencing intimate partner violence when they encounter health care professionals: a meta-analysis of qualitative studies. *Arch Int Med* 2006;**166**:22–37.

9. García-Moreno C, Hegarty K, d'Oliveira AFL, et al. The health-systems response to violence against women. *Lancet* 2015;**385**(9977):1567–9.

10. Feder G, Arsene C, Bacchus L, Dunne D, Hague G, Kuntze S, et al. How far does screening women for domestic (partner) violence in different health care setting meet the UK National Screening Committee criteria for a screening programme in terms of condition, screening method, and intervention? Systematic reviews of nine UK National Screening Committee criteria. *Health Technology Assessment.* 2009; Vol. **13**.17

11. Rivas C, Ramsay J, Sadowski L, Davidson LL, Dunne D, Eldridge S, Hegarty K, Taft A, Feder G. Advocacy interventions to reduce or eliminate violence and promote the physical and psychosocial well-being of women who experience intimate partner abuse. *Cochrane Database Syst Rev.* 2015 Dec 3;**12**:CD005043. doi: 10.1002/14651858. CD005043.pub3.

12. Feder G, Davies RA, Baird K, et al. Identification and Referral to Improve Safety (IRIS) of women experiencing domestic violence with a primary care training and support programme: a cluster randomised controlled trial. *Lancet* 2011;**378**(9805):1788–95.

13. Malpass A, Sales K, Johnson M, et al. Women's experiences of referral to a domestic violence advocate in UK primary care settings: a service-user collaborative study. *Br J Gen Pract* 2014;**64**(620):e151–8.

14. NICE. Domestic violence and abuse: how health services, social care and the organisations they work with can respond effectively. NICE Public Health Guidance 50. February 2014. Available from: http://www.nice.org.uk/guidance/ph50/resources/guidance-domestic-violence-and-abuse-how-health-services-social-care-and-the-organisations-they-work-with-can-respond-effectively-pdf (last accessed 6 October 2015).

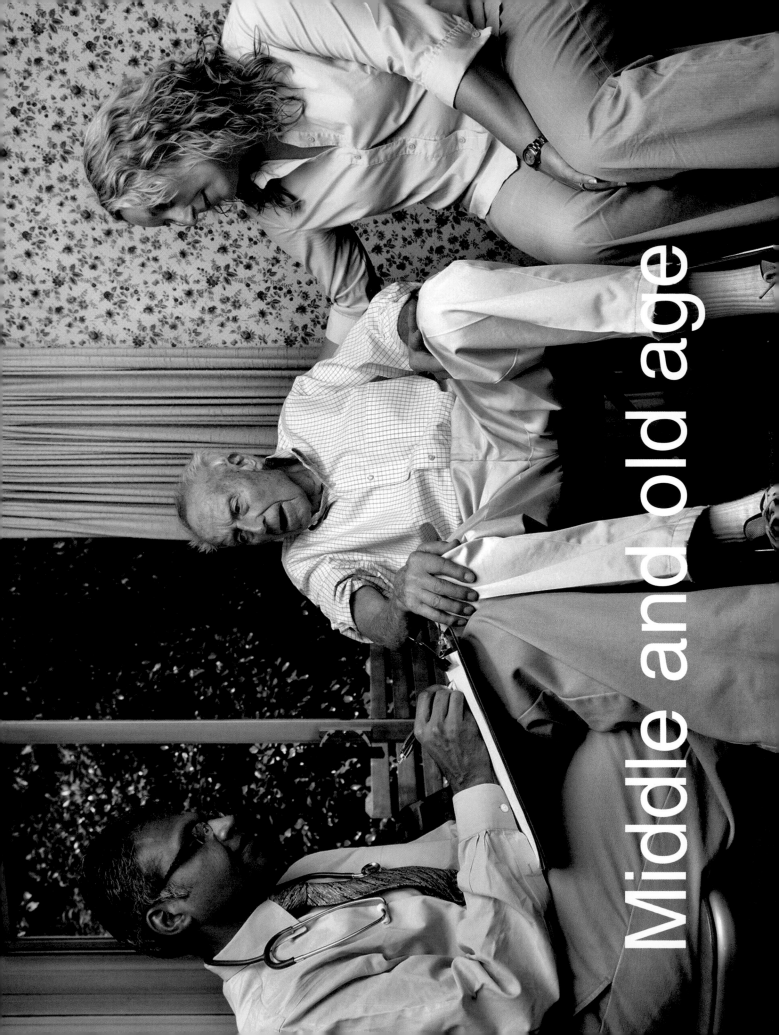

Middle and old age

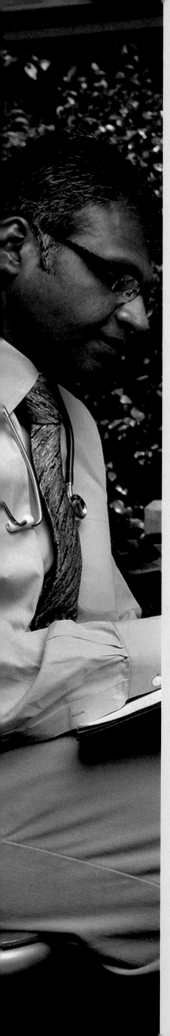

CHAPTER 29
Cardiovascular disease

Andrew Blythe
GP and Senior Teaching Fellow, University of Bristol

Key topics

Learning objectives

- Be able to describe the process for deciding if someone with atrial fibrillation should be started on anticoagulation therapy.
- Be able to identify people who are most likely to have coronary artery disease.
- Be able to advise people who have cardiovascular disease how they can reduce their risk of having another major event, such as a stroke or myocardial infarction.
- Be able to assess someone who presents with symptoms suggestive of a transient ischaemic attack.
- Be able to assess and investigate someone who presents with intermittent claudication.

Essential Primary Care, First Edition. Edited by Andrew Blythe and Jessica Buchan.
© 2017 John Wiley & Sons, Ltd. Published 2017 by John Wiley & Sons, Ltd.
Companion website: www.wileyessential.com/primarycare

Introduction

In Chapter 9, we discussed the role that GPs have in identifying people who are at increased risk of developing cardiovascular disease (CVD) and the work that they do in the primary prevention of CVD. In this chapter, we consider the role of the GP in identifying and treating people with established CVD.

Atrial fibrillation

The prevalence of atrial fibrillation increases with age, such that over the age of 75, 1 in 10 people has atrial fibrillation. Having atrial fibrillation increases a person's risk of having a stroke. This risk can be reduced by antithrombotic therapy, so GPs need to identify atrial fibrillation early and advise those with the condition about antithrombotic therapy.

Identifying patients with atrial fibrillation

We should always check the pulse of anyone who presents with breathlessness, palpitations, chest pain or funny turn, and we should always obtain an electrocardiogram (ECG) for anyone who has had a transient ischaemic attack (TIA) or a stroke. Opportunistic screening is also worthwhile in those over 65; checking someone's pulse is easy and quick, and can be done during any consultation. If the pulse is irregular, feel for 1 minute and then listen to the apex for 1 minute. Is there a discrepancy?

Once we are convinced that the pulse is irregular and we know the apex rate, we need to check the patient's blood pressure. When checking the blood pressure of someone who has an irregular pulse, we should always check it twice, manually.

If they are haemodynamically compromised (their apex rate is over 100 and their systolic blood pressure is low), then they probably need admission to hospital. If they are haemodynamically stable, the next step is to do an ECG. Atrial fibrillation must be diagnosed on an ECG. In atrial fibrillation, there are no P waves (Figure 29.1).

Managing someone with permanent atrial fibrillation

If the patient is young or we suspect an underlying structural abnormality of the heart by virtue of a murmur, then a transthoracic echocardiogram is required.

There has been much debate about what is more important, rate control or rhythm control. If the atrial fibrillation is of recent onset then it may be worthwhile trying to restore sinus rhythm – this can be done by cardioversion or antiarrhythmic medication under the direction of a cardiologist. However, in patients over the age of 65, permanent atrial fibrillation is often managed simply by rate control. In practice, this means prescribing a beta blocker in order to reduce their apex rate to 90 bpm or less.[1]

Much research has been done to establish which patients stand to benefit from anticoagulation. Scoring tools have been devised to identify those patients at greatest risk of thromboembolic events and who should be offered anticoagulation. The National Institute for Health and Care Excellence (NICE) recommends the CHA_2DS_2-VASc score,[2] which has replaced the CHAD2 score.[3] Table 29.1 shows how the CHA_2DS_2-VASc score is calculated.

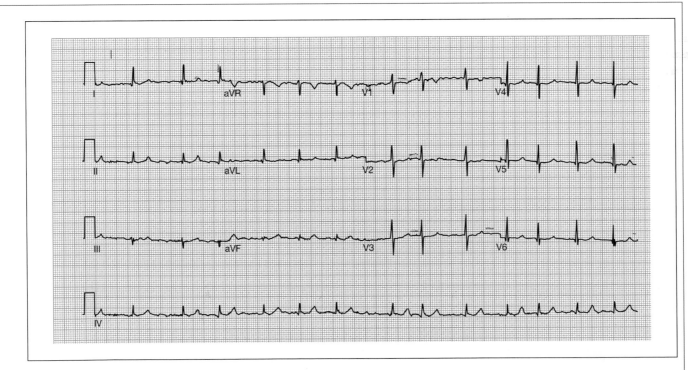

Figure 29.1 ECG showing atrial fibrillation.

Table 29.1 CHA$_2$DS$_2$-VASc score.

Criteria		Score
C	Congestive cardiac failure	1
H	High blood pressure (>140/90 mmHg or on treatment)	1
A	Age 75 or over	2
D	Diabetes mellitus	1
S	Stroke, TIA or other thromboembolism	2
V	Vascular disease	1
A	Age 65–74	1
Sc	Sex category (scores 1 if female)	1

A score of 0 for a man or 1 for a woman indicates that the risk of stroke is low.
A score of 1 for a man indicates an indeterminate risk. The doctor should offer and discuss the possibility of anticoagulation.
A score of 2 of more indicates a high risk of stroke. The patient should be offered anticoagulation in order to prevent a stroke.

Table 29.2 Colours of warfarin tablets in the UK.

0.5 mg	White
1 mg	Brown
3 mg	Blue
5 mg	Pink

Warfarin, a vitamin K antagonist, is the most established anticoagulant drug. Before starting someone on warfarin, we need to discuss in detail with the patient what this involves and check that there are no contraindications.

Patients on warfarin need regular blood tests to ensure that their international normalised ratio (INR) is in the target range. Their dose will need to be varied from time to time in response to their INR. In the UK, warfarin comes in four different strengths of tablet, each of a different colour (see Table 29.2). If a patient has poor eyesight or dementia, they may struggle to take the correct dose. If they are not on the phone, it will be difficult to contact them urgently if their INR turns out to be very high. If they binge on alcohol, this will lead to unpredictable swings in their INR. If they have had falls, they may be at unacceptable risk of developing a cerebral haemorrhage, and if they have had a peptic ulcer recently, this may create an unacceptable risk of having a gastrointestinal bleed. Tools are available for estimating the risk of someone having a major bleed while on oral anticoagulation.[4]

Having regular blood tests is inconvenient for patients, and the cost of phlebotomy (particularly if the patient is too frail to come to surgery and requires visits from a mobile phlebotomist)

is substantial. Newer alternatives, such as dabigatran, which has to be taken twice a day, do not require regular blood tests.

Angina

Anytime that a patient presents to a GP with chest pain, the GP has to think, 'Is this angina?' Angina is most commonly caused by coronary artery disease and is a warning that the patient is at high risk of having a myocardial infarction. But doctors don't always recognise angina when patients describe their chest pain. Why is this?

'Angina' is the name given to a central chest pain that is brought on by exertion, stress or cold weather. It usually lasts for a few minutes and is relieved by rest. Sometimes, people feel short of breath or nauseated with it. As with a myocardial infarction, the pain can radiate to the left arm or jaw. However, angina is not the only cause of episodic central chest pain. The more common and much less serious causes are gastro-oesophageal reflux and musculoskeletal pain. Only by listening carefully to the patient's description of the pain and by considering the patient's background risk of having CVD is it possible for the GP to identify those who are most likely to have coronary artery disease.

Chest pain can be classified by the presence or absence of three features:

1. The pain is central and dull.
2. The pain is provoked by exercise, emotional stress or a heavy meal.
3. The pain is relieved by rest or by a glyceryl trinitrate (GTN) spray.

These features are referred to as the Diamond–Forrester criteria.[5] If the pain has all three features then it is *typical angina*. If the pain has two out of three criteria then it is *atypical angina*. If only one of the three criteria is present then it is said to be *noncardiac*.

Let's consider two examples:

A 35-year-old man complains of intermittent chest pain. Sometimes it's dull, sometimes it's sharp. Usually, it lasts for a few seconds. It can come on at any time, including when he is sitting down feeling relaxed at home. Most often, it comes on after eating or drinking. He does not smoke, but he drinks about two pints of beer most nights. He admits feeling a bit stressed at work. His grandfather, who did smoke, developed angina in his 70s, but no one else in his family has had heart disease.

This man's description is not one of angina. The patient's age, the fact that he does not smoke and the absence of significant family history of heart disease make his background risk of having CVD low. Therefore, it is extremely unlikely that this man has coronary heart disease.

A 55-year-old man complains of intermittent chest pain, which like that of the younger man is sometimes dull, sometimes sharp. He is under threat of redundancy, and when he feels stressed by this fact, the pain can come on; it lasts for up to 5 minutes. He doesn't do any regular exercise. He smokes 20 cigarettes a day and his father had a heart attack, which he survived, sometime in his 50s.

This man's description is not one of typical angina, but the relationship to stress makes angina a possibility. He has atypical angina. His age, smoking status and significant family history of heart disease combine to give him a high background risk of having CVD. So, this man needs investigating to establish whether or not he has coronary artery disease.

In the second case, the GP should prescribe a GTN spray. If this works, it makes angina more likely, but it is does not confirm that the pain is due to coronary artery disease. A GTN spray can also relieve oesophageal spasm. As well as prescribing a GTN spray, the GP needs to make a further assessment. The GP should:

- examine the patient;
- obtain an ECG (to look for arrhythmias, left bundle branch block, evidence of left ventricular hypertrophy and evidence of ischaemia);
- check his haemoglobin (because anaemia is a cause of angina);
- check his lipid profile and fasting glucose (to gain a better understanding of his cardiovascular risk).

If any of the episodes of chest pain have lasted 15 minutes of more, it is possible that the patient has had a myocardial infarction. If the prolonged episode of chest pain has been within the last 3 days, urgent admission to hospital is needed. If this episode has been within the last 12 hours then the patient should be sent to hospital as an emergency.

If the angina is stable (i.e. not increasing in frequency or severity) and there is no evidence of a recent myocardial infarction, further investigation is necessary to establish whether or not the patient has significant coronary artery disease. This is done by a cardiologist, often in a chest pain clinic set up specifically for this purpose.

If the patient's underlying risk of CVD is high and the angina is typical, the probability of the patient having coronary artery disease is high. In such a situation, the cardiologist may proceed straight to a coronary angiogram. However, if the probability of coronary artery disease is less than 60% by virtue of the low background risk or the atypical nature of the angina, then a less invasive test is needed. In this instance, functional imaging or computed tomography (CT) calcium scoring is recommended. These tests are replacing the exercise ECG as a means of excluding coronary artery disease.

Tables are available to help doctors decide what tests should be done on patients with angina, taking into account their background risk (or pretest probability) and the Diamond–Forrester score. The choice of tests has to be tailored to the patient. As we discussed in Chapter 3, the utility of a test depends on the characteristics of the population to which it is applied, as well as its sensitivity and specificity. Furthermore, the tests that are the most accurate, such as a coronary angiogram, often carry

Table 29.3 Deciding whether chest pain is cardiac in origin.

Cardiac cause more likely	Cardiac cause less likely
Patient's 10-year risk of developing CVD is high	Chest wall is tender
Pain triggered by exertion, stress, cold weather or heavy meal	Pain lasts for seconds or hours
Pain severe	
Pain accompanied by nausea or breathlessness	
Pain relieved by rest and/or GTN	
Pain does not respond to antacid	

the greatest risk and are expensive. So, for a lot of patients, the judgement about the cause of their chest pain rests on the 'simplest test of all': taking a good history. Sometimes, this judgement turns out to be wrong, and within a few years of a patient being given the 'all clear', they have a coronary event. To reduce the chances of this happening, the GP needs to keep an open mind and constantly reevaluate the patient's risk of CVD (Table 29.3).

If a GP suspects angina and refers the patient to a chest pain clinic, the GP should consider prescribing three things: a GTN spray, aspirin 75 mg once a day and a statin. In addition, the GP may consider starting antianginal medication: a beta blocker or a calcium-channel antagonist.

Top tip: prescribing a GTN spray

Whenever we prescribe a GTN spray, we should explain to the patient how to use it and what to do if it doesn't work. We might say:

> You should always carry this spray with you. If you get any pain in your chest, you should stop what you are doing and squirt one spray under your tongue. If the pain hasn't gone after 5 minutes, you should take a second spray. If the pain is still there 5 minutes after that, you should dial 999 or call for help and take a third spray. If the pain has lasted this length of time, it's possible that it could be a heart attack and not simply angina.

Remember, coronary artery disease is not the only cause of angina. Other causes that we should look out for include:

- anaemia;
- aortic valve disease;
- thyrotoxicosis;
- cardiomyopathy;
- atrial fibrillation.

Myocardial infarction

Managing a patient with a myocardial infarction

Most people know that if they have prolonged chest pain and feel very unwell, they could be experiencing a heart attack and they should dial 999. But some people phone their GP when this happens, and some people have a myocardial infarction in the GP surgery. If a patient phones to say that they are experiencing chest pain, the GP should make a quick assessment on the phone and, if they suspect a myocardial infarction, tell the patient that they will dial 999. In some situations, the GP may be able to get there before the ambulance, in which case the GP can attend the scene. When confronted with a patient who is likely to be suffering a myocardial infarction, the priorities are to:

- summon help;
- make a brief cardiovascular assessment (this includes pulse, blood pressure, oxygen saturation (SpO2) and auscultation of the chest);
- give pain relief, aspirin 300 mg and GTN;
- give oxygen if SpO_2 < 94% on air;
- perform 12-lead ECG, if available.

Some people, particularly the elderly, don't seek urgent help when they have prolonged chest pain and instead wait, hoping that the pain will settle, and consult their GP the next day or after the weekend. They may do this because they are frightened of going to hospital, because they don't want to cause a fuss or because they think or hope that it's nothing serious. Confronted with such a patient, the GP has to make a thorough assessment. An ECG may confirm what has happened, but if the pain occurred within the last 3 days, the patient still needs urgent admission to hospital in order to establish whether or not they have had a myocardial infarction.

Caring for someone who has had a myocardial infarction

When someone is discharged from hospital after having a myocardial infarction, they should be taking four drugs:[6]

- aspirin;
- statin;
- beta blocker;
- angiotensin-converting enzyme (ACE) inhibitor.

Each of these drugs reduces the risk of the patient having a second myocardial infarction, so the patient needs to be told that they will be on these medicines for life.

The dose of the ACE inhibitor should be titrated up rapidly, checking the patient's serum urea, creatinine and electrolytes after each increase, because ACE inhibitors can affect renal function. If the patient is intolerant of an ACE inhibitor, they should be prescribed an angiotension receptor blocker instead.

The dose of the beta blocker should also be titrated up to the highest dose that the patient can tolerate.

If the patient has a contraindication to aspirin, we can prescribe clopidogrel instead. Patients who have had a non-ST-elevation myocardial infarction, or who have had an ST-elevation myocardial infarction treated with a stent, should be prescribed both aspirin and clopidogrel for the first year after the infarct.

In addition, all patients who have had a myocardial infarction should be encouraged to adopt the following lifestyle measures:[6]

- Take 20–30 minutes of regular exercise a day, to the point of slight breathlessness.
- Adopt a Mediterranean-style diet, with more bread, fruit, vegetables and fish, and less meat.
- Limit alcohol consumption to <21 units/week for men and <14 units/week for women.
- Stop smoking. If they are still smoking, they can halve their risk of having another myocardial infarction by stopping smoking.
- Achieve and maintain a healthy weight.

Anyone who has had a myocardial infarction should be offered cardiac rehabilitation. This consists of a programme of exercises, education and stress management.

Patients with ischaemic heart disease also need an annual flu vaccine and should have a pneumococcal vaccine.

When should someone return to work after a myocardial infarction?

Despite the fact that a third of people who have a myocardial infarction are under the age of 65, there are no clear guidelines about this. Clearly, a period of rest and rehabilitation is needed, but in the long term, not working can precipitate or perpetuate depression and can hinder a return to fitness. GPs need do encourage people back to work with recommendations about modifying what they do there.

Patients are not allowed to drive for at least 4 weeks after a myocardial infarction. The restrictions are greater if the patient drives a heavy goods vehicle (HGV). If the patient holds an HGV licence, they need to inform the Driver and Vehicle Licensing Agency (DVLA). No one should drive if they have unstable angina or if any of their medication causes side effects which interfere with their ability to drive.

The psychological impact of having a myocardial infarction

Having a myocardial infarction has a huge impact on the patient and the patient's family. The GP may need to repeatedly offer them explanation, reassurance and advice. Patients who have had a myocardial infarction are at high risk of becoming depressed. GPs need to be on the lookout for this. If they diagnose depression, they can recommend cognitive behavioural therapy (CBT) or prescribe a selective serotonin reuptake inhibitor (SSRI).

Patients may not initiate a conversation about problems with sex, but sexual activity is often impeded by depression, fear and the side effects of new medication. The GP should make sensitive enquires about this and be prepared to alter the medication regime or prescribe a cGMP-phosphodiesterase-5 (PDE-5) inhibitor (such as Sildenafil). PDE-5 inhibitors cannot be taken with nitrates because the two together can result in severe hypotension.

Strokes and transient ischaemic attacks

Cerebrovascular disease (stroke and TIA) used to be managed much less intensively than coronary heart disease. It was not easy to arrange rapid investigation of someone who had a TIA, and patients who had a stroke were managed on general medical wards or at home by their GP. But things have changed. First, hospitals set up special stroke wards, which meant patients could receive intensive, bespoke rehabilitation from multidisciplinary teams. Then thrombolytic therapy was introduced, offering the possibility of restoring perfusion to the affected part of the brain and minimising the damage and long-term disability.

Stroke

If it's possible that someone is having a stroke, it is important to get them to hospital as soon as possible. The window for thrombolysis is 4.5 hours.[7] In this time, the patient has to have CT or magnetic resonance imaging (MRI) of the head to check that they have not had a haemorrhagic stroke, so there is no time to lose.

Once hospitals had set up systems for scanning people quickly, advertising campaigns were launched to raise people's awareness of the urgency of a stroke. These campaigns encouraged people to phone 999 rather than their GP if they thought that someone might be having a stroke. Three simple questions, known as the face, arm, speech test (FAST), are promoted to help people spot a stroke. FAST has a poor specificity (there are many other causes of weakness and slurred speech), but its sensitivity for detecting stroke is 82%.[8]

As with someone who has had a myocardial infarction, the GP's main roles in caring for someone who has had a stroke are to supervise secondary prevention and keep a watch for depression. Secondary prevention consists of optimising the patient's blood pressure and cholesterol and prescribing antiplatelet therapy. NICE guidelines recommend switching from aspirin to clopidogrel 2 weeks after a stroke; this treatment is lifelong.[9] In the first few days after a stroke, a person's blood pressure can rise, and there is no evidence to suggest that lowering it immediately is of benefit; it may actually be harmful to attempt to reduce the blood pressure at this stage. However, a week or two after the stroke, it is important to bring the blood pressure to target.

If the stroke has resulted in lasting disability then the GP may need to liaise with the community nursing team and social services to ensure that the patient has an adequate package of

---

Case study 29.1

Malcolm Mallory, age 70, is having breakfast when he finds that he can't hold his knife in his right hand. His speech is not affected. At first he doesn't do anything and attributes the weakness to the fact that we was doing a lot of gardening the previous day. But his right arm and hand still feel weak at 11 o'clock. He phones his son, who is a nurse. His son tells him to phone 999.

On arrival in hospital, he has a weakness of his right upper limb. Otherwise, examination is normal. An ECG shows that he is in sinus rhythm and a CT of his head shows no acute intracranial pathology. Carotid Doppler studies shows that he has only mild atheroma. His blood glucose is normal but his serum cholesterol is 6.3 mmol/l.

Mr Mallory has been on amlodipine for his blood pressure for 5 years, and also has a statin on repeat prescription, but he stopped taking the statin earlier this year because of what he read in a newspaper about its side effects. He is an ex-smoker of 30 pack years.

He is admitted to the stroke ward but is not given thrombolysis because he is outside the window. The following day, his weakness is no worse. He is diagnosed with a left lacunar infarct and begins physiotherapy and occupational therapy. The doctors in hospital start him on aspirin 300 mg daily and restart his statin.

He is discharged 4 days later as the strength in his right hand is returning. The discharge letter has the following instructions for his GP:
- Switch from aspirin to clopidogrel after 2 weeks
- Monitor his blood pressure and consider starting ACE inhibitor

He comes to see his GP 1 week later and says he is still having difficulty shaving with his right hand.

Other than follow the hospital instructions, what else should the GP do?
1. The GP should check that Mr Mallory knows what the medication is for.
2. The GP should examine Mr Mallory to make sure there are no new neurological signs. The patient may gain reassurance from this. The strength in his hand may still improve.
3. Patients who have had a stroke are at risk of depression, so the GP should enquire how he is feeling and ask what support he has at home. Is he socialising? How is he sleeping?
4. The GP should advise him not to drive for 1 month. The same is true for someone who has had a TIA.

care. The patient's carer (usually a family member) will need support. If the carer is registered with the same GP then the GP should register them as a carer so that they can access financial support and respite. Carers UK and the Stroke Association are useful sources of information for patients and their carers.

Transient ischaemic attack

After someone has had a TIA, there is a high risk that they will have a stroke. In just the first week after a TIA, the risk of having a stroke is about 5%.[10] Therefore, when someone has a TIA,

Table 29.4 ABCD² rule for assessing patients who may have had a TIA.

		Score
A	Age	60 years or older scores 1 point
B	Blood pressure	Systolic blood pressure > 140 or diastolic > 90 at presentation scores 1 point
C	Clinical features	Unilateral weakness +/– speech disturbance scores 2 points. Speech disturbance alone scores 1 point
D1	Duration	Duration 10–59 minutes scores 1 point. Duration 1 hour or more scores 2 points
D2	Diabetes	Known diabetes scores 1 point

Score 4 or more: request assessment within 24 hours.
Score 3 or less: request assessment within 7 days.

urgent investigation is needed. Within the last few years, hospitals have established TIA clinics to facilitate this investigation. GPs are encouraged to use the ABCD² rule (see Table 29.4) for deciding which patients are at highest risk of stroke. Those with the highest risk should be given aspirin 300 mg immediately and seen in hospital within 24 hours; everyone else should be investigated in the TIA clinic within 7 days.

In the TIA clinic, patients have their blood pressure, cholesterol and blood glucose checked. They have an ECG to look for atrial fibrillation or heart block. They have carotid duplex studies to look for significant atheroma. If a patient has a significant stenosis of the carotid artery on the side which fits with the clinical presentation then they may be a candidate for carotid endarterectomy. In addition, they may have a CT scan to look for nonvascular pathology.

If a patient still has a weakness or dysphasia when they see the GP then the GP has to assume it's a stroke and admit them to hospital. By definition, a stroke is a focal neurological deficit of presumed vascular origin that lasts for more than 24 hours. Until the 24 hours has expired, it could turn out to be a TIA.

Several things can mimic a TIA or stroke; these include:

- migraine;
- hypoglycaemia;
- space-occupying lesion;
- seizure.

Peripheral arterial disease

When someone presents to their GP with symptoms suggestive of peripheral arterial disease (PAD), they often turn out to have CVD elsewhere, causing angina or renal impairment. They need a thorough cardiovascular assessment and a rigorous assault on all their cardiovascular risk factors. This can only be

Case study 29.2

Ann Alder is 80. She comes with her husband to see the GP in the urgent afternoon surgery. This morning, while talking to her husband, her speech became slurred. It returned to normal after 15 minutes. During this time, her husband noted that the right corner of her mouth drooped a little. Her speech is back to normal now and she says she feels perfectly well.

The GP establishes that she has never had anything like this before. She is on treatment for hypertension (ramipril and felodipine), and latterly her blood pressure has been well controlled. She had a knee replacement 2 years ago but has no other significant medical history. She does not have diabetes.

She looks well. Her pulse is 76 and regular. Her blood pressure is 134/56. Examination of her cranial nerves and peripheral nervous system is normal.

What should the GP do?
She is over 65 and the episode lasted for more than 10 minutes and consisted of weakness and speech disturbance, giving her an ABCD² score of 4 (see Table 29.4). The GP should therefore give her 300 mg of aspirin now (providing she is not allergic to this) and request that she is seen in hospital within 24 hours.

Outcome
She is seen in hospital the following morning. An ECG shows sinus rhythm. A carotid duplex scan shows no significant stenosis. A CT scan shows no acute intracranial pathology. She is started on clopidogrel and advised not to drive for 1 month. She remains well 3 months later.

Case study 29.3a

Robert Rudman is 61. He comes to see his GP for the first time in 6 years. He begins the consultation by saying that he's getting pain in his legs. He's had pain in his left calf for about a year, but now his right leg has started hurting, too. The pain comes on when he walks uphill and goes away when he rests. He has stopped walking into town because of this; he gets the bus now. He does not get any pain at rest. He is not on any regular medication. He is a lifelong smoker but, with encouragement from his wife, he has started to cut down; for the last month, he has smoked 10 cigarettes a day.

What is the likely diagnosis and what should the GP do during the consultation?
Mr Rudman's history is typical of intermittent claudication, the most common presentation of peripheral arterial disease (PAD). He needs a through cardiovascular assessment: a focussed cardiovascular history, examination and investigation.

Outcome
Mr Rudman has a 40-pack-year history of smoking. He drinks one or two pints of beer most evenings and admits eating a lot of unhealthy snacks. He doesn't get any pain in his chest on exertion and doesn't get breathless during the day or night. He has never experienced any palpitations.

His blood pressure is 162/92 mmHg. His radial pulse is regular and his heart sounds are normal. He does not have a palpable abdominal aortic aneurysm. His feet feel warm and there are no skin changes. Both dorsalis pedis pulses are palpable, but the GP cannot feel either posterior tibial pulse.

Because Mr Rudman's blood pressure is high, the GP supplies him with a home blood pressure monitor (see Chapter 9). The GP also asks him to have a fasting blood test.

The results of the blood tests are as follows:
- fasting total cholesterol: 5.6 mmol/l;
- fasting blood glucose: 7.4 mmol/mol;
- full blood count (FBC): normal;
- serum urea and electrolytes (U&Es): urea 4.9, creatinine 68, sodium 144, potassium 4.9, eGFR 76.

Mr Rudman returns to the GP with his home blood pressure readings collected over a week; the mean reading is 148/88 mmHg.

What should the GP do now?
The home blood pressure readings confirm that Mr Rudman has stage 1 hypertension. The GP needs to request a baseline ECG and, because the intermittent claudication suggests that Mr Rudman has established CVD, the GP should prescribe antihypertensive medication, preferably an ACE inhibitor. The eGFR of 76 suggests that Mr Rudman has chronic kidney disease stage 2; the GP needs to check his U&Es a week after taking the ACE inhibitor, and periodically thereafter.

Mr Rudman's fasting glucose is high. The GP should ask Mr Rudman if he has any symptoms of diabetes, such as excessive thirst, polyuria or tiredness, and should ask him to have his fasting blood glucose repeated to confirm a new diagnosis of diabetes.

Mr Rudman's cholesterol level is high, so the GP should prescribe a statin. The GP should also prescribe a low dose of aspirin and request Doppler studies. Most importantly, the GP should discuss the benefits of stopping smoking. Mr Rudman has made a start already by cutting down. He may appreciate some information on the options available to help him.

Case study 29.3b

Mr Rudman makes another GP appointment to receive the results of his second fasting blood test, ECG and Doppler studies.
- Fasting glucose: 7.2 mmol/l.
- ECG: normal sinus rhythm, ventricular rate 76.
- Doppler studies: see Figure 29.2 for the full report. The ankle brachial pressure index (ABPI) is 0.63 at rest, but after exercise it falls to 0.34 on the right and rises to 0.79 on the left. The results suggest severe arterial disease on the right and moderate arterial disease on the left.

What should the GP do now?
The GP should inform Mr Rudman that he has diabetes, give him some information about this and refer him to practice diabetic clinic. He should continue taking the ACE inhibitor, statin and aspirin.

The GP should ask Mr Rudman what conclusions he has come to about stopping smoking. What help would he like with this?

In view of the severity of arterial disease in the right leg, the GP refers Mr Rudman to a vascular surgeon.

Outcome
The surgeon performs a duplex scan, which shows a very tight stenosis at the origin of the right superficial femoral artery. The vascular surgeon reinforces the GP's advice to stop smoking and encourages Mr Rudman to keep

walking. The surgeon suggests that Mr Rudman should return to clinic in 6 weeks with a view to discussing surgery.

Meanwhile, Mr Rudman sees the practice nurse for a fuller assessment of his diabetes. He accepts that he is eating too many biscuits and cuts down on these, as well as his evening pint. For the time being, his diabetes is controlled by diet alone. His blood pressure falls to 132/76 mmHg.

He sees the Quit Smoking Counsellor in the practice every 2 weeks and starts nicotine replacement therapy. He succeeds in stopping smoking completely.

He starts going for a walk in the local park every day and loses a bit of weight.

By the time he goes back to see the surgeon, he can walk more comfortably and says he is not keen on having an operation; the surgeon is happy with this and discharges him back to the care of his GP.

Doppler assessment and pressure measurement

		Right				Left	
	Signal	Strength	Pressure	Index	Signal	Strength	Pressure	Index
Arm	Tri	++	142					
PTA	Mono	+			Mono	++	90	0.63
DPA	Mono	++			Mono	++		
ATA	Mono	++	90	0.63	Bi	++		

Tri/bi = normal   Mono = diseased   ++ Normal   + Weak   − Absent

Exercise details

Treadmill speed: **3.0 kph**

10% incline, bilateral calf ache at 20 m, getting worse at 60 m (R>L)

Total distance walked: **85 m**   Reason for stopping: **pain in calves**

Post-exercise pressures

		Right				Left	
	Signal	Strength	Pressure	Index	Signal	Strength	Pressure	Index
Arm			140					
ATA	Mono	++	48	0.34	Mono	++	110	0.79

Figure 29.2 Results of Doppler study for Case study 29.3 (Mr Rudman).

achieved over a series of consultations. In Case study 29.3, Mr Rudman is not on any medication when he first presents to his GP, but he ends up on three different medications: an ACE inhibitor, aspirin and a statin. All of these are recommended by NICE.[11]

A Doppler probe is used to measure the ankle brachial pressure index (ABPI). The patient should be lying down when this is done. First, the systolic blood pressure is measured in one arm, then the highest pressure at which pulses can be detected using Doppler probe in the ankle is recorded.

■ ABPI = highest ankle pressure/highest arm pressure.

In PAD, the index is low, and in severe PAD, the ABPI falls on exercise, rather than rising.

PAD is common in people with diabetes, in people who smoke and in people with coronary artery disease. It can be controlled in primary care by bringing into play all the strategies for reducing cardiovascular risk. Lifestyle measures are important, particularly doing regular exercise and stopping smoking. Only if symptoms do not improve with these measures is surgery necessary.

SUMMARY

Atrial fibrillation is very common and is often picked up incidentally when the GP notices that a patient's pulse is irregular. Patients with atrial fibrillation are at increased risk of stroke, but this risk can be reduced by anticoagulation, which is usually started in primary care. TIAs are a warning sign that a patient is at high risk of having a stroke and require the GP to organise urgent investigation. A patient presenting with chest pain always requires careful assessment. The history gives the best clues about the likelihood of underlying coronary artery disease. Myocardial infarction and stroke are managed in hospital, but the GP has a key role after discharge in reducing the risk of future cardiovascular events. The same principles of secondary prevention are implemented in managing patients with PAD.

Now visit **www.wileyessential.com/primarycare** to test yourself on this chapter.

REFERENCES

1. NICE. Atrial fibrillation: the management of atrial fibrillation. NICE Clinical Guideline 180. June 2014. Available from: http://www.nice.org.uk/guidance/cg180 (last accessed 6 October 2015).

2. Lip GY, Nieuwlaat R, Pisters R, et al. Refining clinical risk stratification for predicting stroke an thromboembolism in atrial fibrillation using a novel risk factor-based approach; the Euro Heart Survey on atrial fibrillation. *Chest* 2010;**137**:262–72.

3. Gage BF, Waterman AD, Shannon W, et al. Validation of clinical classification schemes for predicting stroke: results from the national registry of atrial fibrillation. *JAMA* 2001;**285**:2864–70.

4. Pisters R, Lane DA, Nieuwlaat R, et al. A novel user-friendly score (HAS-BLED) to assess one year risk of major bleeding in atrial fibrillation patients: the Euro Heart Survey. *Chest* 2010;**138**(5):1093–100.

5. Diamond GA, Forrester JS. Analysis of probability as an aid in the clinical diagnosis of coronary-artery disease. *N Eng J Med* 1979;**300**:1350–8.

6. NICE. MI – secondary prevention. Secondary prevention in primary and secondary care for patients following a myocardial infarction. NICE Clinical Guideline 172. November 2013. Available from: http://www.nice.org.uk/guidance/cg172 (last accessed 6 October 2015).

7. Hacke W, Kaste M, Bluhmki E, et al. Thrombolysis with alteplase 3 to 4.5 hours after acute ischaemic stroke. *N Eng J Med* 2008;**359**:1317–29.

8. Whiteley W, Wardlaw J, Thomas R, et al. Oral presentations of 5th UK Stroke Forum. A comparison of stroke screening tools with the clinical diagnosis of emergency room staff: a prospective cohort study. *Int J Stroke* 2010;**5**:3–13.

9. NICE. Stroke: diagnosis and initial management of acute stroke and transient ischaemic attack (TIA). NICE Clinical Guideline 68. July 2008. Available from: http://www.nice.org.uk/guidance/cg68 (last accessed 6 October 2015).

10. Giles MF, Rothwell PM. Risk of stroke after transient ischaemic attack: a systematic review and meta-analysis. *Lancet Neurol* 2007;**6**:1063–72.

11. NICE. Lower limb peripheral arterial disease: diagnosis and management. NICE Clinical Guideline 147. August 2012. Available from: http://www.nice.org.uk/guidance/cg147 (last accessed 6 October 2015).

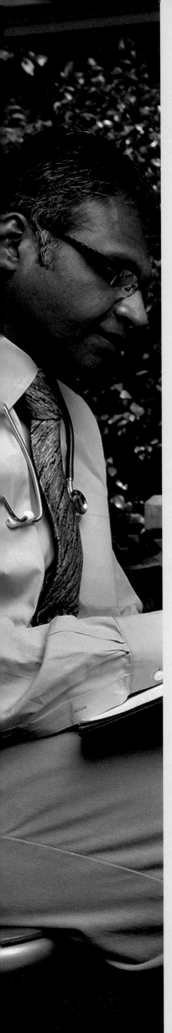

CHAPTER 30
Breathlessness

Jessica Buchan
GP and Teaching Fellow in Primary Care, University of Bristol

Key topics

Learning objectives

- Be able to take a history from a patient who is breathless and plan investigations appropriately.
- Be able to diagnose and manage chronic asthma.
- Be able to diagnose and manage chronic obstructive pulmonary disease.
- Be able to identify people who might have heart failure.

Essential Primary Care, First Edition. Edited by Andrew Blythe and Jessica Buchan.
© 2017 John Wiley & Sons, Ltd. Published 2017 by John Wiley & Sons, Ltd.
Companion website: www.wileyessential.com/primarycare

Introduction

Breathlessness (or dyspnoea) is the sensation that breathing is hard work. In usual circumstances we barely notice our breath. When we do get out of breath, it should be appropriate for the level of exertion; for example, if we are not used to running, we may get out of breath quite quickly if we try to run uphill. Pathological breathlessness occurs in situations that would not normally cause laboured breathing. Patients may describe not getting enough air in with each breath or feeling that they are having to breathe faster or deeper to meet their needs.

Acute breathlessness in primary care

Acute breathlessness comes on over minutes to days, and generally has a different set of causes (see Table 30.1) from those causing chronic breathlessness. Chronic breathlessness typically develops over weeks or months (see Box 30.1). The two

Table 30.1 Causes of acute breathlessness in primary care.

Cause	Feature in the history	Signs
Asthma	Younger patient typical Known history of asthma Trigger, e.g. smoking, exposure to dust, pets or other allergens	Wheeze or silent chest (life-threatening) Tachycardia and tachypnoea Using accessory muscles of respiration, e.g. sitting forward and bracing shoulders
Exacerbation of COPD	Older patient typical History of smoking Symptoms of RTI, e.g. fever, purulent sputum	Wheeze Cyanosis, pursed-lip breathing Scattered or focal coarse crackles Reduced oxygen saturations
Acute left ventricular failure	Older patient typical History of myocardial infarction	Tachycardia Raised jugular venous pressure (JVP) Heart: laterally displaced apex beat with gallop rhythm Bilateral fine crackles over lung fields Fluid retention (leg oedema) Tender, enlarged liver
Pneumonia	Fever Cough Pleuritic pain	Fever and systemically unwell Focal chest signs, e.g. dullness to percussion with coarse crackles
Pulmonary embolism	Sudden onset Sharp pleuritic chest pain, radiation to the left shoulder, syncope	Pulse oximetry <95% Heart rate >100 bpm Absence of wheeze or crackles increases likelihood of pulmonary embolism ECG: right axis deviation, strain or right bundle branch block, nonspecific ST changes or an S1, Q3, T3 pattern
Pneumothorax	Sudden onset Pleuritic pain History of COPD with bullae, or spontaneous in young patient	Tachycardia and tachypnoea Displacement of the trachea Hyper-resonant chest
Pleural effusion	Known malignancy, heart failure, cirrhosis or hypoalbuminaemia	Stony dullness over one or both lung bases, with no air entry
Panic attack	Known anxiety disorder Triggers, e.g. crowded room Associated features, e.g. chest pain, pins and needles	Appears anxious Tachycardia Respiratory examination otherwise normal

Other causes

- Cardiac, e.g. myocardial infarction, arrhythmias, pericardial disease
- Neuromuscular gradual onset, but can be acute as in Guillain–Barré syndrome or myasthenia gravis
- Metabolic acidosis, e.g. ketoacidosis
- Large airway obstruction, e.g. foreign body, anaphylaxis, trauma
- Thyrotoxicosis

Box 30.1 Common causes of chronic breathlessness in primary care

- **Cardiac causes:** Left ventricular disease, heart valve disease (e.g. mitral or aortic stenosis).
- **Pulmonary causes:** COPD, chronic asthma, pulmonary hypertension, pulmonary fibrosis, infiltrates from sarcoidosis or malignancy, multiple pulmonary embolisms.
- **Drugs:** Beta blockers can worsen COPD/asthma; amiodarone can causes pneumonitis or pulmonary fibrosis; local radiotherapy can damage lung tissue.
- **Musculoskeletal:** Obesity or severe kyphoscoliosis.
- **Anaemia:** Gastrointestinal malignancy or haematological condition.
- **Neuromuscular causes**

Box 30.2 Signs indicating need for emergency admission in a breathless patient

Admit any patient by urgent ambulance if they are breathless with:
- altered consciousness;
- systolic blood pressure <90 mmHg;
- tachycardia (>130 bpm);
- respiratory rate of 25 breaths per minute or more;
- reduced oxygen saturations <91%;
- pregnancy, or up to 6 weeks postpartum.

can overlap; conditions can coexist, or patients with chronic breathlessness can have acute exacerbations of their condition; for example, a respiratory tract infection (RTI) can cause a rapid worsening of symptoms in a patient with chronic obstructive pulmonary disease (COPD).

If a patient presents with acute breathlessness, they need urgent assessment. Some of the causes listed in Table 30.1 cause rapid deterioration and, without prompt and effective treatment, death. Although it is not common in a primary care setting, GPs need to recognise a patient in severe respiratory distress who may need intubation and urgent transfer to secondary care (see Box 30.2).

From first seeing the patient, the GP can quickly assess:
- level of consciousness;
- patient distress and ability to talk;
- patient position (e.g. a patient using accessory muscles of respiration or wincing when they breathe in);
- obvious sounds, such as wheeze or stridor;
- breathing pattern (Kussmaul's breathing is a deep sighing breathing classically associated with diabetic ketoacidosis);
- skin colour and cyanosis.

Top tip: normal respiratory rate

A normal respiratory rate in an adult is 12–18 breaths per minute. Expiration should be longer than inspiration, with a ratio of 1 : 2 or 1 : 3.

Examination should include:
- vital signs, including pulse rate and rhythm, respiratory rate, blood pressure and pulse oximetry;
- placement of the trachea, assessment of chest movements, percussion and auscultation of the chest;
- cardiac examination;
- blood glucose;
- electrocardiogram (ECG) to distinguish cardiac from pulmonary causes (this should always be interpreted in the clinical context; for example, a pulmonary embolism can show nonspecific changes on the ECG).

If a history is possible, the GP needs to find out for how long the patient has had breathlessness, how quickly it came on and what precipitated it. For example, sudden onset of acute breathlessness in a young, otherwise healthy adult suggests spontaneous pneumothorax, or a pulmonary embolism if there are risk factors. Finding out if any possible triggers precipitated the episode is important. Exposure to allergens or a very dusty environment can trigger a rapid attack of asthma, or stridor occurring after eating may be due to an inhaled foreign body or anaphylaxis. A more gradual onset with worsening breathlessness occurs in infection, asthma, pulmonary oedema and neuromuscular causes.

Top tip: measuring oxygen saturation

Pulse oximeters use infrared light to measure the amount of oxyhaemoglobin in the blood.
- The probe should be placed on a finger (index is best) that is clean and dry, with nail polish removed.
- Take and record the best reading.
- Oxygen saturation should be >94% on air.
- Falsely low readings can by caused by arrhythmias, haemoglobinopathies, poor perfusion and carbon monoxide poisoning.
- Falsely high readings can be caused by pigmented skin.

Pulmonary embolism

No single risk factor, sign or symptom has been found to be pathognomonic for pulmonary embolism.[1] The biggest risk factors are increasing age (risk is significant at 50 and increases with each year of life) and a previous history of venous thromboembolism (VTE). GPs need a high index of suspicion in patients who are immobile or have had recent surgery, or who have cancer or cardiac disease. Risks are also increased after an infection, such as pneumonia. Obesity becomes a significant risk when body mass index (BMI) exceeds 35 kg/m², but is more likely to be a risk factor when combined with other factors, such as smoking.[1]

Scoring systems such as the Wells score[2] have been designed to help evaluate the probability of a pulmonary embolism. National Institute for Health and Care Excellence (NICE) guidance[3] recommends that the 'two-level PE Wells score' is used. Points are given for specific risk factors, such as a malignancy; symptoms, such as haemoptysis; and signs, such as a deep-vein thrombosis (DVT). Risk is stratified into two levels: a score of more than four makes a pulmonary embolism 'likely'; a score of four or less makes a pulmonary embolism 'unlikely'. For patients falling into the 'unlikely' category in whom signs and symptoms suggest a pulmonary embolism and other causes have been excluded, NICE guidelines recommend a D-dimer level to guide the need for transfer to secondary care for further investigation, such as computed tomography pulmonary angiography (CTPA).

Breathlessness in anxiety and panic attacks

In response to a physical threat, the body undergoes physiological changes to prepare to either face the threat or run away, known as the 'fight-or-flight' response. Hormones such as adrenaline and cortisol are released, which increase the heart rate and blood pressure, tense the muscles and alter the activity of the brain, so that we react on instinct rather than rational thought. Intense feelings of anxiety are experienced alongside negative physical effects, such as chest pain, dry mouth, nausea, diarrhoea, the need to urinate, sweating and trembling. In panic disorder, these hormones are released in response to emotion or fear of a perceived threat – the 'fear of fear' – and can trigger a panic attack. A vicious cycle can emerge when patients hyperventilate and exhale too much carbon dioxide, which in turn causes symptoms of dizziness, confusion and pins and needles. Often the onset of a panic attack is sudden and occurs without a clear trigger, although the patient is usually experiencing generalised anxiety or adverse life stresses.

Top tip: explaining panic attacks to patients

Understanding what is happening during a panic attack can help patients. A GP might say:

When people feel anxious, they start to breathe faster. This means they get rid of too much carbon dioxide. This causes chemical changes in the body that make them feel nauseated and cause frightening tingling sensations.

GPs or emergency services may see patients during a panic attack; the feelings can be intense enough for patients to feel that they are having a heart attack or are going to die. Usually, GPs see patients after the event. Patients may describe

generalised anxiety disorder (GAD), where the physical symptoms (such as breathlessness) are present much of the time, or panic attacks, where the symptoms are intense but short-lived.

Usually, panic disorder is diagnosed by taking a good history. It is more straightforward in a young, otherwise fit patient who describes a clear history of anxiety. Older adults and those with physical comorbidities often need investigating to exclude other cardiac or respiratory causes.

Treating underlying depression or anxiety is helpful, and patients should be assessed for suicide risk. Addressing current stressors, learning relaxation techniques and adopting lifestyle changes are helpful in mild cases. Caffeine and alcohol should be avoided, as they precipitate symptoms similar to anxiety and trigger attacks. GPs often have their own simple breathing or relaxation techniques that they can teach their patients in the consultation. Breathing into a paper (not plastic) bag during an attack can help to rebreathe some of the carbon dioxide and slow the breath rate. In more severe or complex cases of panic disorder, cognitive behavioural therapy (CBT) or antidepressant medication may be needed.

Top tip: a breathing technique for a panic attack

- Try and find somewhere quiet to go.
- Place one hand lightly on your stomach and one hand on your chest.
- Become aware of your breath.
- As you breathe in, feel the hand on your stomach moving out; the hand on your chest should move very little.
- As you breathe out, feel the hand on your stomach sinking in; the hand on your chest should move very little.
- Start to count the length of your breath in…1, 2, 3.
- Count the length of your breath out…1, 2, 3, 4.
- Aim to breathe out for 1 or 2 counts longer than you breathe in.
- Breathing techniques are most effective when practised regularly, and not just when you need them; for example, exercises can be practised when you lie down to sleep at night.

Diagnosing and managing chronic asthma

Asthma is common; 1 in 12 adults in the UK are thought to currently receive treatment for asthma,[4] the vast majority of whom are managed in primary care. The typical symptoms are wheeze, cough, chest tightness and shortness of breath. Symptoms are often worse in the morning, at nighttime, with

Case study 30.1a

Billy Nichols is 24. He was seen at the accident and emergency department one weekend with an acute asthma attack triggered by an RTI. After a period of observation, he was discharged on antibiotics, steroids and a salbutamol (beta-agonist) inhaler. The doctor in accident and emergency suggested he be followed up by his GP, Dr Raj Joshi. Billy is not normally on regular inhalers and is rarely seen at the practice. His records show that he had asthma as a child.

Dr Joshi sees Billy 2 weeks after his hospital visit. Billy is feeling better. He doesn't think he has asthma and he doesn't want to take regular medication. Billy reports he only has a wheeze and cough when he plays football at the weekend. Billy doesn't think this is a problem; until now, he's used his girlfriends 'blue' inhaler, which helps enough for him to carry on playing. He thinks his recent episode was just because he had a chest infection. Billy admits he still has a bit of a dry cough and wheeze in the morning; his inhaler helps these symptoms. He doesn't smoke.

What are Dr Joshi's aims for the consultation?
Dr Joshi explains to Billy that the aim of correct diagnosis of asthma and treatment is to improve quality of life and prevent exacerbations. It is likely Billy will need regular treatment; exercise-induced asthma is often a symptom of poor control, and it is probable that Billy is more symptomatic than he realises or admits.

As well as exercise, what other aggravating factors should be assessed?
- **Occupation:** If symptoms are worse at work, and better at weekends and holidays, consider occupational asthma, which needs specialist management and referral to a chest physician/occupational health.
- **Pets or birds at home:** Atopic asthma can be triggered by allergy to the proteins found in animals' dander (skin flakes), saliva, urine or faeces.
- **Hay fever:** Atopic asthma often coexists with other atopic conditions, such as eczema and hay fever. Managing allergic rhinitis makes asthma treatment more effective.
- **Drugs:** Beta blockers should be stopped. Aspirin and nonsteroidal anti-inflammatory drugs (NSAIDs) may make symptoms worse.
- **Smoking:** Smoking exacerbates symptoms and increases the risk of acute attacks. Patients who smoke should be helped to stop.

What tests does Billy need for diagnosis?
Asthma is a clinical diagnosis based on typical symptoms. It is helpful to document an objective measurement of airway obstruction. Spirometry is the preferred method and is available in most GP practices. Billy can also do serial peak-flow measurements, taken morning and night for 2 weeks and recorded in a visual diary format. A diurnal variation (difference between the morning and evening readings) in peak flow of more than 20% is significant. Other factors can cause this variability, but in Billy's case, Dr Joshi may find a diary useful in assessing Billy's symptoms.

---

exercise and on exposure to cold air. Asthma is a variable and reversible condition characterised by bronchial hypersensitivity. Acute episodes can be life-threatening when the smooth muscles in the airways narrow (bronchospasm) and secretions plug the airways (see Chapter 15).

Peak flow

A peak flow meter is a simple way of measuring the fastest rate at which a patient can expel air from the lungs, measured in litres per minute. It is useful for monitoring asthma, but less so for diagnosing it. Results may be normal when the patient is asymptomatic, so tests do not exclude a diagnosis of asthma. Individuals are given a 'predicted' value based on expected levels for their age, height and sex, which can be read off a normative chart. For monitoring, knowing the 'normal' value for an individual (their best value when they are stable and well) is more useful than knowing their predicted level.

Top tip: how to record peak flow

Explain the device. A peak-flow meter is a tube that the patient blows into as if they were blowing out a candle. It measures the hardness/quickness of the breath, not how long the patient breathes out for.
- Demonstrate the technique yourself.
- Ask the patient to stand up.
- Set the indicator to zero.
- Ask the patient to exhale, then take a deep breath.
- Explain that the patient needs a good seal with their lips around the mouthpiece.
- Ask the patient to blow into the mouthpiece as hard and fast as they can.
- Record the best of three readings.

Case study 30.1b

Spirometry confirms an obstructive picture with good reversibility. Billy agrees to start a regular steroid inhaler. He comes for a review with the practice asthma nurse, Kathy Bailey, 6 weeks later. Billy doesn't think the new 'brown' corticosteroid inhaler works as well as his blue one, so he's stopped using it.

What should an asthma review cover?
Guidelines[5] recommend using the three Medical Research Council (MRC)-defined questions to assess symptoms. This can be done over the telephone:

1. Have you had difficulty sleeping because of your asthma?
2. Have you had your usual asthma symptoms during the day?
3. Have you been prevented from doing your daily activities because of your asthma?

Treatment should be reviewed. Medication should be stepped up or stepped down until a patient is on the lowest possible dose of inhaled steroid that controls symptoms.

Billy should not stop his inhalers suddenly. If his symptoms are controlled, his inhaler can be reduced slowly by 25–50% every few months. If there is poor control, the nurse should assess:

- **Adherence:** A common reason for poor control is that the patient is not taking their inhalers.

- **Inhaler technique:** If the inhaler is not being used properly, it can result in a poor response to treatment.
- **Smoking:** Smoking makes asthma worse, so this should be addressed.

Review the diagnosis in asthma that doesn't seem to respond before increasing doses of medication; 'step back before you step up'.

Patient education
Nurse Bailey explains that in asthma, the airways are sensitive and can 'overreact' at times, causing symptoms. Anyone exposed to enough of a trigger, such as a lot of dust, will react with coughing and wheezing as their airways close up and try to protect the lungs. In asthma, things like household pets, exercise, a chest infection or cold air can be enough to make the airways react.

Nurse Bailey explains that the 'blue' inhaler contains a 'rescue' medication that opens up the airways and makes it easier to breathe. It should be carried at all times and should work in a matter of minutes. The effects should last for 4–6 hours.

Billy's new steroid inhaler is a 'preventer' medicine. It does not work like the rescue inhaler and Billy will not notice any change to his breathing after using it. If used every day, it will prevent the lungs 'overreacting' as much. Billy will know he is on the correct dose of the preventer when he hardly needs to use rescue medicine at all (fewer than three times a week) and can exercise without symptoms.

Treatment and management plans in asthma

UK guidelines[5] advocate a stepwise approach to the management of asthma, where treatment is started at the level appropriate for the patient's symptoms. If symptoms are mild and occasional, it is appropriate to use a short-acting inhaled bronchodilator as required (step 1). If a patient has had an exacerbation in the last 2 years, is waking at night or has symptoms (or uses their inhaler) three times a week or more, they should start inhaled corticosteroids (step 2). If control is still not achieved and the patient is on 400 µg daily of inhaled steroids, a long-acting bronchodilator should be added, but this shouldn't be used without an inhaled steroid (step 3). This step includes the option to increase the steroid inhaler up to 800 µg daily. Combination inhalers that include a long-acting bronchodilator and a low-dose steroid improve adherence. Patients can also use this combination inhaler as a 'rescue' medication, instead of their short-acting bronchodilator.[5] This is especially effective in patients with poor adherence, but risks a high total daily steroid dose. If a GP puts a patient on this regime, the patient should be educated around this issue.

After this, other options include adding in a leukotriene receptor agonist, very high-dose inhaled corticosteroids (or oral steroids) or oral theophyllines (step 4). At this stage, the patient should be under specialist care.

Case Study 30.1 discusses asthma reviews in primary care. Reviews should include an exploration of triggers, education of the patient on recognising when their symptoms deteriorate, a written action plan and a review date. For example, a patient might be told that if their peak expiratory flow rate (PEFR) drops below 80% of their usual level, they should increase or restart inhaled corticosteroids, and they should seek review if they don't improve over 48 hours.

Chronic breathlessness

In chronic breathlessness, finding the underlying cause is not always straightforward. More than one pathology can coexist in the same patient. For example, a patient with underlying COPD may also have anaemia or cardiac failure. Symptoms are also not specific to any one condition. For example, ankle oedema is not a reliable symptom or sign for diagnosing heart failure, as it may result from dependant oedema or venous insufficiency.

Diagnosing and managing left ventricular failure

Heart failure is when the heart is no longer pumping well enough to meet demands. The heart muscle may not contract well, or the resting heart does not fill with enough blood, or there is a combination of these factors. It is caused by:

- damage to the heart muscle (e.g. ischaemic heart disease or cardiomyopathy);
- reduced cardiac output (e.g. valve disease or vascular resistance from hypertension);
- high cardiac output (e.g. anaemia, sepsis or thyrotoxicosis).

GPs need to look for cases where there are risk factors, such as patients with atrial fibrillation or hypertension, or who consume excess alcohol. A previous myocardial infarction greatly increases the chance that a patient's breathlessness is due to heart failure. The prognosis for heart failure is poor; up to 50% of those diagnosed with heart failure die within 4 years, depending on the cause and comorbidities. Early recognition and effective management reduce morbidity and mortality.[6]

Case study 30.2

Amir Hassan is 54. He presents to Dr Louise Clifton with a history of getting more 'puffed out' than usual when walking. Amir works as a taxi driver. He has recently returned from a month-long visit to Pakistan for his mother's funeral. He smokes 20 cigarettes daily. He rarely sees the GP.

What should Dr Clifton assess in the history?
Dr Clifton should assess what Amir means by feeling 'puffed out'. She should examine the duration of his symptoms, what brings on the breathlessness and his exercise tolerance. She should assess associated features such as chest pain, palpitations, light-headedness, cough, sputum and colour, wheeze or other audible noises and ankle swelling. She should review systemic symptoms, including alarm features such as weight loss, haemoptysis, night sweats and fever (suspicious of tuberculosis (TB) or malignancy). She should also review his systems; for example, a change in bowel habit might uncover an undiagnosed gastrointestinal malignancy resulting in breathlessness secondary to anaemia.

Amir describes the sensation of breathlessness as starting during his trip to Pakistan. He was grief-stricken at his mother's funeral and the breathlessness has gradually worsened since then, over a period of about 6 weeks. At first, he was breathless going up hills, or if he hurried. Now, he goes about 200 yards on the flat before he has to stop. He has not noticed any chest pain, palpitations or wheeze. He also tires easily, and his ankles have swollen; his shoes feel really tight. He is sleeping on three pillows. He had a dry, nonproductive cough for a few weeks when he returned from Pakistan, but it has improved. He has not had haemoptysis or night sweats. He has not lost any weight.

What examination should Dr Clifton do?
- Check pulse rate and rhythm for atrial fibrillation and tachycardia.
- Check blood pressure.
- Look for raised jugular venous pressure (JVP).
- Assess for fluid overload (peripheral oedema, bilateral basal crackles and a baseline weight).
- Feel for displaced apex beat and listen for murmurs (valvular heart disease) and third or fourth heart sounds.

On examination, Amir is comfortable at rest. His pulse is regular (88 bpm) and his blood pressure is 162/94. He has pitting oedema of his ankles and fine bi-basal crackles.

What tests should Dr Clifton request?
Investigations help assess the underlying cause of heart failure, find modifiable aggravating factors and exclude alternative causes for the breathlessness. Tests should include:
- ECG;
- biochemical markers (full blood count (FBC), urea and electrolytes (U&Es), eGFR, thyroid function tests (TFTs), liver function tests (LFTs), fasting lipids, HbA1c);
- urinalysis;
- chest X-ray;
- lung function tests, such as spirometry, to exclude COPD.

Dr Clifton may also consider TB in a traveller with a cough who has returned from an area of high prevalence, such as Pakistan. This is investigated with three sputum samples (at least one early-morning sample) for microscopy for acid-fast bacilli, culture for mycobacteria and a chest X-ray. If a GP is highly suspicious of active TB, urgent referral to a specialist clinic is indicated (without waiting for results), or admission if the patient is unwell.

Specific heart failure investigations
- A transthoracic Doppler echocardiogram is needed for diagnosis of suspected heart failure.
- Beta-type natriuretic peptide (BNP) is excreted from the heart muscle. Blood levels can help determine how likely heart failure is, and the need for referral. Raised levels >100 pg/ml are not always due to heart failure, but normal levels make heart failure unlikely unless the

patient is very obese or on cardiac drugs that can lower BNP.[6]

Amir's ECG shows Q waves and T wave inversion in leads II, III and aVF, suggesting an old inferior infarct. On further questioning about his experience of being 'grief-stricken', Amir says he collapsed at his mother's funeral; he felt very sick, sweaty, breathless and unwell, and had to lie down. He was in bed for a couple of days afterwards with exhaustion.

Outcome

Dr Clifton suspects Amir has heart failure secondary to a myocardial infarction. She refers him urgently to a cardiologist, who is able to see him 3 days later. Dr Clifton starts the loop diuretic furosemide for symptom control and organises blood tests to have ready at the cardiology clinic. His echocardiogram confirms myocardial wall damage and impaired systolic ventricular dysfunction. His ejection fraction is 35%.

Top tip: interpreting ejection fraction on echocardiogram

Ejection fraction is a measure of the percentage of blood pumped out with each heartbeat: 60% is normal, 40–55% is not considered significant, <40% is reduced.

Although a reduced ejection fraction indicates impaired systolic function, a patient can still have heart failure with a 'normal' or preserved ejection fraction.

Heart failure treatment[6]

- Stop medicines that may worsen heart failure, such as calcium-channel blockers and NSAIDs.
- Start a diuretic and fluid restriction for symptom control.
- Angiotension-converting enzyme (ACE) inhibitors, beta blockers and aldosterone antagonists such as spironolactone have all been shown to increase life expectancy. Start with an ACE inhibitor (or use an angiotension II-receptor blocker (ARB) if the patient is intolerant of ACE inhibitors).
- Start on low doses of ACE inhibitor and beta blocker, and titrate the doses up gradually (monthly), monitoring blood pressure, pulse and renal function with each increase.
- NICE recommends[6] that newly diagnosed patients are referred to specialist heart failure clinics to be seen within 6 weeks. Refer urgently if the patient has had a previous myocardial infarction, BNP levels are very high (>400 pg/ml) or symptoms are severe; these patients should be seen within 2 weeks.

Review and referral for heart failure

Patients with stable heart failure should be reviewed in primary care at least 6-monthly. This is often done by the GP, in conjunction with a practice nurse who has had additional training in managing patients with heart failure. Table 30.2 outlines what to cover in a primary care review. The GP will also review patients based on clinical need. A sudden worsening of symptoms needs careful assessment and can have numerous causes, including atrial fibrillation or a myocardial infarct, which must not be overlooked. Treatment can cause side effects, such as hypotension, so regular monitoring in primary care is essential. There is often a fine balance to be struck between increasing the dose of diuretics and not making renal function worse.

A patient's condition may deteriorate with disease progression. Part of the purpose of a review is to assess severity. The New York Heart Association (NYHA) has classified the severity of heart failure into four categories:[7]

- **Category I:** Patient has proven heart failure but no symptoms. If a patient can continue their ordinary daily activities without getting breathless, they fall into this category.
- **Category II:** Patient has mild symptoms with limitation of activity. They may be breathless doing light housework or climbing the stairs.
- **Category III:** More severe. A patient with heart failure in this category feels comfortable only at rest, and their activity is impaired by their symptoms.
- **Category IV:** Severe heart failure. Patients are symptomatic even at rest.

Patients with severe symptoms (NYHA category IV) and those who are not responding to usual primary care management should be referred urgently to secondary care. Community heart failure clinics help educate and monitor patients, and provide access to exercise-based rehabilitation programmes. They are a bridge between primary and secondary care services. Community heart failure nurses can advise on symptom control, help provide psychosocial support, aid admission avoidance and help the GP provide palliative care where patients need oxygen therapy and morphine. The life expectancy of those with chronic heart failure remains poor; it is lower than for many cancers.

Diagnosing and managing chronic obstructive pulmonary disease

Huge numbers of people with COPD are undiagnosed. It's estimated that 3.7 million people in the UK have COPD, of which only 900 000 have been diagnosed.[8]

COPD is a disease of smoking. Symptoms are caused by damage to the airways, resulting in narrow airways, which prevent normal airflow into the lungs (hence the term 'obstructive'). The damaged airways also result in air-trapping, making it harder for air to get out of the lungs with each exhalation. Unlike asthma, COPD is progressive and is not fully reversible. It should be suspected on history. The medical records may well show a history of frequent chest infections (especially in the winter months).

Table 30.2 Review of heart failure in primary care.	
Stable heart failure should be reviewed in primary care at least 6-monthly. Patients should also be reviewed if they are symptomatic.	
Educate	Discuss what heart failure is Discuss symptoms, the aims of treatment and prognosis
Lifestyle	Ask about smoking and encourage smoking cessation Aerobic exercise is recommended, especially via a supervised rehabilitation programme
Diet and fluids	A low-salt diet is usually advised. Alcohol should be restricted, and avoided in alcohol-induced cardiomyopathy In severe heart failure, patients may be advised to restrict their fluid intake by secondary care Patients can-self monitor their weight; a sudden gain suggests fluid retention and the need to increase diuretics and seek medical advice (e.g. a gain of >2 kg in 3 days)
Ask about current symptoms and possible medication side effects	Look for underlying causes if symptoms worsen
Ask about sexual function	Patients may not feel comfortable raising this if the GP does not directly ask, but medication can interfere with sexual functioning, or patients may be concerned that sexual intercourse can exacerbate symptoms
Screen for depression	Depression is common in all chronic cardiac and lung conditions
Check pulse rate and rhythm, blood pressure and BMI	Increasing medication doses can be limited by bradycardia and hypotension Raised blood pressure and arrhythmias can worsen heart failure High BMI can worsen symptoms; very low BMI may need input from a dietician
Immunisation	Advise an annual influenza vaccine and a one-off pneumococcal vaccine
Biochemical monitoring	It is essential to monitor renal function on ACE inhibitors and diuretics, and with each dose increase Aldosterone antagonists, such as spironolactone, can contribute to dangerous hyperkalaemia For cardiovascular risk reduction, patients should be monitored for raised cholesterol and diabetes Impaired liver function may suggest congestive hepatomegaly from heart failure or excess alcohol intake Anaemia or thyroid disease can worsen symptoms and should be checked if indicated
Medication	Titrate medication to manage symptoms; review if there are any interactions between current medications
Follow-up and referral	Set next review date Arrange biochemical monitoring, e.g. if medication has been adjusted Consider whether referral is needed for a dietician, exercise rehabilitation programme, community heart failure nurse or secondary care

Screen[9] anyone over 35 who smokes or has smoked by asking if they:

- get breathless on exertion;
- have a cough;
- produce sputum.

Examination findings

Examination may be normal in mild COPD. In longstanding disease, the chest may be hyperinflated and the patient may have obvious dyspnoea with pursed-lip breathing and signs of chronic cyanosis. There may be wheeze or quiet breath sounds on auscultation. Signs of right heart failure (cor pulmonale) may be apparent in severe COPD, where the damage to the lungs results in impairment of right ventricular function.

Spirometry

Spirometry measures the flow of air out of the lungs and compares it with that of an average person of a similar height, weight and gender. A forced expiratory volume in the first second (FEV1) of less than 80% of that predicted shows airflow obstruction, as seen in asthma and COPD. Spirometry also measures the capacity of the lungs (forced vital capacity, FVC). In asthma and COPD, the lungs are usually of normal volume, so the capacity is normal. However, the ratio between the volume the patient can exhale in 1 second and the capacity of their lungs (FEV1/FVC) is reduced (<0.7). In asthma, this is reversible with bronchodilation (using inhaled or nebulised beta-agonists). A diagnosis of COPD is made if the FEV1/FVC ratio is <0.7 after bronchodilation, although in early COPD, changes are often only subtle. FEV1 is used to measure the severity of COPD:[9]

- FEV1 ≥80% indicates mild COPD if there are typical symptoms.
- FEV1 50–79% indicates moderate COPD.
- FEV1 30–49% indicates severe COPD.
- FEV1 < 30% is very severe disease.

A restrictive pattern is seen when the capacity of the lungs is reduced (e.g. in pulmonary fibrosis). Spirometry will show a reduced FVC, and because FEV1 is often reduced too, the FEV1/FVC ratio is normal. A mixed picture is seen when different pathologies coexist or where a disease causes both restriction and obstruction (e.g. cystic fibrosis).

Other investigations

- A chest X-ray is prudent, not so much to diagnose COPD as to exclude other lung pathologies.
- FBC looks for polycythaemia and anaemia.
- Pulse oximetry indentifies those who may need oxygen therapy.
- Sputum culture can be helpful if there is purulent sputum.
- In young patients, lifelong nonsmokers and those with a strong family history, alpha-1-anti-trypsin levels should be measured.
- In patients with symptoms out of proportion to the findings on spirometry, a computed tomography (CT) thorax may be required.

Management

The most important thing a patient can do for their lung function is to stop smoking. GPs must discuss this with them (see Chapter 7). Studies suggest that the fastest rate of lung function decline occurs in the early stages of COPD. GPs should be actively managing mild disease.[10] The challenge is making a diagnosis at a stage where symptoms are subtle and spirometry may be only mildly abnormal.

Treatment of COPD has two aims:

- **Improve symptoms and reduce exacerbations in stable COPD:** Inhaled bronchodilators and corticosteroids or treatment with a long-acting muscarinic agonist aims to reduce symptoms and exacerbations. These medications have not been shown to affect mortality or lung function.[9] They are usually delivered by handheld inhaler devices, although patients with very severe COPD may need to use a nebuliser.
- **Treating exacerbations:** Patients present with worsening breathlessness and purulent sputum. Prompt treatment

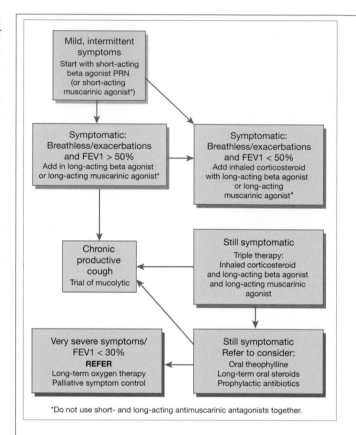

Figure 30.1 COPD treatment flowchart in primary care.

prevents short-term clinical deterioration, but also aims to prevent further damage to lung function. The GP will assess to see if admission is required (see Box 30.2) or if the patient can be managed in the community by doubling the frequency of their short-acting bronchodilators and giving them a course of oral steroids and oral antibiotics.

Inhaled therapy is increased in a stepwise manner (see Figure 30.1). If patients produce copious sputum and have a chronic cough, they can be tried on a mucolytic. These are only continued if there is symptomatic benefit. They are not used for acute exacerbations.

In severe COPD, patients may need continuous low-dose oral steroids or prophylactic antibiotics, but this should be initiated by a specialist. Oral theophylline is also used; there is evidence this improves lung function, but it has a narrow therapeutic window and needs close monitoring. Patients may also need long-term oxygen therapy to reduce the risks of right-sided heart failure and polycythaemia caused by chronic hypoxia. A systematic review[11] found that long-term oxygen therapy improved survival in severe COPD. For a prescription for long-term oxygen, the patient must have been assessed by a specialist. Oxygen is delivered directly to the patient's home from regional suppliers.

Top tip: referral for assessment for home oxygen

GPs should refer anyone with COPD who has:

- symptoms of severe COPD;
- FEV1 < 30%;
- oxygen saturations on air < 92%;
- clinical cyanosis or polycythaemia;
- signs of heart failure with COPD (e.g. peripheral oedema or raised JVP).

Review

As in heart failure, regular review is essential. For COPD, this should be at least annually. The GP should screen for depression and sexual functioning and assess the severity of COPD symptoms. Standard questions in the form of the MRC dyspnoea scale[12] have been developed to assess patients' symptoms from grade 1, where a patient is only breathless on strenuous exercise, to grade 5, where they are breathless on minimal exertion, such as getting dressed. A review should also:

- Check inhaler technique and check whether the patient has the most suitable device for them.

- Adjust treatment according to symptoms (based on the MRC dyspnoea scale and objective measurements of FEV1).
- Assess for pulmonary hypertension and cor pulmonale.
- Measure oxygen saturation. Is referral for home oxygen therapy indicated?
- Measure FEV1 and FVC (spirometry).
- Record BMI and compare to previous readings. A decline in BMI predicts poor prognosis and nutritional supplements and/or indicates referral to a dietician. An underlying lung malignancy should also be considered.
- Consider referral to specialist physiotherapists, who play a large role in helping with breathing dysfunction and pulmonary rehabilitation in patients with chronic lung disease.[13]
- Make sure the patient knows how to manage exacerbations and consider prescribing a 'rescue pack' of antibiotics and steroids that they can keep at home and take at the onset of an exacerbation, until they can be seen at the GP surgery.

COPD is a progressive disease. The natural history varies between individuals. Stopping smoking and preventing exacerbations both help slow the rate of decline in lung function. However, the mortality is still high, and GPs should discuss the prognosis and consider palliative care options with patients who have severe COPD.

SUMMARY

Breathlessness is a frightening sensation for patients. It may come on acutely over a matter of hours or days and present to the GP as an emergency. A sudden onset suggests a pneumothorax or pulmonary embolism. A more gradual build-up occurs in asthma or infection. Anxiety as a cause for breathlessness may be obvious from the history, but investigations to exclude cardiac or pulmonary causes are prudent in the older adult or those with comorbidities. Unravelling the causes behind chronic breathlessness can be a diagnostic challenge. Symptoms of cardiac causes and pulmonary causes can be similar, and different conditions can coexist in the same patient. Diagnosis is therefore a triad of history, examination and investigations, not only to identify the most likely underlying cause for a patient's breathlessness, but also to identify and manage aggravating comorbidities. Regular review of patients with chronic breathlessness is essential. Part of the aim of review is to help patients become partners in their care; they should be taught how to monitor their condition and when to seek medical help.

 Now visit **www.wileyessential.com/primarycare** to test yourself on this chapter.

REFERENCES

1. Kline J, Kabrhel C. Clinical review: emergency evaluation for pulmonary embolism, part 1: Clinical factors that increase risk. *J Emerg Med* 2015;**48**(6):771–80.
2. Wells PS, Anderson D, Rodger M, et al. Excluding pulmonary embolism at the bedside without diagnostic imaging: Management of patients with a suspected pulmonary embolism presenting to the emergency department by using a simple clinical model and D-dimer. *Ann Intern Med* 2001;**135**(2):98–107.
3. NICE. Clinical knowledge summary scenario: managing suspected pulmonary embolism. January 2015. http://cks.nice.org.uk/pulmonary-embolism (last accessed 6 October 2015).
4. Asthma UK. Asthma facts and FAQs, 2014. Available from: http://www.asthma.org.uk/asthma-facts-and-statistics (last accessed 6 October 2015).
5. SIGN. British guideline on the management of asthma. Scottish Intercollegiate Guideline 141. October 2014.

Available from: http://www.sign.ac.uk/pdf/SIGN141.pdf (last accessed 6 October 2015).

6. NICE. Chronic heart failure: management of chronic heart failure in adults in primary and secondary care. NICE Clinical Guideline 108. August 2010. Available from: http://www.nice.org.uk/guidance/cg108 (last accessed 6 October 2015).

7. The Criteria Committee of the New York Heart Association. *Nomenclature and Criteria for Diagnosis of Diseases of the Heart and Great Vessels*, 9th edn. Boston: Little, Brown & Co.; 1994. pp. 253–6.

8. Healthcare Commission. *Clearing the Air: A National Study of Chronic Obstructive Pulmonary Disease*. London: Commission for Healthcare Audit and Inspection; 2006.

9. NICE. Chronic obstructive pulmonary disease: management of chronic obstructive pulmonary disease in adults in primary and secondary care (partial update). NICE Clinical Guideline 101. June 2010. Available from: http://www.nice.org.uk/cg101 (last accessed 6 October 2015).

10. Cooper C. Treatment of COPD: the sooner the better? *Thorax* 2010;**65**(9):837–41.

11. Crockett AJ, Cranston JM, Moss JR, Alpers JH. A review of long-term oxygen therapy for chronic obstructive pulmonary disease. *Respir Med.* 2001;**95**(6):437–43.

12. Fletcher C, Elemes P, Fairbairn M, et al. The significance of respiratory symptoms and the diagnosis of chronic bronchitis in a working population. *BMJ* 1959;**2**:257–66.

13. Bott J, Blumenthal S, Buxton M, et al. Guidelines for the physiotherapy management of the adult, medical spontaneously breathing patient. *Thorax* 2009;**64**(Suppl. 1): i1–51.

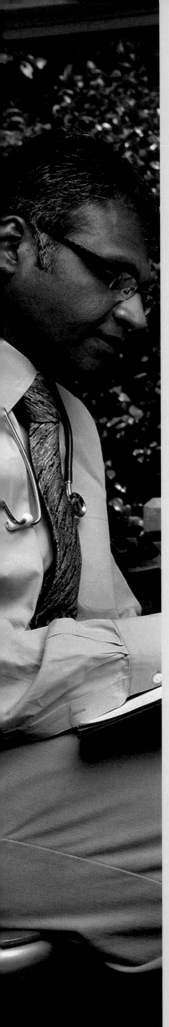

CHAPTER 31
Joint pains and stiffness

Andrew Blythe
GP and Senior Teaching Fellow, University of Bristol

Key topics

Learning objectives

- Be able to conduct a consultation with a person who complains of hip pain.
- Be able to identify someone who may have rheumatoid arthritis.
- Be able to conduct an annual review for someone with rheumatoid arthritis.
- Be able to diagnose polymyalgia rheumatica.

Essential Primary Care, First Edition. Edited by Andrew Blythe and Jessica Buchan.
© 2017 John Wiley & Sons, Ltd. Published 2017 by John Wiley & Sons, Ltd.
Companion website: www.wileyessential.com/primarycare

Osteoarthritis

Osteoarthritis is probably the most common chronic disease in older people. It's so common that we think of being elderly and having osteoarthritis as almost synonymous. On road and bus signs, an elderly person is represented by someone bent over and propped up by a stick. For centuries, walking sticks and ointments rubbed into the affected joint were all we had to offer people with osteoarthritis. Now, we have a huge array of pain-relieving and anti-inflammatory drugs, together with the ability to replace hip and knee joints. In the UK, GPs have responsibility for prescribing most of this potentially hazardous medication and for deciding who should be referred for joint replacement.

Osteoarthritis predominantly affects the large load-bearing joints – the hips and knees – and the small joints of the hands.

A longitudinal study in rural North Carolina estimated the lifetime risk of developing osteoarthritis of the knee as almost one in two, and as high as two in three for those who are obese.[1] More research is published on osteoarthritis of the knee than any other site. We know that it is more common in people who have injured their knee earlier in life, so people who have played a lot of sport tend to develop osteoarthritis at an early age.

People with osteoarthritis complain of pain in the affected joint. The pain is worse on activity, so the sufferer finds it difficult to do certain things at home and work and can start to avoid exercise. This can lead to weight gain, which in turn makes their osteoarthritis worse. The pain can vary from one day to another, and its location can be confusing; osteoarthritis of the hip can cause pain in the thigh and knee, as well as in the groin and buttock. The pain can affect people's sleep, and it can affect

---

Case study 31.1

Raymond Ryder is 79. In his youth, he played rugby, and he sustained a few injuries as a result. He retired from his job as a teacher 15 years ago. He enjoys going for walks with his wife, but his walking is curtailed now because of pain in his right hip. When the pain is bad, he takes paracetamol. More recently, he's had difficulty going up and down stairs and putting his shoes and socks on. After putting up with this for about 4 months, he decides to consult his GP, Dr Hussain. The pain is getting him down a bit. He wants Dr Hussain to confirm his suspicion that this is osteoarthritis, and he wants to know what he can do about it, but he isn't very keen on having an operation.

After clarifying this history, what are the important things for Dr Hussain to check on examination?
Dr Hussain will probably have made a quick assessment of Mr Ryder's gait as he came into the consulting room. If not, it would be useful to observe this. People with osteoarthritis are described as having an 'antalgic gait', meaning that that while walking, they spend less time putting weight on their painful joint. Dr Hussain should look at Mr Ryder's hands (people with osteoarthritis often have Heberden's nodes – painless nodules on the distal interphalangeal joints) and should weigh and measure him in order to calculate his body mass index (BMI).

Dr Hussain should then examine Mr Ryder on the couch, looking first for any deformity. If he can't put his leg flat on the bed, this may be because of a loss of range of movement in the hip or knee. Dr Hussain should assess all ranges of movement in the hips and knees and check for crepitus in the knees. He should examine the feet too. Does the patient have any deformities of his feet? Is the skin intact? Are his peripheral pulses palpable?

Findings
Mr Ryder's BMI is 32. His hands are normal. He does not walk with a limp. He can lie supine with his right leg straight, but when lying on his left side he cannot extend his right leg – there should be 10° of extension. Back in the supine position, passive flexion of his right hip (with his knee flexed to 90°) is limited to 90°, compared to 110° on the left. Internal rotation of his right hip is restricted to 10°, compared to 30° on the left, and there is only 20° of external rotation, compared to 40° on the left. Abduction and adduction of his hips are not restricted. He has a full range of movement in both knees, and examination of his feet is normal. Table 31.1 shows the range of movement in a normal hip.

Should Dr Hussain request an X-ray?
Maybe not at this stage. The restricted range of movement in Mr Ryder's right hip indicates osteoarthritis, and the appearance of a plain radiograph is unlikely to alter his management at this stage, although it may provide a useful comparison for radiographs taken in the future. A systematic review has shown that, in osteoarthritis of the hip, there is an inconsistent relationship between the appearance of the joint on a plain radiograph and the clinical diagnosis.[2]

What advice should Dr Hussain give Mr Ryder?
Weight loss is crucial. Mr Ryder is obese, and this is a key factor in the development of his osteoarthritis. If he does not lose weight, his osteoarthritis is likely to get worse. Dr Hussain should encourage him to keep exercising, to strengthen his muscles and to maintain his aerobic fitness. Dr Hussain could refer him to a physiotherapist to be taught how to do these things. The physiotherapist could also assess him for a walking stick (see Top tip box). Supportive, well-padded footwear will help; trainers are good.

Providing there are no contraindications, Dr Hussain could suggest some stronger analgesia, in the form of codeine or a nonsteroidal anti-inflammatory tablet.

Table 31.1 Normal range of movement in hip.	
Supine (lying on back)	**Degrees**
Flexion	110–120
Abduction	30–50
Adduction	20–30
Internal rotation	30–40
External rotation	40–60
Lateral decubitus (lying on side)	
Extension	10–15

their mood. People with osteoarthritis also complain of stiffness, but if this lasts more than half an hour or if it is the predominant symptom, we should think of an alternative explanation – such as polymylagia rheumatica or rheumatoid arthritis.

Pain relief for osteoarthritis

Conservative measures such as weight loss and exercise are extremely important and should always be the first step in the management osteoarthritis. People with osteoarthritis of the knee who are given at least 12 sessions of exercise supervised by a health professional see an improvement in their pain and function.[3] Unfortunately, adherence with exercise regimes is often poor, and patients find it difficult to lose weight, so we turn to medication.

For osteoarthritis of the hip, paracetamol is the first drug to try for pain relief, because it is the safest, but its efficacy is in doubt. For osteoarthritis of the knee, topical nonsteroidal anti-inflammatory preparations are a reasonable and safe alternative.[4] Topical capsaicin can also be helpful for people with osteoarthritis of the knee or hand.

The problematic area is what to prescribe when paracetamol and/or topical nonsteroidal anti-inflammatory preparations prove inadequate. Codeine and other opioids can cause constipation and drowsiness, which in turn run the risk of the patient falling. Oral nonsteroidal anti-inflammatory drugs (NSAIDs), on the other hand, run the risk of gastrointestinal bleeding, anaemia and renal impairment. For these reasons, GPs have to be very careful when prescribing NSAIDs on a regular basis, particularly to older people, who are likely to have several other chronic illnesses. It is prudent to co-prescribe a proton-pump inhibitor (PPI) to protect against gastrointestinal bleeding. It is also important to monitor the patient's blood pressure, haemoglobin and renal function.

Top tip: pain relief for osteoarthritis

If someone is on low-dose aspirin, try to avoid prescribing NSAIDs for their osteoarthritis – it makes the aspirin less effective and increases the risk of gastrointestinal bleeding.

If the GP cannot control the patient's pain with these medications, or if the patient's ability to function at home or work is persistently affected by their osteoarthritis, the GP should offer referral for joint replacement.[5] Hip and knee replacements are very effective at relieving pain, and improve function, too. But having a joint replacement is a frightening prospect for some, and comorbidities can make surgery more risky. A longitudinal study of patients referred by their GP for primary joint replacement showed that only half of those referred for osteoarthritis of the hip had a total hip replacement within 1 year, and only a third of those with osteoarthritis of the knee had a total knee replacement in this time.[6] The best predictor of whether or not someone ends up having a joint replacement is their desire to have surgery. Many patients, like Mr Ryder (Case study 31.1), do not want surgery. For these patients, an intra-articular injection of corticosteroid can be helpful. At most practices, there is a GP who can give injections into the knee. An injection can give pain relief for several weeks, although a Cochrane review showed that on average the benefit is for just 1–2 weeks[7]. It's a useful thing to try while someone is waiting for surgery of if they want to postpone surgery for a while because they have a big holiday or family celebration coming up. Injections can be repeated.

Once a joint is replaced, what effect does this have on the other load bearing joints? We don't really know the answer to this, but many people end up having both knees replaced, or hip and knee replacements. Perhaps the abnormal gait caused by the osteoarthritis in one joint puts undue pressure on the opposite or adjoining joint.

Top tip: walking sticks

Walking sticks help because they improve stability and they transfer some of the weight from the affected load-bearing joint to the arm.

A walking stick needs to be the correct length. If it is too long, less force is transferred to the arm. If it is too short, it will make the patient stoop. The correct length for a walking stick is the distance from the flexor crease of the wrist to the ground, measured with the patient standing straight, in their shoes, with their arms by their side.[8]

The stick should be held in the hand opposite the painful joint. However, people often prefer to hold it their dominant hand.

Rheumatoid arthritis

Rheumatoid arthritis is much less common than osteoarthritis. It can develop at any age, but the peak incidence is around the age of 70. It is twice as common in women as it is in men. Table 31.2 highlights the main differences between osteoarthritis and rheumatoid arthritis.

Table 31.2 Comparison of osteoarthritis with rheumatoid arthritis.

	Osteoarthritis	Rheumatoid arthritis
Age of onset	50s onwards	Any age, peak age 70
Joints affected	Knees, hips and hands	Small joints of hands, feet, wrists and ankles
Association with movement	Pain worse on activity	
Stiffness	Lasts <30 minutes	Lasts >30 minutes

Rheumatoid arthritis tends to affect the small joints in a symmetrical distribution. The hands and feet are most commonly affected, together with the wrists and ankles; but any joint can be affected. Patients come to their GP complaining of pain and stiffness, and sometimes report a warm swelling of the joints. The stiffness is worse in the morning, and typically lasts an hour or more.

Rheumatoid arthritis tends to develop over several weeks, and if untreated it produces a series of flare-ups, characterised by increased pain, tiredness and swelling of the affected joints. It is an autoimmune condition (and so is often seen in conjunction with other autoimmune diseases and runs in families). The swelling of the joints is caused by synovitis. The repeated inflammatory processes within the joint eventually lead to destruction of the joint and rupture of the tendons, which together produce a disabling deformity. Early treatment can prevent damage to the joints, so the task for the GP is to identify possible cases and make a referral to the rheumatologist as soon as possible.

In the early stages of the disease, there may be little to find on examination. The synovitis is transient and may have gone by the time that the patient sees their GP. However, if there is any warm, boggy swelling over the joint lines, this is a strong indicator of rheumatoid arthritis. No blood test is particularly helpful for GPs in diagnosing rheumatoid arthritis. GPs usually request an erythrocyte sedimentation rate (ESR) or C-reactive protein (CRP) to look for evidence of inflammation and check the rheumatoid factor (RF) or anticyclic citrulinated peptide (anti-CCP), but patients can be negative for both and still have rheumatoid arthritis.[9] These tests are more useful in hospital settings. Therefore, the GP's decision about whether to refer the patient to a rheumatologist rests primarily on the site and number of joints for which the history or examination suggests synovitis. Current National Institute for Health and Care Excellence (NICE) guidelines[10] recommend referral if:

- there is evidence of synovitis in a small joint of the hands or feet; or

- more than one joint is involved; or
- the patient has put up with possible synovitis for more than 3 months before coming to see their GP.

If a rheumatologist confirms the diagnosis of rheumatoid arthritis, they usually start the patient on a combination of disease-modifying drugs: methotrexate plus another disease-modifying drug and a low-dose steroid.[10] Although there are many new disease-modifying drugs, there is still a role for steroids. A systematic review has confirmed that low-dose steroids provide extra benefit above that of other disease-modifying drugs in terms of slowing radiological progression of the disease.[11] Methotrexate is taken in a single weekly dose, and, because it is a folate antagonist, on other days of the week the patient should take folic acid supplements. Methotrexate is a highly effective drug but has many potential side effects (see Chapter 4) and requires close monitoring. Initially, patients require fortnightly blood tests to check for neutropenia, hepatitis and renal impairment. Once stabilised, the frequency of blood tests can be reduced to once a month. At this stage, the GP can take over responsibility for prescribing the methotrexate. However, the rheumatologist may retain responsibility for prescribing the newer disease-modifying drugs, particularly the biological therapies.

From the point of diagnosis onwards, the GP and rheumatologist have to work closely to support the patient with rheumatoid arthritis. The disease can have a profound impact on the patient's ability to function at home and at work. The patient may have to change their job or stop work altogether and become dependent on welfare benefits. They may become depressed. GPs need to be on the lookout for this (the Whooley questions are useful here; see Chapter 11) and be proactive in offering psychological support, as well as directing them to charities like the National Rheumatoid Arthritis Society and Arthritis UK, which are useful sources of support and information.

Conducting an annual review for someone with rheumatoid arthritis

Patients with rheumatoid arthritis also need a comprehensive annual review; this is necessary not just because of the polypharmacy associated with rheumatoid arthritis, but also because of the significant physical, psychological and social complications of the disease. Table 31.3 lists the key components of an effective annual review.

In order to track the progress of the disease and monitor the effectiveness of the treatments that they give for it, doctors need validated, reliable methods of rating the activity of the disease and the disability that it inflicts. The most widely used method of rating disease activity is the Disease Activity Score 28 (DAS28). The score is calculated from four components:

1. The number of joints (out of 28 specified joints) that are tender.
2. The number of joints (out of the same 28 joints) that are swollen.

3. A blood marker of inflammation: CRP or ESR.

4. The patient's rating of their well-being on a visual analogue scale.

A quick and easy-to-use online tool allows a health professional and patient to calculate this score together.[12] Table 31.4 shows how the score is interpreted. If the score suggests the disease is active, the GP may need to request an urgent review with the rheumatologist. On the other hand, if the score indicates remission, it may be possible to reduce the dose or stop some therapies.

Table 31.3 Annual review for patients with rheumatoid arthritis.

Component of review	Assessment tool/investigation
Assess activity of disease	Disease Activity Score (DAS28) CRP
Assess functional ability	Health Assessment Questionnaire (HAQ)
Assess impact on work	Are any adaptations needed?
Assess psychological well-being	Whooley questions (see Chapter 11)
Review pain control	
Review disease-modifying medication	Check blood tests (full blood count (FBC), urea and electrolytes (U&Es) and liver function test (LFT), if on methotrexate)
Ask about possible extra-articular manifestations	See Table 31.5
Estimate risk of fragility fracture	FRAX +/– DEXA scan

Table 31.4 Interpretation of DAS28 CRP score.

Score	Interpretation
<2.6	In remission
2.7–3.2	Disease well controlled
3.3–5.1	Disease moderately active
>5.1	Active disease

The Health Assessment Questionnaire (HAQ)[13] is the most widely used method of measuring functional ability and self-reported level of disability. It was devised at Stamford University specifically to monitor patients with rheumatoid arthritis. The full HAQ takes a long time to complete and is used mainly for research purposes, but a component of it, the HAQ Disability Index, is short enough to be useful in everyday practice and has been adopted for monitoring of many different diseases, not just rheumatoid arthritis. It asks the patient to rate the difficulty that they have in several domains: washing, going to the toilet, dressing, eating, getting up (from a chair or bed), walking, reaching for things, gripping things and doing daily household chores. It also asks what aids and gadgets they require to help them with these things and whether they require assistance from another person. As well as tracking the impact of the disease, the HAQ Disability Index can be a useful guide when thinking about what other agencies might need to be contacted: physiotherapists and occupational therapists, in particular.

Patients with rheumatoid arthritis have reduced bone mineral density, for two reasons: the effect that the inflammatory processes have on the bones and the effect of prolonged treatment with prednisolone. Therefore, the GP should estimate their risk of developing a fragility fracture (see Chapter 35) and consider the need for bone protection.

There are several extra-articular manifestations of rheumatoid arthritis (see Table 31.5) for which the GP and rheumatologist need to keep a constant lookout. If a patient with rheumatoid arthritis presents with a new symptom, stop and think. Could this be a complication of rheumatoid arthritis, or could it be a side effect of their treatment? Patients with rheumatoid arthritis often become anaemic, either as a direct result of their chronic disease or because of gastrointestinal bleeding caused by NSAIDs. Responsibility for investigating this anaemia and, if necessary, requesting a gastrointestinal endoscopy usually falls to the GP.

An annual review can help to reduce the impact of rheumatoid arthritis, but the disease is not predictable: it can flare up at any time, and when it does so, patients still need prompt access to their GP or rheumatologist. In the event of flare-up, GPs can offer a short course of oral NSAIDs and opioids, and maybe a fit note; rheumatologists often offer a depot injection of corticosteroid.

Polymyalgia rheumatica

Polymyalgia rheumatica usually presents with pain and stiffness in the shoulders, the hips or both. It is a disease of old age and is rare under age 60. Most cases are managed exclusively in

Table 31.5 Extra-articular manifestations of rheumatoid arthritis.

Systemic	Heart	Lung	Kidney	Eyes	Nerves
Fever	Pericardial effusion	Pleural effusion	Renal impairment due to vasculitis	Scleritis	Carpal tunnel syndrome
Tiredness	Pericarditis	Pulmonary fibrosis		Sjögren's syndrome	

Table 31.6 Example of steroid regime for treating polymyalgia rheumatica.

	Dose of prednisolone
Weeks 1–3	15 mg daily
Weeks 4–6	12.5 mg daily
Weeks 7–52	10 mg daily
1 year onwards	Reduce by 1 mg every 4–8 weeks

Table 31.7 Differential diagnosis of shoulder pain and stiffness.

Diagnosis	Clues
Polymyalgia rheumatica	Sudden onset, age > 60, pain in pelvic girdle
Osteoarthritis	Pain worse on movement, gradual onset
Rotator cuff injury, supraspinatus tendinitis	History of trauma
Late-onset rheumatoid arthritis	Family history, other autoimmune diseases, other joints affected
Malignancy (myeloma, lung or bony metastasis from other cancer)	Existing cancer, weight loss
Myositis	On statin
Hypothyroidism	Weight gain, tiredness
Hypercalcaemia	Polyuria, polydipsia

primary care. The pain tends to come on quite suddenly. Typically, the patient says that their shoulders are painful in bed and they can't lift their arms fully. They may have difficulty getting in and out of a chair.

If we suspect polymyalgia, we should request an urgent ESR. If the patient has polymyalgia, this usually shows a modest elevation. Patients respond quickly to steroids and express profound thanks to their GP because they feel so much better.

A retrospective cohort study conducted in GP practices in Staffordshire showed that the diagnosis is made most commonly on the basis of three things: bilateral shoulder pain, a modestly raised ESR (around 50 mm/hour) and a response to steroids within 1 week.[14] Typically, patients have to stay on prednisolone for 1–2 years; in the Staffordshire study, the mean duration was 14 months. With this length of time on steroids, it is important to co-prescribe medication to prevent osteoporosis. Table 31.6 shows how the dose of prednisolone is gradually reduced. Sometimes, patients relapse, and if this happens, we simply increase the dose of prednisolone to the previous dose.

Polymyalgia rheumatica is not the only cause of painful, stiff shoulders. Table 31.7 lists the other causes; clues that point to one or more of these causes will come from the history. A history of falling on to the arm, for instance, raises the possibility of a rotator cuff injury. We must always be alert to the possibility of cancer: lung cancer can present with shoulder pain, as can myeloma or bony metastasis from breast, bowel or the kidney. If this is a possibility, we request a plain X-ray or a bone scan.

If any of the following features are present, we should question the diagnosis of polymyalgia and refer the patient:

- under 60 years old;
- chronic onset;
- shoulders not involved;
- systemic features;
- ESR very high or normal;
- recurrent relapses;
- treatment has been needed for over 2 years.

> **Top tip: think about giant-cell arteritis**
>
> Many patients with polymyalgia rheumatica also have, or go on to develop, giant-cell arteritis. If we suspect someone has polymyalgia, we must ask if they have a headache, scalp tenderness or jaw pain on chewing and check that they have not experienced any visual loss. Chapter 22 has more information about giant-cell arteritis.

SUMMARY

Osteoarthritis of the hips and knees is extremely common in old age and causes substantial disability. Rheumatoid arthritis is much less common, but causes even greater disability; it causes pain and swelling, mainly in the small- and medium-sized joints and has many extra-articular manifestations. Weight loss and regular exercise aimed at strengthening muscles are the best ways of preventing osteoarthritis. For rheumatoid arthritis, early diagnosis and prompt initiation of intensive disease-modifying therapy offers the best hope of controlling the disease. Pain-relieving medication, particularly NSAIDs, which are used for both osteoarthritis and rheumatoid arthritis, can cause serious harm and must be monitored. Joint replacement has revolutionised the treatment of advanced osteoarthritis, and GPs have to decide who and when to refer for surgery. Polymyalgia rheumatica responds well to treatment with steroids, but it is important to be sure of the diagnosis.

Now visit **www.wileyessential.com/primarycare** to test yourself on this chapter.

REFERENCES

1. Murphy L, Schwartz TA, Helmick CG, et al. Lifetime risk of symptomatic knee osteoarthritis. *Arthritis Rheum* 2008;**59**:1207–13.

2. Kinds MB, Welsing PMJ, Vignon EP, et al. A systematic review of the association between radiographic and clinical osteoarthritis of hip and knee. *Osteoarthritis Cartilage* 2011;**19**(7):768–78.

3. Fransen M, McConnell S. Land-based exercise for osteoarthritis of the knee: a meta-analysis of randomised controlled trials. *J. Rheumatol* 2009;**36**:1109–17.

4. Dieppe P. Osteoarthritis of the knee in primary care. *BMJ* 2008;**336**:105–6.

5. NICE.Osteoarthritis: care and management in adults. NICE Clinical Guideline 177. February 2014. Available from: http://www.nice.org.uk/guidance/cg177 (last accessed 6 October 2015).

6. McHugh GA, Campbell M, Luker KA. GP referral of patients with osteoarthritis for consideration of total joint replacement: a longitudinal study. *Br J Gen Pract* 2011;**61**(589):e459–68.

7. Bellamy N, Campbell J, Welch V, et al. Intra-articular corticosteroid for treatment of osteoarthritis of the knee. *Cochrane Database Syst Rev* 2009;**2**:CD005328.

8. Mulley GP. Everyday aid and appliances: walking sticks. *BMJ* 1988;**296**:475–6.

9. Mahtani, KR, Miller A, Rivero-Arias O, et al. Autoimmune markers for the diagnosis of rheumatoid arthritis in primary care: primary care diagnostic technology update. *Br J Gen Pract* 2013;**63**:553–4.

10. NICE. Rheumatoid arthritis: the management of rheumatoid arthritis in adults. NICE Clinical Guideline 79. 2009. (Modified August 2013.) Available from: http://www.nice.org.uk/guidance/cg79 (last accessed 6 October 2015).

11. Kirwan JR, Bijlsma JWJ, Boers M, Shea BJ. Effects of glucocorticoids on radiological progression in rheumatoid arthritis (review). *Cochrane Database Syst Rev* 2007;**1**:CD006356.

12. Fries JF, Spitz P, Kraines G, Holman H. Measurement of patient outcome in arthritis. *Arthritis Rheum* 1980;**23**(2):137–45.

13. Health Assessment Questionnaire (HAQ). Available from: http://www.4s-dawn.com/HAQ/HAQ-DI.html (last accessed 6 October 2015).

14. Helliwell T, Hider SL, Mallen CD. Polymyalgia rheumatica: diagnosis, prescribing and monitoring in general practice. *Br J Gen Pract* 2013;**63**(610):e361–6.

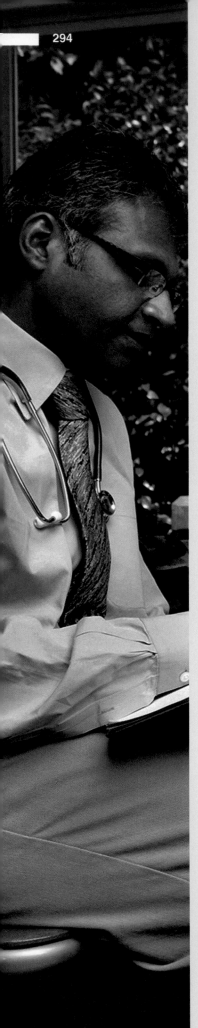

CHAPTER 32

Urinary problems and prostate disease

Simon Thornton
Academic Clinical Fellow, University of Bristol

Key topics

Learning objectives

- Be able to assess, investigate and manage patients who have visible and nonvisible haematuria.
- Be able to describe how to assess, investigate and manage patients presenting with lower urinary tract symptoms.
- Be able to differentiate between storage and voiding symptoms and understand the different causes.
- Be able to describe what should be done if a patient presents with a lump or pain in their scrotum.
- Be able to conduct a consultation with a man who presents with erectile dysfunction.

Essential Primary Care, First Edition. Edited by Andrew Blythe and Jessica Buchan.
© 2017 John Wiley & Sons, Ltd. Published 2017 by John Wiley & Sons, Ltd.
Companion website: www.wileyessential.com/primarycare

Haematuria

Visible haematuria is a frightening symptom and normally prompts patients to seek an urgent appointment with their GP. Nonvisible haematuria is often an incidental finding made when the urine is dipped as part of a routine review or as part of the investigation of abdominal pain, hypertension or urinary symptoms. Nonvisible haematuria is further subdivided into symptomatic nonvisible haematuria (e.g. with pain or a feeling of needing to pass urine more frequently) and asymptomatic nonvisible haematuria.[1]

Haematuria has many causes (Table 32.1). In the absence of infection, visible haematuria requires urgent referral to urology for further investigation to exclude kidney or bladder cancer. This usually involves cystoscopy and imaging, which in the first instance is often an ultrasound scan of the renal tract. Nonvisible haematuria is much more common and does not always require investigation, but sometimes it does (see Figure 32.1).

Table 32.1 Causes of haematuria.

Cause	Examples
Infection	Cystitis, prostatitis, pyelonephritis
Tumour	Kidney, bladder, prostate, ureter
Inflammation	Glomerulonephritis, IgA nephropathy, Henoch–Schönlein purpura, systemic lupus erythematosus
Surgery	Cystoscopy, prostate biopsy (usually up to 3 days after biopsy)
Structural	Calculi, polycystic kidney disease
Toxins	NSAIDs, sulphonamides
Trauma	Renal trauma, pelvic trauma

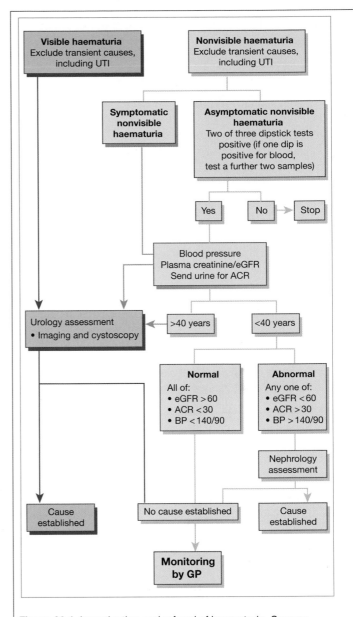

Figure 32.1 Investigation and referral of haematuria. *Source*: Adapted from BAUS/RA guidelines.

Case study 32.1

Mrs Jane Oldham, age 46, makes an appointment to see Dr Louise Whyte in surgery. Mrs Oldham noticed a bit of stinging when she was passing urine yesterday evening, and when she woke this morning she saw bright red blood in her urine. She is very anxious, as this has never happened before. She has no past medical history of note and is a nonsmoker. On examination, she has a temperature of 38 °C and mild suprapubic discomfort.

What is the most likely diagnosis?
Mrs Oldham's history of dysuria with a high temperature is most suggestive of a lower urinary tract infection

(UTI). Stones (calculi) are another common cause of haematuria in this age group, and classically present with colicky 'loin-to-groin' pain. Although nonvisible haematuria is more common with a UTI, visible haematuria can occur.

Urinalysis shows leucocytes, nitrites and blood, consistent with a UTI. Dr Whyte prescribes a 3-day course of trimethoprim and sends a midstream specimen of urine (MSU) to the laboratory; this confirms an *Escherichia coli* infection sensitive to trimethoprim. When Dr Whyte reviews Mrs Oldham 2 weeks later, she reports her symptoms have settled. Repeat urinalysis does not show any blood.

2 years later

Mrs Oldham returns to see Dr Whyte 2 years later, age 48. She has not had any further episodes of haematuria. However, as part of a routine medical at work, her urine was dipped and showed some blood. She was asked to come to see her own GP.

How should Dr Whyte proceed?

First, Dr Whyte should reassure Mrs Oldham that she is very unlikely to have a bladder tumour on the basis of a one-off positive urinalysis. She should ask about any symptoms, such as pain on passing urine (dysuria) or an increased frequency of passing urine. She should repeat the urinalysis, looking for blood.

Repeat urinalysis does not show any blood. Dr Whyte asks Mrs Oldham to drop another urine sample in to the surgery in 2 weeks' time and advises her to come back sooner if she sees any blood. Her urine sample 2 weeks later again shows nonvisible haematuria.

How should Dr Whyte manage the patient?

Dr Whyte should look for potential renal causes of her haematuria: check her blood pressure, request a blood test to check her kidney function (urea and electrolytes, U&Es) and send a urine sample for an albumin/creatinine ratio (ACR). This is to assess whether her kidneys are more 'leaky' and are losing protein as well as blood. Given her age, Dr Whyte should also refer her to a urology clinic for imaging and cystoscopy (see Figure 32.1).

Flexible cystoscopy is completely normal. Mrs Oldham is discharged back to the care of Dr Whyte.

Should Dr Whyte continue to monitor Mrs Oldham?

Yes. Patients who have persistent nonvisible haematuria should have their blood pressure, creatinine and ACR measured every year. If Mrs Oldham develops visible haematuria or starts to develop symptoms with persistent nonvisible haematuria, Dr Whyte should re-refer her to the urologist. If her renal function deteriorates or if she has increasing proteinuria, Dr Whyte should refer to a nephrologist.

Table 32.2 Storage versus voiding symptoms.

Storage		Voiding	
Frequency	The need to pass urine frequently	Poor stream	A weak stream of urine
Urgency	Having a sudden urge to pass urine; often incontinent if unable to reach toilet quickly	Hesitancy	Having to wait a while for the urine to start flowing
Dysuria	Pain on passing urine	Terminal dribbling	The leakage of a small amount of urine after urination has finished
Nocturia	Having to get up frequently at night to pass urine		
Stress incontinence	Involuntary loss of urine with raised intra-abdominal pressure, e.g. coughing		

Haematospermia

Haematospermia (blood in the ejaculate) is another alarming symptom. Its incidence is difficult to gauge, as most ejaculates go unnoticed during intercourse.[2] It has a peak incidence in men aged 30–40. It is usually a benign and self-limiting condition, analogous to a 'nose bleed of the prostate'. Nevertheless, the prostate should be examined, as haematospermia can rarely be a presentation of prostate cancer. Urinalysis should be done to exclude infection as a cause.

Lower urinary tract symptoms in men

Increased urinary frequency, urgency, nocturia, difficulty initiating and ending micturition and poor urinary flow can all significantly reduce a man's quality of life and may point to serious underlying pathology.[3] These symptoms used to be referred to loosely as 'prostatism', but in fact there is often a combination of pathological processes at play, not all of them confined to the prostate, so now the term 'lower urinary tract symptoms' (LUTS) is preferred. LUTS are extremely common, and show increasing prevalence with age. At the age of 45, 30% of men get up at least once at night to pass urine, and by the age of 80 it is around 80%.[4]

When taking a history, it is important to distinguish between 'storage' and 'voiding' symptoms (Table 32.2). Storage symptoms relate to problems with storage of urine in the bladder. This is commonly due to an overactive bladder that contracts involuntarily, resulting in the feeling of an urge to pass urine with small volumes. Symptoms may be made worse by stress and caffeine, which as well as being a diuretic, is also an irritant to the bladder. Storage symptoms may also be a result of serious underlying bladder pathology, such as a tumour, hence the importance of performing a urinalysis on any patient presenting with LUTS to check for blood and exclude an infection.

Voiding symptoms relate to problems with the passage of urine from the bladder out through the urethra. The most common cause of this in men is benign prostatic hyperplasia (BPH). The prostate gland sits below the neck of the bladder (see Figure 32.2) and produces around 70% of the volume of seminal fluid. As men age, the prostate gland gradually enlarges under the influence of hormones, although other factors such as vascular and inflammatory processes are also important. The prostatic section of the urethra runs through the middle of the prostate gland and is susceptible to narrowing as the prostate enlarges.

Prostate cancer may also give similar symptoms to BPH, and this is often a major concern of men who present with LUTS. However, prostate cancer usually starts in the periphery of the prostate gland, and so in its early stages it is less likely to cause voiding symptoms than benign prostatic hypertrophy, which usually starts in the centre of the prostate gland, around the urethra.

In a man presenting with fever and LUTS, consider the possibility of a UTI or acute prostatitis (a bacterial infection of the prostate).

Managing benign prostatic hypertrophy

In some circumstances, the best option is to do nothing. Sometimes, when patients are reassured that they don't have cancer, they don't feel their symptoms are troublesome enough to warrant medication. It's worth teaching patients with troublesome terminal dribble about urethral milking by exerting a firm upward pressure from the perineum. For patients like Mr Gentle (Case study 32.2) who are bothered by their symptoms, we can prescribe an alpha blocker such as tamsulosin to relax the smooth muscle within the prostate gland, as well as a 5-alpha reductase inhibitor such as finasteride to slowly shrink the prostate. Tamsulosin takes around a month to have its full effect, whereas finasteride takes around 6 months.

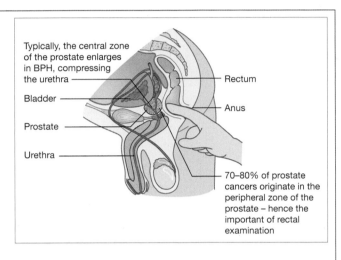

Typically, the central zone of the prostate enlarges in BPH, compressing the urethra — Rectum — Bladder — Anus — Prostate — Urethra — 70–80% of prostate cancers originate in the peripheral zone of the prostate – hence the important of rectal examination

Figure 32.2 Prostate examination.

Case study 32.2a

John Gentle, a 59-year-old Afro-Caribbean man, sees his GP in surgery. He is troubled by difficulty passing urine. It often takes him quite a while to get going, and he has to stand at the toilet for quite a while before he finishes. He's also rather embarrassed that occasionally he thinks he has finished and done his trousers up only to find a small amount of urine trickles down his leg and marks his trousers.

What should the GP's differential diagnosis be?
Mr Gentle is describing voiding symptoms, suggesting that something is interfering with the outflow of urine from the bladder. The commonest cause in a man of his age is BPH, but the GP should consider the possibility of prostate cancer.

What are the common risk factors for prostate cancer?
Family history, Afro-Caribbean ethnicity.

What examination and investigations should the GP do?
The GP should examine Mr Gentle's abdomen to check for evidence of urinary retention. They should perform a rectal examination to examine the size and texture of the prostate gland. Any abnormality other than symmetrical smooth enlargement should prompt an urgent 2-week-wait urology referral. They should perform urinalysis: the presence of blood could indicate an underlying bladder/prostate malignancy. They could consider measuring his serum prostate-specific antigen (PSA), a protein produced by the prostate gland. The PSA level is a useful guide in deciding if a prostate biopsy is needed. Measuring the serum PSA is one way in which we monitor patients with established prostate cancer, but its utility as a screening test for men without LUTS is yet to be established (see Chapter 38). If a man is found to have a PSA level above the age-specific normal range, the GP is obliged to make a referral to a urologist for a prostate biopsy. This carries a risk of prostatitis.

Outcome
Mr Gentle's urinalysis is normal. Rectal examination reveals a smooth, symmetrically enlarged prostate. His PSA comes back below the age-specific cut-off (<4 IU/l for a man aged 50–59). Therefore, the most likely explanation for his symptoms is BPH.

Case study 32.2b

Mr Gentle returns to see the GP 2 years later because he's passing urine much more frequently and finds he has to rush to the toilet. He admits that on a couple of occasions he has not been able to make it to the toilet on time and has wet his trousers.

What might the diagnosis be?
Mr Gentle is describing storage symptoms. The involuntary loss of urine associated with urgency is known as 'urgency urinary incontinence'. He may well have developed an overactive bladder. However, we still need to exclude potential serious causes, including diabetes and bladder/prostate cancer.

What examination and investigations should the GP perform?
It is important to repeat the urinalysis and rectal examination, given that there has been a change in the nature of his symptoms. The GP could also consider asking him to keep a bladder diary: measuring what and how much he drinks, as well as how frequently and how much he urinates. The passage of frequent small or variable volumes of urine is suggestive of an overactive bladder.

How should the GP manage Mr Gentle's symptoms now?
It is important to discuss lifestyle measures, including cutting back on caffeine and smoking, which are both known bladder irritants. He may benefit from anticholinergic medication, such as oxybutynin, although patients often complain of a dry mouth.

Top tip

Perform a urinalysis and prostate examination in any man presenting with LUTS.

Urinary incontinence

Up to 55% of women suffer from urinary incontinence.[5] It is a common and costly problem that can cause embarrassment and significant impairment of quality of life. It contributes to depression, falls and admission to nursing homes. Risk factors include childbirth, hysterectomy, higher body mass index (BMI) and advancing age.

Incontinence is classified into urgency urinary incontinence, stress urinary incontinence (the involuntary loss of urine with raised intra-abdominal pressure) and mixed urinary incontinence (a mix of both stress and urgency urinary incontinence). The type of incontinence is usually identified through

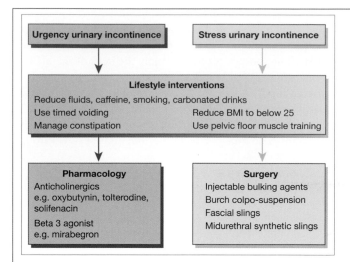

Figure 32.3 Treatment options for women with urinary incontinence.

the history, and the use of a bladder diary may help diagnosis. All types of urinary incontinence are more common in women than men. Urgency urinary incontinence is still encountered relatively frequently in men, but any man with stress incontinence should be referred for specialist assessment.[3]

Figure 32.3 summarises the treatments for urinary incontinence in women. For all types of urinary incontinence, pelvic floor muscle training has been shown to be superior to placebo in women who are able to contract their pelvic floor muscles.[6] This should be confirmed by asking the patient to squeeze on digital examination of the vagina. Pelvic floor muscle training consists of strengthening the muscles of the pelvic floor (to reduce stress urinary incontinence) and contracting them in isolation to inhibit detrusor contractions (reducing urgency urinary incontinence).[7] Other conservative measures include weight loss to reduce BMI below 25, timed voiding, reduction of fluids, caffeine and smoking and managing constipation.

If conservative measures fail, the next step for urgency urinary incontinence is usually drug treatment in the form of anticholinergics such as oxybutynin. In stress urinary incontinence, the next step is often surgery, such as a mid-urethral sling.

Top tip

Remember to discuss conservative and lifestyle measures in a woman presenting with urinary incontinence.

Testicular problems

The two most common testicular problems encountered in primary care are testicular pain and the discovery of a lump in the scrotum. Either or both of these symptoms make men concerned about the possibility of testicular cancer.

Testicular pain

If a patient presents with testicular pain, the key diagnoses to consider are testicular torsion, epididymo-orchitis and testicular cancer.

Epididymo-orchitis

Epididymo-orchitis (inflammation of the epididymis and testis) is the commonest cause of acute scrotal pain. The onset is usually more gradual than that of torsion. Typically, the pain is unilateral, and there may be associated urinary symptoms. It is important to take a sexual history (see Chapter 25), as this may point to a sexually transmitted infection (STI) as the underlying cause. Initial investigation should include:

- urinalysis;
- urine for microscopy and culture;
- urine sample for nucleic acid amplification testing (NAAT), looking for chlamydia and gonorrhoea.[8]

Under the age of 35, the most common causative organisms are the STIs *Chalmydia trachomatis* and *Neisseria gonorrhoea*. Over 35, the most common organisms are the non-sexually transmitted Gram-negative enteric organisms, such as *Esherischia coli*. We should consider mumps as a possible (although rare) cause in someone who has had a viral illness during the preceding days.

Leucocytes may be present on urinalysis for both STIs and non-STIs. However, the presence of nitrites and the absence of a urethral discharge suggest a non-STI.

Treatment should be started immediately, before the results of lab tests are known, on the basis of what cause seems most likely. If it's an STI, treatment is usually with a stat dose of ceftriaxone followed by a course of doxycycline for 10–14 days with abstinence from intercourse, and partner-tracing and notification once the diagnosis is confirmed. If a non-STI is more likely, the usual treatment is a quinolone antibiotic such as ciprofloxacin for 10–14 days. The patient should return for review if there is no improvement after 72 hours.

Testicular torsion

Testicular torsion most commonly affects boys aged 7–12 but can occur in any age group. It occurs when the spermatic cord twists, cutting off the blood supply to the testicle. It is a surgical emergency and it is vital that the diagnosis is not missed as delayed management results in testicular ischaemia and necrosis.

> **Top tips**
>
> In anyone with suspected epididymo-orchitis, ask yourself two questions:
>
> 1. 'Am I sure this is not testicular torsion?' *If in doubt, refer.*
> 2. 'Is it likely to be caused by an STI, or not?'
>
> Examine the scrotum in any young male complaining of abdominal pain, as it may be a symptom of torsion.

Scrotal lumps

When a young man consults his GP looking slightly awkward, it's often because he has discovered a lump in his scrotum which he wants checking out. Usually, these turn out to be harmless epididymal cysts, but the GP always has to exclude the possibility of testicular cancer and explain to the patient what features of a lump should prompt a consultation in the future. It's also a good opportunity to give sexual health advice. A list of common causes can be found in Table 32.3.

Table 32.3 Differential diagnoses of testicular lumps.

Lump	Pain	Features
Epididymal cyst	Sometimes	Separate from testis Can be pressed between fingers
Varicocoele	Aching sometimes	Above and around testicle More prominent on standing 'Bag of worms' feel
Testicular cancer	Usually not	Arises from testis Hard and irregular
Epididymo-orchitis	Yes	Scrotum may be too tender to examine testicle with confidence
Testicular torsion	Yes	Usually young Very painful Often horizontal lie of testis
Hydrocoele	Usually not	Smooth, fluctuant, enveloping a testis Transilluminates
Inguinal hernia	Sometimes a dragging sensation Pain on strangulation	Reducible Bowel sounds may be present

Epididymal cysts are common in men of all ages. They are usually painless. They feel smooth and are separate from the testis, lying above or behind it. An ultrasound scan confirms the diagnosis, but is not always needed.

Testicular cancer is the most common malignancy in men aged 20–34. It creates a hard, irregular lump that arises directly from the testicle. The discovery of such a lump should prompt an urgent referral. Testicular cancer is usually painless, although occasionally pain or a hydrocele may be the only presenting feature. Ultrasound may aid the diagnosis of a patient with unexplained unilateral testicular pain, but we mustn't wait for investigations if we suspect testicular cancer on examination.

A hydrocele (a collection of fluid in the tunica vaginalis) may be a presentation of testicular cancer and should be referred for ultrasound examination. A hydrocele has a smooth surface and transilluminates when a pen torch is held against it. The testis is within the swelling, and not palpable separately.

A varicocele is a collection of varicose veins in the pampiniform plexus of the cord and scrotum. It is typically described as having a 'bag of worms' feel when the scrotum is palpated with the patient standing. Rarely, it can be associated with obstruction of the testicular veins in the abdomen, although it is usually idiopathic, occurring in around one in seven men. There is an association with infertility. However, patients can be reassured that the overwhelming majority of men with varicoceles are not infertile. Supportive underwear can be advised if discomfort is a presentation, although treatment is very rarely indicated and surgery does not improve pregnancy rates.[9]

Erectile dysfunction

Erectile dysfunction is the inability to achieve and maintain an erection adequate for satisfactory sexual intercourse.[10] It affects up to 50% of men aged 40–70 years. It is often considered to have two components: a psychological component and an organic component. The psychological component may be attributable to stress or performance anxiety and is suggested by the preservation of morning erections or the ability to maintain an erection for masturbation. Prostate cancer can

Top tips

Patients are often embarrassed to raise the subject of erectile dysfunction. Ask at-risk patients such as those with diabetes whether it is something they experience. If successfully treated, these will be some of your most grateful patients.

If a man has stopped taking his antidepressant or antihypertensive drug, consider the possibility that it's because it's causing erectile dysfunction; he may be reluctant to volunteer this information.

present with erectile dysfunction. Other organic causes may relate to neurological, vascular, structural or hormonal abnormalities. It can also result from commonly prescribed drugs, such as antihypertensives and antidepressants, as well as recreational drugs, such as alcohol.

Examination should include looking for any structural abnormality of the penis, assessment of secondary sexual characteristics, digital rectal examination, measurement of blood pressure and a PSA test. Erectile dysfunction is considered an early marker of cardiovascular disease (CVD), so in order to complete the patient's cardiovascular risk assessment, it is important to check his lipid profile and fasting glucose or HbA1c. Consider measuring an early morning testosterone.

Phosphodiesterase-5 (PDE-5) inhibitors have revolutionised the treatment of erectile dysfunction and work for patients who have a psychogenic or an organic cause of their dysfunction, but the patient still needs to be sexually stimulated. There are many types of PDE-5 inhibitor; some have a faster onset of action than others. They come in a range of doses. Viagra (sildenafil) was the first to come on the market. The patient should be advised to take it 1 hour before they are intending to have sex and should be warned that it can cause a headache and stuffiness of the nose.

It's also important to address any risk factors discovered during the cardiovascular assessment, such as hypertension or hyperlipidaemia.

SUMMARY

Once a UTI has been excluded, patients of any age who have visible haematuria need urgent referral to a urologist to look for renal-tract cancer. Patients over 40 with recurrent nonvisible haematuria need referral to a urologist. In men, nocturia is common from middle age; difficulty voiding is usually due to prostatic hypertrophy, but prostate cancer needs to be excluded. Problems with urinary storage in both sexes are most commonly due to an overactive bladder. Urinary incontinence is very common in women and can be helped by pelvic floor exercises. Haematospermia rarely has a serious cause. In contrast, a lump arising from the testicle requires urgent referral to exclude testicular cancer. Erectile dysfunction is a side effect of many medicines and can indicate the presence of CVD. GPs must be proactive in asking about this embarrassing symptom and can help by prescribing phosphodiesterase inhibitors and by making a full assessment of cardiovascular risk.

Now visit **www.wileyessential.com/primarycare** to test yourself on this chapter.

REFERENCES

1. Anderson J, Fawcett D, Feehally J, et al. Joint consensus statement on the initial assessment of haematuria. BAUS/RA Guidelines 2008. Available from: http://www.renal.org/docs/default-source/what-we-do/RA-BAUS_Haematuria_Consensus_Guidelines.pdf?sfvrsn=0 (last accessed 6 October 2015).

2. Kumar P, Kapoor S, Nargund V. Haematospermia – a systematic review. *Ann R Coll Surg Engl* 2006;**88**(4):339–42.

3. NICE. Lower urinary tract symptoms: the management of lower urinary tract symptoms in men. NICE Clinical Guideline 97. May 2010. Available from: http://www.nice.org.uk/guidance/cg97 (last accessed 6 October 2015).

4. Malmsten UG, Milsom I, Molander U, Norlen LJ. Urinary incontinence and lower urinary tract symptoms: an epidemiological study of men aged 45 to 99 years. *J Urol* 1997;**158**:1733–7.

5. Thom D. Variation in estimates of urinary incontinence prevalence in the community: effects of differences in definition, population characteristics and study type. *J Am Geriatr Soc* 1998;**46**:473–80.

6. NICE. Urinary incontinence: the management of urinary incontinence in women. NICE Clinical Guideline 171. September 2013. Available from; http://www.nice.org.uk/guidance/cg171 (last accessed 6 October 2015).

7. Wood L, Anger JT. Urinary incontinence in women. *BMJ* 2014;**349**:g4531.

8. British Association for Sexual Health and HIV. United Kingdom national clinical guideline for management of epididymo-orchitis. 2010. Available from: http://www.bashh.org/documents/3546.pdf (last accessed 6 October 2015).

9. NICE. Fertility: assessment and treatment for people with fertility problems. NICE Clinical Guideline 156. Available from: http://www.nice.org.uk/guidance/cg156 (last accessed 6 October 2015).

10. Muneer A, Kalsi J, Nazareth I, Arya M. Erectile dysfunction. *BMJ* 2014;**348**:g129.

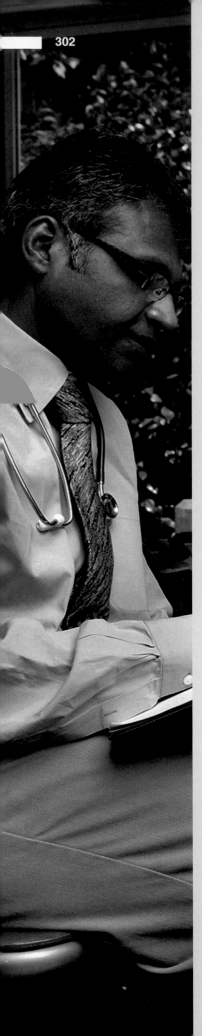

CHAPTER 33

The menopause

Jessica Buchan
GP and Teaching Fellow in Primary Care, University of Bristol

Key topics

Learning objectives

- Be able to appreciate the range of symptoms caused by the menopause and advise on management options.
- Be able to identify symptoms in the menopause that might indicate gynaecological cancer and know when to investigate and refer.

Essential Primary Care, First Edition. Edited by Andrew Blythe and Jessica Buchan.
© 2017 John Wiley & Sons, Ltd. Published 2017 by John Wiley & Sons, Ltd.
Companion website: www.wileyessential.com/primarycare

Symptoms of the menopause

The menopause is a normal physiological process. Declining levels of the hormones of reproduction cause symptoms of menopause, which begin before the last menstrual period (perimenopause) and can continue for a few years. Women vary both in the severity of symptoms and in the impact their symptoms have on them. Some women barely notice the transition, while others seek medical input.

Symptoms include hot flushes or night sweats (vasomotor), urogenital symptoms such as vaginal dryness and psychological issues such as anxiety or low mood. Perimenopausal women may attribute somatic symptoms such as headaches and joint pain to the decline in fertility, but these symptoms can be harder to untangle from other causes. A longitudinal cohort study carried out in the UK questioned a cohort of 695 women who had gone through a natural menopause and showed that vasomotor, sexual dysfunction and psychological symptoms had a clear relationship to the timing of the menopause, whereas somatic symptoms showed a flat trajectory throughout midlife.[1]

Sometimes, GPs may need to make the link between symptoms and the menopause for their patients. For example, post-menopausal women may present with urinary symptoms only for the GP to find atrophic vaginitis (thinning of the vulval and vaginal mucosa) on examination. The evidence for whether topical oestrogen reduces the risk of urine infections is mixed,[2] but it is often tried as it does improve urogenital symptoms such as vaginal dryness and it has fewer risks than systemic hormone-replacement therapy (HRT).

Identifying the menopause

The average age for menopause in the UK is 51. Women do not need investigations if they get typical symptoms at the expected age, and they may need reassurance that what they are experiencing is normal. Hormone levels are useful if premature menopause is suspected, or if a woman presents with atypical symptoms. Follicle-stimulating hormone (FSH) of 30 IU/l or more indicates ovarian failure.

Managing menopausal symptoms

HRT was initially seen as the answer to menopausal symptoms. The Women's Health Initiative[3] was published in 2002 and the Million Women Study[4] in 2003; these studies raised concerns about the risks of breast cancer, thrombosis and cardiovascular disease (CVD) with HRT, and many women who might have benefitted from HRT were put off. Recent evidence[5, 6] is more reassuring. It is now recommended that symptomatic women may benefit from HRT in the years around the menopause, depending on their individual risk profile.

Women with a premature menopause (under 40 years of age) or early menopause (under 45 years of age) should be offered HRT until they are 51. HRT is not usually initiated after the age of 60 as the risks start to outweigh the benefits and a topical route may be preferable. HRT should be used at the lowest dose for the shortest time needed to control symptoms.

Top tips: contraindications to HRT

- Pregnancy and breastfeeding.
- Undiagnosed abnormal vaginal bleeding. Investigate before starting.
- Previous thrombosis (deep-vein or pulmonary thrombosis). Gel or patches may be suitable.
- Cancer: current, past or suspected breast, endometrial or other hormone-dependent cancer. Refer for specialist advice.
- Cardiovascular: uncontrolled hypertension, recent angina or myocardial infarction or high risk of cardiovascular or cerebrovascular disease. Refer for specialist advice.

Case study 33.1

Melanie James, age 49, has had increasingly heavy, irregular periods for the past year. She visits her GP, Dr Liz Walters, as she is now bleeding every fortnight. Her current period has lasted 4 weeks. She is feeling quite tired and is wondering if she is becoming anaemic.

What should the Dr Walters do first?
Although some women do experience heavy irregular bleeding prior to the menopause, if this happens the GP still needs to exclude pelvic pathology. If a period has been missed then the possibility of pregnancy needs to be considered. Dr Walters will do a pelvic examination, check a full blood count (FBC) and organise a pelvic

ultrasound scan. The ultrasonographer can assess the endometrial thickness. Evidence of endometrial hyperplasia, polyps or a woman at high risk (unopposed oestrogen or tamoxifen use or family history) requires further investigation with an endometrial biopsy or hysteroscopy.

After investigation, Melanie's symptoms are confirmed as perimenopausal dysfunctional uterine bleeding, meaning that no suspicious pathology is found to account for the change in her bleeding pattern that can be attributed to the change in hormone levels. Her iron levels are low. Melanie declines a Mirena intrauterine system (IUS) (see Chapter 26), so she is started on iron replacement and tranexamic acid to reduce the bleeding.

Case study 33.2

Sarah Webb, age 51, works as a bed manager in the local hospital. She has frequent hot flushes and sweating, which she finds embarrassing, and which are making it difficult to concentrate on her busy job. Night sweats are interfering with her sleep and her symptoms are getting her down. She comes to discuss the pros and cons of HRT with her GP, Dr Liz Walters.

What should Dr Walters discuss with Sarah?
Dr Walters should:
- Assess menopausal symptoms and their impact on Sarah's sleep, mood and quality of life.
- Assess contraindications (see Top tip box on Contraindications to HRT) and specific risks from Sarah's personal medical history and from her family history.
- Assess her expectations. HRT may improve sleep and low mood if secondary to the menopause, but not if there is pre-existing anxiety or depression.

Sarah wants to know the evidence behind some of the risks and benefits – she has heard that HRT can reduce thinning of the bones but may increase her risk of cancers and heart disease, and this puts her off.

What can Dr Walters tell her about this?
Osteoporosis is reduced by HRT for the time that it is taken, but HRT should not be used just for this purpose.

The Women's Health Initiative showed an increase in coronary heart disease events in the first year of use, but a more recent study suggests HRT may reduce the risk of **CVD** if started under 60 and within 10 years of menopause.[6] It is not licensed for prevention, however. If Sarah has no identifiable risks for CVD then Dr Walters can advise her that, if used for a short duration to manage her symptoms, HRT is unlikely to increase her risk of CVD.

Colorectal cancer risks may be reduced, but Dr Walters should take individual risk factors into consideration.

Breast cancer risks are slightly increased by HRT. Dr Walters should discuss individual risk with Sarah and take a family history. Sarah's maternal aunt (her mother's sister) died from secondary breast cancer aged 73, so Sarah is particularly worried about increasing her risk of this.

Should Sarah avoid HRT?
Women who take HRT, particularly combined HRT (containing oestrogen and progesterone), have a small increased risk of breast cancer. The actual risks are small. For every 1000 women who take HRT, one extra woman will develop breast cancer; this is a similar risk to that in women who are obese, who have never had children or who drink more than the weekly recommended level of alcohol. Sarah's personal risk would be higher than this if she had a family history suggestive of familial breast cancer (e.g. a first-degree relative with breast cancer younger than 40) or if she met any of the criteria that would indicate the need for referral to a specialist genetic clinic.

Are there any alternative treatments Sarah could use to manage her hot flushes and sweating?
Night sweats and hot flushes may be helped by regular exercise and by reducing stress, although the evidence is conflicting.[7] It makes sense to wear lighter clothing and to keep her bedroom cool for sleeping, but it is also worth trying to identify and avoid common triggers, such as alcohol and spicy food. See also Table 33.1 and the Top tip box on Alternatives to HRT.

What else should Dr Walters cover in this consultation?
A consultation for menopause symptoms is a good chance to discuss lifestyle advice and primary prevention. Is she up to date with breast and cervical screening? The GP should check she is covered for contraception (see Top tip box on Contraception in Perimenopause).

Table 33.1 Alternatives to HRT for vasomotor symptoms.

Prescribed medications	Comments	Herbal preparations	Comments	Dietary
Progesterones Selective serotonin reuptake inhibitors (SSRIs) Gabapentin	Can help vasomotor symptoms (can return on stopping)	Red clover[a]	Contains phyto-oestrogens and coumarins (avoid if on anticoagulants)	Food rich in phyto-oestrogens: • Soya beans • Nuts • Wholegrains
Clonidine	Side effects can be problematic	Black cohosh[a]	Small risk of liver damage	

[a] The evidence for nonprescribed alternatives to HRT is equivocal. They may help hot flushes, but the placebo effect is high and it is difficult to be sure of the efficacy or quality of the ingredients.

Top tips: contraception in the perimenopause

- If a woman's last period occurs before she is 50, she should use contraception for another 2 years after this.

- If a woman's last period occurs after she is 50, she should use contraception for another 1 year after this.

- HRT does not provide contraception; additional methods should be employed.

- The progesterone-only Mirena IUS is licensed for use as endometrial progesterone protection in women taking oestrogen-only HRT.

- If a woman opts for combined HRT, a nonhormonal method of contraception should be used, such as condoms.

- An alternative to HRT for menopausal women younger than 50 who need contraceptive cover is a low-dose combined oral contraceptive (COC) pill. These patients should be free of all risk factors.

Hormone-replacement therapy preparations

Women with an intact uterus need to take progesterone to protect the lining of the womb, as unopposed oestrogen risks development of endometrial carcinoma. Cyclical HRT is where progesterone is given in the last 12–14 days of the cycle, which causes a monthly withdrawal bleed. The Mirena IUS has been licensed to protect the endometrium; it also reduces heavy periods and provides contraception. Continuous combined HRT (a 'no-bleed' formulation) is given to woman more than 12 months after their last period and is a daily dose of oestrogen and progesterone. It can cause some light bleeding in the first few months of use. If this doesn't settle in 6 months, it should be investigated as postmenopausal bleeding.

There are different routes of administration of HRT. It can be taken orally, it can be delivered transdermally via a patch applied to the skin every week (or twice weekly) or it can be applied to the skin as a gel (away from the breast tissue). Transdermal options are useful for women who get side effects with oral tablets, are lactose intolerant or have migraines (there is less of a hormone spike compared to tablets), or where there is potential malabsorption, such as in inflammatory bowel disease. Using a patch or gel also avoids the first-pass metabolism by the liver, so it is useful for women with gallstones or high triglycerides.

Sometimes, women have to switch to different types of HRT because of side effects. Women on HRT should be reviewed annually. See Table 33.2 for an outline of what to cover in the HRT annual review.

Table 33.2 Annual review of HRT.

Check effectiveness	After 3 months of use, persistent symptoms may indicate the dose is too low or there is an alternative cause
Ask about side effects	Breast tenderness and nausea tend to be oestrogenic effects. They may resolve with use, reduction of the oestrogen dose or change of the formulation Headaches, acne or mood swings tend to be progesterone side effects and can resolve with use or on change of the formulation
Ask about abnormal bleeding	
Ask about any change in risk profile	Personal and family history of thromboembolic disease, hormone-dependent cancers, CVD
Check blood pressure and body mass index (BMI)	
Ask about breast awareness	Encourage mammogram screening programme (if in age range)
Discuss options	Continuing, changing, reducing or stopping therapy If it is 12 months from the last menstrual period, the patient can switch to continuous combined HRT

Top tip: alternatives to HRT

The plethora of advice about managing menopausal symptoms without hormones can be confusing. The alternative market is big and it can be difficult for women to get accurate, up-to-date evidence and advice.

Women may find the following sources of information helpful:

- **www.menopausematters.co.uk**

- **www.patient.info**

- 'Alternatives to Hormone Replacement Therapy for Symptoms of the Menopause' (available from http://www.rcog.org.uk/globalassets/documents/patients/patient-information-leaflets/gynaecology/pi-alternatives-to-hormone-replacement-therapy-for-symptoms-of-the-menopause.pdf)

Using topical hormone-replacement therapy

Menopausal atrophic vaginitis can be treated with a vaginal oestrogen pessary or cream used daily for 2 or 3 weeks until symptoms improve, then twice weekly, or with a vaginal ring left in place for 3 months. GPs should review at 3–6-monthly intervals and examine with a view to stopping treatment. Topical treatments are often used in older women, where the risk–benefit ratio of using systemic HRT is less favourable.

Postmenopausal bleeding

Bleeding that occurs 6 months after the last menstrual period or persistent bleeding on HRT that continues when it is stopped should be investigated. Most bleeding is benign and can be from vaginal atrophy or endometrial polyps or hyperplasia. However, the vast majority of endometrial cancers present with postmenopausal bleeding, so postmenopausal bleeding is treated as cancer until proven otherwise and needs urgent referral to a gynaecology clinic, to be seen within 2 weeks. Often, this will be a 'one-stop' clinic, where transvaginal ultrasound can assess endometrial thickness, endometrial sampling can biopsy the endometrium and hysteroscopy can be organised, if necessary.

SUMMARY

Although the menopause is a normal physiological phase of a woman's life, symptoms can have a significant effect on quality of life. Studies have raised concern about the risk of exogenous hormones, but the benefits often outweigh the risks for many symptomatic women near the menopause, if used at the lowest dose for the shortest time required to control symptoms. Patients on hormone replacement need regular review and reassessment of the risks and benefits. Women may be unable or unwilling to take hormones, so GPs must be aware of lifestyle strategies and alternative treatments that might help the transition though the menopause.

Now visit **www.wileyessential.com/primarycare** to test yourself on this chapter.

REFERENCES

1. Mishra G, Kuh D. Health symptoms during midlife in relation to menopausal transition: British prospective cohort study *BMJ* 2012;**344**:e402.

2. Ewies AA, Alfhaily F. Topical vaginal estrogen therapy in managing postmenopausal urinary symptoms: a reality or a gimmick? *Climacteric* 2010;(**5**):405–18.

3. Rossouw JE, Anderson GL, Prentice RL, et al. Risks and benefits of estrogen plus progestin in healthy postmenopausal women: principal results From the Women's Health Initiative randomized controlled trial. *JAMA* 2002;**288**(3):321–33.

4. Beral V. Breast cancer and hormone-replacement therapy in the Million Women Study. *Lancet* 2003;**362**(9382):419–27.

5. Langer RD, Manson JE, Allison MA. Have we come full circle-or moved forward? The Women's Health Initiative 10 years on. *Climacteric* 2012;**15**(3):206–12.

6. Schierbeck LL, Rejnmark L, Tofteng CL, et al. Effect of hormone replacement therapy on cardiovascular events in recently postmenopausal women: randomised trial. *BMJ* 2012;**345**:e6409.

7. Daley A, MacArthur C, Mutrie N, et al. Exercise for vasomotor menopausal symptoms. *Cochrane Database Syst Rev* 2007;**4**:CD006108.

CHAPTER 34
Multimorbidity and polypharmacy

Polly Duncan[1] and Andrew Blythe[2]

[1] Academic Clinical Fellow, University of Bristol
[2] GP and Senior Teaching Fellow, University of Bristol

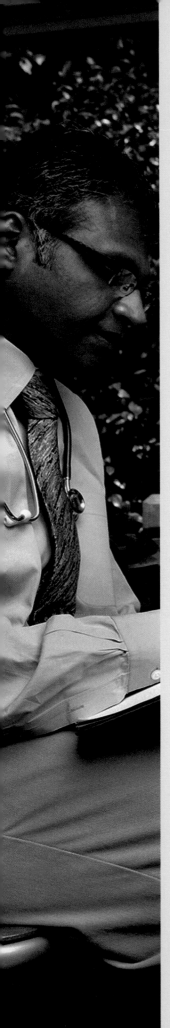

Key topics

Learning objectives

- Be able to describe how common multimorbidity is and who is most at risk.
- Be able to describe the impact of multimorbidity on patient well-being.
- Be able to outline some of the challenges that GPs face when consulting with patients with multimorbidity.
- Be able to outline changes to primary health care services that might improve the management of patients with multimorbidity.
- Be able to describe the problems caused by polypharmacy.
- Be able to describe the key steps to rationalising a patient's medications.

Essential Primary Care, First Edition. Edited by Andrew Blythe and Jessica Buchan.
© 2017 John Wiley & Sons, Ltd. Published 2017 by John Wiley & Sons, Ltd.
Companion website: www.wileyessential.com/primarycare

Epidemiology of multimorbidity

Over the past few decades, advances in medicine and public health have led to increased life expectancy, so that more and more people are now living with multiple long-term conditions. Multimorbidity is defined as the coexistence of two or more unrelated long-term conditions in one person. Over half of the UK population over the age of 65 has multimorbidity.[1] Amongst the elderly, multimorbidity is the norm rather than the exception, and as such it represents a major challenge for patients and clinicians. Figure 34.1 shows how people accumulate chronic diseases as they get older. It also shows that multimorbidity is by no means restricted to the elderly population. Due to the current population demographics, more people below the age of 65 years have multimorbidity than those aged over 65.[1]

The prevalence of multimorbidity increases with deprivation, so that people in the most deprived quintile are almost twice as likely to have multimorbidity as those in the least deprived quintile, after adjusting for age and sex.[2] Multimorbidity also occurs earlier in deprived populations, with the same prevalence of multimorbidity occurring 10–15 years earlier in the poorest communities compared with the most affluent in society.[1] Figure 34.2, taken from the work of Barnett et al. in Scotland,[1] shows the likelihood of having other conditions alongside each of four common chronic conditions: coronary heart disease, diabetes, chronic obstructive pulmonary disease (COPD) and cancer. For each condition on this chart, the chance of having another condition is greater if the patient is from a deprived sector of society.

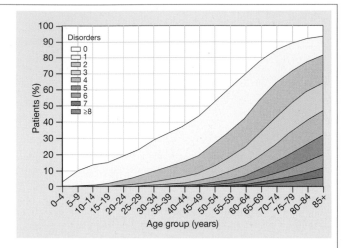

Figure 34.1 Number of chronic disorders by age group. *Source*: Barnett, K et al. *The Lancet* 2012; **380**: 37–43. Reproduced with permission of Elsevier.

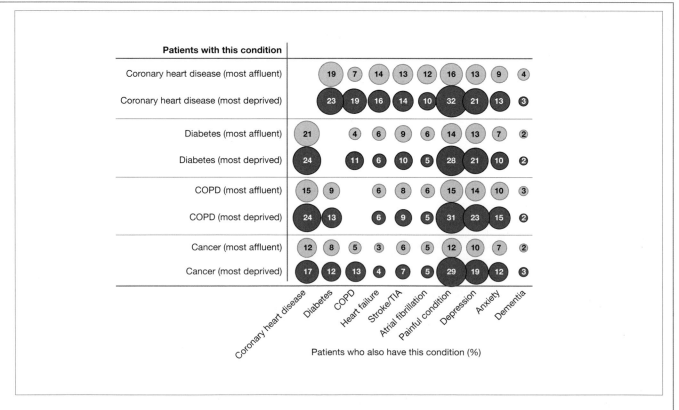

Figure 34.2 Selected comorbidities in people with four common important disorders, from the most affluent and most deprived decile. *Source*: Barnett, K et al. *The Lancet* 2012; **380**: 37–43. Reproduced with permission of Elsevier.

The impact of multimorbidity on patients, GPs and the health system

The patient

To cope with the demands of an elderly population, the responsibility for managing medical conditions is shifting to the patients themselves. For example, patients are responsible for coordinating their appointments, for monitoring their conditions and for finding ways to incorporate complex medical regimens into their everyday lives. A patient's perception of the effort required to self-manage their medical conditions and the impact that this has on their general well-being is known as *treatment burden*.[3] This can in itself be overwhelming for patients, and it has been shown that those with a high treatment burden comply less with treatment and either under- or overuse health care services, resulting in an increased use of unscheduled care and more frequent and longer hospital admissions. Patient-reported barriers to self-management include financial constraints, having symptoms and treatments that interfere with one another, physical limitations and the 'hassles' of interacting with the health care system.[4]

Illness burden describes the impact that a medical condition has on a patient's physical and mental well-being. As multimorbidity encompasses a range of medical conditions of varying severity, the illness burden experienced by patients with multimorbidity varies from patient to patient. In general, however, patients with multimorbidity have poorer health outcomes than those without multimorbidity, including a worse life expectancy, poorer quality of life and higher rates of mental health problems, such as depression.[1]

The GP

Patients with multimorbidity consult their GP more frequently than their non-multimorbid counterparts, such that almost 8 out of 10 GP consultations involve patients with multimorbidity.[5]

In a 10-minute consultation, GPs are expected to explore the patient's agenda (ideas, concerns and expectations) for each problem; to apply their clinical knowledge to work out probable diagnoses and treatment options; and to form a shared management plan with the patient. The latter requires them to weigh up and communicate the risks and benefits of treatment in view of the patient's long-term medical conditions and current medications.

Continuity of care can improve consultation satisfaction, both for the GP and for the patient.[6] It gives the GP the opportunity to familiarise themselves with the patient's medical history, drug history, preferences and social background. If a patient has lots of different conditions, it seems intuitive that the patient should have one GP who can provide an overview and continuity of care. In fact, the evidence shows that patients with multimorbidity are less likely to receive continuity of care than their non-multimorbid counterparts.[2]

The health system

Multimorbidity is associated with huge health care costs in both primary and secondary care. Expenditure on health care rises exponentially with the number of chronic disorders an individual has. A study in Ireland found that the average total health care cost over the previous 12-month period for patients with more than four chronic conditions was €4097, compared to €760 for those with no chronic conditions.[7]

Managing patients with multimorbidity

Disease-centred care versus patient-centred care

At present, patients are usually invited to attend separate appointments in order to review each of their chronic diseases. This applies to both primary and secondary care. It means patients attend many different hospital clinics and several appointments at the GP surgery, sometimes all within a short period of time. Increasingly, these appointments are with nurses who have specialist training in certain chronic diseases.

Case study 34.1

Malcolm Mumford is 78. He has type 2 diabetes treated with insulin, glaucoma, prostate cancer, osteoarthritis and hypertension.

He was diagnosed with diabetes in his early 60s. He was started on insulin 3 years ago because his HbA1c was consistently high despite triple oral therapy (metformin, gliclazide and sitagliptin). The practice nurse supervised the initiation of his insulin therapy. She sees him every 6 months in the practice diabetic clinic. He is also invited to diabetic retinopathy screening at the GP surgery once a year.

He was diagnosed with glaucoma 10 years ago and is on eye drops to control this; he has a check-up at the eye hospital once a year.

His prostate cancer was diagnosed 4 years ago and is treated with a gonadotrophin-releasing hormone analogue (goserelin), given as an injection at the GP surgery every 3 months. Once a year, he attends the urology and oncology clinics.

He had his left knee replaced 2 years ago and he sees the orthopaedic surgeon once a year for review. His right knee is painful now and may have to be replaced soon.

He takes 10 different medicines:
- insulin and metformin for his diabetes;
- atorvastatin to keep his cholesterol to target;
- ramipril and amlodipine to keep his blood pressure to target;
- latanoprost and timolol eye drops for his glaucoma;

- goserelin for his prostate cancer;
- co-codamol for the pain in his right knee;
- senna, to treat the constipation caused by the co-codamol.

There are a few things that are worrying Mr Mumford at present. He has intermittent pains in his legs and feet that he thinks may be a side effect of the statin, or possibly his cancer. He is also very worried about what will happen if his eyesight gets worse. Will he have to give up driving? He's struggling to read the numbers on his insulin pen. What if it gets to the stage where he can't read at all? His worries get on top of him sometimes and he is not sleeping well.

In October, he attends two separate hospital appointments – the glaucoma clinic and orthopaedic clinic – and he attends the GP surgery for his annual flu vaccine. At the glaucoma clinic, the optometrist says his glaucoma is under control but mentions something about an early cataract, which makes him more worried. The orthopaedic surgeon tells him his new knee is fine, but doesn't offer any opinion on the pain in his feet.

In November, he sees the practice nurse for his 3-monthly goserelin injection. She reminds him that he's due to have his prostate-specific antigen (PSA) checked again in January and books him an appointment for his next goserelin injection in February.

In December, he has some routine blood tests at the surgery in advance of his diabetic review with the practice nurse. When he comes to the diabetic clinic, he mentions to the nurse that he's bothered by pain in his legs and feet. His pedal pulses are strong and sensation is intact, so the nurse suggests he makes an appointment to see his GP about his pain.

When he sees the GP at the end of December, he is unhappy because despite having answered lots of questions and having attended several examinations and blood tests over the last 3 months, none of *his* concerns have been addressed. This is one problem with a disease-centred approach. The other main problem, which is apparent in this case, is the treatment burden for Mr Mumford: he has to attend numerous appointments, none of which seem to connect very well.

An alternative approach is patient-centred care, whereby the management of a patient's conditions is guided by the patient's agenda and their medical conditions are reviewed simultaneously. The obvious advantages of this approach are that it is much more patient-focussed and that, in reviewing the chronic conditions simultaneously, the likelihood of causing adverse drug events is reduced. Since each patient will have a different combination of medical conditions and will come from a different viewpoint and social background, following a set protocol becomes difficult, and clinicians are required instead to apply their experience. This may require a longer consultation with a fairly experienced and skilled practitioner. The fact that patients are required to attend fewer reviews counterbalances the longer consultation length and is likely to be time-saving overall.

Some GP practices have begun introducing this new model of care and inviting their patients with multimorbidity to a single annual review, sometimes coinciding with the month of their birthday. The length of this review is determined by the mix of chronic diseases. Patients are encouraged to write down in advance of the consultation issues that they want to discuss. If any blood tests need to be done, these are scheduled before the review, so that the results are available. Usually, most of the review is done by the practice nurse, but some of it, particularly the prescribing component, is likely to be done by the GP. The outcome of the review should be a care plan with a set of clear goals for the patient and a list of medication that has been reviewed.

For patients who are at high risk of admission, care plans are particularly important. If these care plans contain a summary of the patient's usual status (their cognitive state, mobility and oxygen saturation), this can be extremely useful if the patient requests a home visit out of hours and sees a

health professional who is not familiar with them. For instance, knowing that the patient's oxygen saturation is normally around 93% might make the difference between deciding to admit them and keeping them at home.

Carers

Many patients with multimorbidity rely on help from a carer – often a relative or close family friend who helps the patient with day-to-day activities, including taking multiple medications and attending various health care appointments. As well as having a duty of care to the patient, GPs have a duty of care to the patient's carer, and if someone is a carer, this should be flagged up by the computer system. Having an awareness of the impact that being a carer can have on day-to-day life is a start, and GPs should be proactive in checking whether carers are coping and whether they need any extra support.

Polypharmacy

'Polypharmacy' is defined as being prescribed four or more medications. It is a common problem that has increased in recent decades. It is estimated that one in five patients prescribed regular medication takes five or more medications, and that one in six patients over the age of 65 years is prescribed 10 or more medications.[8]

Polypharmacy can be categorised as being appropriate or problematic.[9] 'Appropriate polypharmacy' describes a situation where a patient's medications have been optimised to extend their life expectancy and to improve their quality of life. In contrast, 'problematic polypharmacy' refers to the increased risk of adverse drug events, interactions between medications,

Table 34.1 The 'NO TEARS' mnemonic for rationalising a patient's medications.[10]

N	**Need**
	• Is there a clear indication for the medication?
	• Does the patient know what it is for?
	• Is the dose appropriate for the indication?
	• Is long-term therapy appropriate?
	• Are there any alternative nonpharmacological treatments? (e.g. weight loss or physiotherapy for knee osteoarthritis)
O	**Open questions**
	• Give the patient a chance to have their say. (e.g. 'I realise a lot of people have difficulty taking all their medicines. Do you have any problems at all?')
	• Does the patient have any concerns about taking the medication? (e.g. worries about side effects or interactions with other medications)
	• How are they taking the medication?
	• Are they taking any over-the-counter medications or complementary medications?
T	**Tests and monitoring**
	• Is any monitoring required? (e.g. urea and electrolytes (U&Es) for patients taking angiotensin-converting enzyme (ACE) inhibitors)
	• Is the medical condition progressing? Is the medication working? (e.g. monitoring of the HbA1C and for cardiovascular complications in patients with diabetes)
E	**Evidence and guidelines**
	• Has the evidence changed?
	• Does the evidence apply to this patient? (Many randomised controlled trials (RCTs) exclude elderly patients with multimorbidity)
A	**Adverse events**
	• Any side effects?
	• Check for possible interactions. Avoid high-risk combinations (e.g. nonsteroidal anti-inflammatory drug (NSAID), ACE inhibitor and diuretic). These should be flagged up by the computer system
R	**Risk reduction**
	• Does the medication increase the patient's risk of falls (e.g. benzodiazepines), fractures (e.g. long-term steroids), stomach ulcers (e.g. NSAIDs) or renal impairment (e.g. NSAIDs, diuretics)?
	• Are additional medications required to reduce this risk? (e.g. bone protection for patients on long-term steroids)
S	**Simplification**
	• Can the treatment be simplified? (e.g. changing to a modified-release medication to reduce the daily frequency from four times a day to once or twice a day)

prescribing errors and pill burden associated with being prescribed multiple medications. This can lead to a poorer quality of life for the patient, reduced compliance with treatment and an increase in morbidity, mortality and hospital admissions.

GPs are under pressure to adhere to guidelines.[9] Indeed, part of their pay is determined by it. However, since most randomised controlled drug trials exclude both elderly patients and patients with multimorbidity, the evidence base upon which the guidelines are written is not as robust as one might hope and should be interpreted with caution when reviewing patients with multimorbidity. Most patients who have one chronic disease have at least one other chronic condition.

How to manage patients with polypharmacy

Undertaking regular medication reviews with patients can help reduce problematic polypharmacy. The 'NO TEARS' mnemonic provides a useful systematic approach to rationalising

medications (see Table 34.1).[10] Each medication should be reviewed in turn. The advantages of using this tool are that it encourages the patient's involvement and that it should allow the medication review to be completed within a 10-minute GP consultation.

In practice, however, GPs will seldom spend a whole consultation reviewing a patient's medication. A common scenario is that a patient will receive a letter asking them to come in for a medication review and this will act as a trigger for something else. So they might come into the consulting room saying, 'You wrote to me about my medication. That reminded me, I wanted to see you about...' Then there's a decision: should the GP try to meet the patient's agenda of their new problem or their own agenda of reviewing the patient's medications? Invariably, the GP will focus on the patient's new problem and squeeze a medication review in at the end by saying something like, 'No problems with your medication? Great.' An alternative approach is for the GP to review the medications once the patient has left the consultation, but this means the patient has no say in any changes made to their medications. One solution to this problem is for the GP to signpost the patient to the pharmacist, who can undertake a thorough patient-centred medication review using a special form. Practice pharmacists also undertake paper reviews of patients' medications.

One area that GPs find particularly difficult is rationalising preventative medications in elderly patients. It can be hard to know whether a patient will live long enough to benefit from preventative medication, and this must be weighed against any potential ill effects of the medication. A study in the Netherlands found that GPs were concerned about raising this topic with patients and worried that by stopping preventative medications they might make their patients feel that they were giving up on them.[11] The same study found that GPs tended to underestimate the burden that polypharmacy causes for patients.

Patient decision aids are becoming increasingly popular with GPs and patients, and can play an important role in deciding whether or not to start or to continue a particular medication. For example, patients with atrial fibrillation can work through a decision aid to weigh up the risks and benefits of taking anticoagulant medication, such as warfarin. The limitations of patient decision aids are that they are only available for a small number of medications and medical conditions and that the evidence they are based on is drawn from trials that often exclude elderly patients and patients with multimorbidity.

Top tips: managing patients with multimorbidity

- Be aware of how treatment can impact on patient well-being (e.g. having to take multiple medications and attending multiple appointments).

- Try to find out the patient's agenda and treatment goals.

- Involve the patient in treatment decisions, where possible. This way, they are more likely to comply with treatment and the doctor–patient relationship will be strengthened.

- Try to review a patient's medical conditions simultaneously, rather than individually.

- Encourage patients to book for a separate medication review appointment so that you can spend time reviewing each medication with them using 'NO TEARS'.

- Encourage patients to use patient decision aids where appropriate.

- Be aware that patients with multimorbidity are often excluded from trials, so the evidence base is not always as robust as one might think.

- Be aware of medications and combinations of medications that are most likely to cause adverse drug reactions.

SUMMARY

'Multimorbidity' describes the coexistence of two or more long-term medical conditions. Consulting with patients with multimorbidity has become the norm in UK general practice, and this presents several challenges to GPs, not least having to manage an average of 2.5 problems per 10-minute consultation. Multimorbidity also has a significant impact on patient well-being and is associated with higher rates of mental illness such as depression, higher rates of hospital admission and significant health care costs. Attending multiple appointments and taking complex medication regimens can also cause a significant burden for patients. A shift is needed away from the current disease-centred model of general practice, whereby patients attend individual reviews for each of their medical conditions, towards a patient-centred approach, whereby efforts are made to find out the patient's agenda and goals, and their conditions are reviewed simultaneously.

 Now visit **www.insertwebaddress.com** to test yourself on this chapter.

REFERENCES

1. Barnett K, Mercer SW, Norbury M, et al. Epidemiology of multimorbidity and implications for health care, research and medical education: a cross-sectional study. *Lancet* 2012;**380**:37–43.

2. Salisbury C, Johnson L, Purdy S, et al. Epidemiology and impact of multimorbidity in primary care: a retrospective cohort study. *Br J Gen Pract* 2011;**61**:212–21.

3. Eton DT, Ramalho de Oliveira D, Egginton JS, et al. Building a measurement framework of burden of treatment in complex patients with chronic conditions: a qualitative study. *Patient Relat Outcome Meas* 2012;**3**:39–49.

4. Bayliss E A, Ellis JL, Steiner JF. Barriers to self-management and quality-of-life outcomes in seniors with multimorbidities. *Ann Fam Med* 2007;**5**(5):395–402.

5. Salisbury C, Procter S, Stewart K, et al. The content of general practice consultations: cross-sectional study based on video recordings. *Br J Gen Pract* 2013;**63**(616):e751–9.

6. Adler R, Vasiliadis A, Bickell N. The relationship between continuity and patient satisfaction: a systematic review. *Fam Pract* 2010;**27**:171–8.

7. Glynn LG, Valderas JM, Healy P, et al. The prevalence of multimorbidity in primary care and its effect on health care utilization and cost. *Fam Pract* 2011;**8**(5):516–23.

8. Shiner A, Ford J, Steel N, et al. Managing multimorbidity in primary care. *InnovAIT* 2014;**7**(11):691–700.

9. Duerden M, Avery T, Payne R. Polypharmacy and medicines optimization: making it safe and sound. The King's Fund. 2013. Available from: http://www.kingsfund.org.uk/publications/polypharmacy-and-medicines-optimisation (last accessed 6 October 2015).

10. Lewis T. Using the NO TEARS tool for medication review. *BMJ* 2004;**329**:434.

11. Schuling J, Gebben H, Veehof LJG, Haaijer-Ruskamp FM. Deprescribing medication in very elderly patients with multimorbidity: the view of Dutch GPs. A qualitative study. *BMC Family Practice* 2012;**13**:56.

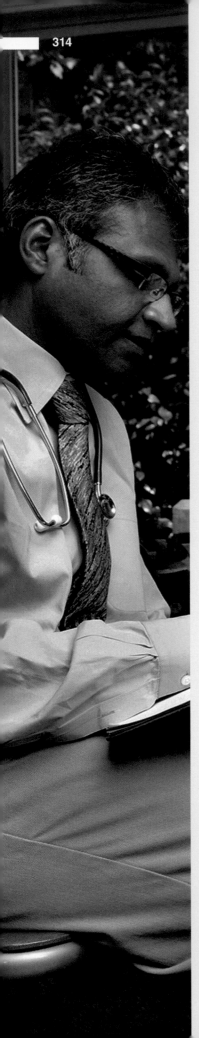

CHAPTER 35
Falls and fragility fractures

Andrew Blythe
GP and Senior Teaching Fellow, University of Bristol

Key topics

Learning objectives

- Be able to identify someone who is at risk of falling.
- Be able to assess someone who has a history of falls.
- Be able to identify people who are at high risk of having a fragility fracture.
- Be able to give advice to someone about bone protection.

Essential Primary Care, First Edition. Edited by Andrew Blythe and Jessica Buchan.
© 2017 John Wiley & Sons, Ltd. Published 2017 by John Wiley & Sons, Ltd.
Companion website: www.wileyessential.com/primarycare

Falls

Falls are common, and become more common with advancing age, due to the deterioration of several physiological functions, including muscle strength, proprioception and vision. Some medicines that we prescribe for elderly people, particularly those that lower blood pressure, opioid-based painkillers and hypnotic drugs, can make patients even more susceptible to falls. Over half of everyone over the age of 80 has at least one fall a year.

Not only are older people more likely to fall, but they are more likely to sustain a serious injury as a result of falling. They may not be able to get up again, and if they are unable to summon help, they may develop hypothermia and renal failure. If they bang their head, they may develop a subdural haematoma. Many elderly people are on anticoagulant medication, so if they fall, they are at high risk of having an intracranial bleed. If they fracture their femur, they will need admission to hospital, where they face potential complications including pneumonia and deep-vein thrombosis (DVT). All of these things carry a substantial risk of death. Even less serious injuries such as dislocations and sprains can have a profound effect on an individual if they prevent them from carrying out everyday tasks such as washing, dressing and cooking.

Given that falls can have such catastrophic consequences and are responsible for so many hospital admissions, it seems sensible to try to identify those at risk of falling and take action to reduce this risk. All primary care health professionals have a role in identifying these people. The strongest indicator of risk is a previous fall, and discovering that someone has fallen should prompt further assessment. In a hospital setting, the Physiological Profile Assessment (PPA)[1] can be used to identify people at high risk of falling. This measures five indices: visual contrast sensitivity, proprioception, quadriceps strength, reaction time and sway. The scores on these indices indicate what sort of interventions might prove fruitful in reducing the risk of falling. But this assessment is too time-consuming for use in primary care. A quicker tool for identifying those at risk of falling is the timed-up-and-go test.[2] Ask the patient to:

- stand up from a seat (46 cm high);
- walk forward 3 m;
- turn 180°;
- return to their seat.

This test doesn't require any equipment and can be done in the patient's home or the GP surgery. Whitney and colleagues conducted this test on patients referred to a falls clinic at King's College Hospital London from GPs and accident and emergency.[3] They found that there was a positive correlation between the time taken to do this test and the PPA falls risk score. Using a cut-off time of 15 seconds created optimal sensitivity and specificity for identifying people who are at high risk of falling, as judged by the more sophisticated PPA.

People who have recurrent falls need a careful multifactorial assessment (see Table 35.1). We start by exploring the circumstances surrounding the fall, symptoms that might suggest a cardiac cause, the patient's medical problems and the patient's medication. Alcohol misuse and dependence are common in all age groups (see Chapter 8) and often cause falls, but may be concealed by the patient, so we should consider using the AUDIT questionnaire. We check the patient's vision and think about environmental hazards that might cause falls, such as rugs that slip and poorly lit rooms or staircases. We focus our examination on the cardiovascular, musculoskeletal and neurological systems and remember that several different pathologies may be contributing to the risk of falls. For instance, the patient may have a peripheral neuropathy due to diabetes, poor vision due to cataracts and postural hypotension aggravated by an angiotensin-converting enzyme (ACE) inhibitor. Depression, memory problems and fear of falling can compound the problem, so we need to do a mental state examination, too. It's unlikely that a GP will have time to complete this assessment in one go. We might ask a practice or community nurse to complete parts of the assessment or else refer the patient to a falls clinic at the local hospital. The benefit of a falls clinic is that a comprehensive assessment can be made in a single visit, culminating in an action plan.

There are four key interventions that can reduce the risk of falls which are not due to cardiac events, epilepsy or intoxication. They are listed here in order of efficacy:

1. **Strength and balance training:** There is evidence from meta-analysis that this reduces the risk of falling.[4]
2. **Rationalising medication:** Stopping psychotropic medication, in particular, reduces the risk of falling.
3. **Prescribing calcium and vitamin D:** These supplements have a role in preventing osteoporosis, but they also improve muscle strength and reduce the risk of falls by 26%.[5] See the Top tip box for tips on giving patients advice about calcium and vitamin D.
4. **Conducting a home assessment:** This should be done by an occupational therapist (OT), who can remove hazards, such as rugs, and request the installation of aids and appliances, such as a second stair rail and a grab rail by the toilet.

Using these interventions, falls clinics can make a substantial reduction to the risk of falls.[6] All four interventions can be initiated by a GP, however. The GP has control of what is prescribed, can make a referral to physiotherapy for strength and balance training and can refer a patient to an OT.

It's also important to think about what would happen if the patient did have a fall. It's essential that they can summon help. A personal alarm, which the patient wears round their neck or on their wrist, is a good way of ensuring this. Pressing the button triggers an automatic phone call to a call centre or carer. If the patient also has a phone with a speakerphone system, the alarm can permit them to speak to a person in the call centre. Paramedics often attend to people who have fallen, and for this purpose they carry special lifting equipment.

Table 35.1 Assessment of someone who has recurrent falls.

Component of assessment	Specific things to check	Tests
History of falls	Frequency, context, nature	
Symptoms	Warning, palpitations, loss of consciousness	
Continence	Symptoms of urge or stress incontinence, prolapse	Midstream specimen of urine (MSU), fasting glucose
Alcohol and smoking		AUDIT-C
Medication	Sedatives, psychotropic drugs, analgesia	
Body mass index (BMI)		
Muscle bulk and strength	Quadricep bulk	
Joints	Hips, knee and ankles	
Feet	Deformities, nails, sensation, footwear	Vibration sense, proprioception, monofilament test
Gait and balance	Walking into the room. Do they use any aid? Romberg's	Timed-up-and-go test Functional reach Dynamic gait index Berg balance
Cardiovascular exam	Pulse, blood pressure (lying and standing)	
Vision	Acuity and visual fields	Report from optician
Mental state	Evidence of dementia, low mood, anxiety, fear	Abbreviated Mental Test (AMT)/Folstein/ Montreal Cognitive Assessment (MoCA), Patient Health Questionnaire-9 (PHQ-9)
Home assessment	*Hazards*: rugs, steps	
Bone mineral density (BMD)		Use the Fracture Risk Assessment Tool (FRAX) to decide whether to request a dual-energy X-ray absorptiometry (DEXA) scan

Items highlighted in ***bold italics*** are considered by NICE to be the most predictive of falls amongst older people living in the community.[9]

Hip protectors are padded shields that fit into special underwear to reduce the force transmitted to the most vulnerable part of the femur. They can reduce the risk of someone fracturing their femur should they fall, but they are tricky to put on and are uncomfortable. There is most evidence in support of their benefit in nursing and residential homes, where assistance is available. At the time of writing, the National Institute for Health and Care Excellence (NICE) does not recommend their use.[7]

Osteoporosis and bone protection

A fall is more likely to cause a fracture if the bones are fragile. So another strategy for reducing the risk of fractures is to identify people with low bone mineral density (BMD) and offer them treatment to prevent a further decline in their BMD, or possibly to increase it. Within industrialised countries, this strategy has attracted far more attention

and resources than falls prevention; some authors have questioned the wisdom of this.[8] The most significant risk factor for having a fracture is, after all, falling – not having a low BMD.

Bone mineral density

BMD declines with age, and declines most quickly in post-menopausal women. Table 35.2 lists the other factors that are associated with a reduction in BMD. It is measured using dual-energy X-ray absorptiometry (DEXA) and is not uniform throughout the skeleton. When interpreting the value at a given site, we can consider how many standard deviations this is from the mean value of a healthy young person of the same sex (referred to as the T score) or of the same age and sex (referred to as the Z score). If the T score is between –1.0 and –2.5, the patient is said to have osteopenia. If the T score is less than –2.5, they are said to have osteoporosis.

Table 35.2 Risk factors for low bone mineral density.

Age	BMD begins to decline after the age of 35
Female sex	BMD falls most rapidly in women after the menopause
Smoking	
Alcohol	Men >3 units/day; women >2 units/day
Low BMI	<18.5
Coeliac disease	
Prolonged corticosteroid use	Equivalent to prednisolone 5 mg daily for >3 months
Family history of osteoporosis	

Table 35.3 Fragility fractures.

Common		Other
Wrist	Distal radius	Humerus
Hip	Proximal femur	Pelvis
Spine	Vertebral wedge fracture	Ribs

Fragility fractures

The lower the T score, the more likely a person is to sustain a fracture if they fall. Fractures that occur following a fall that we wouldn't expect to cause a fracture in a healthy young adult are referred to as 'fragility fractures'. Typically, these fractures occur when someone falls from standing height, such as when slipping on an icy pavement. The most common fragility fractures are listed in Table 35.3. People with osteoporosis can also develop fractures following apparently minimal trauma, such as sneezing. In the case of the spine, fractures can develop spontaneously purely as the result of the bone being unable to withstand the body's weight.

If someone has a fragility fracture, we might assume they have osteoporosis and give them treatment to maintain their BMD. NICE says this is reasonable approach if they are over 75, but if they are younger we should do a DEXA scan and then use their BMD to calculate their risk of having another fracture.[9]

The most widely used tool for estimating the risk of developing a fracture is the Fracture Risk Assessment Tool (FRAX).[10] FRAX was developed by the World Health Organization (WHO) in conjunction with the University of Sheffield. It takes into account many of the independent risk factors for fragility fracture: age, sex, body mass index (BMI), use of glucocorticoids, alcohol consumption, smoking status, personal history of fractures, family history of fractures and the presence of rheumatoid arthritis.

Case study 35.1a

Katya Kaufman is 58. While walking from her office to the carpark, she slipped and fractured her right distal radius. Her GP, Dr Phil Jones, receives a letter from the orthopaedic surgeon informing him of the fracture. This prompts Dr Jones to invite Mrs Kaufman to the surgery to discuss what can be done to prevent her having another fracture. Mrs Kaufman smokes 10 cigarettes a day and has mild chronic obstructive pulmonary disease (COPD), for which she is on an inhaler (a long-acting muscarinic agonist). This is her only regular medication, but last winter she had a course of antibiotics and prednisolone for an infective exacerbation of her COPD. She drinks about 6 units of alcohol a week. Her mother fractured her hip sometime in her 70s and died a few years ago. Mrs Kaufman is 1.66 m tall and her weight is 59.2 kg, giving her a BMI of 21.5.

Dr Jones explains that the fracture is a warning sign that her bones may have become more fragile. A scan may reveal more information about their strength and will give them a better idea of what can be done to avoid another fracture. The results of the DEXA scan are shown in Table 35.4.

Dr Jones enters all the information he has gathered, including the BMD at the femoral neck, into the FRAX tool (http://www.shef.ac.uk/FRAX/tool.jsp). FRAX offers two estimates of Mrs Kaufman's risk of having another fracture over the next 10 years:

- Her 10-year risk of having a major osteoporotic fracture is 20%.
- Her 10-year risk of having a hip fracture is 3.3%.

Should Dr Jones offer Mrs Kaufman medication to strengthen her bones?

There is no fixed threshold of risk above which we should intervene, but the National Osteoporosis Guideline Group (NOGG) has developed a chart which can be used in conjunction with FRAX to guide our decision about whether or not to offer bone protective medication.[11] For a woman aged 58, the NOGG chart recommends intervening if the 10-year risk of an osteoporotic fracture is above 10% and/or the 10-year risk of having a hip fracture is above 2%. Mrs Kaufman exceeds both thresholds of risk. Therefore, Dr Jones should offer her bone protection.

Table 35.4 Results of Mrs Kaufman's DEXA scan (Case study 35.1).

Site		BMD g/cm³	T score	Z score
Left hip	Total hip	0.802	−1.2	−0.3
	Femoral neck	0.673	−1.6	−0.4
Right hip	Total hip	0.804	−1.1	−0.3
	Femoral neck	0.643	−1.9	−0.6
Lumbar spine	L1–L4	0.748	−2.7	−1.4

Table 35.5 Groups in which to consider calculating 10-year fracture risk.

Age	Women	Men
50–65	Smoker, low BMI (<18.5), drinker (>2 units/day), on long-term steroids, history of falls, previous fragility fracture or family history of hip fracture	Smoker, low BMI, drinker (>3 units/day), on long-term steroids, history of falls, previous fragility fracture or family history of hip fracture
65–75	All	
>75	All	All

In Case study 35.1, even though most of Mrs Kaufman's T scores are greater than −2.5, we give treatment. What we are weighing up is not whether or not someone has osteoporosis, but whether bone protection might prevent a future fracture. Half of all hip fractures occur in people with a T score above −2.5. There is a close analogy here with how we approach the prevention of cardiovascular disease (CVD). In the case of CVD, the outcomes that we want to prevent are a myocardial infarction and stroke; cholesterol and blood pressure are risk factors for these. In the case of bone health, the outcome we are seeking to prevent is a fragility fracture, and the T score is a risk factor for this. In Chapter 9, we saw that the decision of whether or not to offer a statin is based not on the absolute cholesterol level, but on the 10-year risk of developing CVD. It is the same with the T score: the decision whether or not to offer bone protection is based not on the BMD, but on our estimation of the 10-year risk of the patient having a major osteoporotic or hip fracture. In the case of CVD, a fixed threshold of risk is applied to the patient regardless of their age. In the case of fragility fractures, there is a sliding threshold of when to start treatment that changes with age.

Assessing the risk of fracture in someone who has not had a fracture

FRAX can still be used even if we don't know the patient's BMD as they have not yet had a fracture. We can also use QFracture,[12] developed by a team in Nottingham. QFracture takes into account more risk factors than FRAX; specifically, it takes into account ethnicity, the presence of a larger number of conditions causing secondary osteoporosis, whether the patient has a history of falls and whether they live in a nursing home. The majority of residents in nursing homes have osteoporosis, and 40% of all hip fractures occur amongst people living in long-stay residential care.

NICE recommends that health professionals should consider using one of these tools to calculate the fracture risk for any woman over 65 and any man over 75. In addition, it recommends calculating the risk for certain categories of younger people (see Table 35.5). At present, most GPs do not actively seek out all these patients to calculate their risk, and

---

Box 35.1 Groups for whom FRAX may underestimate the risk of fracture

- Age > 80.
- High alcohol intake.
- On high dose of glucocorticoid (>7.5 mg/day).
- Multiple fractures.
- Previous vertebral fracture.
- Living in residential care.
- On a drug which inhibits bone metabolism: anticonvulsant, proton-pump inhibitor (PPI), selective serotonin reuptake inhibitor (SSRI), antiretroviral, thiazolidinedione.

---

instead adopt an opportunistic approach, using the guidance when patients consult about related problems. The groups of people for whom screening is most worthwhile are those who have been on long-term steroids and those with rheumatoid arthritis.

With FRAX, the percentage probability of developing a fracture over the next 10 years can be interpreted as giving low, intermediate or high risk. If the risk is intermediate or high, it is recommended that we request a DEXA scan to assess BMD. Once we have a result for the BMD, we can feed this back into FRAX to recalculate the 10-year risk and then use the NOGG chart to decide whether bone-protection treatment is warranted. There are some groups of people for whom FRAX may underestimate the risk of having a fragility fracture (see Box 35.1). The disadvantages of QFracture are that it doesn't let us incorporate BMD into the risk calculation and it doesn't offer a chart giving guidance about the level of risk that should prompt treatment.

Reducing the risk of a fragility fracture

If someone has had a fragility fracture and their T score is low, we should consider whether or not there might be a secondary cause of osteoporosis. These are more common in men. Table 35.6 lists the secondary causes of osteoporosis and the simple tests that we can do to screen for them.

Table 35.6 Investigating possible secondary causes of osteoporosis.

Cause of osteoporosis		Investigation
Endocrine	Hyperthyroidism	Thyroid-stimulating hormone (TSH)
	Secondary hyperparathyroidism (caused by vitamin D deficiency)	Serum calcium, phosphate and vitamin D
	Diabetes	Fasting glucose or HbA1c
	Hypogonadism (caused by hormonal treatment for breast or prostate cancer)	
	Cushings syndrome (caused by oral glucocorticoids)	
Gastrointestinal	Coeliac disease	Antitissue transglutaminase
Rheumatological	Rheumatoid arthritis	History +/− inflammatory markers
Respiratory	COPD	Spirometry + CXR
Haematological	Multiple myeloma	Serum calcium, inflammatory markers, serum electrophoresis, urinary Bence Jones protein
Liver	Chronic liver disease	Liver function tests (LFTs)
Renal	Chronic kidney disease	Urea and electrolytes (U&Es), urinary albumin/creatinine ratio

There are several medicines that have shown to decrease the risk of fragility fractures; these include bisphosphonates, selective oestrogen receptor modulators, strontium, hormone-replacement therapy (HRT) and the monoclonal antibody therapy Denosumab.[13] Out of these, bisphosphonates are the most widely prescribed at present, and NICE recommends them as first-line treatment. They work by reducing the rate of bone destruction. There is good evidence that they reduce the risk of vertebral fractures in women, but the evidence that they prevent hip fractures and benefit men is less good. A major problem is their side effects. They often cause dyspepsia, which is a common reason for people to stop taking them. A rarer but serious side effect is osteonecrosis of the jaw, which causes dental problems. Some types are prescribed weekly, some monthly, some annually. All of the major studies of bisphosphonate treatment have been done on people who were simultaneously prescribed calcium and vitamin D or who had adequate blood levels of these chemicals. Therefore, it is standard practice to co-prescribe supplements of vitamin D and calcium with a bisphosphonate.

Ideally, patients should be advised to continue the bisphosphonate for 5 years.[14] At this stage, they should have another DEXA scan and their FRAX score should be recalculated. If they decide to stop treatment at this stage, the decision should be reviewed after a while, because we don't know how long the benefit of bisphosphonates lasts after the patient stops taking them. If someone cannot tolerate bisphosphonates, one of the alternative agents can be tried.

Nonpharmacological treatment also has a role. Systematic reviews have demonstrated that regular exercise improves BMD at the neck of femur.[15] Non-weight-bearing exercise of the lower limbs against increasing resistance is best. It is safe, but there is no evidence yet that it prevents fractures. We should also give smoking-cessation advice and warn the patient about the harm caused by exceeding the recommended weekly intake of alcohol. We should recommend a balanced diet containing calcium-rich foods. All of this lifestyle advice is important not just for people who have had a fragility fracture, but for anyone with whom we discuss the risk of having a fracture.

Case study 35.1b

Having established that Mrs Kaufman is at high risk of developing an osteoporotic fracture, Dr Jones requests a battery of blood tests to exclude secondary causes of osteoporosis. All of these are normal, apart from her total 25-O vitamin D level, which is slightly low (52 nmol/l).

Dr Jones explains that smoking is known to reduce bone strength. If Mrs Kaufman were to stop smoking, her bone density would decrease at a slower rate and her COPD would improve. Dr Jones finds out that last year Mrs Kaufman cut down from 20 to 10 cigarettes a day, and she would like to stop smoking altogether. After discussing the options available to her, she says that she would like to try nicotine-replacement therapy, and says she will make an appointment to see the smoking-cessation advisor.

Dr Jones checks that Mrs Kaufman is not about to have any dental work; she says not and reports that her teeth are in good condition. Knowing this, Dr Jones suggests that she starts taking alendronic acid – a bisphosphonate that is taken once a week. Because it can cause heartburn, he recommends that she take it with a full glass of water, when upright, at least 30 minutes before her breakfast.

Dr Jones also prescribes calcium and vitamin D supplements to take every day.

He advises her to keep active in order to maintain her muscle strength, balance and coordination. Exercise, he says, will help to keep her bones strong, too. Mrs Kaufman decides to join a gym.

Top tips: advice to give patients about calcium and vitamin D

- The daily recommended intake of calcium is at least 700 mg. This is contained in a full glass of milk. There's just as much calcium in low-fat milk as there is in full-fat.

- Exposing the skin to sunlight for 10 minutes twice a day during the summer provides you with enough vitamin D to last throughout the year.

- Vitamin D is also present in milk, eggs and oily fish.

- Some types of calcium and vitamin D tablets are chewable. People with dentures find these difficult to take.

- Don't take calcium tablets at the same time as thyroxine or bisphosphonates; it affects their absorption.

SUMMARY

Fractures caused by falls cause substantial morbidity and mortality, especially amongst the elderly population, and are costly to treat. The whole primary care team has a role to play in identifying people who are at risk of falling. Some simple measures can reduce the risk of falling and thereby reduce the risk of fractures. Reduced BMD is another risk factor for fractures. It can be modified with lifestyle advice and medication.

Now visit **www.wileyessential.com/primarycare** to test yourself on this chapter.

REFERENCES

1. Lord SR, Menz HB, Tiedemann A. A physiological profile approach to falls risk assessment and prevention. *Phys Ther* 2003;**83**:237–52.

2. Padsiadlo D, Richardson S. The timed 'up and go' a test of basic functional mobility for frail elderly persons. *J Am Geriatr Soc* 1991;**39**:142.

3. Whitney JC, Lord SR, Close JC. Streamlining assessment and intervention in a falls clinic using the timed up and go test and physiological profile assessments. *Age Ageing* 2005;**34**:567–71.

4. Robertson MC, Campbell AJ, Gardner MM, Devlin N. Preventing injuries in older people by preventing falls: a meta-analysis of individual-level data. *J Am Geriatr Soc* 2002;**50**:905–11.

5. Pfiefer M, Begerow B, Minne HW, et al. Effects of a long term vitamin D and calcium supplementation on falls and parameters of muscle function in community dwelling older individuals. *Osteoporosis Int* 2009;**20**:315–22.

6. Close J, Ellis M, Hooper R, et al. Prevention of falls in the elderly trial (PROFET): a randomised controlled trial. *Lancet* 1999;**353**:93–7.

7. NICE. Falls: assessment and prevention of falls in older people. NICE Clinical Guideline 161. June 2013. Available from: http://www.nice.org.uk/cg161 (last accessed 6 October 2015).

8. Jarvinen TLN, Sievanen H, Khan KM, et al. Shifting the focus in fracture prevention from osteoporosis to falls. *BMJ* 2008;**336**:124–6.

9. NICE. Osteoporosis: assessing the risk of fragility fracture. NICE Clinical Guidance 146 August 2012. Available from: http://www.nice.org.uk/cg146 (last accessed 6 October 2015).

10. WHO. FRAX: Fracture Risk Assessment Tool. Available from: http://www.shef.ac.uk/FRAX/ (last accessed 6 October 2015).

11. Compston JE, Cooper A, Cooper C, et al. Guidelines for the diagnosis and management of osteoporosis in postmenopausal women and men aged 50 years and over in the UK. *Maturitas* 2009;**62**:105–8.

12. Hippsley-Cox J, Coupland C. Derivation and validation of updated QFracture algorithm to predict risk of osteoporotic fracture in primary care in the United Kingdom: prospective open cohort study. *BMJ* 2012;**344**:e3427.

13. NICE. Alendronate, etidronate, risedronate, raloxifene and strontium ranelate for the primary prevention of osteoporotic fragility fractures in postmenopausal women (amended). TA160. 2011. Available from: http://www.nice.org.uk/guidance/ta160 (last accessed 6 October 2015).

14. Black DM, Bauer DC, Schwartz AV, et al. Continuing treatment for osteoporosis – for whom and for how long? *N Engl J Med* 2012;**366**(22):2051–3.

15. Howe TE, Shea B, Dawson LJ, et al. Exercise for preventing and treating osteoporosis in postmenopausal women. *Cochrane Database Syst Rev* 2011;7:CD000333.pub2.

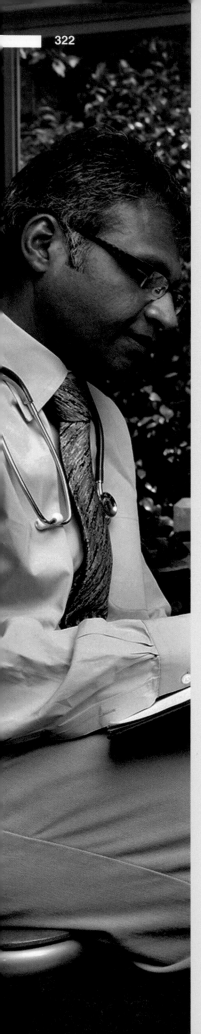

CHAPTER 36
Visual and hearing loss

Andrew Blythe
GP and Senior Teaching Fellow, University of Bristol

Key topics

Learning objectives

- Be able to assess someone who has experienced disturbance of their vision.
- Be able to assess someone who has a cataract in order to make a referral to an ophthalmologist.
- Be able to describe the common causes of preventable sight loss.
- Be able to assess someone's hearing using the whisper and tuning-fork tests.
- Be able to advise someone on the benefits and risks of having their ears syringed.
- Be able to adapt your consultation technique to someone who has a visual and/or hearing loss.

Essential Primary Care, First Edition. Edited by Andrew Blythe and Jessica Buchan.
© 2017 John Wiley & Sons, Ltd. Published 2017 by John Wiley & Sons, Ltd.
Companion website: www.wileyessential.com/primarycare

Identifying people with visual problems

Visual loss becomes increasingly common with advancing age. In most cases, it is preventable or treatable. One in five people over the age of 75 in the UK lives with visual loss.[1] Alongside optometrists, GPs can play a key role in identifying people who are at risk of developing visual loss and can refer patients who have started to lose their sight for treatment. There are some conditions which demand immediate attention in order to prevent blindness, and GPs must be able to spot these.

People who have diabetes are at particular risk of losing their sight. Retinal screening, often done by optometrists within GP surgeries, is offered to everyone with diabetes on an annual basis. Patients with learning disabilities are much more likely to have sight problems than other people and may not realise that they have them, so the GP should encourage them to have regular eye tests.

Visual loss is a common cause of falls. It can cause social isolation and depression, and it can complicate the management of other chronic conditions, particularly when it comes to taking medication. People with visual loss often experience visual hallucinations – they may see birds, people or coloured patterns. This does not mean that they have any sort of mental illness. These hallucinations are referred to as 'Charles Bonnet syndrome' after the Swiss philosopher, who described the condition in his grandfather.

The simplest way of screening for visual loss is by asking the patient three questions:

1. 'Do you have any difficulty reading a book or newspaper?'
2. 'Have you fallen?'
3. 'When did you last have your eyesight checked?'

When seeing any elderly person, it is worthwhile asking these questions. If visual loss is suspected, further questioning and examination is necessary. Most GPs' equipment for examination of the eye is limited to a Snellen chart, pen torch, ophthalmoscope and fluorescein drops. What can a GP do with these things?

Snellen chart

The standard Snellen chart (see Figure 36.1) is designed to be read at a distance of 6 m and is used to record visual acuity, first in each eye individually and then with both eyes together. A result of 6/6 means that that the patient can read at 6 m what a person with normal eyesight can read at 6 m. A result of 6/12 means that the smallest line the patient can read at 6 m can be read by a normally sighted person at 12 m. Many GPs use modified Snellen charts that are designed to be read at 3 m. If the patient cannot read the lowest line of the Snellen chart, visual acuity can be recorded as the ability to count fingers, sense hand movements in front of the eye or just detect light.

The confrontation visual field test

The confrontation visual field test doesn't require any equipment and can be used to assess the outer boundaries of the patient's visual field in each eye. The doctor sits 1 m in front of the patient

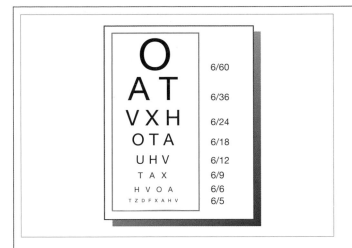

Figure 36.1 Snellen chart.

and asks the patient to cover one eye. The doctor covers their opposing eye and then moves one finger within a plane that is equidistant between the doctor and patient, bringing it from the point of furthest reach into the middle of each quadrant. The doctor asks the patient to identify when they first glimpse the finger moving into each quadrant. While doing this, the patient must keep looking straight ahead at the doctor's opposing eye. The confrontation field test can reveal a hemianopia, such as that caused by stroke. It is not sensitive enough to detect a scotoma – an area of visual loss within the visual field – which can develop as a result of glaucoma. Optometrists can map a person's visual field more accurately using an automated perimetry test, in which the person sits in front of a screen and presses a button each time they see a light flash anywhere in front of them.

Examining the eyelids

As a person ages, the muscles of their eyelids get weaker. Sometimes, the eyelid starts to turn inwards (an entropion) and the lashes brush against the cornea. Sometimes, the eyelid starts to turn outwards (an ectoprion), so that the tears are not contained and the person complains of a watery eye. In combination with either of these things, the eyelashes can become encrusted and matted and the conjunctivae can become inflamed (blepharoconjunctivitis). All of these changes can be seen with the light of a torch. A torch can also be used to inspect the everted eyelids to look for foreign bodies and to inspect the surface of the eye. Fluorescein drops can be used to reveal corneal abrasions and ulcers. These drops concentrate in areas of corneal damage and show up as luminescent green when viewed with a blue filter over the torch.

The ophthalmoscope

As well as inspecting the fundus, the ophthalmoscope can be used to view each part of the eye by adjusting the focal length of the lens. Cataracts, for instance, are visible as black silhouettes that obscure part or all of the red reflex. To make full use of the ophthalmoscope, we need to dilate the pupil. We should warn the patient that their vision will be blurred afterwards and they will not be able to drive home. An ophthalmoscope can reveal cupping of the optic disc (a feature of glaucoma) and areas of ischaemia, neovascularisation and haemorrhage, all of which cause visual loss.

> **Top tip**
>
> Always check the blood pressure and blood glucose of someone with visual loss. Hypertension is linked to many causes of visual loss, such as stroke and retinal vein occlusion. Diabetes is linked to glaucoma and cataracts, and can result in diabetic retinopathy.

Assisting people with visual loss

People can be certified as sight-impaired (partially sighted) or severely sight-impaired (blind) if their visual acuity and/or visual fields are below certain thresholds (see Table 36.1). Certification, which has to be done by an ophthalmologist, not a GP, entitles the patient to certain benefits, as well as access to a variety of visual aids.

Since visual loss is so common, almost every day a GP will conduct at least one consultation with a person who has poor eyesight. Consulting with someone who has a visual impairment requires extra care. The patient may not be able to recognise the GP's face, so the GP should introduce themselves. The patient may need assistance entering the room and finding the chair in the consulting room. The GP should describe the lay-out of the room to them and explain any equipment before using it. The patient may like to hold and feel the equipment (such as a peak flow meter) before it is used. When a management plan is agreed on, rather than writing down the key points (as for a fully sighted person), the GP might dictate something for the patient on their mobile phone. When writing a prescription, the GP can ask for the label to be printed in large font or in braille.

> **Top tips: guiding people with impaired sight**
>
> - Ask them if they want to hold your arm/shoulder.
> - If they have a guide dog, approach them from the side opposite the dog.
> - Say which way the door opens; make sure they are on the hinge side and open the door with your guiding arm.
> - Never back them into a seat; guide them to it, tell them if it has armrests, ask them to let go of your guiding arm and place their hand on the back of the seat.
> - Don't leave the room without telling them you are going.

Common causes of visual loss

Cataracts

If part of the lens becomes opaque, it is referred to as a 'cataract'. Depending on the position of the opacity within the lens, reading and recognising faces can be difficult, colours can seem duller, driving at night can be difficult because of glare and, when the sun is low in the sky, vision can be hazy. Smoking, diabetes, use of systemic steroids and exposure to ultraviolent light are all risk factors for the development of cataracts. Cataracts are the major cause of reversible sight loss, and they get more common with advancing age. Removing the cataract and replacing it with an artificial lens restores normal vision. In the UK[2] and other developed countries, cataract extraction is the most commonly performed operation. In developing countries, there is a huge unmet need for cataract extraction, which means that people are living unnecessarily with visual loss.

Only one eye is operated on at a time, because cataract extraction carries a tiny risk of losing all sight in the eye as a

Table 36.1 Certification of visual impairment.

	Visual acuity	Visual field
Sight-impaired (partially sighted)	3/60 to 6/60	Full
	Worse than 6/24	Moderate restriction
	Worse than 6/18	Large field defect
Severely sight-impaired (blind)	Worse than 3/60	Full
	3/60 to 6/60	Very contracted visual field
	Better than 6/60	Very constricted visual field

> **Case study 36.1**
>
> David Dallimore, age 74, wears spectacles to correct myopia. He sees his optician for an annual eye check and tells them that his vision has been a bit blurred recently. His optician detects bilateral cataracts (the left one being worse) and sends a report to his GP, Rachel Johnson, recommending referral to an ophthalmologist.
>
> Mr Dallimore is on warfarin for atrial fibrillation, amlodipine for hypertension and tamsulosin (an alpha

blocker) for benign prostatic hypertrophy. His wife has dementia. Dr Johnson is aware of all of this.

When Mr Dallimore comes to see her, what further assessment does Dr Johnson need to make before referring him to an ophthalmologist?
Simply having uni- or bilateral cataracts is not sufficient reason for having a cataract extraction. Dr Johnson needs to find out if the cataracts are affecting Mr Dallimore's functional capacity. Is his vision impeding his ability to care for his wife? Does he drive? Is he still able to read? Does he want an operation? Before deciding this, Mr Dallimore may want Dr Johnson to tell him what is involved in the operation. In particular, he may be anxious about leaving his wife for too long and may be worried about having to stay in hospital overnight.

The ophthalmologist will want to know if his blood pressure is under control and will need to know about all his medication, including how closely his international normalised ratio (INR) has been kept within the target range. If Mr Dallimore hasn't been checked for diabetes recently, Dr Johnson should request a fasting blood glucose test.

Outcome
Mr Dallimore says he is finding it difficult to read labels and he has problems with driving due to glare. This is significant because he needs to take his wife to a day centre twice a week and he has to drive to the supermarket. His blood pressure is 146/72 and his heart rate is 82 and irregular.

Dr Johnson explains that the operation is usually done as a day case under local anaesthetic. A tiny incision is made in the cornea, through which an instrument is inserted to emulsify and 'mash up' the lens (a process known as 'phaecoemulsification'), before the lens is sucked out of the capsule. The capsule is left in the cornea and acts as a casing for the new lens. After the operation, Mr Dallimore will have to apply steroid eye drops for 1 month. Mr Dallimore is relieved to hear that he will not have to stay in hospital overnight and decides that he would like to be referred.

Dr Johnson forwards the optician's report to the local ophthalmologist, together with a referral letter outlining the impact of Mr Dallimore's visual loss on his role as a carer and highlighting the fact that Mr Dallimore is on warfarin and tamsulosin. The latter is important because alpha blockers can cause intraoperative floppy iris syndrome, which makes surgery difficult.

Mr Dallimore has a phaecoemulsification of his left cataract and insertion of an intraocular lens 2 months later. He has the right cataract removed 6 months after that, and is able to resume driving.

result of infection (endophthalmitis), haemorrhage or retinal detachment. Endophthalmitis typically presents with pain, and sometimes loss of vision, a week or two after surgery. To reduce the chances of this happening, the surgeon injects the anterior chamber with antibiotics at the time of the operation.

A few years after a cataract extraction, the patient's vision can deteriorate again as the result of opacification of the posterior capsule. If this happens, the ophthalmologist can perform laser treatment.

Age-related macular degeneration

Macular degeneration accounts for over half of all the cases of preventable sight loss in the UK. It is often discovered late, but is something that can be picked up at an early stage by an optometrist. Macular degeneration makes it difficult for the sufferer to read and recognise faces. Patients may present to their optometrist or GP with sudden distortion of their central vision. Typically, patients see straight lines, like window- and doorframes, as curved. If a patient describes this, they should be referred urgently to an ophthalmologist.

The early stages of macular degeneration are characterised by the formation of Drusen bodies and focal depigmentation of the macula. The later stages are characterised by the growth of new blood vessels (neovascularisation), and it is this growth that causes visual distortion. Diagnosis is confirmed by fluorescein angiography. The causes of macular degeneration are not well understood, but there is a definite link with smoking, so this is yet another reason for GPs to give smoking-cessation advice. Vitamin supplements do not help prevent macular degeneration.

The treatment of neovascular macular degeneration has been revolutionised by the advent of monoclonal antibody therapy, which inhibits vascular endothelial growth factor. The drug has to be injected into the eye by an ophthalmologist. Patients usually need several injections. Good though this treatment is, one in five patients still ends up losing their sight.

Glaucoma

After age-related macular degeneration, glaucoma is the second most common cause of preventable sight loss in the UK. It runs in families and is very common, and its incidence increases with age, such that over the age of 75, 1 in 10 people has glaucoma. Unlike other common chronic conditions, such as chronic obstructive pulmonary disease (COPD), diabetes and hypertension, it is diagnosed and monitored in secondary, not primary care. This is because diagnosis requires expertise and equipment that most GPs do not have. The role of the GP is therefore limited to prescribing medication on the instructions of optometrists and ophthalmologists.

The commonest type of glaucoma is primary open-angle glaucoma, in which the outflow of aqueous fluid is impeded without any obstruction being visible. 'Primary' refers to the absence of other pathology. Secondary closed-angle glaucoma is the result of other pathology, such as rubeosis (the proliferation of blood vessels), causing visible obstruction. In both types of glaucoma, the rise in intraocular pressure (IOP) causes damage to the optic nerve head, which in turn causes patches of field loss, referred to as 'arcuate scotomas'. People may have several scotomas without being aware of them, because the good eye fills in the gaps. Thus, many patients present late in the course of the disease.

People who have a family history of glaucoma should visit an optometrist every year from the age of 40 to have their IOP measured and their fundi examined. There is some debate about what level of IOP should prompt further assessment. Most optometrists will request assessment by an ophthalmologist if the pressure is consistently above 21 mmHg. Sometimes, they refer the patient directly to an ophthalmologist; sometimes, they do so via the GP.

In order to make a diagnosis of glaucoma, an ophthalmologist considers five factors:

1. IOP, measured with a Goldman tonometer;
2. presence of visual field defects;
3. appearance of the optic discs, viewed with a stereoscopic slit lamp through a dilated pupil;
4. appearance of the peripheral anterior chamber, viewed with a gonioscope;
5. central corneal thickness.

Many people referred to an ophthalmologist because of raised IOPs turn out not to have glaucoma, but they do require ongoing observation because they are at increased risk of developing it.

If someone is diagnosed with primary open-angle glaucoma, their risk of developing visual loss can be reduced by lowering their IOP. Mostly, this is done with eye drops (see Table 36.2). Often, combinations of different eye drops are needed to achieve adequate control. This is a particular problem, because the people who are most likely to have glaucoma – the elderly – are those who are most likely to have difficulty applying drops, due to arthritic fingers, dementia and polypharmacy, not to mention visual loss.

The National Institute for Health and Care Excellence (NICE) recommends different thresholds of IOP for starting treatment, depending on age and central corneal thickness.[3] Prostaglandin-analogue drops are used first-line because they can be given once a day and are the most effective at reducing IOP. If two agents are needed, adherence can be improved by prescribing combination drops. Sometimes, patients are allergic to preservatives and require preservative-free preparations.

Conditions that require immediate action to prevent sight loss

There are several ophthalmic problems for which GPs must be particularly vigilant in order to prevent rapid sight loss.

Acute-angle closure glaucoma

Acute-angle closure glaucoma occurs when there is sudden obstruction of the aqueous humour from the anterior chamber of the eye, resulting in a rapid rise in IOP. It is more common in older people. It presents with pain in and around the eye, in association with blurriness of vision. It can also cause headache, vomiting and abdominal pain, and as a result it can be mistaken for many other diagnoses. Usually, the eye is red and the pupil is mid-dilated. Visual acuity is reduced. Acute-angle closure glaucoma is an emergency; the patient needs to be assessed by an ophthalmologist in order to prevent permanent sight loss. Management consists of constricting the pupil with drops (to increase the drainage angle) and reducing the IOP with acetazolamide, and sometimes surgery. Acute-angle closure can be precipitated by several drugs, notably anticholinergic drugs and selective serotonin reuptake inhibitors (SSRIs).

Anterior uveitis (iritis)

Another serious cause of an acutely painful red eye is inflammation of the iris (iritis), which is linked to several autoimmune conditions. The pain of iritis is usually worse in bright light. Without treatment, there is a risk of glaucoma or a cataract developing. Prompt treatment with topical steroids can prevent this. Sufferers of iritis can experience recurrent attacks, so they often have a good idea of what the diagnosis is before they see their GP. It can be tempting for the GP to oblige the patient by prescribing another course of steroid drops. However, the diagnosis of iritis cannot be confirmed without a slit lamp, and herpes simplex keratitis, which is made worse by

Table 36.2 Medication for lowering IOP in glaucoma.

Mode of action	Medication	Example	Notable side effects
Reduces production of aqueous humour	Beta blocker	Timolol	May make COPD and heart failure worse
	Carbonic anhydrase inhibitor	Brinzolamide	
Increases outflow of aqueous humour	Prostaglandin analogue	Latanoprost	Makes eyelashes grow
	Parasympathomimetic	Pilocarpine	
Both of the above	Alpha blocker	Brimonidine	

steroids, presents in much the same way. Overuse of topical steroids can also cause complications, including glaucoma. For both reasons, GPs should refer patients with suspected iritis to an ophthalmologist the same day.

It's important not to mistake acute iritis or acute-angle closure glaucoma for conjunctivitis. Patients with conjunctivitis can have a red eye, but they describe the affected eye as itchy or sore, not painful, and their visual acuity is not reduced. In iritis or glaucoma, the pupils may be of unequal size.

Flashes and floaters

After the age of 40, it is common for people to see occasional translucent shapes or shadows 'float' across their visual field as the result of ageing processes within the vitreous humour. The appearance of a new, large floater or an increase in the number of floaters can herald a posterior vitreous detachment (PVD) or a retinal detachment. In PVD, the vitreous gel that fills the orbit shrinks and separates from the retina. When the vitreous gel tugs at the retina, the patient can experience a flashing light. PVD does not cause sight loss. In contrast, retinal detachment does cause sight loss, because when the retina peels away from the choroid, it loses its vascular supply. Retinal detachment also causes flashing lights. The moment of detachment is often described by the patient as like a curtain or cobweb being drawn across their eye.

If a patient reports flashing lights, the GP must make an immediate assessment and refer the patient urgently to an ophthalmologist in order to ascertain whether there has been a PVD or a retinal detachment.

Retinal vein occlusion

The central retinal vein, or more commonly a branch of the retinal vein, can become occluded by a thrombus. This can occur at any age, and is more common in people with high blood pressure and those who smoke. A branch retinal vein occlusion presents with painless distortion and loss of vision in one eye. When presented with someone who has a suspected retinal vein occlusion, a GP should request that an ophthalmologist sees them the same day.

Assessing someone who complains of poor hearing

As we get older, our hearing deteriorates as a result of the death of sensitive hair cells in the cochlea. Our ability to hear high-pitched noises deteriorates first. Thus, age-related deafness is characterised by a bilateral high-frequency sensorineural hearing loss. GPs can assist older people with age-related hearing loss by referring them to an audiologist for confirmation of the diagnosis and fitting of a hearing aid. Age-related hearing loss is the most common cause of hearing loss. GPs also need to be on the lookout for other causes of hearing loss that require urgent or routine referral to an ear, nose and throat (ENT) specialist.

Table 36.3 lists the important and common causes of deafness. The first step in identifying the cause is taking a simple history. A sudden onset of hearing loss in one ear is worrying and should prompt an urgent referral. Fluctuating hearing loss, especially if associated with tinnitus or vertigo, suggests

Table 36.3 Causes of hearing loss.

	Prevalence and history	Examination and audiogram
Age-related	Extremely common Gradual onset	Bilateral sensorineural loss at high frequencies
Noise-related	History of exposure to loud noise Bilateral tinnitus	Bilateral sensorineural loss Dip at 4000 Hz
Meniere's	Episodes of vertigo and tinnitus in association with periods of hearing loss	Low-frequency sensorineural loss
Otosclerosis	Onset in early adulthood	Bilateral conductive loss
Accoustic neuroma	Unilateral loss +/− ipsilateral tinnitus	Unilateral sensorineural loss (Weber tests localise to contralateral ear)
Cholesteatoma	Smelly discharge Unilateral hearing loss +/− vertigo and tinnitus	Retraction pocket in tympanic membrane or 'aural polyp' (granulation tissue) Unilateral conductive loss
Pagets	Bone pain	Mixed conductive/sensorineural loss
Medication	Chemotherapy, aminoglycosides, high-dose furosemide, quinine, salicylates	Bilateral sensorineural loss
Nasopharyngeal tumour	Rare	Middle ear effusion Unilateral conductive loss

Meniere's disease. Otorrhoea raises the possibility of a cholesteatoma. Always ask what jobs the patient has done, whether they have been exposed to loud noise and if there is a family history of deafness. Find out what medicines they have taken; certain types of chemotherapy, salicylates, high doses of loop diuetics and aminoglycosides can all cause a sensorineural deafness.

Hearing tests

GPs have two simple tests by which to assess a patient's hearing: using their voice (the whisper test) and using a 512 Hz tuning fork (the Rinne and Weber tests).

The whisper test

The whisper test is as good as a portable audiometry in detecting hearing loss and can accurately pick up patients who have a hearing loss of 30 dB;[4] this is the degree of loss at which patients may gain benefit from a hearing aid.

To do the whisper test, the GP stands behind the patient (so that they can't lip-read) and occludes one ear by pressing on the tragus. In their quietest whisper, the GP says a combination of three letters and numbers (such as '6, C, 8') at arm's length from the other ear. One can produce one's quietest whisper by exhaling completely before speaking. The GP then asks the patient to repeat the triplet back to them. If they get the complete triplet correct, they have passed the test. If they get one or more letters/numbers wrong, the GP repeats the test with another triplet. If the patient cannot hear at least three out of the six letters and numbers correctly, they have failed the test and may have a hearing loss. This is the method described by Swann and Browning.[5] There are other methods, which vary by virtue of the number of digits whispered and the distance at which they are whispered.

The whisper test is a screening test for hearing loss, but it can be modified to gauge the level of hearing loss. To do this, we start with a normal spoken voice, then gradually make our voice quieter until the patient can no longer discern what letters and numbers we are saying.

Tuning-fork tests

If the whisper test reveals a hearing loss in one ear, the GP can use the tuning-fork tests to ascertain whether this loss is conductive or sensorineural. They should start with the Weber test: they hold the vibrating tuning fork on the centre of the patient's forehead and ask them where they hear the noise. If their hearing is normal, they will say the middle. If they hear it on the same side as the hearing loss then they have a conductive deafness. If they hear it on the opposite side then they have a sensorineural loss.

To do the Rinne test, the GP holds the vibrating tuning fork on the patient's mastoid process (position 1) and then a few centimetres in front of their external auditory meatus (position 2). They ask the patient in which position the noise

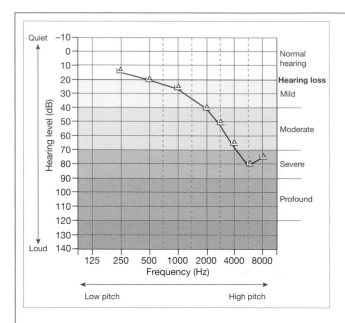

Figure 36.2 Audiogram showing age-related hearing loss in the right ear.

is loudest. If the patient has normal hearing, it will be louder in position 2, because air conduction is better than bone conduction. This is referred to as 'Rinne positive' (normal). If they have a conductive loss, such as otosclerosis, then it will be louder in position 1, because their bone conduction will be better ('Rinne negative').

Audiograms

The best way of assessing hearing is with an audiogram. Figure 36.2 shows an audiogram of someone who has a typical age-related hearing loss. The triangular symbols indicate the bone-conduction threshold in the right ear, while the corner symbols indicate the air-conduction thresholds: ∟ (right).

Wax and ear-syringing

Any hearing loss may be aggravated by a build-up of wax, which occludes the tympanic membrane and can cause a conductive hearing loss. Many patients consult their GP to request removal of earwax. It is not just the hearing loss that concerns them; it is also the feeling of blockage and discomfort. If the GP finds that the tympanic membrane is completely occluded by wax, they will normally recommend that the patient applies an earwax softener for anything from 1 to 2 weeks and then has the ear syringed by the practice nurse. Health professionals recommend all sorts of different wax softeners: olive oil, sodium bicarbonate and preparations sold over the counter. A systematic review[6] has shown that they are all equally effective. Sometimes, softening the wax, without syringing, provides adequate relief for the patient.

Ear-syringing is one of the most frequently performed procedures undertaken by practice nurses, but for many people the measurable improvement that it produces in their hearing is negligible. A randomised study undertaken in primary care showed that one-third of patients who had their ears syringed experienced a 10 dB or more improvement in their hearing, but two-thirds had no improvement.[7] Ear-syringing also carries risks. Patients can develop otitis externa after syringing. If the procedure is not done correctly, it can cause a perforation of the tympanic membrane. Most audiology clinics insist that patients are free of earwax before they attend.

ENT surgeons use microsuction, not syringing, to remove wax. Microsuction is safer, but most GP surgeries lack the necessary equipment.

Conducting a consultation with someone who has a hearing loss

Hearing loss is something we should consider in any consultation with an older person, not just when the presenting complaint is about an ear symptom. If we do not establish that the person in front of us has a hearing loss and fail to make suitable adjustments then the consultation is likely to be dysfunctional and frustrating for both parties. People don't mind being asked if they have any difficulty hearing. If they do have some difficulty, we should ask what form of extra help they need. They might just say that they want us to speak clearly, or they might say they have a hearing aid. Some people use lip-reading; others might request a sign interpreter.

A hearing aid amplifies all the noise that reaches the ear. This can be a problem if someone is trying to focus on a particular voice in a room with lots of background noise. To overcome this problem, we can use an induction loop. This consists of a microphone sited next to the person who is speaking and a device which converts the input into a signal that is transmitted from a wire loop via a magnetic field. Hearing aids have a special 'T' (telecoil) setting that enables them to detect this signal, thereby allowing the listener to hear the voice without

the background noise. The loop can be contained in a small portable box, or it can be fitted inconspicuously beneath a reception counter or desk. In cinemas and theatres, a loop can be installed around the perimeter of the whole auditorium.

Finally, remember that many older people have dual sensory loss: sight and hearing loss. When consulting with them, we need to take extra special care.

Top tips: consulting with someone who has a hearing loss

- Make sure the room is well lit and that there is as little background noise as possible (shut the window to block out traffic noise, switch off fans and printers).

- Face the patient whenever you are speaking to them. Remember to explain what you are doing before you examine them or turn to the computer. They won't hear you when you are standing behind them to listen to their chest.

- Try not to distort your words by speaking too slowly or by exaggerating your lip movements.

- Don't shout. It's uncomfortable for someone who has a hearing aid and it makes you look aggressive.

- Lip-reading is hard work. An expert lip-reader can only pick up half of the words they see spoken. If the patient doesn't pick up a word first time, it may be helpful to say it again. If they still can't understand, try rephrasing what you are saying.

- Write down key bits of information and words that may be unfamiliar, like the name of a disease or medication.

- If there is a sign interpreter, be sure to face and talk to the patient, not the interpreter.

- Above all, be patient and check that the patient has understood what you have said.

SUMMARY

At the start of a consultation, it may not be apparent that the patient has a visual or hearing loss. Unless we discover this and take precautions to facilitate communication, the consultation is likely to be dysfunctional. Hearing and visual problems are very common and can be identified using simple strategies. Visual problems may come to light using three questions: (1) 'Do you have any difficulty reading a book or newspaper?' (2) 'Have you fallen?' (3) 'When did you last have your eyesight checked?' The whisper test will identify most people who might benefit from a hearing aid. Early identification and treatment of the commonest visual problems can save a person's sight. GPs should encourage patients with diabetes to have retinal screening and should be alert to the conditions that demand an urgent referral to an ophthalmologist. By addressing the factors that increase cardiovascular risk, they can also improve eye health. Many patients are bothered by a build-up of earwax. Ear-syringing (a very common procedure in primary care) can improve the hearing in some of these patients.

 Now visit **www.wileyessential.com/primarycare** to test yourself on this chapter.

REFERENCES

1. Access Economics. Future Sight Loss UK 1: the economic impact of partial sight and blindness in the UK adult population. RNIB. 2009. Available from: http://www.rnib.org.uk/sites/default/files/FSUK_Report.pdf (last accessed 6 October 2015).

2. HESonline. Main procedures and interventions: 2000–2008. Available from: http://www.hscic.gov.uk/hes (last accessed 6 October 2015).

3. NICE. Glaucoma: diagnosis and management of chronic open angle glaucoma and ocular hypertension. NICE Clinical Guideline 85. April 2009. Available from: http://www.nice.org.uk/guidance/cg85 (last accessed 6 October 2015).

4. Pirozzo S, Pinczak, Glasziou P. Whispered voice test for screening for hearing impairment in adults and children: systematic review *BMJ* 2003;**327**:967.

5. Swan IR, Browning GG. The whispered voice as a screening test for hearing impairment. *Br J Gen Pract* 1985;**35**:197.

6. Loveman E, Gospodarevskaya E, Clegg A, et al. Ear wax removal interventions: a systematic review and economic evaluation. *Br J Gen Pract* 2011;**61**(591):e680–3.

7. Memel D, Langley C, Watkins C, et al. Effectiveness of ear syringing in general practice: a randomised controlled trial and patients' experiences. *Br J Gen Pract* 2002;**52**:906–11.

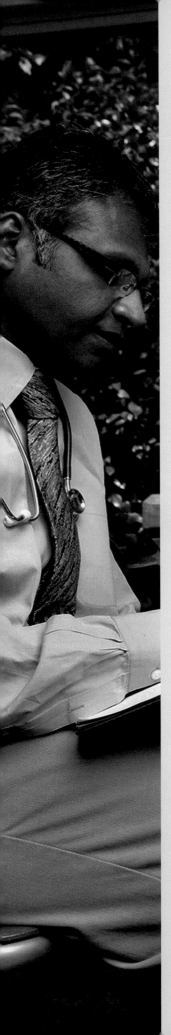

CHAPTER 37
Dementia

Andrew Blythe
GP and Senior Teaching Fellow, University of Bristol

Key topics

Learning objectives

- Be able to conduct an assessment of someone's cognitive function.
- Be able to describe the features that help to distinguish between the different types of dementia.
- Be able to offer support and advice to the carer of someone who has dementia.

Essential Primary Care, First Edition. Edited by Andrew Blythe and Jessica Buchan.
© 2017 John Wiley & Sons, Ltd. Published 2017 by John Wiley & Sons, Ltd.
Companion website: www.wileyessential.com/primarycare

Diagnosing dementia

Our memories define us, so the thought of losing our memory is a frightening one. Dementia is common, and is becoming more common as people live longer. Approximately 700 000 people in the UK have dementia.[1] Most of us know someone in our family who has dementia.

What is dementia?

Dementia is more than just memory loss. It is a long-term progressive condition which affects the sufferer's cognitive (thinking) skills and their ability to perform everyday tasks. People with dementia find it difficult to plan and execute tasks; they may have difficulty finding their way around and they may find it difficult to operate gadgets. They have difficulty remembering conversations and friends, and as a result, their ability to interact with others is diminished. Their behaviour changes, too, but consciousness is preserved. In the late stages of the disease, people with dementia become increasingly immobile, and they may become incontinent.

Studies of GP computer records in the UK suggest that the annual incidence of dementia rises from 0.5 per 1000 in those aged 60–69 to 12 per 1000 in those aged 80–89, but other studies have shown that the true annual incidence is three times greater than this in each age group.[2,3] Why are GPs not diagnosing more cases? Perhaps it's because GPs do not feel confident about diagnosing dementia. Alternatively, it may be that they are reluctant to diagnose or record it for fear of causing distress to the patient and their family. A lot of stigma has been attached to dementia, and there are two commonly held false beliefs: that it's a normal part of ageing and that nothing can be done about it.

While the risk of developing dementia certainly does increase with age, it is not inevitable, and there is increasing evidence that there are interventions which can help to prevent or slow the progression of dementia. Stopping smoking and treating cardiovascular disease (CVD) can help; if it is diagnosed early, patients can be kept in their own home with an appropriate package of care and support; and cholinesterase inhibitors can slow the progression of Alzheimer's disease.

There is a national initiative to increase the detection rate of dementia in the UK and to diagnose it earlier in primary care. GPs are being encouraged to ask people if they would like to be tested for dementia, and patients who are concerned about their memory are being encouraged to consult their GP. This creates a challenge, because it turns out that being concerned about your memory is not a good predictor of whether or not you develop dementia.[4]

What tests should a GP do to screen for dementia?

GPs need a quick test that they can incorporate easily into their consultations. One such test that is growing in use is the General Practitioner assessment of Cognition (GPCOG), which was devised in Australia.[5] The GPCOG has two parts: the patient interview and the informant interview (see Box 37.1). The informant is normally the partner or a friend who knows the patient well. A score of 4 or less out of 9 on the patient interview indicates cognitive impairment, as does a score of 3 or less out of 6 on the informant interview. Informants tend to be better at spotting the symptoms of dementia than the patient themselves.

Box 37.1 GPCOG

Patient interview
- 'I'm going to give you a name and address: John Brown, 42 West Street, Kensington. Can you repeat that for me? Then remember it, because I'm going to ask you to repeat it later.'
- 'What is the date?' – day, month and year (1 point if correct)
- 'Please draw all the numbers around the clockface' (1 point if correct). 'Now put on the hands to show the time as ten past eleven' (1 point if correct)
- 'Can you tell me something that's in the news at the moment?' (1 point if correct)
- 'Can you repeat that address I asked you to remember?' (maximum of 5 points if correct)

Informant interview
These six questions relate to how the patient is now, compared to 5–10 years ago:

1. 'Do they have more difficulty remembering things that happened recently?'
2. 'Do they have more difficulty remembering conversations from a few days ago?'
3. 'When talking, do they have more difficulty finding the right word?'
4. 'Do they need assistance managing money and their financial affairs?'
5. 'Do they need assistance remembering to take their medication?'
6. 'Do they need assistance using transport?'

Each of these questions earns 1 point if the answer is 'no', so a score of 6 means the person has not got a problem.

Official website for GPCOG: http://www.gpcog.com.au/info.php.

Even quicker than the GPCOG is the mini-COG.[6] This consists of asking the patient to remember just three words and, between telling them the words and asking them to recall them, asking them to draw a clockface. This takes just 3 minutes. The patient's ability to draw a clockface and indicate the time on it is a particularly informative part of these two tests. Figure 37.1 shows an attempt by a patient with dementia to draw a clockface showing the time at half past four.

The longer and best known test of cognitive function is the Mini-Mental State Examination (MMSE), also known as the Folstein test. This has been used for long time both in general practice and in hospitals, but it is now under patent, and as a result many clinicians in the UK have started using other tests, such as the Montreal Cognitive Assessment (MoCA) or the Addenbrooke's Cognitive Examination (ACE)-III. The value of all three of these tests is that they have subsections which test different aspects of cognitive function, such as orientation, attention, language, visuospatial memory, execution, registration and recall. The total scores of the MMSE, MOCA and ACE-III provide a rough gauge for describing the severity of someone's dementia, and they are useful for monitoring the progression of dementia. However, a lot of information comes from the way in which patients answer each question, so it is important to record each answer in full, not just note it as being correct or incorrect. The disadvantage of these tests is that they take much more time to complete than the GPCOG, so they are not so useful as screening tests in primary care. Table 37.1 compares the different tests. All of them need to be interpreted in the light of the individual's baseline IQ and level of functioning. For instance, someone who has never been able to read very well or do mental arithmetic may never have been able to score full marks, whereas for someone who used to be a barrister, a loss of any point on the MMSE may be significant.

It is often difficult to differentiate dementia from depression. We can get some clues from the way in which a patient answers the questions in the MMSE. If we ask someone with depression to spell the word 'WORLD' backwards or to copy a diagram, they may say, 'I can't do that', but then, with a bit of encouragement, and given time, be able to do it accurately.

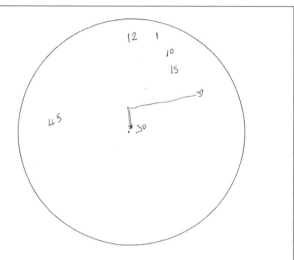

Figure 37.1 Attempt by a patient to draw a clockface showing the time at half past four.

Table 37.1 Comparison of different tests of cognitive function.

Test	Components	Score out of
Mini-COG	Ask patient to repeat and remember three words Ask them to put the numbers on a clockface then draw the time Ask them to recall the three words • Negative (normal) if all three words are correct or if one or two words are correct and the clockface is accurate • Positive (impairment) if no words are correct or if one or two words are correct and the clockface is inaccurate	3
GPCOG	Patient interview • Negative if >4	9
	Informant interview • Negative if >3	6
MMSE	Subsections on orientation/attention, language, visuospatial abilities, registration and recall • Negative if >26	30
MoCA	Subsections on visuospatial abilities, memory, language, attention, abstraction, delayed recall and orientation • Negative if ≥26	30
ACE-III	Subsections on attention, memory, fluency, language and visuospatial abilities	100

Source: Brodaty, H et al. *J Am Geriatr Soc* 2002; **50**: 530–4. Reproduced with permission of John Wiley & Sons.

Case study 37.1a

Mrs Miller is 77 and is well known to Dr Coulson. She has glaucoma and osteoarthritis, she had a myocardial infarction 9 years ago and she had her left knee replaced last year. She takes paracetamol, an angiotensin-converting enzyme (ACE) inhibitor, a statin, aspirin, a beta blocker and travoprost eye drops. She used to be a heavy smoker, but she stopped immediately after her myocardial infarction. Her husband died a year ago from bladder cancer and she lives alone now.

She has come to see Dr Coulson today for a review of her medication. Dr Coulson notices that she failed to attend her last appointment at the eye hospital for a review of her glaucoma, so this has been rescheduled. Also, he notes that she has not been requesting her repeat medication as often as she should and asks if she is still taking it regularly. 'I forget sometimes', she says. 'I've not been keeping on top of things since John died.'

What should Dr Coulson do next?

He should ask what problems Mrs Miller's memory is causing her and ask if anyone else has commented on this. It may be that friends and family have expressed concern, or it may be that she has just had the occasional lapse of memory that we are all prone to from time to time.

He should find out how she is functioning. Is she still able to do things about the house? How often does she get out of the house and how does she get around? Is she doing the shopping, and is she able to manage her finances? Is she maintaining contact with friends and family?

He should ask about mood. Her forgetfulness may be a manifestation of depression. The self-deprecating manner in which she describes her inability to 'keep on top of things' hints at depression. He should ask her about sleeping pattern and appetite, and consider doing a Patient Health Questionnaire-9 (PHQ-9).

To assess her cognitive function further, he could conduct the patient interview section of the GPCOG or the MMSE.

He should request some routine blood tests to look for reversible causes of memory loss: thyroid function tests (TFTs) (to look for hypothyroidism), serum B12 (to check for deficiency), serum urea and electrolytes (U&Es) (mainly to check for hyponatraemia), a full blood count (FBC) and liver function tests (LFTs) (to look for evidence of alcohol misuse).

Outcome

Mrs Miller says she has been concerned about her memory for about a year. She used to be a school teacher, and prided herself on her memory. Now, she has to rely on lists. Sometimes she feels a bit down about this, and a couple of times she has forgotten where she has parked her car. She does her own housework and cooking, and keeps in touch with a couple of close friends and her daughter, who visits twice a week and helps with the heavy shopping.

She scores 28/30 on the MMSE. She loses 1 point for getting the date wrong (she knows the day, month, year and season) and loses 1 point for failing to remember one of three words. She is able to put the numbers round a clockface accurately, but slowly, and is able to represent the time as asked. On the PHQ-9, she scores 12/27, indicating mild to moderate depression.

All the blood tests are normal. When she returns to see Dr Coulson to get the results, he concludes that does not have dementia, but thinks she may have mild depression. He suggests that she attend a club for people who have suffered bereavement or try a course of antidepressants, but she declines both of these. He offers to prescribe her medication weekly so that the chemist can dispense it in a dosette box; she thinks this is a good idea. Dr Coulson also advises her not to drive, because her poor short-term memory puts her at much greater risk of having an accident. Finally, he suggests that they review the situation together in 3 months.

Someone who comes to their GP to talk about their memory is less likely to have dementia (and more likely to be suffering from depression) than someone whose relative is expressing concern about their memory. This is a generalisation, though. Sometimes, the GP is really not sure whether it is depression or early dementia, and in this situation a trial of antidepressants can be helpful.

The other mimic of dementia is delirium, also known as an 'acute confusional state'. Like dementia, delirium causes problems with memory, loss of language skills and difficulty executing tasks. But the cardinal features of delirium, which make it different from dementia, are its rapid onset (over hours), the patient's clouded consciousness and the patient's inability to focus and concentrate. It may present with someone behaving oddly, talking incoherently or becoming agitated at home. If there is no history of memory impairment or no previous suspicion of dementia then it is prudent to assume that the patient has delirium and begin an urgent search for a cause, of which there are many (see Table 37.2). This investigation often has to be done in hospital. Sometimes, delirium is superimposed on dementia. For instance, it is common for patients with dementia to develop a urinary tract infection (UTI), which results in a rapid worsening of their mental state.

Box 37.2 lists some of the important questions that we should ask when considering a diagnosis of dementia. Making a diagnosis of dementia takes a long time (in the order of months). Clues come from repeated visits to the GP surgery, backed up by the observations of other support workers and family.

Table 37.2 Causes of delirium.

Cause	Example	Investigation
Infection	Urinary tract infection (UTI), pneumonia	Midstream urine microscopy, culture and sensitivity (MC&S), chest X-ray
Pain	Back pain	X-ray or magnetic resonance imaging (MRI) of the spine and blood tests
Hypoxia	Pulmonary embolus	D-dimer, computed tomography (CT) pulmonary angiogram
Electrolyte imbalance	Hyponatraemia	Serum U&Es
Drugs	Anticholinergic drugs, opiates	Collateral history
Drug and alcohol withdrawal	Withdrawal from benzodiazepine	
Liver failure	Hepatic encephalopathy	LFTs
Brain injury	Subdural haematoma, stroke	CT of head
Urinary retention		Bedside scan

Box 37.2 Important questions to ask when considering a diagnosis of dementia

- How long has this been going on?
- What was the first symptom?
- Does the patient have any difficulty finding words?
- Has there been any change in their personality?
- Have they experienced hallucinations?
- Have they become less mobile?
- Are they depressed?
- Are they taking any anticholinergic drugs?
- Are they drinking alcohol to excess or taking illegal drugs?

Case study 37.1b

It is 6 months since Mrs Miller's last visit to the GP surgery. Today, she is accompanied by her daughter, Jane.

Dr Coulson invites Mrs Miller to sit next to him and moves another chair from the side of the room for Jane. Dr Coulson looks at Mrs Miller first, to ask how he can help. Before she can answer, Jane says, 'I'm a bit worried about mum's memory. I'm always having to remind her to do things. I've asked her to mention it to you before but I'm not sure if she has, so that's why I've come today…I hope that's ok. My aunt (my mum's older sister) was diagnosed with Alzheimer's 3 years ago. I'm not sure if she's told you that.' Dr Coulson hadn't been aware of this last bit of information and feels a bit guilty for not establishing this earlier. He turns to Mrs Miller again. Her face doesn't convey much emotion. He asks her what she's worried about, and slowly she starts talking.

What information should Dr Coulson collect during this consultation?

This is an excellent opportunity to reassess the situation and get a good collateral history from the daughter.

Depression is still a possibility, but dementia is looking more likely.

Dr Coulson should find out how much help Mrs Miller needs now with everyday tasks.

With her osteoarthritis in mind, he should ask if she is in pain (maybe her other knee is painful now) and enquire what painkillers she is taking. Has there been any deterioration in her mobility?

Has Jane noticed any change in her mother's personality or any evidence that she is hallucinating?

With Mrs Miller's permission, Dr Coulson should conduct a full GPCOG or repeat the MMSE.

Outcome

Mrs Miller says she is managing ok, but she appears to lack insight, because Jane reports that she is having difficulty sorting out her bills and rarely cooks for herself now. She has stopped driving her car (a good thing), and Jane does all her shopping. Sometimes, she phones Jane several times during the day to check various minor things. She still gets herself washed and dressed, and walks normally. She denies having any joints pains. She says she doesn't feel down, but she comes across as rather flat and her speech is slow. There is no evidence that she's experiencing hallucinations, and she denies drinking more than the occasional glass of wine.

She scores 24 out of 30 on the MMSE: 6/10 for orientation, 3/3 for registration, 1/3 for recall, 5/5 for

attention and 9/9 for language. She has some difficulty with putting the numbers on the clockface: rather than beginning with 12, 3, 6 and 9 around the circle, she bunches up the numbers, then realises they need spacing out.

The length of her symptoms, her family history of Alzheimer's disease, her loss of function, her apparent lack of insight and her deteriorating score on the MMSE in the domains of recall and orientation all point towards a diagnosis of dementia.

Finding the cause of dementia

Although it is unlikely that a reversible cause will be found for a patient's dementia, it is always important to do some routine blood tests to check for one. The important tests are listed in Table 37.3. When neurosyphilis was more common, the standard battery of tests used to include a venereal disease research laboratory (VDRL) test. Today, it's worth thinking about doing a human immunodeficiency virus (HIV) test in a younger person with dementia or in someone in a high-risk group. It's probably useful to check the serum cholesterol, too, because if it turns out the patient has vascular dementia, we might want to optimise their cholesterol level.

If all the blood tests are normal, the next step is to request a computed tomography (CT) scan of the head with coronal views. Together with the history and the results of any cognitive tests, the appearance on the CT scan can assist us in diagnosing the type of dementia.

Most cases of dementia are of the Alzheimer's type or have mixed aetiology (Alzheimer's and vascular dementia). The next most common types are Lewy-body dementia and pure vascular dementia. Frontotemporal dementia accounts for about 5% of cases. Then there are several rare causes, including Creutzfeldt–Jakob disease (CJD) and HIV. It's important to try to find out what type of dementia the patient has, because each has a different natural history (this should be explained to the patient and their carers) and each is treated differently.

Alzheimer's-type dementia

Typically, in Alzheimer's dementia, the first reported symptom is memory loss. Then the patient loses insight and their level of functioning gradually deteriorates. A CT scan shows atrophy and shrinkage of the hippocampus and medial temporal structures.

Vascular dementia

People with vascular dementia usually have other evidence of CVD, such as hypertension or ischaemic heart disease, or maybe a stroke. In contrast to patients with Alzheimer's dementia, those with vascular dementia display a stepwise deterioration in their function, which may be the result of new cerebral infarcts. Loss of executive function tends to predominate. They can recall facts when they are prompted, and their personality tends to be preserved. A CT scan shows lacunar infarcts, white-matter ischaemia, leukoencephalopahty and cerebral small vessel disease.

Table 37.3 Blood tests that should be done to exclude reversible causes of memory loss.

Cause	Test
Pernicious anaemia	FBC, serum B12 and folate levels
Acute renal failure Hyponatraemia	Serum U&Es
Jaundice	Serum bilirubin
Hypercalcaemia	Serum calcium
Hypothyroidism	TFTs
Diabetes	Plasma glucose

Lewy-body dementia

People with Lewy-body dementia demonstrate a marked variability in their mental state and level of alertness from day to day. They may experience visual hallucinations, and they have Parkinsonian features: notably, stiffness and slowness of movement, which makes them less mobile. There are no characteristic features on a CT scan. A special single-photon-emission computed tomography (SPECT) scan used with a radioactive iodine isotope (known as a DaTscan) can be useful in making the diagnosis, but this is only available in specialist clinics.

Frontotemporal dementia (Pick's disease)

If behavioural or personality changes are the dominant feature then we should consider the possibility of frontotemporal dementia. This tends to start at an earlier age than Alzheimer's. The change in behaviour may be quite dramatic; the patient might make a sudden decision to give all their money to charity, or switch from being placid to outspoken and start making rude or racist remarks. A CT scan may show frontal and temporal atrophy, but to differentiate frontotemporal dementia from Alzheimer's it is sometimes necessary to do a SPECT scan.

As the incidence of dementia rises, new pathways are being developed for coping with the need to investigate more people. A decade ago, most GPs would refer a patient to a specialist memory clinic after doing some blood tests. Now that many GPs can request CT scans, there is pressure on GPs to take on the whole diagnostic phase. With a typical history, the results of cognitive tests and a characteristic appearance on CT scan, a

GP is in a position to confirm a diagnosis of Alzheimer's or vascular dementia. However, if a GP is not certain about the diagnosis or suspects a rarer cause of dementia (including Lewy-body and frontotemporal dementia), they should refer the patient to a specialist clinic. Anyone who develops dementia before the age of 65 or who demonstrates a rapid decline also needs specialist investigation. GPs who do not have direct access to CT still need to refer all patients to a specialist clinic.

Giving the diagnosis

Once the diagnosis of dementia is confirmed, this news has to be explained carefully and sensitively to the patient and their family. A diagnosis of dementia is just as devastating as a diagnosis of cancer. Everyone needs time to absorb the information. In the first days and weeks after the diagnosis, the carers will turn to the GP for advice and support.

When giving a new diagnosis of dementia, many GPs give information packs to the patient and their carers, listing the contact details of all the various agencies that might be useful. These include:

- The Alzheimer's Society.
- Adult social services: to make an assessment and provide support at home.
- Admiral nurse: a mental health nurse who specialises in caring for people with dementia.
- Age UK: a charity that provides financial and legal advice.
- Day-care centres for people with dementia.
- Local clubs for people with dementia, where the emphasis is on activity, such as singing or exercise.

Creating a power of attorney and a will

One of the benefits of making an early diagnosis of dementia is that it gives the patient time to make plans for their future while they still have the ability to consider it. They can create an advance directive, in which they make clear how they would like to be treated in the event that their health deteriorates to such an extent that they can no longer make or communicate decisions. They can also make a will, and they can appoint one or more people to be their attorney(s). In England and Wales, there are two forms

---

> **Top tip: assessing capacity to make a decision**
>
> Under the Mental Capacity Act,[7] there are four aspects that the GP has to consider when deciding if a patient has the capacity to make a decision:
> - Can the patient understand the information that they need to make this decision?
> - Can they retain this information long enough to make the decision?
> - Can they weigh up this information in order to make the decision?
> - Can they communicate their decision?

---

that they can complete: one to give lasting power of attorney for decisions about their health and welfare and one to give lasting power of attorney for decisions about their property and financial affairs. Usually, the patient will decide to give power of attorney to their partner and/or their children. The GP or another health professional has to sign the forms to confirm that the patient has the mental capacity to bestow each power of attorney.

Once the forms are signed, they have to be registered with the Office of the Public Guardian (OPG). A lasting power of attorney for property and financial affairs can be used as soon as it is registered, but a lasting power of attorney for health and welfare can only be used once a patient is no longer able to make their own decisions.

Supporting the family and carers of those with dementia

Being a carer for someone who has dementia is an exhausting and, at times, frustrating responsibility. The GP can ease this burden by giving advice to the carer, by ensuring they get support and by making sure that the carer's own health is not neglected. Carers are often elderly and have their own chronic illnesses. They may be registered with the same GP. In this situation, the GP should consider creating longer appointments when the patient with dementia comes to the surgery with their carer so that there is time to address the health needs of both. If the GP has to visit the patient at home, this may be a good opportunity to check up on the health of their carer too.

The carer may worry what will happen to the patient in the event that they, the carer, have to be admitted to hospital. To allay this worry, the GP can recommend that they carry a Carer's Emergency Card in their wallet. This card alerts the emergency services to the fact they are a carer. Ringing the telephone number on the card activates a contingency plan for looking after the person with dementia.

It is important for the carer to have breaks. Sometimes, other family members can take over for a short time. If not, then social services might help to arrange an admission to a residential home in order to provide some respite.

All carers are entitled to a carer assessment conducted by their local authority. This gives them access to a pot of money, which they can use as they see fit to pay for equipment or for help at home. The carer and the patient may also be eligible for certain state benefits, such as the carer's allowance and attendance allowance. These benefits may make it possible to employ someone else to do the caring for a few hours each week. There are several voluntary agencies (national and local) which can provide practical support, too.

Creating the right environment at home

One of the challenges of caring for someone who has dementia is keeping them safe in their own home. They may wander or fall. It's helpful to remove things on which they might slip (such as rugs), make sure they have good lighting and provide a night light in the bedroom and toilet. If they do wander outside, it's useful for them to have an identity bracelet. Removing clutter about the house makes things less confusing for them. Putting labels on cupboards and drawers can help them find things. Sometimes, people with dementia no longer recognise their own face and are frightened when they see their reflection in a mirror; it can be worthwhile putting a roller blind over the mirror. People with dementia often need regular reassurance, and they can benefit from having a routine. They may find family photos and scrapbooks comforting. Music can help, too.

Even if the carer follows all this advice, the person they are caring for can still become agitated or even aggressive, sometimes with little warning.

Medication for dementia

There is a limited but increasing role for medication in treating patients with certain types of dementia.

Cholinesterase inhibitors

People with Alzheimer's disease have a deficiency of the neurotransmitter acetylcholine. This contributes to their loss of memory, because it impedes neurotransmission in the hippocampus and limbic structures within the temporal lobe. Cholinesterase inhibitors work by boosting the level of acetylcholine. They are useful for people with Alzheimer's or mixed Alzheimer's/vascular dementia who have an MMSE score under 25; someone with a high premorbid IQ might benefit from cholinesterase inhibitors even if their score is 25 or more.

At the time of writing, there are three cholinesterase inhibitors in use in the UK: donepezil and galantamine, which both come in tablet form, and rivastigmine, which comes as a patch. They can all cause a bradycardia and should be used with caution in someone who has sick-sinus syndrome, asthma, chronic obstructive pulmonary disease (COPD) or a history of peptic ulcers. If the patient has heart disease, a baseline electrocardiogram (ECG) should be requested to look for conduction defects before one of these drugs is started.

If someone is started on a cholinesterase inhibitor, they should be monitored regularly and should have cognitive testing at regular intervals. If their score on cognitive testing improves or if there is an improvement in function then it is worth continuing.

If the patient is on an anticholinergic drug (see Table 37.4), the dose should be lowered or the drug should be stopped, because it will work in the opposite direction to the cholinesterase inhibitor and it is very likely to be contributing to the patient's dementia.

NMDA-type receptor antagonists

N-methyl-D-aspartate (NMDA)-type receptor antagonists such as memantine are an alternative to cholinesterase inhibitors. They are useful in treating patients with advanced Alzheimer's disease, especially those who have behavioural problems.

Table 37.4 Anticholinergic drugs.	
Drug	**Indication**
Amitriptyline	Adjunct to pain relief
Ipratropium bromide (inhaler)	COPD
Oxybutynin and trospium	Irritable bladder/ urge incontinence
Paroxetine	Anxiety/depression
Risperidone	Psychosis

Secondary prevention of CVD

For patients who have vascular dementia or mixed Alzheimer's-type/vascular dementia, it would seem sensible to reduce their overall risk of CVD by reducing their blood pressure and cholesterol. However, in someone with advanced dementia who is on many different medicines, the benefits of taking a statin may be marginal.

Antipsychotic medication

Antipsychotic medication used to be prescribed to control behavioural problems in people with dementia. However, these drugs increase the risk of stroke, so they should no longer be prescribed for this purpose.[8] If medication is needed then a small dose of a short-acting benzodiazepine, such as lorazepam, can be helpful.

Monitoring patients with dementia

GPs have responsibility for monitoring their patients with dementia. This means monitoring all aspects of their health and reviewing their medication. A review is also an opportunity to find out about the particular concerns of the patient and their carer. Table 37.5 lists the things that need to be checked. Action taken as a result of the review may prevent the development of a crisis, such as a fall or an emergency admission.

The median survival of patients diagnosed with dementia is less than that of people without dementia.[3] It depends on the age at diagnosis: the median survival of people diagnosed with dementia in their 60s is 6.7 years, whereas that of people diagnosed at the age of 90 or older is 1.9 years. Mortality rate peaks in the first year following the diagnosis of dementia, reaching three times that of other people of the same age. This may be because some patients present at a time of crisis, relatively late in the progression of the disease.[3]

As dementia progresses, the physical manifestations become more apparent. The person's mobility declines, they can become incontinent and they develop upward plantar reflexes (Babinski sign) and other primitive reflexes. Ultimately, they can become bedbound and require full nursing care, but the aim should always be to support the patient in their own home for as long as possible.

Table 37.5 Components of an annual review of someone with dementia.

Component		Action that might be necessary
Update from patient and carer	Memory change	Review medication and/or package of care
	Function: are there things they can no longer do?	Refer to occupational therapy and/or social services
	Mood	Start antidepressant
	Behaviour	Refer to mental health team (psychiatrist)
	Wandering	Ensure patient has got an identity bracelet
	Appetite	Review diet
	Sleep	Review bedtime routine
	Continence	Refer to continence advisor
General health	Falls	Examine feet Check balance, gait and sensation. Refer to occupational therapist and physiotherapist Refer to podiatrist
	Hospital admissions	Alert out-of-hours GP service Review admission avoidance plan
	Hearing and vision: impairment of either sense may compound problems of dementia	Refer to audiology for hearing aid Refer to optician/ophthalmologist
	Other chronic diseases	
Medication	Adherence with dementia medication	Provide compliance aid, e.g. dosette box
	Side effects	Reduce dose/stop
	Medicines that can be stopped	Keep total number of medicines to a minimum
Examination	Repeat cognitive assessment (MMSE)	
	Pulse	Stop anticholinesterase, if too slow
	Blood pressure	Prescribe antihypertensive
	Weight	Prescribe fortified drinks if body mass index (BMI) low Recommend exercise classes if BMI high
Review support for carer	Benefits	
	Power of attorney	
	Carer's Emergency Card	
	Help from social services	
	Help from voluntary agencies	
	Carer's mental and physical health	Make appointment with carer's own GP

Case study 37.1c

Mrs Miller's history and performance on the MMSE suggest that she has dementia. No treatable cause is identified by the routine blood tests. Her CT scan shows extensive low-attenuation white matter, consistent with severe small vessel ischaemic changes. In addition, it reveals small lacunar infarcts within the lentiform nuclei. These findings are consistent with vascular dementia. There is some cerebral volume loss, with more focal volume loss within the hippocampus on the left. This latter finding is consistent with early Alzheimer's disease.

Dr Coulson concludes that she has a mixed vascular and Alzheimer's dementia. Remember, her sister was diagnosed with Alzheimer's disease 3 years ago. After obtaining an ECG, which shows normal sinus rhythm, Dr Coulson decides to start her on donepezil (an anticholinesterase) to treat the Alzheimer's component. She is already on full secondary prevention for CVD because of her myocardial infarction.

Following advice from Dr Coulson, Mrs Miller's daughter, Jane, registers as her carer and obtains a Carer's

Emergency Card. Jane also helps her mother to apply for both lasting powers of attorney.

When Dr Coulson reviews her 6 weeks later, neither Mrs Miller nor her daughter has noticed much change in her memory, but Mrs Miller has started going to an exercise class once a week and has started to meet up with one of her old friends for coffee. Her score on the MMSE has improved; it is now 26 out of 30. Her pulse is 58 (not too slow), so Dr Coulson increases the dose of donepezil to the full treatment dose.

After 6 months on donepezil, Mrs Miller's MMSE has risen to 27. After 18 months on treatment, her level of function is much the same and her MMSE is still 27, but she spends more time sleeping and she doesn't walk as far. She goes to a day centre once a week, and Jane calls in every evening after coming home from work to help prepare a meal and check that she has taken her tablets. Jane and her mother have talked about what they will do if the dementia gets worse. In the first instance, Mrs Miller will move in to live with Jane and Jane will reduce her hours of work.

SUMMARY

Dementia is more than just memory loss. It is a long-term progressive condition which affects the sufferer's cognitive skills and their ability to perform everyday tasks. GPs can use a variety of cognitive tests to assist them in making a diagnosis. The different types of dementia (Alzheimer's, vascular, mixed, Lewy-body and frontotemporal dementia) can be identified by the pattern of cognitive and behaviour changes, together with the appearance on CT scan. Reversible causes of dementia should always be excluded by performing blood tests. Delirium can be mistaken for dementia, but it differs in that it has a rapid onset and causes clouding of consciousness. Depression is another mimic of dementia; if there is doubt, a trial of antidepressants can be helpful. Cholinesterase inhibitors offer some hope for people with dementia, but what people with dementia and their carers need more is information from their GP and advice about where to get practical support. In the early stages of dementia, it is helpful to make a lasting power of attorney and write an advanced directive.

Now visit **www.wileyessential.com/primarycare** to test yourself on this chapter.

REFERENCES

1. Department of Health. *Living Well With Dementia: A National Dementia Strategy*. London: HMSO; 2009.

2. Rait G, Walters K, Bottomley C, et al. Survival of people with clinical diagnosis of dementia: cohort study. *BMJ* 2010;**341**:c3584.

3. Matthews F, Brayne C, Medical Research Council Cognitive Function and Ageing Study Investigators. The incidence of dementia in England and Wales: findings from the five identical sites of the MRC CFA study. *PLoS Med* 2005;**2**:e193.

4. Iliffe S, Pealing L. Subjective memory problems. *BMJ* 2010;**340**:c1425.

5. Brodaty H, Pond D, Kemp N, et al. The GPCOG: a new screening test for dementia designed for general practice. *J Am Geriatr Soc* 2002;**50**:530–4.

6. Borson S. The mini-cog: a cognitive 'vital sign' measure for dementia screening in multi-lingual elderly. *Int J Geriatr Psychiatry* 2000;**15**(11):1021–7.

7. Office of Public Guardian. Making decisions: a guide for people who work in health and social care. OPG603. 1 April 2009. Available from: https://www.gov.uk/government/uploads/system/uploads/attachment_data/file/348440/OPG603-Health-care-workers-MCA-decisions.pdf (last accessed 6 October 2015).

8. Douglas IJ, Smeeth L. Exposure to antipsychotics and risk of stroke: self controlled case series study. *BMJ* 2008:**337**:a1227.

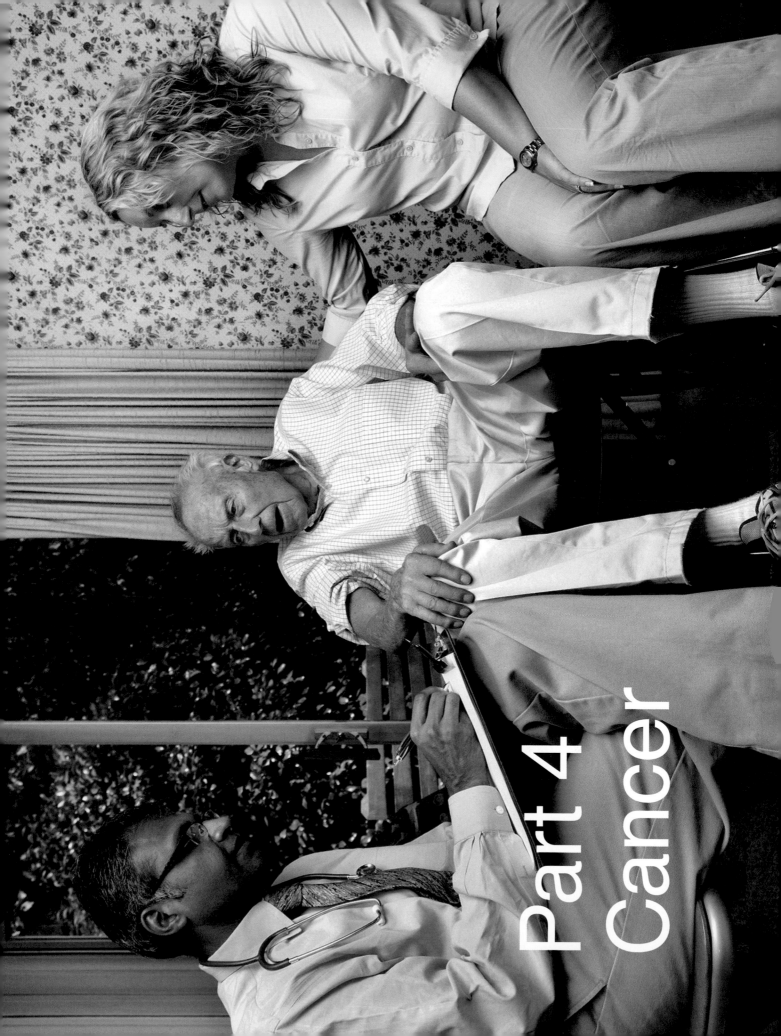

Part 4
Cancer

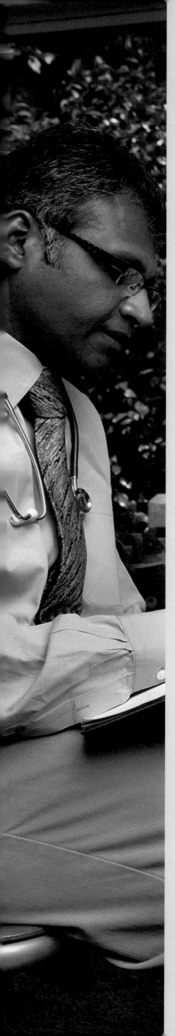

CHAPTER 38

Spotting patients with cancer

Andrew Blythe
GP and Senior Teaching Fellow, University of Bristol

Key topics

Learning objectives

- Be able to explain the role of the GP in reducing the incidence of cancer.
- Be able to weigh up the benefits and disadvantages of screening for cancer.
- Be able to recognise when a patient needs urgent investigation for the possibility of cancer.
- Be able to describe methods for making the diagnosis of cancer earlier.

Introduction

In his semiautobiographical novel *Sons and Lovers*, D.H. Lawrence tells the story of the Morel family from Nottingham. Towards the end of the novel, Mrs Morel's health deteriorates. She is staying with her daughter in Sheffield when she develops severe abdominal pain. Her daughter summons the local doctor, Dr Ansell, who visits her at home. The next day, her son, Paul, goes to speak to Dr Ansell to find out what's happening to his mother.

> The doctor looked at the young man, then knitted his fingers.
>
> 'It may be a large tumour which has formed in the membrane', he said slowly, 'and which we *may* be able to make go away.'
>
> 'Can't you operate?' asked Paul.
>
> 'Not there', replied the doctor.
>
> 'Are you sure?'
>
> '*Quite!*'
>
> Paul meditated a while.
>
> 'Are you sure it's a tumour?' he asked. 'Why did Dr Jameson in Nottingham never find out anything about it? She's been going to him for weeks and he's treated her for heart and indigestion.'
>
> 'Mrs Morel never told Dr Jameson about the lump', said the doctor.
>
> 'And do you know it's a tumour?'
>
> 'No, I am not sure.'
>
> 'What else might it be? You asked my sister if there was cancer in the family. Might it be cancer?'
>
> 'I don't know.'

D.H. Lawrence, Sons and Lovers, 1913

Identifying patients who might have a cancer is an important part of every GP's work. A hundred years on from Lawrence's account, many patients are still diagnosed with cancers at a late stage when they cannot be operated on or cured with chemotherapy and radiotherapy. Ovarian cancer, which may well be what Mrs Morel had, is often diagnosed late, as is lung cancer. Partly as a result of late diagnosis, the survival rates for cancer in the UK lag behind those in many other European countries. In this chapter, we will discuss how GPs can spot patients with cancer at an early stage and explore what they can do to help patients reduce their risk of developing cancer.

The common risk factors for cancer

Most people know that smoking can cause lung cancer and that exposure to the sun is linked to skin cancers, but their awareness of the other risk factors for cancers is hazier. Alcohol is linked to several cancers, and the rise in alcohol consumption in the UK has been accompanied by an increase in oral and

Table 38.1 Risk factors for cancers.

Risk factor	Cancers
Obesity	Breast, bowel, endometrium, oesophagus
Smoking	Lung, larynx, mouth, pharynx, oesophagus, stomach, pancreas, liver, bowel, kidney, bladder, cervix
Alcohol	Mouth, pharynx, larynx, oesophagus, breast, bowel, liver
Ultraviolet exposure	Melanoma
Viruses:	
• Hepatitis B	Liver
• Human papilloma virus (HPV)	Cervix
Genes:	
• BRCA1, BRCA2	Breast, ovary
• APC	Bowel

oesophageal cancers. Four cancers are linked to obesity, and as we become a more obese nation, the incidence of these cancers may increase. Table 38.1 lists the risk factors for common cancers.

GPs have a role in helping patients to reduce all these risks. GPs can help people to lose weight, moderate their alcohol consumption and stop smoking. They can refer patients to other support services, such as weight-loss and smoking-cessation clinics, and they can prescribe drugs to help people make these changes to their lifestyle. Out of all these lifestyle risks, smoking is the most important. Professor Mike Richards, the UK's first National Cancer Director, says that tackling smoking is the single most important intervention that can reduce the number of deaths from cancer in the UK (see Chapters 7 and 9 for a discussion of behaviour change and smoking-cessation therapies).

Some viruses increase the risk of cancer. Cervical cancer, the 20th most common cancer in the UK, is caused in part by the human papilloma virus (HPV). At the age of 13, all girls in the UK are vaccinated against HPV in schools. If a girl misses one or more of the doses, she can have the vaccination at her GP surgery.

Some people carry genes that put them at increased risk of developing certain cancers. The BRCA1 and BRCA2 genes cause breast and ovarian cancer, and the APC gene causes familial adenomatous polyposis, which can lead to bowel cancer. GPs are in a good position to obtain a detailed family history and identify patients who might need to be tested for these genes. However, these genes only cause a small proportion of all cases of bowel and breast cancer.

When should women be referred to assess their risk of familial breast cancer?

Breast cancer is very common (affecting one in nine women at some stage in their life), so a large proportion of women have someone in their family who has had breast cancer. Not everyone who has a close relative with breast cancer needs to be referred to a genetic clinic. To decide whether a woman needs referral, we take a detailed history of her first- and second-degree relatives: her siblings, parents, aunts, neices and grandparents (on both her paternal and maternal sides). If she has two or more first- or second-degree relatives who have had breast cancer, we should refer. If she has just one first- or second-degree relative with breast cancer, we should refer only if she has other risk factors, such as being Jewish or having a family history of ovarian cancer, male breast cancer or bilateral breast cancer.

When a woman is seen in a genetic clinic, her probability of developing breast cancer is reassessed, and at this stage she may be offered genetic screening. Women who are found to carry a gene that increases their risk of developing breast cancer can be kept under surveillance using magnetic resonance imaging (MRI) or mammography. If a woman is judged to be at high risk of developing breast cancer, she can be offered a selective oestrogen receptor modulator such as tamoxifen.

The role of screening

The commonest cancers in the UK are breast, bowel, prostate and lung cancer. Between them, these four cancers account for about half of all the new cases of cancer diagnosed each year. Screening programmes exist for two of these 'big four': breast and bowel cancer. There is also a screening programme for cervical cancer.

Screening for cervical cancer using cervical smears began in the 1960s, but it was not until 1988 that screening was systematised by introducing a robust mechanism for inviting and recalling women for their smears. In the same year, breast screening was introduced following the publication of the Forrest report,[1] which concluded that screening could save the lives of women over the age of 50.

Breast screening

Today, all women between the age of 50 and 70 years are invited to have a mammogram every 3 years (see Table 38.2). Two views are obtained of each breast, and if anything suspicious is seen, the woman is invited to a breast clinic, where an ultrasound scan and fine-needle aspiration can be performed. Mammograms can reveal ductal carcinoma in situ as well as cancers. We don't know which of these will cause harm so some women end up having unnecessary treatment. Overall, one in three patients with breast cancer is detected by screening; the majority of cases still come to light because a woman detects a breast lump herself and goes to her GP.

Table 38.2 Screening timetable.

	Start (age)	End (age)	Screening interval (years)
Cervix	25	64[a]	3–5
Breast	50	70[a]	3
Bowel	60	69	2

[a] Can continue beyond this at patient's request.

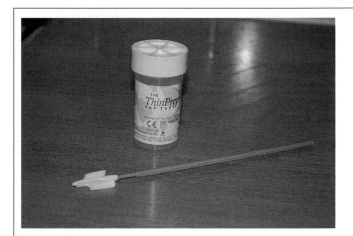

Figure 38.1 Brush and pot used for cervical screening.

Cervical screening

The process of cervical screening has changed over the years. Initially, a sample of cervical cells was obtained using a wooden spatula, which was swept over the surface and then 'smeared' on to a glass slide. In 2003, laboratories switched to liquid-based cytology, which requires the collection of cells using a brush, which is then agitated in a pot of liquid (see Figure 38.1). The collection of these samples is done in GP surgeries, usually by a practice nurse, but sometimes by a GP. However, the invitation to attend for this test is sent by the screening service, not the GP.

In 2011, the cervical screening process was enhanced by testing for HPV. If cytology is negative, HPV testing is not done and the woman is invited for routine recall. If cytology is reported as showing borderline or low-grade dyskaryosis, HPV testing is used to decide if the woman needs referral for colposcopy. Women who are reported as having high-grade dyskaryosis are referred to colposcopy immediately, without HPV testing (see Figure 38.2). Colposcopy involves examination of the cervix under a high-power lens, which allows biopsies to be taken for definitive diagnosis. Cervical screening begins at the age of 25 and automatic recall continues every 3 years until the age of 49, then every 5 years until the age of 64.

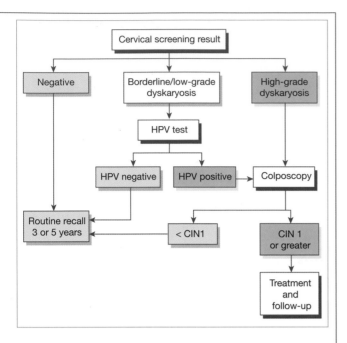

Figure 38.2 Flow chart for dealing with the result of cervical screening in England.

Bowel screening

Bowel screening is the newest cancer screening programme in the UK. As with breast and cervical screening, there is a centralised administration system. Every 2 years from the age of 60 to 69, patients are sent a pack for collection of a small sample of faeces on some blotting paper, which they have to return in the post. These samples are tested for occult blood. If this test is positive, the patient is invited for a colonoscopy.

Of the three national screening programmes, bowel screening has the poorest uptake. Nationally, fewer than 60% of people return the faecal occult blood test kit the first time that they are sent it, but with each of the subsequent invitations, the uptake rate improves.[2]

The problems with screening

Current screening programmes do not provide a solution to the challenge of detecting cancers at an early stage.

Only 10% of all cancers in the UK are detected through screening, and the detection of these cancers comes at the cost of harm to others. There is a mismatch between the public perception that 'it's good to catch things early' and the evidence on the benefits and harms of screening programmes. The programmes create a great deal of anxiety. The vast majority of people who do not receive the 'all clear' on the first test (cervical cytology, mammography or faecal occult blood testing) do not turn out to have cancerous or precancerous abnormalities; the next round of tests that these people undergo (colposcopy and colonoscopy in particular) are unpleasant and invasive, and at each stage in the screening process, cancers can be missed.

Pilot studies on bowel screening using faecal occult blood tests show that out of 100 000 men and women, 1936 (2%) were offered investigation because their faecal occult blood test was positive.[3] Out of these 1936 worried people, 35 were found to have bowel cancer, and their life was prolonged because they received treatment early. However, a further 82 were diagnosed with bowel cancer and did not see an increase in their survival; and up to 540 people were treated for benign tumours. Out of the people whose faecal occult blood test was negative, 55 were diagnosed with bowel cancer within the next 2 years. So, when someone in their 60s presents with possible symptoms of bowel cancer, we cannot reassure them that they don't have cancer on the basis of a negative result from their last screening test.

Expanding the screening programmes

At present, bowel cancer screening stops at 69, but there are plans to increase it up to the age of 74. Women stop receiving invitations for cervical screening at 64 and for breast screening at 70, but if they want to go on having tests, they can do so on request.

There is not a screening programme for prostate cancer. Although it is possible to measure the serum level of prostate-specific antigen (PSA), the utility of the PSA as a screening test is controversial. At present, the compromise offered by the NHS is that men can have their PSA level checked if they request it. Many men do visit their GP for this reason.

Case study 38.1

William Wakeman, age 72, comes to see his GP to request a prostate check. He has had two basal cell carcinomas removed recently and has osteoarthritis in his right knee.

What should the GP ask him before doing any test or examination?
Before advising him on what test would be best, the GP needs to find out a bit more information. They should

ask him why he would like a check. Does he have any symptoms that are worrying him? What is his health like generally? Does he have any lower urinary tract symptoms that might indicate prostatic hypertrophy? What has he heard about prostate checks? Does he know anyone who has had a prostate problem?

Mr Wakeman tells the GP that a friend of his has just been diagnosed with prostate cancer, so he thought he should get checked out himself. He gets up twice a night to pass urine. During the day, his urinary stream is quite strong. He never has to wait more than a few seconds before starting to pass urine, but very occasionally he dribbles urine at the end of micturition. Generally, he's quite well; he walks into town every day and his weight is steady. Another of his friends has just had a blood test to check his prostate and has been given the 'all clear'.

What would the GP do next?
The GP should explain to Mr Wakeman that the blood test measures something called the 'prostate-specific antigen' (PSA). This is not a foolproof test for picking up prostate cancer; it comes up with a number. In general, the lower

the number, the less likely you are to have prostate cancer. If the blood test produces a high number, the GP will refer Mr Wakeman to a urologist to have a prostate biopsy – this has to be done by inserting needles inside his bottom. If the blood test comes up with a low number, the GP will want to do a digital rectal examination, too, because this is the only way of feeling the prostate gland. If the gland feels abnormal, the GP will recommend a referral.

Mr Wakeman says he didn't realise it was so complicated but that he wants to go ahead with the blood test. His PSA is reported as 6.5 IU/l (the suggested normal range for a man over 70 is less than 5.0 IU/l). After explaining this to him, the GP refers him to a urologist. The urologist performs a digital rectal examination, which reveals a moderately enlarged prostate and a slight area of nodularity on the right lobe. The urologist books him in for a prostate biopsy under guidance of a transrectal ultrasound scan. This is done 2 weeks later. Several samples are taken, but none shows any cancer. Mr Wakeman is discharged to the care of his GP with a diagnosis of benign prostatic hypertrophy.

Large, multicentre trials are in progress to explore the possibility of screening for ovarian cancer using a blood test to measure the Ca 125 antigen or using transvaginal ultrasound scanning.

The National Awareness and Early Diagnosis Initiative

If we cannot rely on screening for a solution, how else can we diagnose cancer at an earlier stage?

In 2008, the National Awareness and Early Diagnosis Initiative (NAEDI)[4] was launched. Its aim was, and still is, to make diagnoses earlier by:

- making people aware of the symptoms that can be a pointer to cancer;
- encouraging people to see their GP as soon as they are concerned about worrying symptoms;
- improving GPs' ability to spot patients who might have cancer;

- speeding up the process of investigation of someone who might have cancer.

Why don't people go to their GP?

Many people do not know what symptoms are worthwhile bringing to their GP's attention. People tend to be alarmed by lumps and bleeding, but many are unaware that a persistent cough can be due to lung cancer, that diarrhoea can be due to bowel cancer or that a persistent mouth ulcer can be cancerous. NAEDI has commissioned a series of advertising campaigns to overcome this problem. People now therefore come to their GP saying things such as, 'My husband told me that I should see you because he's heard that if you've had a cough for 3 weeks, you should have a chest X-ray'.

Detection of three of the four commonest cancers involves having an intimate examination: a breast or rectal examination. The embarrassment caused by this examination is another deterrent to people consulting their GP. Finding the time to go to the GP can be a problem, too.

Case study 38.2

Eileen Edgecombe, age 72, comes to see her GP because she has discovered a lump in her right breast. She discovered it 4 weeks ago, when she was lifting some furniture and knocked herself there. It was sore at the time, and she hoped the lump would go away. The pain did go, but the lump persisted, so last week she booked this appointment. She doesn't check her breasts for lumps very often. She is the main carer for her husband, who has

mild dementia and severe chronic obstructive pulmonary disease (COPD), so she doesn't have a lot of time for her own health. She made this appointment a week ago.

What should the GP do?
The GP should get a bit more information. Has she noticed any discharge from her nipple? Has she been investigated for breast lumps before? When did she last have a

mammogram? Has anyone in her family had breast cancer? Does she have any children? If yes, did she breastfeed them (nulliparity and not breastfeeding increase the risk of breast cancer). The GP should ask about her general health and then, with an offer of a chaperone, suggest that he examines her.

Outcome

Mrs Edgecombe hasn't noticed any discharge from the nipple. She hasn't been investigated for any lumps before, but has only ever had one mammogram. She never got round to going for mammograms after the age of 60 because that's when her husband's health deteriorated. She has two daughters and she breastfed both of them; one lives nearby. Her aunt on her father's side had breast cancer in her 50s.

On examination, the GP notices the there is a slight dimpling of the skin in the upper outer quadrant of her right breast. At that site, he can feel a hard, fixed, irregular lump about 15 mm in diameter. He cannot feel any other lumps and cannot palpate any axillary or supraclavicular lymph nodes.

Mrs Edgecombe asks the GP if he thinks the lump is cancerous. The GP says that it might be and that she needs

to have further tests to find out whether it is. He tells her that he will make a referral today and that she should expect to receive an appointment within the next 2 weeks. Under the 2-week rule introduced in 2001, all patients with suspected cancer should be referred by their GP within 24 hours and the hospital should offer an appointment within 2 weeks of this referral. The GP tells her that at the clinic, she is likely to have an ultrasound scan and to have a sample of the lump taken through a long needle. Remembering that she is the carer for her husband, he asks how she will get to clinic. She says she can ask one of her daughters to look after her husband for the day so that she can get to hospital. That means she'll have to explain things to her daughter. So far, she hasn't told anyone else about the lump.

At the end of morning surgery, the GP completes an online referral form to the local breast clinic. The next day, Mrs Edgecombe receives a phone call from the hospital inviting her to a clinic in 4 days' time. At the clinic, she has an ultrasound scan and a fine-needle aspiration of the lump. Cytology confirms that she has an invasive adenocarcinoma of the breast. She has a lumpectomy and axillary node sampling 2 weeks later.

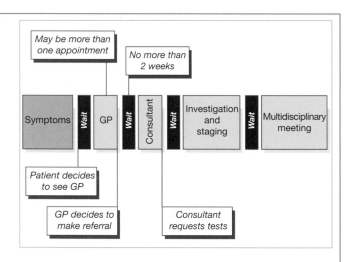

Figure 38.3 Possible causes of delay in cancer diagnosis.

Delays to referral

The steps in the route to a patient's diagnosis of breast cancer are illustrated in Figure 38.3. The final stage in this journey is the multidisciplinary team meeting, when the hospital specialists review all the results and decide on the treatment plan. Delays in making a diagnosis can occur at any of these stages. In Case Study 38.2, the whole process is fairly swift. The longest delay was because the patient didn't go to her GP as soon as she found the lump and, when she did decide to see her GP, she waited a week for an appointment. The GP referred

her immediately; that's because, for breast lumps, the decision about what to do is normally straightforward. For other symptoms suggestive of other cancers, the GP might want to do some tests before making a decision about referral. For patients who end up being diagnosed with cancer, the median length of time from being seen by a GP to being referred is 4 days.

The introduction of the 2-week rule in the UK has helped to minimise delays, but only 60% of patients who end up being diagnosed with cancer are referred under this rule.[5] When the 2-week wait scheme was introduced for breast cancer, resources were diverted from other clinics in order to meet this target, and as a consequence the waiting time for non-urgent referrals increased. So, for patients with breast cancer who were not on the 2-week pathway, the time to diagnosis increased. When this came to light, a 2-week target was applied to all breast clinic referrals.

Defining the predictive value of symptoms, signs and tests

Among patients who are diagnosed with cancer, 80% present themselves to their GP with a related symptom. This gives GPs the opportunity to identify most new cases of cancer. To do this effectively, GPs need to know what symptoms and signs warrant urgent investigation. Coughing up blood (haemoptysis) is a relatively good predictor of lung cancer, but it is a symptom of advanced disease and only very few cases of lung cancer are made on this basis. To pick up cases early, GPs must act on more subtle symptoms, such as a persistent cough or pain in the shoulder.

Table 38.3 Symptoms, signs and test results requiring urgent investigation for suspected cancer

Cancer	Symptom/sign/test result	Action
Lung	Age ≥40 with unexplained haemoptysis	Refer 2 week wait (2ww)
	Abnormal chest X-ray (CXR) that suggests cancer	Refer 2ww
	Age ≥40 with 2 of the following symptoms (or 1 if they have ever smoked): cough, chest pain, short of breath, tiredness, weight loss, appetite loss.	Urgent CXR
	Age ≥40 with any of following signs:, finger clubbing, cervical &/or supraclavicular lymphadenopathy, thrombocytosis, chest signs consistent with cancer/persistent chest infection	Urgent CXR
Breast	Age ≥30 with unexplained breast lump with/without pain	Refer 2ww
	Age ≥50 with any of the following symptoms in one nipple only: discharge, retraction, other changes of concern	Refer 2ww
	Age ≥30 with unexplained lump in axilla	Consider 2ww
	Skin changes that suggest breast cancer	Consider 2ww
Bowel	Age ≥40 with unexplained weight loss and abdominal pain	Refer 2ww
	Age ≥50 with unexplained rectal bleeding	Refer 2ww
	Age ≥60 with iron-deficiency anaemia or change in bowel habit	Refer 2ww
	Occult blood test positive	Refer 2ww
	Rectal or abdominal mass	Consider 2ww
	Age <50 with rectal bleeding + 1 of following: abdominal pain, change in bowel habit, weight loss, iron-deficiency anaemia	Consider 2ww
	Age ≥50 with abdominal pain or weight loss	Occult blood test
	Age <60 with change in bowel habit or iron-deficiency anaemia	Occult blood test
	Age ≥60 with anaemia (even if not iron-deficient)	Occult blood test
Prostate	Prostate-specific antigen (PSA) >age related reference range	Refer 2ww
	Prostate gland feels hard/irregular on digital rectal examination	Refer 2ww
	Lower urinary tract symptoms, erectile dysfunction, visible haematuria	PSA & digital rectal exam

Table 38.3 lists the symptoms, signs and test results for each of the big four cancers which the National Institute for Health and Care Excellence (NICE) says should prompt a GP to make urgent investigation or referral.[6]

Much research has been done in recent years to refine the predictive value of certain symptoms, singly and in combination. For example, rectal bleeding in isolation carries a risk of bowel cancer of about 0.6–1.0%, and weight loss on its own carries a risk of bowel cancer of just under 1%. However, when present together, these two symptoms carry a risk of bowel cancer in the region of 8–22%.[7]

As with cardiovascular disease (CVD), age is one of the best predictors of cancer. Thus, while a man under the age of 60 who presents with rectal bleeding has a less than 1 in 100 risk of having bowel cancer, a man in his 80s who presents with rectal bleeding has a 1 in 20 risk.

The guidelines developed by NICE reflect the predictive value of age, symptoms and test results. They make decisions more evidence-based, but there is a still a role for instinct and professional judgement.

Rarer cancers

So far, we have concentrated on the four commonest cancers: lung, breast, bowel and prostate. These cancers account for about half of all new cases of cancer each year. A full-time GP can expect to diagnose eight new cases of cancer a year. Four of these will be lung, bowel, breast or prostate; the other four will be rarer cancers. Figure 38.4 shows the 10 most common cancers in men and women in the UK. On average, a GP will see one case of the rarer cancers, such as ovarian cancer, every 5 years.[8]

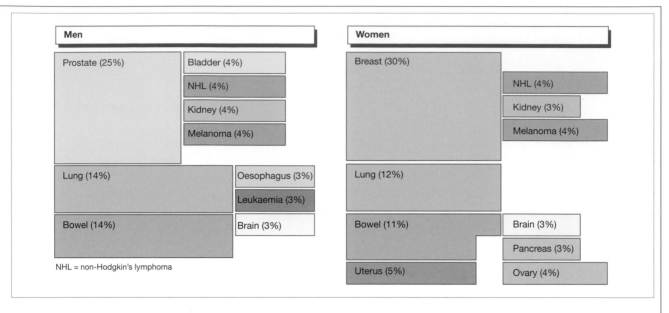

Figure 38.4 Top 10 cancers in men and women in the UK (by incidence). *Source*: Data from Cancer UK: http://www.cancerresearchuk. org/cancer-info/cancerstats/incidence/commoncancers.

GPs have access to most of the first-line tests that are needed to diagnose these cancers: blood tests, chest X-rays, ultrasound scans, computed tomography (CT) of the head and endoscopy. A negative test may provide all the reassurance needed to eliminate some types of cancer (such as a brain tumour), but for others, such as lung cancer, the GP may have to be more tenacious. Not all lung cancers show up on a chest X-ray, so, if a GP strongly suspects that a patient has lung cancer and the chest X-ray is reported as normal, the GP may need to refer the patient for a CT of the thorax or a bronchoscopy.

Missing a diagnosis of cancer in primary care

Case study 38.3 illustrates a number of common reasons for missing a diagnosis of cancer. The GP is misled by the existing known pathology: a hiatus hernia. Instead of looking for alternative explanations for the chest discomfort, she attributes it to the hiatus hernia. Perhaps she was falsely reassured by the absence of any abnormal findings when she examined the patient at the first consultation. A mesothelioma is a relatively rare cancer, but this patient's occupation provides the key to his diagnosis. People who worked in the construction industry in the 1960s and 1970s are at high risk of developing a mesothelioma because of their exposure to asbestos; if they smoked,

their risk is even higher. Perhaps if the GP had asked about the occupation at the first consultation, she might have requested a chest X-ray then.

As part of NAEDI, practices in one area of the UK were asked to conduct an audit of all the cancer diagnoses made amongst their patients over a 1-year period and to conduct significant event analyses on cases in which the diagnosis was delayed. A review of these significant analyses revealed several common reasons for delay:[9]

- pre-existing pathology that might explain the symptoms;
- reluctance to challenge a diagnosis if the patient gets worse or the symptoms don't fit;
- vague symptoms;
- stoical and uncomplaining patients;
- falsely reassuring examinations or X-ray results.

Reflecting on our practice, conducting audits and significant event analyses is a powerful way of improving our ability to make swift, accurate diagnoses. Without inventing any new treatments, up to 6000 lives could be saved in the UK each year if the diagnosis of cancer was made earlier.

Returning to Mrs Morel in *Sons and Lovers*, how might things be different for her now? Might she have been persuaded by a public advertising campaign to tell her GP about the lump? Might her GP have been less ready to attribute her symptoms to 'heart and indigestion'? We shall learn more about the fate of Mrs Morel in Chapter 40.

Case study 38.3

Jeff Jacobs, age 77, presents to his GP with discomfort in his chest. He says it has been going on for a few weeks but only bothers him at night. It is usually relieved by getting up and moving around. He has not felt breathless. He hasn't had a cough and has not experienced any nausea. His weight is steady and he has not experienced any difficulty swallowing. He had a duodenal ulcer 25 years ago and takes omeprazole 20 mg every day. An endoscopy 12 years ago showed that he has a sliding hiatus hernia. When he was younger, he drank quite heavily. He only drinks modest amounts. He has never smoked.

The GP examines him and cannot find any abnormality. On this basis, she attributes the discomfort to the hiatus hernia and advises the patient to double the dose of his omeprazole.

A month later, the patient returns and says that things are no better. It hurts to lie on his right side now, and he has noticed that when he goes upstairs, he gets a bit short of breath.

At this stage, the GP reviews the history and this time asks what job the patient used to do. He was a roofer for most of his life. The only new finding on examination is dullness and reduced air entry over the base of the right lung. The GP requests a chest X-ray. This reveals a right-sided pleural effusion. She makes an urgent referral to the respiratory team. The next day, the patient has his effusion drained and a CT scan and biopsy. The final diagnosis is a mesothelioma.

GPs can reduce deaths from cancer by targeting risk factors, encouraging participation in screening and making the diagnosis of cancer at an early stage in the disease. Smoking, alcohol consumption, exposure to sun and obesity are all important risk factors for cancer that can be addressed in primary care. In the UK, screening programmes exist for breast, bowel and cervical cancers; these have the potential to identify 10% of all cancers, but they can cause harm. Breast, lung, bowel and prostate cancers account for half of all new cancer diagnoses in the UK. NAEDI is attempting to educate the public about the symptoms of cancer that should prompt them to consult their GP. Meanwhile, much research is being done to define the predictive value of symptoms and signs, singly and in combination, to assist GPs in identifying patients who might have cancer. The onus is on GPs to refer patients with suspected cancer promptly. GPs should be wary of attributing new symptoms to existing pathology, and if patients return with the same symptoms, they should be willing to reconsider their diagnosis. A normal examination does not rule out cancer.

SUMMARY

Now visit **www.wileyessential.com/primarycare** to test yourself on this chapter.

REFERENCES

1. Forrest P. *Breast Cancer Screening: Report to the Health Ministers of England, Wales, Scotland and Northern Ireland*. London: Her Majesty's Stationary Office; 1986.

2. Steele RJC, Kostourou I, McClements P, et al. Effect of repeated invitations on uptake of colorectal cancer screening using faecal occult blood testing: analysis of prevalence and incidence screening. *BMJ* 2010;**341**:C5531.

3. Raffle A. Honesty about new screening programmes is best policy. *BMJ* 2000;**320**:872.

4. Richards MA. The National Awareness and Early Diagnosis Initiative in England: assembling the evidence. *Br J Cancer* 2009:**101**(Suppl. 2):S1–4.

5. Potter S, Govindarajulu S, Shere M et al. Referral patterns, cancer diagnoses and waiting times after introduction of two week wait rule for breast cancer: prospective cohort study. *BMJ* 2007;**335**:288.

6. NICE. Suspected cancer: recognition and referral. June 2015. NICE guideline NG12. Available from http://www.nice.org.uk/guidance/ng12 (last accessed 7 January 2016)

7. Astin M, Griffin T, Neal RD, et al. The diagnostic value of symptoms for colorectal cancer in primary care: a systematic review. *Br J Gen Pract* 2011:**61**(586):e231–43.

8. Hamilton W, Menon U. Easily missed? Ovarian cancer. *BMJ* 2009;**340**:96–7.

9. Wint A. Common pitfalls in the diagnosis of cancer in primary care. 2010. Poster presentation at the Annual Conference of the Royal College of General Practitioners 2010, Harrogate.

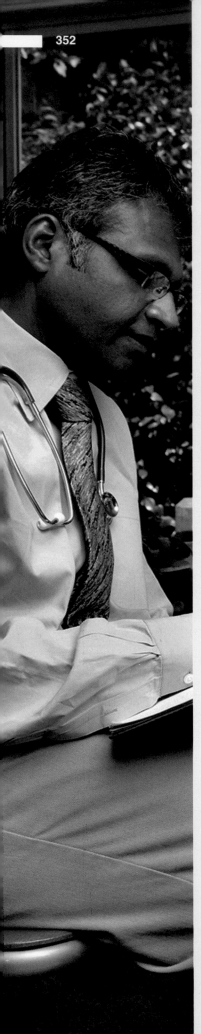

CHAPTER 39

Looking after patients with cancer

Andrew Blythe

GP and Senior Teaching Fellow, University of Bristol

Key topics

Learning objectives

- Describe the role of the GP in managing patients with the common types of cancer.
- Describe some of the common side effects of cancer treatment.
- Recognise a possible presentation of neutropenic sepsis.
- Recognise when a patient needs investigation to look for a recurrence of their cancer.

Essential Primary Care, First Edition. Edited by Andrew Blythe and Jessica Buchan.
© 2017 John Wiley & Sons, Ltd. Published 2017 by John Wiley & Sons, Ltd.
Companion website: www.wileyessential.com/primarycare

The role of the GP in the treatment of patients with cancer

Once a patient has been diagnosed with cancer, their care is delivered and coordinated by consultants (usually the relevant organ specialist and an oncologist). Many hospital cancer teams also have nurse specialists to whom the patient can turn for advice. So what role does the GP have once a patient embarks on their treatment for cancer?

Chemotherapy

Chemotherapy may be given at various stages of treatment for cancer. Sometimes it's the first-line treatment, with an intention to cure the cancer; sometimes it's given to shrink the tumour before surgery (neoadjuvant chemotherapy); sometimes it is given after surgery to reduce the risk of recurrence (adjuvant chemotherapy); and sometimes it is given as a palliative treatment to buy the patient a bit more time. The chemotherapy can be given in hospital or, increasingly, by specialist nurses working in the community. The patient's GP needs to ensure that the patient has the necessary blood tests before each cycle of chemotherapy and must be prepared to treat the side effects of chemotherapy (see Tables 39.1 and 39.2). Most importantly, the GP and the patient need to be alert to the possibility of neutropenic sepsis.

Anyone on chemotherapy who has a temperature of 38.0 °C or higher for more than an hour should be admitted immediately to receive intravenous antibiotics and to exclude the possibility of neutropenic sepsis.

Table 39.1 Side effects of treatment for breast cancer.

Treatment	Early side effects	Prevention/treatment of side effect	Late complications	Prevention/treatment of complication
Surgery	Infection	Antibiotic	Lymphoedema	Referral to lymphoedema clinic; compression sleeve
Radiotherapy	Sore, dry, red skin	Moisturisers	Lymphoedema	Referral to lymphoedema clinic
	Tiredness	Adjust level of activity	Pulmonary toxicity	
	Hair loss	Scalp cooling, wig, head scarf	Cardiac toxicity	
			Other cancers	Screening
Chemotherapy	Tiredness	Adjust level of activity	Renal failure	Adjust dose of medication
	Nausea	Antiemetic (domperidone, cyclizine)	Pulmonary fibrosis	
	Mucositis	Artificial saliva	Neuropathy	Gapapentin, amitriptyline
	Hair loss	Scalp cooling, wig, head scarf	Hand–foot syndrome	Emollients, e.g. Udder cream
	Neutropenia	Check full blood count (FBC)	Menopause	
Hormone therapy: tamoxifen	Climacteric symptoms		Menopause	
	Vaginal bleeding		Increased risk of endometrial cancer	
			Increased risk of cerebrovasular events and thrombotic event	Control of other risk factors: blood pressure and cholesterol
Aromatase inhibitors	Climacteric symptoms		Osteoporosis, fractures	Calcium supplements, bisphosphates
Biological therapy: trastuzumab (Herceptin)	Arrhythmias		Heart failure	
	Tiredness		Infertility	
	Diarrhoea			
	Rashes			

Table 39.2 Side effects of treatment for prostate cancer.

Treatment	Early side effects	Prevention/treatment of side effect	Late complications	Prevention/treatment of complication
Surgery: radical prostatectomy	Infection	Antibiotics	Erectile dysfunction	Phosphodiesterase inhibitor
	Inability to produce ejaculate		Infertility	Sperm storage
			Urinary incontinence	Bladder training
Orchidectomy	Hot flushes and sweats			
Hormone treatment: gonadotrophin-releasing hormone analogues	Hot flushes and sweats	Bicalutamide	Osteoporosis	Bisphosphonate
	Tiredness		Weight gain	
			Increased risk of diabetes and cardiovascular disease (CVD)	Control of other risk factors: blood pressure and cholesterol
			Memory and mood problems	
Radiotherapy	Dysuria and increased frequency of micturition (radiation cystitis)		Erectile problems	Phosphodiesterase inhibitor
			Urethral strictures	Self-catheterisation
			Urinary incontinence	Bladder training
			Looser stools, proctitis	Loperamide

Case study 39.1

Jane Spencer, age 65, was diagnosed with metastatic adenocarcinoma of the oesophagus 1 month ago. Her cancer was deemed inoperable, so she was referred to an oncologist, who offered palliative chemotherapy, consisting of cisplatin, capecitabine and herceptin. The oncologist warned her about the possible side effects, including tiredness, nausea, vomiting, diarrhoea, a sore mouth, a peripheral neuropathy, kidney damage and a rash affecting the hands and feet. She accepted these risks and went ahead with the chemotherapy.

When she was given the first cycle of chemotherapy, the oncology nurse sent a letter to the GP with information about the possible side effects and gave Mrs Spencer an antiemetic to take for the first few days after chemotherapy.

The GP phones Mrs Spencer 1 week after the first cycle of chemotherapy to check how she is getting on. Mrs Spencer reports losing her appetite for a few days but says it is improving again. The oncology nurse told Mrs Spencer

that she would need baseline blood tests the day before the next cycle, so Mrs Spencer makes an appointment for the practice nurse to do this and books an appointment to see the GP for a review in 1 month.

On the day of her scheduled review with the GP, Mrs Spencer phones the practice receptionist to say she feels too unwell to come to the surgery.

What should the GP do?
The GP should review her notes and any recent correspondence from the hospital and out-of-hours GP service. Then the GP should contact Mrs Spencer to establish whether she needs to be reviewed at home or in hospital.

Outcome
The GP phones Mrs Spencer immediately and ascertains that she has been feeling generally unwell for the last 10 days. She feels tired, her tummy feels 'tight' and she is

short of breath. She had her third cycle of chemotherapy 6 days ago. She has not felt hot.

Mrs Spencer lives a few blocks from the surgery, so the GP decides to visit immediately. The GP's first impression is that Mrs Spencer has lost a considerable amount of weight since their last encounter. She is not jaundiced and is alert. Her temperature is 38.0 °C, her pulse is 100 bpm and regular and her blood pressure is 110/50 mmHg. Her oxygen saturation is 96% on air. Both lung bases are dull to percussion, and air entry is reduced in these zones. Her abdomen is distended but not tender.

What should the GP do now?
The GP should arrange immediate admission to hospital. Mrs Spencer has a fever, fatigue and abdominal pain; these are all possible presentations of neutropenic sepsis. Typically, neutropenic sepsis develops 7–10 days after a dose of chemotherapy. Other presenting symptoms

include a sore throat and rigors. Neutropenic sepsis is an emergency.

Mrs Spencer also has signs of bilateral pleural effusions, and her abdominal distension suggests ascites. It appears that her cancer has advanced, and this may be another reason why she feels generally unwell.

Outcome
The GP dials 999 and phones the oncology team to request urgent admission. On admission, her neutrophil count is $26 \times 10^9/l$ (normal range $1.5–7.5 \times 10^9/l$). So, thankfully, this is not neutropenic sepsis. However, she does have a chest infection requiring treatment with antibiotics. A chest X-ray shows bilateral pleural effusions and an ultrasound scan confirms the presence of ascites; this is drained. Her plans for future chemotherapy are modified and she is discharged home with a request to the GP to monitor her renal function and analgesia.

Hormone therapy

The growth of some cancers – breast and prostate cancer in particular – is mediated by hormones. Breast cancer is often sensitive to oestrogen, and prostate cancer is sensitive to testosterone.

Breast cancers that are sensitive to oestrogen can be controlled with two types of drug: aromatase inhibitors (which block the production of oestrogen) and tamoxifen (which blocks the oestrogen receptors on breast cancer cells). Both types are given orally and are prescribed by GPs under the instruction of an oncologist. Most of the time, they are given after surgery, to reduce the risk of recurrence, and are continued for 5 years. During this time, they can cause osteoporosis, so this is something the GP needs to look for.

Antiandrogen treatment is one of the principle treatments for prostate cancer and is administered in primary care. The most common therapy is a gonadotrophin analogue, which is given as a depo injection, lasting up to 3 months at a time. For many patients, this is the only treatment needed to control their prostate cancer. The success of treatment can be monitored by measuring the prostate-specific antigen (PSA); GPs are normally asked to check this

every 3 months so that the consultant can make decisions about the patient's treatment.

Biological therapy, surgery and radiotherapy

GPs have less of a role in the other therapies for cancer – biological therapy, surgery and radiotherapy – although they often have to arrange baseline investigations and manage side effects (see Tables 39.1 and 39.2).

Other problems encountered by patients with cancer

Throughout their treatment for cancer, patients will need help with the management of their other health problems, and they are likely to need emotional support. The GP can maintain an overview of all of this care. A single consultation with a GP may include a review of the patient's medication (ensuring the patient has sufficient supply of everything), a discussion of how treatment is going and how they are coping generally and some form-filling (sick notes and insurance forms).

Case study 39.2

Michael Carpenter is 52. He underwent a high anterior resection 4 months ago to remove a carcinoma of the rectum. He is now receiving adjuvant chemotherapy (oxaliplatin and capecitabine) and comes to see his GP, Dr Fiona Nicholson, to obtain a prescription for more antiemetics and to obtain a fit note.

Dr Nicholson finds out that Mr Carpenter is doing reasonably well. The only side effects that he's noticed from the chemotherapy have been nausea and numbness in his hands. He works as an engineer, operating machinery, and this numbness is preventing him from returning to work. This is getting him down a bit and is causing financial problems. Mr Carpenter's wife, Susan, had to stop work 2 years ago to look after her mother, who has dementia. Dr Nicholson looks after Susan, too, and knows that she is finding things a struggle right now. Last week, Dr Nicholson referred Susan for psychological therapy for mild depression.

Dr Nicholson listens to Mr Carpenter and, without breaching his wife's confidentiality, acknowledges the various problems he faces. She gives him a prescription for more cyclizine and a fit note, then asks if there is anything else that she can help with. At this point, Mr Carpenter says that his left leg has been swollen for a few days; it is not painful.

What should Dr Nicholson do now?
Foremost in Dr Nicholson's mind is the possibility of a deep-vein thrombosis (DVT). Anyone who has cancer is at increased risk of thrombosis. Dr Nicholson enquires about other risk factors for thrombosis and discovers that a week ago Mr Carpenter went on a 6-hour return car journey to visit his father. Examination reveals pitting oedema of the left leg; its circumference is 2 cm larger than that of the right. Dr Nicholson refers Mr Carpenter to hospital for a Doppler study.

Outcome
The Doppler study confirms the presence of a left common femoral-vein thrombosis. Dr Nicholson starts him on daily enoxaparin injections and informs the oncologist. The oncologist advises her that Mr Carpenter should stay on enoxaparin and not switch to warfarin, because the warfarin might interact with his chemotherapy.

Cancer survivorship

For some patients, such as Mrs Spencer in Case study 39.1, cancer may be diagnosed too late to allow them to receive curative treatment; they may progress directly from diagnosis to palliative care. Sadly, this is still often the case in patients diagnosed with lung cancer. But most patients with cancer are offered curative care; once this is complete, they are kept under surveillance, usually for 5 years.

There are 2.5 million survivors of cancer in the UK. This number is increasing every year, because the incidence of cancer is rising and the death rate is falling. One-quarter of these are survivors of breast cancer; 12% have had colorectal cancer; 11% have had prostate cancer; and 3% have had lung cancer.

So, although each GP may only diagnose eight new cases of cancer every year, they care for a lot more patients who have cancer or who have been treated for cancer. Amongst those over the age of 65, 1 in 10 people has had a cancer. Some people have two or even three cancers in their lifetime. The risk of having another cancer increases once you've had one cancer, because of the side effects of chemo- and radiotherapy.

Spotting patients who have a recurrence of their cancer

If a patient has had cancer, there is always the fear that it may come back. Any new symptom is viewed by the patient in this light. Patients may assume that their GP is aware of their history of cancer, but sometimes this piece of information is overlooked because the patient is seeing a new GP and the diagnosis of cancer does not appear at the front of their notes or on the list of active problems. The first step to spotting a patient with a recurrence of their cancer is recognising that they have been treated for cancer in the past.

Top tip

When talking to someone who presents with back pain, breathlessness, a cough or unusual persistent symptoms, check whether they have ever had cancer.

What cluster of symptoms should cause concern?

A recurrence can cause almost any symptom. It can cause a symptom at the site of origin of the cancer or elsewhere. There are patterns to the spread of each cancer, and it is important for the GP to bear these in mind.

- Breast cancer commonly spreads to the bones (causing pain), the lungs (causing breathlessness or a cough), the brain (causing a variety of neurological symptoms) and the liver (causing jaundice).
- Lung cancer spreads to the bones and the liver.
- Bowel cancer spreads to the liver, lung and peritoneum.
- Prostate cancer spreads to the bones (typically causing back pain) and to the liver and lung.

The symptoms that are most likely to suggest that a patient has metastatic cancer are groin pain and pleural symptoms, but these symptoms are rare[3]. The more common symptoms of low back pain, vomiting, shoulder pain and loss of appetite

Case study 39.3

Samantha Middleton is 56. She was diagnosed with invasive ductal carcinoma of the breast 4 years ago, which was treated with wide local excision and chemotherapy, followed by anastrazole (an aromatase inhibitor), which she is still taking. She consults her GP because she has pain in her right hip and is finding going up- and downstairs particularly difficult. The pain has come on gradually over the last month or so. She has tried taking paracetamol; this helps a bit. Other than anastrazole, she is not on any other medication.

Ms Middleton suspects that this is the start of osteoarthritis. She has always been a bit overweight and is conscious of the fact that her mother, who was also overweight, developed osteoarthritis in her knees in her 50s. Ms Middleton was divorced 3 years ago and lives alone. She is a school teacher.

Her GP examines her hip and notes that flexion of the hip beyond 90° is painful, as is internal rotation. The GP requests a plain X-ray of the right hip. This is normal, apart from a possible small area of lucency around the acetabulum. The radiologist suggests that the GP request a bone scan. The GP sees Ms Middleton in surgery and explains that there are other things that this might be than osteoarthritis. Ms Middleton asks if it could be the cancer and the GP says that this is one possibility.

Outcome

The bone scan is done a week later and shows several areas of activity, one of which coincides with the area of lucency in Ms Middleton's acetabulum. The other hot spots are in the sixth thoracic vertebrae and two ribs. The report of this scan states that this looks like bony metastasis.

The GP sees Ms Middleton in surgery the next day and explains the findings of the scan. The GP refers her back to the oncologist and, a few weeks later, she begins some chemotherapy.

---

have a weaker association with metastatic disease. However, these symptoms also warrant investigation to look for possible recurrence of a cancer.

Surveillance of patients with cancer

Once a patient has completed their treatment for cancer, it is usual practice to follow them up in hospital for at least 5 years. Visits to the hospital may involve a review of the patient's symptoms, an examination and various investigations: blood tests and scans. The aim of this is to identify early signs of recurrence and check for the late side effects of treatment. Patients value these check-ups and gain reassurance from them.[1] However, if there is a recurrence of the cancer, this may cause symptoms in the period between check-ups, and the patient is then likely to consult their GP.

Should patients who have had cancer receive their routine follow-up in primary care?

A systematic review has shown weak evidence that follow-up of patients with breast cancer can be done in primary care without any detriment to the recurrence rate or survival.[2] However, most GPs lack the expertise to be able to answer patients' specific questions about treatment, side effects and prognosis.

Where GPs can usefully contribute to the follow-up is in providing continuity and emotional support. They can check the patient's understanding of what has been said in clinic and help to clarify misunderstandings. They provide a safety net between hospital appointments and ensure that the patient is not lost in the system.

For some cancers, where treatment is not considered necessary after diagnosis, GPs do have an important role in surveillance. Early prostate cancer, for instance, is often managed by active monitoring; this means 6-monthly or yearly visits to the GP to have the PSA level checked. Likewise, chronic lymphatic leukaemia often doesn't need treatment immediately after diagnosis. A haematologist may advise the GP to review the patient every 6 months to ask them about any symptoms suggesting activation of the leukaemia (sweats and weight loss), examine them to look for splenomegaly, hepatomegaly and lymphadenopathy and check their full blood count (FBC).

As treatments for cancer become more complex and patients survive for longer, GPs will have to spend more time helping patients to manage the problems created by the long-term side effects of treatment. Patients may be discharged from follow-up in hospital but still face disabling symptoms of treatment, such as peripheral neuropathy, breathlessness and urinary incontinence, as well as the psychological impact. GPs are in the best position to assess these problems and refer patients to other services when necessary.

SUMMARY

GPs have to monitor and manage many of the side effects of cancer treatment. Under the direction of oncologists, they prescribe hormone treatment for breast and prostate cancer. GPs must be alert to the possibility of neutropenic sepsis in someone who is receiving chemotherapy; this is an emergency. There are 2.5 million survivors of cancer in the UK. Amongst this group of patients, GPs need to be on the lookout for symptoms and signs that might indicate a recurrence, and they need to manage the long-term side effects of cancer treatment. This includes providing psychological support.

Now visit **www.wileyessential.com/primarycare** to test yourself on this chapter.

REFERENCES

1. Lewis RA, Neal RD, Henry M, et al. Patients' and healthcare professionals' views of cancer follow-up: systematic review. *Br J Gen Pract* 2009;**59**:e248–59.

2. Lewis RA, Russell D, Hughes DA, et al. Follow-up of cancer in primary care versus secondary care: systematic review. *Br J Gen Pract* 2009;**59**:e234–47.

3. Hamilton W, Barret J, Stapley S, Sharp D, Rose P. Clinical features of metastatic cancer in primary care: a case controlled study using medical records. *Br J Gen Pract* 2015;**65**:e516–522.

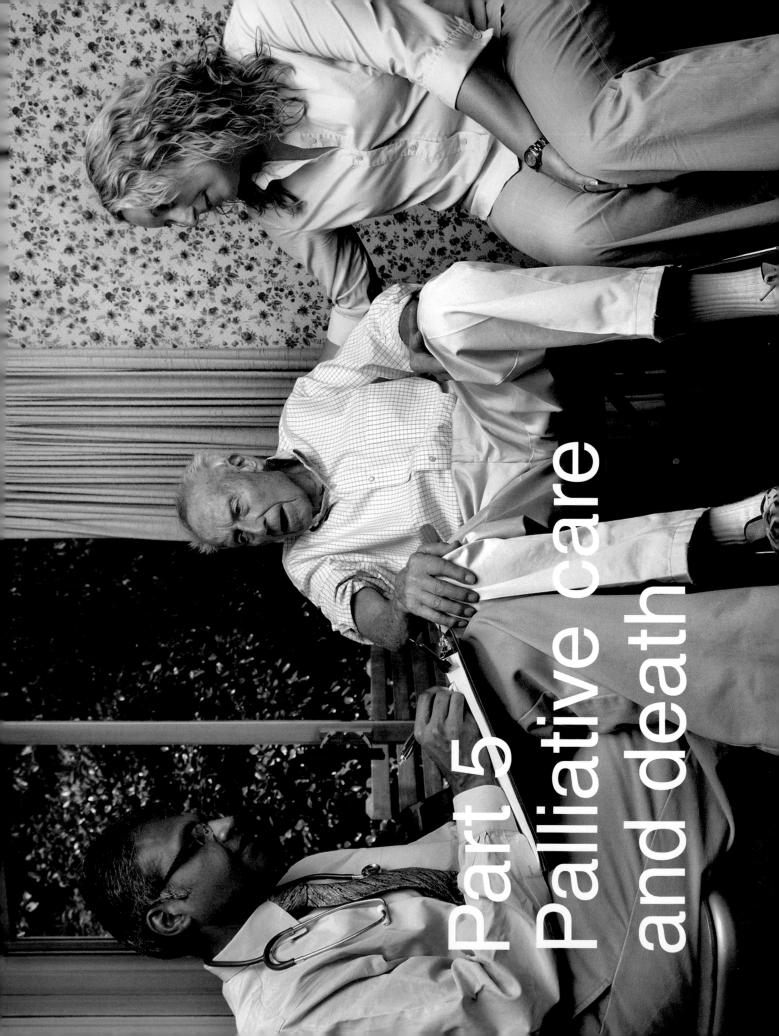

Part 5 Palliative care and death

CHAPTER 40
Palliative care and death

Andrew Blythe

GP and Senior Teaching Fellow, University of Bristol

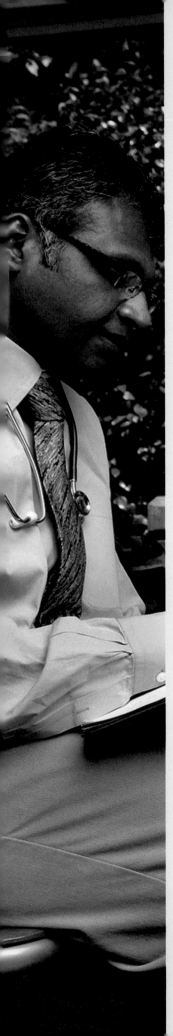

Key topics

Learning objectives

- Be able to describe the transition from active to palliative care.
- Be able to describe some common scenarios in palliative care.
- Be able to describe how a doctor confirms death.
- Be able to identify cases that need referral to the coroner.
- Be able to provide support to someone who is bereaved.

Essential Primary Care, First Edition. Edited by Andrew Blythe and Jessica Buchan.
© 2017 John Wiley & Sons, Ltd. Published 2017 by John Wiley & Sons, Ltd.
Companion website: www.wileyessential.com/primarycare

What is palliative care?

You matter because you are you, and you matter to the end of your life. We will do all we can not only to help you die peacefully, but also to live until you die.[1]

Dame Cicely Saunders,
founder of the hospice movement

The term 'palliative care' embraces a philosophy that aims to maximise the quality of a person's remaining life when they face a terminal illness. It is not a means of hastening or postponing death; it is about helping the person to live in comfort and die with dignity. The delivery of palliative care is not confined to hospices. Excellent palliative care can be provided wherever the patient is: in their home or in hospital. Coordinating and giving palliative can be one of the most rewarding aspects of being a GP. There is a great sense of satisfaction that comes from providing practical and emotional support to the patient and their family. The bond that this creates between the GP and the family can last for years.

Identifying those in need of palliative care

Sometimes a person's final illness can come out of the blue and there is little time to plan and prepare for death, but in developed countries death usually comes at the end of a chronic illness. In the UK, one-quarter of all deaths are from cancer, one-third from chronic organ failure such as heart failure or chronic obstructive pulmonary disease (COPD) and one-third from dementia and general frailty (see Figure 40.1). Each of these classes of terminal illness has a different trajectory. Patients with incurable cancer often seem to be fairly stable for a while, then all of a sudden their condition deteriorates rapidly and within a few weeks or days they are dead. Patients with diseases like COPD often have a long, slow decline, punctuated by a series of exacerbations; they recover from each exacerbation but never quite return to their previous level of functioning. Patients with dementia also experience a gradual decline, but often without any exacerbations (see Figure 40.2).

When a life-threatening illness is first diagnosed, the focus is on active treatment and prolonging life, but at some stage the priority has to switch to easing suffering: providing palliative care. Recognising when it is appropriate to make this transition is tricky, but GPs are in a good position to judge this because in most cases they have known the patient over a long time and have oversight of all the patient's care. Often, perhaps because of increasingly frequent consultations, repeated hospital admissions or just a general sense of decline, it is apparent to the GP that a patient is unlikely to survive for much longer. This is the time to start palliative care. The Macmillan Gold Standards Framework for palliative care recommends the use of the surprise question:[2] 'Would you be surprised if this patient were to die in the next few months, weeks or days?' If the answer is 'no' then it's time to start planning palliative care.

Most people want to die at home, but a large proportion end up dying in hospital instead.[3,4] In 2012, 52% of all deaths

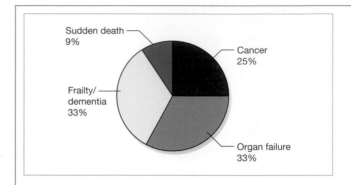

Figure 40.1 Causes of death.

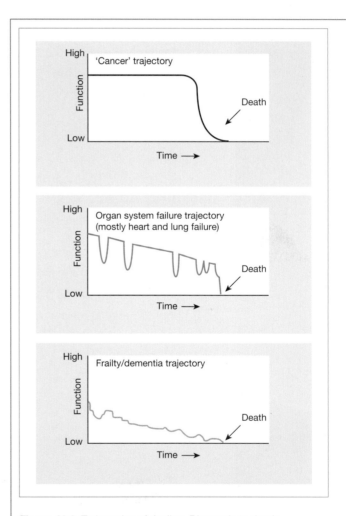

Figure 40.2 Trajectories of decline. Diagnosis to death.

amongst men and 48% of all deaths amongst women occurred in hospital; 40% of men and 45% of women died in their usual residence (their own home or a care home). The Macmillan Gold Standards Framework encourages GPs to support palliative care at home and ensure that more people are able to die

Case study 40.1

Patricia Porter is 82. She was diagnosed with incurable non-small-cell carcinoma of the lung 6 months ago. She has been receiving chemotherapy as a palliative measure, and today she attends the oncology clinic for review. She is feeling breathless. She appears jaundiced and her oxygen saturation is 87% on air. The oncologist does some blood tests, which show a deterioration of all parameters, including a substantial rise in her serum bilirubin. This leads the oncologist to conclude that the treatment is proving ineffective and that the cancer is continuing to spread. The consultant phones the GP, Dr Adam Fletcher, to say that he is not going to recommend any more chemotherapy, and asks Dr Fletcher to take over Mrs Porter's management and provide palliative care.

Dr Fletcher visits Mrs Porter the next day, makes his own assessment and explains the situation to her and her husband. Dr Fletcher organises home oxygen for Mrs Porter and puts in place a package of care at home, which includes visits from the district nurse. The following weekend, despite the oxygen therapy, Mrs Porter becomes much more breathless. Her daughter, who is visiting at the time, phones for an ambulance. The paramedics take her to hospital and the next day she dies in hospital.

Her widow, John, comes to see Dr Fletcher 2 weeks later. John says he is still shocked at Patricia's death. He can't understand how it is that she died so quickly and he feels guilty that he wasn't able to look after her at home. They had lived in the same house for over 40 years and Patricia had told him that she wanted to die there. She hasn't left a will.

What could Dr Fletcher have done to support Mrs Porter in the lead-up to her death?
Non-small-cell carcinoma of the lung is often diagnosed at a late stage and carries a very poor prognosis. The 1-year survival rate in the UK is about 30%. Usually, it's not possible to offer curative therapy, but sometimes, as in this case, the patient is offered chemotherapy and radiotherapy in order to slow the progression of the disease. To the patient and the family, this can give a sense of hope, and the subject of death is avoided. But the fact remains that the patient is likely to succumb to the cancer within a year, so in this case plans for all aspects of palliative care could have started much earlier.

As soon as Dr Fletcher knew that Mrs Porter had advanced lung cancer, he could have informed the district nurses. The nurses might have made contact with Mrs Porter simply to introduce themselves and to tell Mr and Mrs Porter what sort of help they could offer, now and in the future. Dr Fletcher might have made an appointment to review Mrs Porter in the surgery or at her home to answer any questions that she and her husband had and to open up a conversation about future care.

While Mrs Porter was having her course of chemotherapy, Dr Fletcher might have talked with her and her husband about where she would like to be looked after when her condition got worse. Would she like to go to hospice or stay at home? If she was interested in the idea of going to a hospice, an early meeting with a hospice nurse might have been helpful. At the same time, while Mrs Porter was relatively well, Dr Fletcher might have suggested that she set up an advance directive and lasting power of attorney so that when the time came, her husband could easily take over her financial affairs. Dr Fletcher could have checked Mrs Porter had a will. Talking about these things is difficult and has to be done at the patient's pace, often over a series of encounters.

When the oncologist decided to stop the chemotherapy, it might have been prudent to think about what symptoms might develop and get worse. Dr Fletcher could have prescribed medication to relieve breathlessness and could have explained to Mrs Porter and her family how to use it. Alerting the out-of-hours GP service about her condition might also have been helpful.

---

where they want to. The first step is identifying patients at an early stage who may be in need of palliative care. The other key features of the framework are:

- Assessing the patient's needs and making a plan for their care.
- Discussing and recording the patient's preferred place of death.
- Sharing information with everyone in the primary care team, so that they are all familiar with the situation and with the wishes of the patient.
- Making sure that important medicines are available when needed. This means prescribing medication in advance so that it is in the patient's home and ready for immediate use should the situation demand it.

The transition from active treatment to palliative care should be as seamless as possible (Figure 40.3).

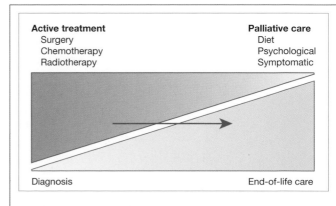

Figure 40.3 Transition from active treatment to palliative care.

Symptom relief in palliative care

In Case study 40.1, the most distressing symptom for Mrs Porter, and the one that resulted in hospital admission, was breathlessness. Morphine, in oral or injectable form, can be effective in relieving breathlessness in those who have advanced cancer, severe heart failure or end-stage respiratory disease. Sometimes, the breathlessness is aggravated by anxiety, so a benzodiazepine can be useful. Excessive secretions in the upper airways can also cause problems with breathing; hyoscine butylbromide can help to relieve this.

Table 40.1 list the drugs that can be used to relieve the common symptoms experienced by someone who has a terminal illness. The introductory chapter in the British National Formulary (BNF) gives an excellent overview of this important area of prescribing. As a patient gets weaker, they may no longer be able to take medicine by mouth. In this situation, the route of delivery is usually switched to subcutaneous infusion delivered continuously over a 24-hour period. Whether it is during normal daytime hours or at night, this switch has to be made quickly, so the injectable drugs need to be there and ready in the patient's home just in case, together with a prescription chart written by the GP, which gives the district nursing team authority to set up the syringe driver.

Assessing a patient's need for pain relief can be difficult, particularly when the patient is stoical and uncomplaining. Simply asking the patient if they have any pain often yields an answer like, 'I'm all right'. Many people are afraid of morphine and are worried that they might get dependent on it.

The person who is with the patient for most of the time, usually a close family member, often has the best sense of the situation. In Chapter 38, we recalled the case of Mrs Morel in *Sons and Lovers*, who is cared for by her son, Paul. When she is very ill, Paul comes to live with her.

Paul and she were afraid of each other. He knew, and she knew, that she was dying. But they kept up a

Table 40.1 Symptom relief in palliative care.

Symptom	Class of drug	Specific drug	Indication
Breathlessness	Morphine	Oramorph	End-stage cardiac and respiratory disease
	Benzodiazepine	Diazepam – oral Lorazepam – sublingual Midazolam – subcutaneous injection	When anxiety is contributing to breathlessness
	Hyoscine butyl bromide		Excessive secretions in upper airway
Nausea	Antihistamine	Cyclizine	Movement-induced nausea, gastric obstruction and nausea due to raised intracranial pressure
	Dopamine blocker	Haloperidol	Opiate-induced nausea, metabolic-induced nausea (such as hypercalcaemia) and post-radiotherapy nausea
		Levomepromazine	Opiate-induced nausea and metabolic-induced nausea
	5HT receptor antagonist	Ondansetron	Useful after abdominal radiotherapy, which causes release of a large amount of serotonin from the gastrointestinal tract
	Steroid	Dexamethasone	Vomiting due to raised intracranial pressure
Pain	Morphine	MST – modified release Oramorph – immediate release Diamorphine – injection or subcutaneous infusion	Regular dose Breakthrough pain When unable to take oral medication
	Oxycodone	OxyContin – modified release OxyNorm – immediate release	Regular dose Breakthrough pain
Restlessness	Benzodiazepine	Midazolam – subcutaneous infusion	
		Levomepromazine – subcutaneous infusion	

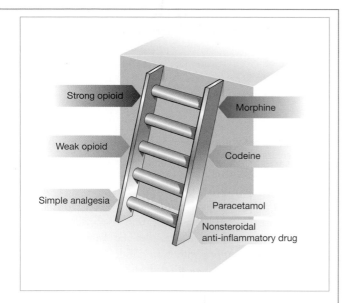

Figure 40.4 The analgesic ladder.

Table 40.2 Features of opioid toxicity.	
Symptoms	**Signs**
Confusion	Pinpoint pupils
Drowsiness	
Hallucinations, seeing things out of the corner of the eye	
Myoclonic jerks (twitches)	

pretence of cheerfulness. Every morning, when he got up, he went into her room in his pyjamas.

'Did you sleep, my dear?' he asked

'Yes', she answered.

'Not very well?'

'Well, yes!'

Then he knew that she had lain awake. He saw her hand under the bedclothes, pressing the place on her side where the pain was.

D.H. Lawrence, Sons and Lovers, 1913

In the novel, Mrs Morel is prescribed morphine by her GP, and today, 100 years on, morphine is still the most widely used drug for the control of severe pain in advanced disease. It sits at the top of the analgesic ladder (see Figure 40.4). The first things to try for pain are simple analgesic drugs such as paracetamol and nonsteroidal anti-inflammatory drugs (NSAIDs). If these prove ineffective, weak opioids such as codeine may help. And if these are ineffective, morphine is the next thing to try. Patients need a dose of morphine to take regularly (every 12 hours, if it's a slow-release preparation) and a supply of morphine solution to take as a 'top-up' if they get breakthrough pain in between the regular doses. The breakthrough dose should be one-sixth of the total regular dose prescribed over a 24-hour period. So, if the patient is on morphine sulphate 30 mg slow-release every 12 hours, the correct dose of morphine sulphate solution for breakthrough pain is 10 mg. The patient should keep a record of all the top-up doses that they take, so that the GP can use this to calculate the total amount of morphine that the patient actually needs and titrate up the regular dose.

Morphine sulphate should not be used in patients who have renal failure; these patients can be given hydromorphone

instead. All opiates cause constipation and nausea as side effects, so patients need a regular laxative and an antiemetic when required. If the dose is too strong, patients can experience opioid toxicity (Table 40.2).

Allowing natural death

Witnessing death is part of the GP's working life, and all GPs will tell you that there is such a thing as a 'good death'. What are the features of a good death? Tranquillity is one, and the other is being surrounded by close family. Both of these things are prevented if an attempt is made at cardiopulmonary resuscitation (CPR). If CPR is commenced, the family has to move to one side, often to another room; the patient is surrounded by health professionals and equipment, and the scene resembles an accident and emergency unit. In someone who has an acute illness but is otherwise reasonably well, CPR offers some hope of saving life, but in someone who is terminally ill and whose condition has been getting worse, CPR is likely to be futile – and if the person does survive, they will need intensive treatment, which is unlikely to give them many more days of life. For someone who is terminally ill, cardiac or respiratory arrest is the natural end of their illness.

The General Medical Council (GMC) recognises that there are situations in which CPR is not appropriate.[5] The default position (and one that has to be adopted by paramedics and health professionals who do not know the patient) is that in the event of a cardiac or respiratory arrest, CPR should be commenced. However, in its guidance on treatment and care towards the end of life, the GMC states that it is permissible not to attempt resuscitation if it is not in the patient's best interests and if the harm of treatment outweighs the benefits. The harm of treatment is not just broken ribs from chest compression, but the intensive treatment that is always needed if CPR is successful. The decision not to attempt resuscitation cannot be left until the time that cardiac or respiratory arrest occurs; it must be made in advance, and documented and discussed with the patient and their family. If the doctor senses that it is inappropriate to talk about this with the patient, they can make a decision about it themselves, but it is always good practice to discuss it with the family. If the family disagrees with the doctor, an attempt should be made to reach a consensus, but ultimately it is the doctor's decision. The GMC is clear that doctors are not compelled to provide treatment which in their view is likely to be futile; this applies as much to resuscitation as it does to surgery or prescribing medication.

If it's decided that it would be inappropriate to attempt resuscitation, this has to be communicated to all those who are involved or who may become involved in the patient's care. A form known as a 'Do Not Attempt Resuscitation' or 'Allow Natural Death' form[6] is left in the patient's house, and copies are sent to the ambulance service, the out-of-hours GP service and the community nurses.

Watching someone die, especially if you have not witnessed a death before, can be frightening. The GP and community nurses can take some of this fear away by explaining to the family members what is likely to happen. The patient's conscious level will fall and their breathing will become erratic In *Sons and Lovers*, Mrs Morel dies at home, watched over by her son and her daughter:

> His mother lay with a cheek on her hand, curled up as she had gone to sleep. But her mouth had fallen open and she breathed with long, hoarse breaths, like snoring, and there were long intervals between…The sound, so irregular, at such wide intervals, sounded through the house…
>
> He watched. Sometimes he thought the great breath would never begin again. He could not bear it – the waiting. Then suddenly, startling him, came the great harsh sound.
>
> *D.H. Lawrence, Sons and Lovers, 1913*

This is Cheyne–Stokes breathing. It can last a few hours, and to the onlooker it can appear as if the person is distressed. However, this is not the case, and the doctor can reassure the family of this.

After death

When death comes, it has to be confirmed by a health professional – at home, this is usually the GP. If the death is expected, there is no rush to do this; sometimes, the family appreciate an hour or so to themselves.

Confirming death

Diagnosing death at home requires a series of detailed observations, and the GP needs to explain this to the relatives. They should ask the relatives if they want to stay in the room when they confirm death. Most of the time, the relatives will want to leave, but sometimes they will stay; if so, the GP should make sure they explain what they are doing as they go along. Many GPs speak to the deceased person as they are confirming death. The relatives will often want to speak to them but will worry whether this is ok. If they see the doctor speak to their loved one then it gives them permission to do the same.

The body may still be warm, but the skin is pale and the limbs are floppy. Later on, a marbled-type bruising appears and the limbs stiffen. It may seem obvious that the patient is dead, but every so often mistakes are made, so it is important to be systematic in the examination.[7] According the code of practice of the Academy of Medical Royal Colleges,[8] the GP should check and record the following things:

- **Lack of motor response to stimuli:** 'Mrs Morel, can you feel this?' Speaking the patient's name and pressing on the supraorbital ridge should not provoke any response.
- **Absence of circulation:** 'I'm listening to your heart now.' Verifying that there is no circulation entails feeling for a carotid pulse and listening over the precordium with a stethoscope continually for 1 minute, and thereafter at intervals for a total of 5 minutes.
- **Absence of respiratory effort:** 'I'm checking your breathing.' We do this by holding the back of our hand over the mouth and observing the chest wall with our head close to the deceased person's chest for one minute. Observations should be continued for 5 minutes.
- **Changes to the eyes:** 'I'm going to look at your eyes now, and shine a torch in them.' The eyes may be wide open and their cornea may appear cloudy and dull. The corneal reflex is absent. The pupils are dilated and do not constrict in response to light. In two-thirds of cases, examination with an ophthalmoscope shows that the red blood cells are stacked up in short, stationary segments within the retinal arteries; this is referred to 'palisading' of the red blood cells and is an absolute indicator of death.

Once the examination is complete, the GP should note the time. This is the time at which death is confirmed. They should finish by closing the patient's eyes and checking what medical equipment is around them. If a syringe driver is in place, this will need to be removed, and the remaining ampoules of medicines disposed of safely. The community nurses will arrange this, but someone needs to contact them as soon as possible.

Having told the family that they have confirmed death and expressed their condolences, there are some other important things for the GP to consider and discuss. Are they in a position to issue a death certificate? Is the body going to be cremated or buried? Which undertaker is the family going to contact?

Issuing a death certificate

The statistics quoted earlier in this chapter about the proportion of patients who die at home and from what cause come from death certificates. Death certificates can only be issued by a doctor or the coroner. If the patient has died at home then it is the GP's duty to ensure that the death certificate is issued. The doctor who writes the death certificate must have seen the patient within 14 days of their death.[9] Therefore, the doctor who visited the patient at home and confirmed death may not be the doctor who issues the certificate. When a patient dies at night or the weekend, it is the out-of-hours GP who confirms death, but they leave it to the patient's usual GP to sort out a death certificate the next day.

The GP can issue a death certificate if they are confident of the cause of death; if not, they must refer the patient to the coroner by speaking to the coroner's officer. In the case of someone who has been receiving palliative care, the cause is rarely in doubt. However, even then it may be necessary to refer the case to the coroner.

Case study 40.2a

Gloria Goodman was 79 when she was diagnosed with a mixture of vascular dementia and Alzheimer's disease. She had previously enjoyed good health; the only medication she took was for hypertension. Her dementia came to light when her husband died and she struggled to live alone. Once the diagnosis was made, she went to live with her daughter. Her dementia got worse and, 2 years later, she had a fall when trying to get to the toilet at night. She was admitted to hospital and treated for a fractured neck of femur. She had several postoperative complications, but eventually she was discharged to a nursing home. She's been at the nursing home for 8 months now, and in that time her condition has continued to deteriorate. She needs help with eating and spends most of her time sitting in a chair next to her bed; she cannot walk. She can no longer hold a conversation, but she can make her wishes known by her expression and the tone of her voice. Since being at the nursing home, she has had several courses of antibiotics for chest and urine infections.

Last week, she became a bit more sleepy and started coughing. After examining her, the GP who visits the nursing home regularly diagnosed Mrs Goodman with another chest infection and talked with the staff and her daughter about her future care. Everyone was in agreement that Mrs Goodman was continuing to decline and that it would not be long before she succumbed to an infection and died. No one thought that it would be in her best interest to be admitted to hospital for intravenous antibiotics, and there was consensus that in the event of a cardiac arrest, CPR would be futile. The GP signed a 'Do Not Attempt Resuscitation' order, alerted the out-of-hours GP service and prescribed a course of amoxicillin suspension for her chest infection.

This morning, the staff are concerned that she is worse and ask the GP to visit again. The GP notes that she has Cheyne–Stokes breathing. Her temperature is 38.5 °C, her pulse is 124 and her oxygen saturation is 92% on air. The GP concludes that she has sepsis as the result of pneumonia. He anticipates that death is near and phones Mrs Goodman's daughter to say that her mother is seriously ill. Mrs Goodman is given rectal paracetamol to lower her temperature. She is unable to take anything by mouth and is unable to communicate; her eyes are closed. Later this afternoon, with her daughter and one nurse by her side, she dies. The GP visits again, confirms death, and then speaks to Mrs Goodman's daughter.

Can the GP issue a death certificate?
The GP saw Mrs Goodman the day before she died, saw her after death and has an explanation for her death. However, the fact that she had a fractured neck of femur fixed means that the GP needs to inform the coroner. Referral to the coroner doesn't mean that the patient will have a post mortem (although this can be the outcome); it simply gives the coroner the opportunity to investigate the death further. The situations in which a doctor should refer a death to the coroner are listed in Box 40.1.

Outcome
The GP phones the coroner's officer and outlines the case. The coroner's officer asks a few questions and concludes that the death is linked neither to the fall 9 months ago nor to the operation to fix her fractured neck of femur. The coroner's officer agrees with what the GP will write as a cause of death on the certificate: 'I(a) Pneumonia, I(b) Vascular dementia and Alzheimer's disease' (Figure 40.5).

Box 40.1 Situations in which death has to be referred to the coroner

- Cause of death not known.
- Patient has not seen a doctor within 14 days of death.
- Patient had an accident which may be linked to their death.
- Patient may have had an industrial-related disease.
- Death was violent or circumstances of death were suspicious.
- Evidence of neglect.
- Suicide.
- Death during or after an operation.
- Death while detained by the state (e.g. in prison).

Cause of death (the disease or condition thought to be the underlying cause should appear in the lowest completed line of part I)		
I	(a) Disease or condition leading directly to death	Pneumonia
	(b) Other disease or condition, if any, leading to I(a)	Vascular dementia and Alzheimer's disease
	(c) Other disease or condition, if any, leading to I(b)	
II	Other significant conditions **contributing to death** but not related to the disease or condition causing it	

Figure 40.5 Cause of death on a death certificate.

About one-third of all deaths in England and Wales are referred to the coroner, but only in one-fifth of cases (about 100 000 a year) does the coroner request a post mortem and end up issuing the death certificate. Only 15% of the referrals that are made when death follows a fractured neck of femur (as in Case study 40.2) proceed to a coroner's inquest.[9]

The death certificate has two parts in which the doctor can record the cause of death. The first part is for the immediate cause of death and the conditions underlying it. The second part is for other significant disease that does not have direct bearing on the cause of death but is related to it. A doctor does not have to write anything in part II, but must write something in part I. In Case study 40.2, the immediate cause of death is pneumonia, so this goes in part I(a) (see Figure 40.5). The pneumonia was caused by the immobility of Mrs Goodman's advanced dementia, so her vascular dementia and Alzheimer's disease go in part I(b). The lowest completed line of part I identifies the underlying cause of death, which causes all the conditions above it. In this case, the lowest completed line is 'I(b) Dementia'. The GP could also have written 'I(a) Pneumonia, I(b) Immobility, I(c) Mixed vascular and Alzheimer's dementia'.

Case study 40.2b

Gloria Goodman wrote in her will that she wanted to be cremated. Her daughter knows this and relays this information to the GP after her death.

What does the GP need to do to ensure that the cremation can go ahead?

If the deceased is to be cremated, an extra form has to be completed. This is because there will not be another opportunity to review the evidence (after a burial, a body can be exhumed). The cremation form has to be completed by two doctors. Part 1 is completed by the doctor who looked after the patient during their last illness (in this case, the GP) and Part 2 is completed by a doctor who had no involvement at all in the patient's care. This second doctor acts as a monitor, to check that the cause of death is correct. The murders by the GP Harold Shipman came to light because the doctors from a nearby practice were concerned about the number of Part 2 cremation certificates they were being asked to complete for his patients. The doctor signing Part 2 must speak to the GP who has completed Part 1 of the cremation form and to another person who was with the patient during their last illness, to check that they have no reason to doubt the cause of death. Both doctors must examine the body. Getting all this done can take a few days, and the GP needs to warn the family of this before they make plans for the funeral.

Once the GP has completed the death certificate, it needs to be collected by the deceased's family and taken by them to the registry office.

Bereavement

The bereaved family members are often registered at the same practice as the deceased, and they may require their GP's help in the days and weeks after the death. They may seek comfort simply by talking to the GP. They may have an ailment of their own that they bring to a consultation, but underlying this is just a need to talk. They may want things explained: 'I don't understand why he got bowel cancer; he was always such a fit man', or, 'Do you think he could hear us when we were sitting next to him in those last few hours?'

Bereavement can cause a mixture of emotions: disbelief, sadness at the loss, anger that the deceased has been 'taken' from them and sometimes guilt that they did not do more to help. There may be things that the bereaved person wishes they had said to their loved one, or things they wish they hadn't said. Talking to the deceased and imagining that they are still in the house is normal. Sometimes, the bereaved person feels angry with the deceased for abandoning them. For any or all of these things, the person may need reassurance from their GP.

Other sources of support are the charity CRUSE, which offers counselling, and Age UK, which provides an excellent leaflet on bereavement.[10] The most important support may be the bereaved person's faith. Sometimes, the bereaved and the GP will share the same faith, but often they will not, and so the GP has to tread carefully and not impose their own beliefs.

When does bereavement become depression? It's difficult to answer this, but it's something that GPs often have to consider. If bereavement does turn into depression then psychological therapies or antidepressants can be helpful.

The death of someone close to you can heighten worries about your own health. The widow of a man who died from lung cancer will naturally be concerned next time she gets a cough. 'Have I got lung cancer too?', she may think, 'I smoked more than him'. Often, when someone comes to their GP, the trigger that made them book the appointment was some shocking news about the death or serious illness of a friend, colleague or family member.

Self-care

Doctors are not immune to these worries and emotions. Caring for a patient over a long period of time and seeing them die takes its toll. Patients can become friends, and when they die, the GP can feel shaken and tearful. The death of a patient may rekindle other upsetting memories and emotions. GPs need to be aware of this and ask themselves – not just their patients – 'Am I ok?'

Case study 40.3

Claire Cookson is a 42-year-old GP. She works at the surgery 3 days a week and is at home the other 2 days; she is married and has two young children. Her husband is working away this week. Her mother, who lives 2 hours' drive away, was diagnosed with breast cancer last month. Today, Claire is the duty doctor at the surgery. Just before the start of her afternoon surgery, she receives a phone call from the daughter of one of her patients, Janet Jakeman, who has metastatic breast cancer. Janet has been on a syringe driver delivering morphine for the last 4 days; she has just died at home.

Claire tells the receptionists that she will be a bit late starting afternoon surgery and then goes to Janet's house. Janet's daughter takes her upstairs and there, in Janet's bedroom, Claire examines Janet and confirms death. Janet looks peaceful.

Back downstairs, in the front room, Claire sits with Janet's daughter. On the mantelpiece is an old family photo, taken when Janet's daughter was still at school. As they are talking, Claire feels her tears building up; she is thinking of her own mother. In a year's time, will she be in the position of Janet's daughter?

What should Claire do?
Claire could explain to Janet's daughter that her own mother has just been diagnosed with breast cancer. If Claire has got to know Janet's daughter well, it may be very natural to talk openly like this. But Janet's daughter may be so overwhelmed with grief that it would be inappropriate for Claire to discuss her own worries.

Outcome
Claire settles herself and says to Janet's daughter that she will have a death certificate ready for collection in the morning. Back at the surgery, the receptionists can see that Claire is upset; they make her a cup of tea and tell her that one of her first patients has rebooked for another day (it wasn't that urgent) and one of the other GPs has seen another couple of patients. She will therefore not be starting her surgery too much behind schedule. Claire gets through the rest of the surgery, and when she gets home, she asks a neighbour to look after the children for an hour so that she can go for a run. Running is one of her ways of relaxing. After this, she phones her mother and arranges to visit her at the weekend.

SUMMARY

Providing palliative care is an important and rewarding part of a GP's work. Most people want to die at home. The proportion of people who actually do so is increasing, and GPs can support people in this wish using the Macmillan Gold Standards Framework. GPs can prescribe medication to provide relief of the common symptoms experienced in the last weeks and days of life, and can help patients and their families prepare for death. The legal duties of GPs include confirming death and completing medical certificates of the cause of death and cremation certificates. After a patient's death, GPs are often in a good position to support those who are bereaved. At the same time, GPs should not ignore their own emotional well-being.

 Now visit **www.wileyessential.com/primarycare** to test yourself on this chapter.

REFERENCES

1. Saunders C. Care of the dying. 1. The problem of euthanasia. *Nurs Times* 1976;**72**(26):1003–5.
2. Gold Standards Framework. The GSF Prognostic Indicator Guidance: the National GSF Centre's guidance for clinicians to support earlier recognition of patients nearing the end of life. Available from: http://www.goldstandardsframework.org.uk/cd-content/uploads/files/General%20Files/Prognostic%20Indicator%20Guidance%20October%202011.pdf (last accessed 6 October 2015).
3. Hunt KJ, Shlomo N, Addington-Hall J. End-of-life care and achieving preferences for place of death in England: results of a population-based survey using the VOICES-SF questionnaire. *Palliat Med* 2014:**28**(5);412–21.
4. Office for National Statistics. Mortality statistics: deaths registered in England and Wales (Series DR), 2012. Available from: http://www.ons.gov.uk/ons/publications/re-reference-tables.html?edition=tcm%3A77-325289 (last accessed 6 October 2015).

5. General Medical Council. Treatment and care towards end of life: good practice in decision making. 2010. Available from: http://www.gmc-uk.org/guidance/ethical_guidance/end_of_life_care.asp (last accessed 6 October 2015).

6. Resuscitation Council (UK). Model form: do not attempt cardiopulmonary resuscitation. 2009. Available from: http://resus.org.uk/pages/DNARrstd.htm (last accessed 6 October 2015).

7. Charlton R. Diagnosing death. *BMJ* 1996;**313**:956–7.

8. Academy of Medical Royal Colleges. A code of practice for the diagnosis and confirmation of death. 2008. Available from: http://www.aomrc.org.uk/doc_details/42-a-code-of-practice-for-the-diagnosis-and-confirmation-of-death (last accessed 6 October 2015).

9. Office for National Statistics' Death Certification Advisory Group. Guidance for doctors completing medical certificates of cause of death in England and Wales. Revised 2010. Available from: http://www.gro.gov.uk/images/medcert_July_2010.pdf (last accessed 6 October 2015).

10. Age UK. Bereavement: support after death. July 2014. Available from: http://www.ageuk.org.uk/health-wellbeing/relationships-and-family/bereavement/emotional-effects-of-bereavement/ (last accessed 6 October 2015).

Index

Essential Primary Care, First Edition. Edited by Andrew Blythe and Jessica Buchan.
© 2017 John Wiley & Sons, Ltd. Published 2017 by John Wiley & Sons, Ltd.
Companion website: www.wileyessential.com/primarycare

diabetes (*cont'd*)
  type 1 126
  type 2 99–104
  visual problems 99, 323
diagnosis 22–9
  defining 23
  errors (misdiagnosis/missed diagnosis) 12, 27
    cancer 349–50
    prevention 28
  information at discharge on 48
  learning disability and overshadowing a 88
  making/reaching a 23–9
    labelling in 23
    learning 29
    prescribing and 34
    processes for 25–6
  revision failure 27
  science and art 23
Diagnostic and Statistical Manual of Mental Disorders 5 (DSM5) 211, 216
diarrhoea 178–82
  child 126
dietary modification/management 60
  menopausal symptoms 304
  type 2 diabetes 101
digoxin, monitoring 37
disc, intervertebral
  inflammation (discitis) 166
  non-inflammatory pathology 166
discharge from hospital 47–8
disclosure of domestic violence and abuse 258
  responding to 258, 259
Disease Activity Score 28 (DAS28) 290–1
disease-centred vs patient-centred care in multimorbidity 309–10
disease-modifying drugs in rheumatoid arthritis 37, 290, 291
dissatisfaction, good communication reducing 12
dissonance 53
diuretics
  in diarrhoea, temporarily ceasing 181
  monitoring 37
  thiazide 82, 83
dizziness 206–8
doctor *see* GP
domestic violence and abuse 254–61
donepezil 338
Doppler studies, peripheral arterial disease 272, 273
dose of drug 34
Down's syndrome (trisomy 21) 86, 87, 88, 89
  antenatal screening 345
  case study 90–1
drinking *see* alcohol
driving
  and epilepsy 206
  and myocardial infarction 269
drug-induced disorders (and adverse reactions/side effects) 33
  asthma aggravation 279
  breathlessness 277
  diarrhoea 180
  heartburn 171
  hypothyroidism 98

osteoarthritis 289
psoriasis 186
reporting 40
specific drugs/drug types
  antimigraine agents 196
  chemotherapeutics 353
  combined oral contraceptive pill 236
  opioids 365
  statins 83
drug misuse 74–6
  teenagers 151
drug therapy *see* medications/drugs
DSM5 (Diagnostic and Statistical Manual of Mental Disorders 5) 211, 216
DTaP/(diphtheria; tetanus; pertussis) 115
dual-energy X-ray absorptiometry (DEXA) scan 316, 317, 318, 319
duodenal ulcer 24, 175
duration of drug therapy 35
dysfunctional uterine bleeding 235
dysmenorrhoea (painful periods) 235
  case study 237
dyspepsia 171, 173–6
dyspnoea *see* breathlessness
dysuria 220–2

ear
  infection, middle *see* otitis media
  pain (earache) 130
  wax, and syringing 328–9
  see also hearing loss
ear, nose and throat (ENT), over-the-counter medicines 32
eardrum/tympanic membrane
  children
    in chronic otitis media 142
    with earache 130
  occlusion by wax 328
  perforation 130
eating disorders 148, 153, 232
ECG *see* electrocardiogram
echocardiography, ejection fraction measurement 282
ectopic pregnancy 247
eczema *see* dermatitis
EEG, epileptic fit 205
ejection fraction, echocardiographic measurement 282
elderly *see* older people and the elderly
electrocardiogram (ECG)
  atrial fibrillation 266
  breathlessness 277
  hypertension 81
  syncope 204
electroencephalogram (EEG), epileptic fit 205
'elicit– provide–elicit' model 63
embolism, pulmonary 27, 277, 277–8
emergency admission to hospital *see* admission to hospital
emergency contraception (postcoital) 239
emollients 142
emotional abuse, children 117
empathy 13
  alcohol misuse 71

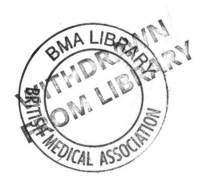

Hands On

Setting Up a Discovery Room in Your Museum or School

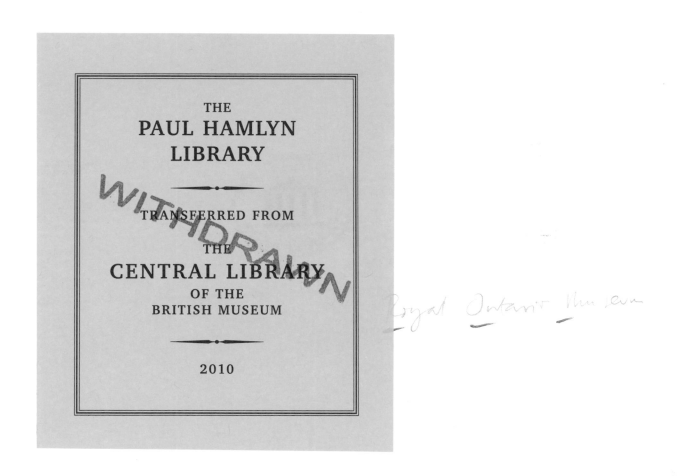

RŌM
Royal Ontario Museum
1979

© the Royal Ontario Museum, 1979
100 Queen's Park, Toronto, Ontario M5S 2C6

ISBN 0-88854-241-0

Printed and bound in Canada

Cover photo: the Stumper shelf in the ROM Discovery Room,
with the Tree Unit in the background

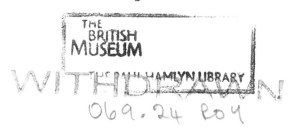

Contents

APPENDIX B: EVALUATION

Plates and Figures

Plates

Figures

Tables

Foreword

It is fairly common knowledge that infants and young children use all their senses, including the tactile sense, in learning about their new environment. Children are constantly touching and feeling objects and even placing them in their mouths in this process of learning about the world that surrounds them. Large segments of Western society, however, have traditionally introduced the child, very early in his development, to the "don't touch" syndrome. By the time we are adults, most of us have long lost the ease with which a young child uses the tactile sense to explore his environment, to gather data about the world around him, and to learn through his sense of touch.

For a variety of reasons, most museums in the Western world also accepted the social limitations on the methods by which people are expected to learn. Visitors to museums were to learn by looking, by reading, and sometimes by listening. Only under very special conditions were objects or specimens to be touched by the general museum visitor during the learning process.

Over the past ten years there have been discussions and deliberations at the Royal Ontario Museum as to how the institution might provide a variety of opportunities for its visitors to use all of their senses in learning within the museum context. Coupled with this concern was a desire to share with the visitor some of the sense of discovery which museum staff members constantly experience in working with the museum collections. This movement towards the introduction of "discovery" learning approaches at the ROM was accelerated by the opening of the Discovery Room at the Smithsonian Institution in Washington, D.C. In the spring of 1976, a small work group was set up in the Royal Ontario Museum under the chairmanship of Mr. Riley Moynes, Head of the Education Services Department, to investigate the feasibility of establishing a test Discovery Room in the ROM. The individuals in this work group, listed in the introduction to this book, set to work on this task with enormous energy and enthusiasm.

In September 1976, the Discovery Room Working Group came under the general supervision of the Exhibits Communication Task Force, which was established at that time to consolidate all gallery planning in the Museum into a master plan to be implemented over the next twenty years. The ECTF subsequently approved the Discovery Room Working Group's recommendation that the Museum should test a prototype Discovery Room in order to learn how much of the discovery approach could be introduced into its galleries and whether a specialized Discovery Room could work at the ROM. The soundness of this recommendation has been overwhelmingly attested by the acclamation of the 100,000 visitors who have used the prototype Discovery Room during the first year and a half of its existence. It has also been validated by the results of an evaluation of the prototype Discovery Room carried out by Urban Design Consultants, under contract. An account of the objectives of this evaluation, the methodology used, the results, and the analysis of the data has been very deliberately included in this publication. We feel that this evaluation can show readers, more vividly than anything else, what is likely to be successful and what to avoid in setting up their own discovery approaches or discovery facilities. The evaluation, whose results are printed as Appendix B in this volume, was carried out over the first six months of the prototype Discovery Room's operation. As a result of it, some components have been removed and others added. The process of evaluation, of course, is on-going as a basis for the development of a new and enlarged Discovery Room.

The report produced by the Discovery Room Working Group has had a strong impact on the Museum's gallery plans described in *Mankind Discovering*, Volume I.* It has also affected the planning for other educational facilities and programmes within the Museum.

It was felt that the report, which was originally written for internal use, should be shared with other museums and schools which might also be interested in re-introducing the tactile sense to the learning process and the sense of discovery to education. The production of this handbook, from

---

*Obtainable from Publication Services, Royal Ontario Museum.

the original Discovery Room report, has been carried out by
Dr. Ross James, Mr. David Newlands, Mr. John Campsie, Mrs.
Alison Glennie, and myself.

We, in the Royal Ontario Museum, hope that the process described in this report and the conclusions presented will
be found useful and stimulating in helping you to set up a
Discovery Room in your own museum or school.

Joseph Di Profio
Chairman,
Exhibit Communication Task
Force

January 18, 1979

Hands On

Setting Up a Discovery Room
in Your Museum or School

Introduction

The Royal Ontario Museum (ROM) is centrally located in Toronto.
It is a large museum with more than twenty curatorial departments and approximately 14,000 m² (150,000 square feet) of galleries, and it has acquired an international reputation for
its collections and its research.

The original Museum building was started in 1910, and a major
addition was undertaken in 1932. Apart from the addition of
the McLaughlin Planetarium and a cafeteria in 1970 and 1971
respectively, no major alterations have been made to the building since 1932. The ROM is currently (1979) in the midst of
an expansion and renovation project which will include an increase of approximately 4,700 m² (50,000 square feet) of gallery
space and will provide improved facilities for the production
of exhibits for these galleries.

In preparation for expansion and renovation, the Museum has
undertaken a comprehensive planning programme, as part of
which the Exhibits Communication Task Force (ECTF) was established in 1976 to formulate an overall plan for the re-organ-
ization and development of galleries. Early in its deliberations, the ECTF decided to formulate and test a "Discovery
Room" concept as a possible component of the plan. A memorandum from the Director in September 1976 outlined this concept in the following terms:

> The discovery room concept is one in which a large room would be
> provided in the Museum, open to the public, and stocked with
> materials from and about the ROM collections. Visitors to the
> room would be able to handle and interact with these materials
> under minimum supervision. The underlying educational concept
> is that the visitors would discover new levels of knowledge
> through this interaction with the materials. The manipulation
> of materials, closer observation afforded by this, and curiosity
> aroused, would deepen the learning of the visitors to this room.

The same memorandum announced the formation of the Discovery Room Working Group (DRWG), a sub-group of the ECTF charged with the design and testing of a discovery room for the ROM, and assigned it three specific tasks:

(1) To prepare recommendations for the Exhibits Communication Task Force on the development of a "discovery room" for the ROM.

(2) To pre-test the underlying educational principles for such a room, and to determine the best way of implementing those principles.

(3) To make recommendations to the Task Force on the use of discovery approaches in the regular galleries of the Museum.

Staff assistance was provided from the outset to assist the DRWG in defining its objectives and in designing and carrying out an evaluation programme (Appendix B) based on these objectives, which were formulated as follows:

The Discovery Room should be a place with an informal atmosphere where people can become more actively involved with the ROM and its collections. This objective is defined by the following criteria which are ranked in order of priority:

- *The Discovery Room will provide an enjoyable learning experience.*

- *The components of the Discovery Room should be oriented to discovery learning. It is more important that the components of the Room be interrelated by their common demonstration of the discovery learning approach than by their content. The Room should supply the visitor with a place to work, and books, equipment, and labelled specimens which he/she can actively examine and study. Replicas will only be used where necessary in the Room. Static displays should be of minimum importance.*

- *The Discovery Room should experiment with the discovery learning concept and with various approaches to determine its applicability elsewhere in the ROM and outside of the Museum.*

- *The Discovery Room should be designed for everyone, but experience has shown that family groupings tend to be the primary audience; therefore, components should be designed with that in mind. Also, where possible, the text should be presented multilingually and in Braille.*

- *The use of all senses interacting together should be encouraged.*

● *The components of the Discovery Room should relate to the galleries and departmental collections. In this way the content of the Discovery Room will reflect the ROM content. However, attempts to make the Room representative of all divisions and departments should be secondary to the criteria for developing the best examples.*

The DRWG included a wide range of specialists from within the Museum as well as a representative from the Ontario Teachers' Federation. The members were:

Dr. David Barr, Entomology Department

Miss Jane Court, Public Relations Department

Dr. Gordon Edmund, Vertebrate Palaeontology Department

Dr. Helmut Fuchs, Ethnology Department

Miss Nancy Gahm, Education Services Department

Dr. Ross James, Ornithology Department

Ms. Mary Jones, Extension Services Department

Mr. Robert Madeley, Education Services Department

Mr. Tim Moore, Exhibit Design Services Department

Mr. Riley Moynes, Education Services Department

Mr. David Newlands, Museum Studies Department

Mr. John Richardson, Ontario Teachers' Federation

In an effort to gather new ideas and to learn from the experience of other institutions, some members of the group and Discovery Room staff visited other discovery rooms at the American Museum of Natural History in New York, the National Museum of Natural History at the Smithsonian Institution in Washington, the Florida State Museum in Gainesville, and the Brooklyn Children's Museum, the last named of which is entirely devoted to the "discovery" concept. The group also conducted research in museum literature and worked closely with the curatorial departments at the ROM to develop the components of the new Room. The following general recommendations were then presented to the DRWG.

(1) Staffing There should be a full-time manager for the supervision and further development of the Room and for the care of its materials. This individual should have good communication skills and enthusiasm for the concept of a discovery room.

Discovery Room staff must be well-trained and able to encourage and stimulate visitors without interfering in the "discovery" experience.

(2) <u>Room design</u>   The physical design of the Room should in-corporate bright lighting, attractive colours for dec-oration, ample space, materials that absorb sound, tables for work space, and an adequate amount of seating. The disruptive effects of audio-visual equipment should be carefully studied before any decision is made about the permanent installation of any audio-visual materials.

(3) <u>Room components</u>   Materials that are either in boxes or in drawers or are free-standing should be the main fea-tures   Large display cases have little place in a dis-covery room.

The boxes, drawers, and their contents must be attract-ively presented, easily accessible, and capable of being used by children and adults alike. Construction mater-ials must be carefully chosen for durability and visual appeal, and labelling and illustrations for clarity, legibility, and interest.

Live exhibits, such as plants and aquaria, are assets to the Room only if they are well maintained and attract-ively presented. Dying plants or dirty fish tanks in-dicate insufficient care or improper room conditions.

(4) <u>Discovery Room policies</u>   Guidelines should be established to restrict the number of visitors in the Room at one time. Too great a number of visitors in the Room, es-pecially unaccompanied young children, can often result in tension, theft of materials, or damage to the Room's components.

The security measures must be adequate to deter theft and damage. Volunteers should check the contents of any box or tray that has been used.

(5) <u>Range of interest</u>   Discovery Room activities and printed materials should appeal to a variety of ages, interests, and educational backgrounds. Most of the material should be aimed at a grade eight education level. Children be-low school age should not be admitted to the Room because their activities interfere with the use of the Room by other people.

The multicultural nature of Toronto should be reflected in multilingual printed material.

Wherever possible, the Room should attempt to appeal to handicapped visitors. Some labels could be printed in Braille. Large print is helpful for the very young or elderly visitor.

(6) <u>Outreach programmes</u> Because of the interest that the Discovery Room is expected to generate, several extension activities should be considered.

During the year after its formation, the DRWG met regularly to develop the goals of the Room and to choose components that would realize these goals. Its members were encouraged to listen to one another and to weigh each issue so that the group could reach a consensus. The group submitted a formal report to the ECTF at five stages of the process. Day-to-day reporting was the task of the DRWG's chairman. Usually, the DRWG submitted proposals with estimated budgets to the ECTF. After the proposals were approved, the responsibility for making further decisions rested principally with the group.

The goals of the DRWG provided a framework for the development of the contents of the Room as well as for the design and layout of facilities. In addition to the main goals already enumerated, it was intended that the Room should provide a limited identification resource, should encourage the visitor to visit other ROM galleries, and should create an interest in museum work in general and the work of the Royal Ontario Museum in particular.

The time and effort expended by members of the Discovery Room Working Group were generously supplemented by assistance from the Museum staff and from the community at large, which is here gratefully acknowledged. Many curators provided objects for the Room and gave expert advice on related technical matters. Each component was developed in cooperation with curatorial staff so that the natural link between the knowledge of the Museum staff, the collections of the ROM, and the contents of the Room was maintained. Mrs. Bette Shepherd and Miss Nancy Willson worked full time for six months to plan, assemble, and test all components before the Room was opened to the public. The hundreds of small but nonetheless important tasks that were performed by all those people are reflected in this report. Leila Gad, Harold Vanstone, Georgia Guenther, Robin Shepherd, Andrea Rankin-Cameron, and Frances MacArthur also provided much-needed assistance prior to the opening of the Room. A special vote of thanks should be given to Ms. Jan Schroer, Assistant Co-ordinator of the Exhibits Communication Task Force, who was in daily contact with the DRWG, and who provided most of the necessary support and coordination. Her assistance enabled the Room to be opened without long and costly delays.

The Discovery Room Working Group would further like to thank the Members' Committee of the Museum and the Museum Volunteers, who helped in assembling the components and who are still the main source of staff for the operation of the Room.

The ECTF has also been helpful and has supported the Discovery Room. Urban Design Consultants (UDC), under contract with the Museum, have assisted in scheduling the work on the Room and testing its effectiveness by studying the responses of visitors.

A number of groups and institutions that have helped with preparations must also be mentioned. They include: the Public Affairs Branch of the Metro Toronto Postal District, Canada Post Office; the Abitibi Paper Company; the Toronto East General Hospital; Wellesley Hospital; the Hospital for Sick Children; the Toronto Entomological Society; the Botany and Metallurgy Departments of the University of Toronto; and the Canadian National Institute for the Blind. Without their support, various components in the Room could not have been prepared.

The Museum would like to express its appreciation to the many individuals, both from the ROM and from other institutions, who have given freely of their time and experience to help make the Discovery Room such a success.

Creating an Environment

Because the Discovery Room is located on the lower level of the Museum, apart from other exhibits and in an area most visitors do not use, it was important that the entrance be attractive. The vestibule was painted in a dark colour and a low light level was used as a contrast to the brighter light inside. The light in the vestibule was focussed on the "Touch Wall" and on two large "Stumpers". By placing the touch wall and stumpers right at the entrance, the designers hoped not only that people would be drawn to the Room but also that, once inside, they would be encouraged to handle the exhibits. The doors had glass panels installed so that visitors would be attracted into the Room by the sight of the exhibits. A large sign was mounted over the entrance to indicate that this room was one of the Museum's galleries.

The walls of the Room were painted a bright colour, but the high ceiling was painted in a dark shade in order to make it appear lower. Air conditioning was installed to make the atmosphere as comfortable as is possible in a small area continuously filled with people. Carpeting was laid to muffle sounds and to enhance the Room's appearance.

Because the Discovery Room has an area of only 150 m^2 (approx. 1,600 square feet), it was necessary to make the optimum use of space. Many components had to be mounted on the walls, while some Stumpers were placed on top of tables or on other units, and mobiles were suspended from the ceiling. Originally, the Room was intended to accommodate up to twenty-five people (this limit has since been lowered to twenty), but only one table and eight chairs were installed, because of limited space. Raised carpeted areas could also be used for seating. However, the need for another table and several chairs soon became apparent and these had to be added.

Stools, carpeted areas, and chairs were placed in different parts of the Room to lessen congestion and to encourage visitors to work near the components. Tables provided work areas for family groups and were placed near the most frequently used boxes.

In order to encourage visitors' involvement, the contents of the Room differ in many ways from those of a conventional gallery. Boxes and identification units are easily moved from shelves to work areas. Stumpers are placed on open shelves as well as on tables and other surfaces throughout the Room so that they can be used freely. The Tree Unit has components on open shelves, and the skeleton can be approached and touched without any hindrance. Brightly coloured boxes with large clear lettering and identification units with colour photographs on the front help attract attention to these items.

The heights of components are varied. The Tree Unit and Stumper shelves are on different levels, and the touch wall extends nearly to the floor. Components were made as durable as possible to withstand the extensive use that would be made of them by visitors of widely varying ages. Cards are laminated and held together with leather thongs; boxes, made of wood, have lids secured by long piano hinges; carpeted floors soften the impact of items that might be dropped; pieces of equipment such as hand lenses are secured by chains.

Materials used in the Room come from ROM departments. Instead of purchasing commercially available display boxes of a standard size, the Discovery Room boxes are constructed according to the designers' specifications, a practice which allows a greater range of materials to be displayed. Soft padding in the boxes reduces damage and lessens noise. Carpeting on shelves and unit tops further helps to absorb sound.

Many of these features can be seen on the accompanying floor plan or in the photographs.

Components

Initially, a large part of every Discovery Room meeting was spent discussing components. All suggestions were considered in the light of the established goals of the Room, and from a practical and financial standpoint. Each component received preliminary approval from the DRWG. After the staff had prepared a detailed outline, final approval for the development of the component was given by the DRWG.

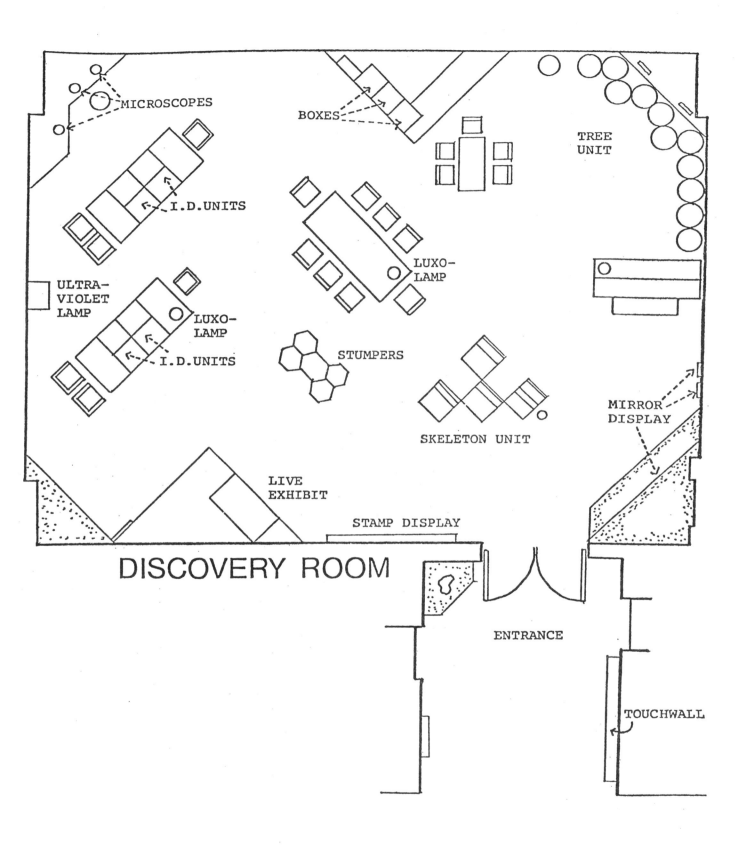

The types of components that were chosen can be grouped under six headings: discovery boxes; stumpers; identification units; fixed exhibits; live exhibits; and support components. Photographs of many of these units are to be found on pages 13, 14, 19, and 20.

DISCOVERY BOXES

The most popular component in the ROM Discovery Room, as in other museum discovery rooms, is the discovery boxes. The ones in the ROM are made of brightly stained wood and are approximately 40 cm square and 10 to 15 cm high. "Letra-sign" titles are written on the sides in French and English. The lids, supported with strong piano hinges, are chained to the bases to hold them upright when open. Light-weight plastic was not used in construction because it could not be made sufficiently colourful nor was it strong enough for the lids.

The boxes are lined with corduroy-covered foam and the interiors are divided into compartments by wooden slats to house the contents properly. Photographs or diagrams are mounted on the inside of the lids where appropriate. Each box is self-contained and usually comprises a few objects lying loosely in the separate compartments. A magnifying glass may be included. A numbered sequence of laminated 12 x 20 cm cards is available in French and English. Some sets of cards have been translated into Portuguese, Chinese, Italian, Spanish, German, and Braille.

The boxes are designed to be used by one person or by a family, and the cards lead the reader through a carefully planned series of questions and activities that involve the objects in the box. The contents of the boxes vary in difficulty according to the subject treated and to the number of boxes about each subject. Most were intended to be completed in less than ten minutes, but the interest time for each depends upon the visitor.

Although every box is designed as a complete unit, some deal with different aspects of the same topic. If boxes relate to each other, to other objects in the Room, or to a gallery exhibit elsewhere in the ROM, the relationship is indicated on the cards. Open shelving provides accommodation for twenty-two boxes against one wall. Since over thirty boxes have been developed, and more are being prepared, they are not all in circulation at the same time.

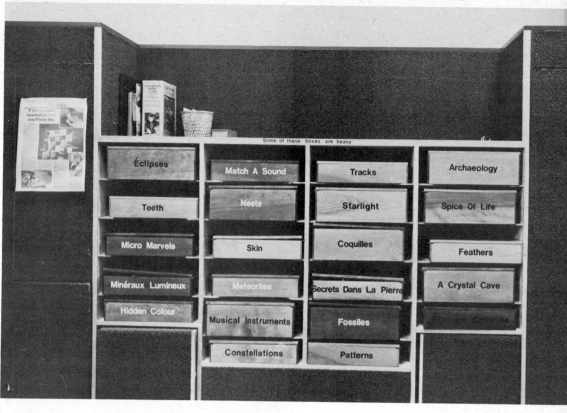

1. Box Shelf

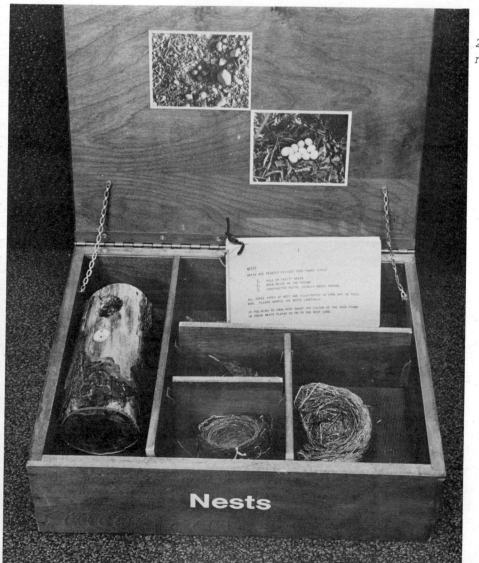

2. Nests Box, showing nests and cards

14

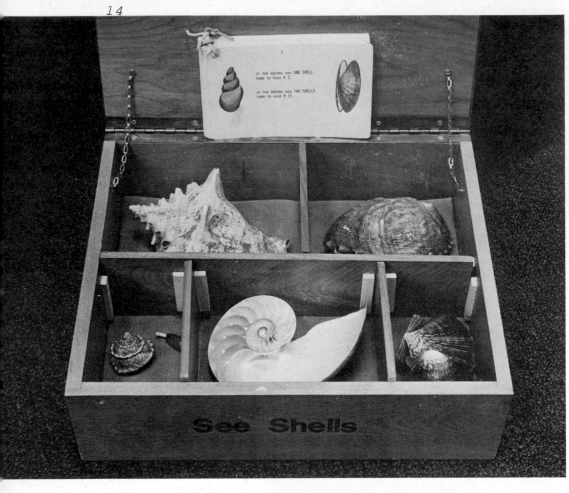

3. *Sea Shell Box*
showing shells and
illustrated cards

4. *Glowing Rocks Box,*
showing rocks and
cards

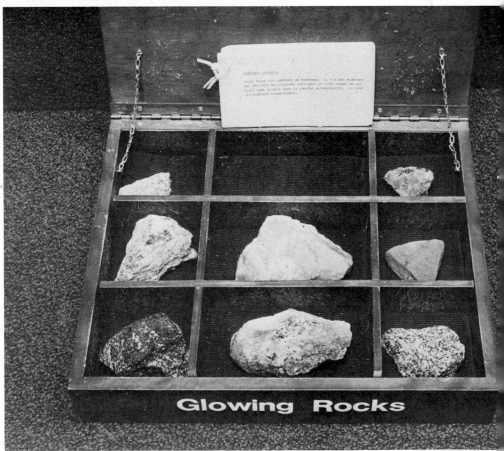

The following boxes were in circulation at the end of 1977:

(1) Micro-Marvels	(13) Patterns
(2) Spice of Life	(14) Feathers
(3) Meteorites	(15) Hidden Colour - fluores-cent objects
(4) Starlight - colours and brightness	(16) Shells
(5) Fossils	(17) Tracks
(6) Skin	(18) Chinese Writing
(7) Constellations	(19) Eclipses
(8) Teeth	(20) Musical Instruments
(9) Nests	(21) Glowing Rocks
(10) Match-a-Sound (2 boxes)	(22) Moonlight
(11) Archaeology - potsherds	(23) Bean Bag
(12) Crystal Cave	

STUMPERS

Though the Room is designed for the reading public, many visitors to a museum only wish to look. "Accidental dis-covery" plays a very important role in arousing visitors' interest. About thirty unrelated objects called "Stumpers", are arranged on a five-tiered glass and chrome shelving unit. Some of the Stumpers are accompanied by a card which asks a question and gives the answer. Others are simply identified. These Stumpers are in the Room to catch the attention of visitors, to stimulate their curiostiy, and to invite them to touch an exotic or unusual item.

The following items have proved to be among the most popular Stumpers:

Ostrich egg	Mammoth tooth
Cinnamon bark	Ammonite fossil
Cocoa pod and beans	Tamarind seed necklace
Wooden winter horseshoe	Large glass marble
Gar skin	Nickernut pod
Spittoon	Brazil nut pod

Brook trout in alcohol   Yellow perch in alcohol

Egyptian stone weight   Seabean pod

Wooden corn planter

Fossiliferous limestone slab   English "pot" helmet

Seychelle Island palm nut   Grinding stone

Wasp nest   Section of a tree trunk
                                     chewed by a beaver

Crock which collapsed   Mounted Great-horned Owl
     in the kiln

Mounted Spotted Sandpiper   Mounted Red-tailed Hawk

Pilot whale skull   Model of Canada's largest
                                     meteorite

Interesting objects brought in by visitors or volunteer staff
can become new Stumpers. Skeletons of a squirrel, a crow,
two bats, and a pigeon have recently been donated to the
Room.

IDENTIFICATION UNITS

Visitors have always brought material to the Museum for identification. Thus, it seemed logical to set up identification
units that would enable visitors to answer their own questions. The specimens are housed in four ten-drawer units,
with study tables at either end, and in an accessible location to encourage visitors' involvement. Each drawer is 42
cm square and 7.5 cm deep, made of wood, and stained a light
blue. The entire structure is carpeted on the top where a
selection of reference books is kept (see plate on page 19).

Lists are provided showing the location of further study
specimens in the galleries. A wide range of magnifying
glasses, microscopes, and lamps, together with special
lighting for the removable drawers, helps to make the experience pleasant for both the collector and the general
visitor.

When the Room opened, two problems emerged almost immediately.
The printing in the drawers was difficult to read, and the
public had to be encouraged to open drawers and touch the
objects. The unit was therefore improved by adding coloured
photographs to the drawer fronts, by using more legible print,
and by including directions for the unit's use.

At the end of 1977, the unit contained ten drawers of Ontario butterflies and moths, ten of insects embedded in plastic or dried and pinned in small plastic jewellery boxes, five of Canadian stamps, six of Ontario arrowheads and spear points, and four of prehistoric Ontario potsherds.

The butterfly drawers have non-removable glass tops and bottoms. Fixed glass lids protect the stamps, arrowheads, and potsherds, but the glass lids on the fossil drawers are removable. The drawers that contain insects set in plastic have no lids.

FIXED EXHIBITS

(a) Human Skeleton

An articulated, adult human skeleton is a constant source of interest to a large number of visitors to the Room. The skeleton is mounted in an upright position and there are no barriers to prevent people from touching the bones or from carefully "shaking hands". An illuminated panel presents a labelled diagram of a skeleton as well as radiographs of a variety of bone fractures and diseases. A human skull cut open to expose the cranial cavity, a femur with an imperfectly set fracture, and a series of tubercular vertebrae lie on three carpeted cubes. Three panels displaying photographs of human remains from past cultures hang above the exhibit.

(b) Tree Display

A large, 152-year-old red oak tree that had been removed from the ROM garden because it was diseased became the focus of a component which deals with Ontario wood. The parts of a cross-section of the trunk are labelled on one side. On the other, several growth rings have been indicated, along with the year of their formation and an important event of that year.

Carpeted cylinders act as pedestals for small labelled sections of the trunks of fourteen species of Ontario tree. The sections are cut both lengthwise and in cross-sections so that the characteristic grain of each can be examined. A selection of wooden objects, some modern and some from pioneer times in Canada, are housed in a wooden barrel or are lying on the cylinders. These objects include:

a hockey stick

a rolling pin

a butter paddle

a maple sugar mould

a carpenter's plane

With each type of wood are cards that name and describe it, outline its uses, and show a silhouette of the tree and its leaf shape. A folder containing pressed leaves and colour photographs of the tree, its leaves, and its bark is provided for each of the fourteen species.

Although the unit is attractive, it has proved to be less successful than anticipated and plans for condensing the physical layout are being considered.

(c) Stamp Display

A Stamp Display mounted on the wall contains panels of stamps illustrating Indians of Canada and human evolution. A selection of first day covers, photographs of a few early Canadian stamps, and samples of Canadian postmarks complete the unit. Three magnifying glasses attached to a shelf in front of the unit invite closer examination.

(d) Mirror Display

A display of mirrors from different ages, which includes a piece of obsidian, an Egyptian copper mirror, Palestinian, Greek, Chinese, and Japanese bronze mirrors, and European Rococo and American Sheraton glass mirrors is to be found in one corner of the Room. An information panel records important stages in the development of mirror glass.

As there is little opportunity for the visitor to involve himself with this unit, the Mirror Display has not been popular and plans are being made to remove it.

(e) Mobiles

Specimens of a Sandhill Crane, a Canada Goose, a Ring-billed Gull, and a Silver-haired Bat are suspended from the ceiling and mounted in flying positions. These mobiles add an upper dimension to the Room and provide resource material for use in conjunction with the boxes.

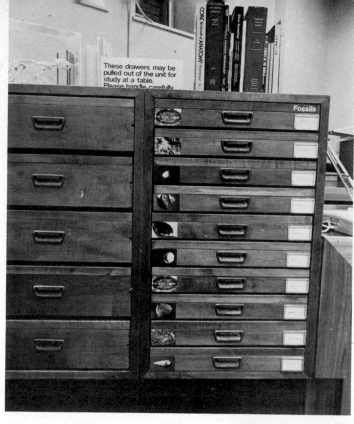

5. Fossil Identification Unit

6. Skeleton and bone X-rays

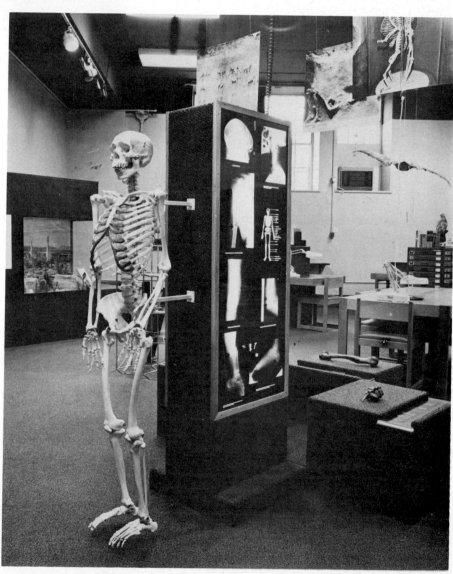

20

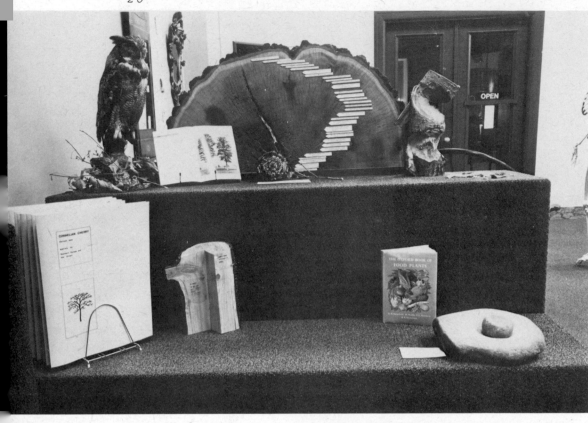

7. Tree Unit: labelled tree ring; owl; and tree folders in rack

8. Canada Goose, with Tree Unit in background

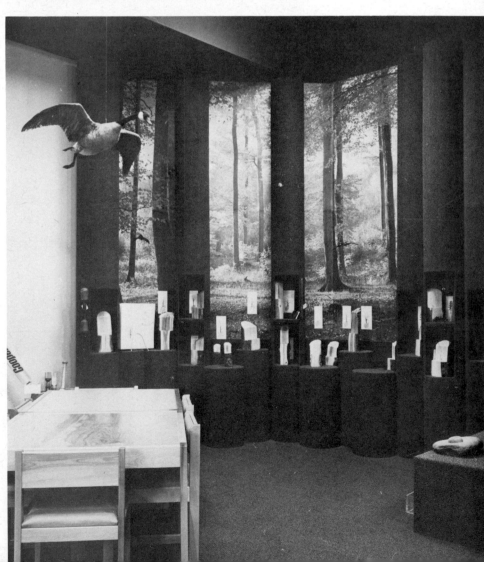

(f) Touch Wall

One of the most innovative components - a Touch Wall with
thirty-two squares of tactile material - is located in the
vestibule of the Room. The wall, composed of samples mounted
on a large panel, introduces the visitor to a major aim of
the Discovery Room, namely, to provide a tactile as well as a
visual experience with Museum objects. Beside the wall is a
list of the materials which comprises:

Coarse chain mail	Fine chain mail
Lace	Mummy bandages
Silk, cotton, flax, wool	Woven materials
Grass matting	Sandpaper squares
Corrugated cardboard	Egg crating
Kidney beans	Cork bark mosaic
Bark samples	Fur mosaic I
Fur mosaic II	Reindeer fur
Hog bristle hide	Feathers
Feather goose breast	Snake skin
Shadow grill	Plastic bubbles
Metal squares	Nails
Sponge	Braille sheet
Horse hide	Fossils: tree bark, bees nest, coral, dinosaur skin cast, fern

LIVE EXHIBITS

Against one wall of the Room is a 90 x 90 cm glass terrarium
containing about fifteen species of cactus growing under the
appropriate heat, light, moisture, and soil conditions. An
information panel briefly describes the major adaptations of
a cactus to its dry environment and displays photographs of
the two species of cactus native to Ontario.

A similar terrarium containing live turtles was initially
included next to the cactus display, but it had to be removed
because of the difficulty in meeting environmental requirements and in keeping the unit clean.

Although live exhibits have proved popular in other museums, they do not permit as much involvement as other components and are therefore less attractive. Despite the fact that the Cactus Unit requires only minimal care, it will be removed from the Room.

SUPPORT COMPONENTS

(1) Three stereo microscopes with simple instruction cards are placed at a work bench in a corner of the Room.

(2) An ultraviolet light source is built into a wall unit.

(3) A luxo-lamp (a ring light around a large magnifying glass) is provided at the two wooden tables that seat six people each.

(4) Books containing additional information are located in several spots throughout the Room, so that reference materials are close to the appropriate objects. Texts or reference books on each of several broad subjects are available.

AUDIO-VISUAL EQUIPMENT

Although one of the boxes employs a cassette tape-recorder, other audio equipment has not been included in the Discovery Room. Museum materials, rather than electronic equipment, have been used wherever possible. Furthermore, considerations of cost and possible distractive influences have discouraged the use of audio-visual equipment even though several different units were considered during the planning.

Launching the Discovery Room

The Discovery Room was promoted wherever and whenever possible, through radio, television, and newspapers, in an attempt to reach all of Toronto and the rest of the province. Articles in newspapers with provincial distribution described the nature and contents of the Room, and the media were invited to a special preview on July 14, 1977. The description of the Room "the only one of its kind in Canada" because of its size and the extent of its materials, helped to ensure a good attendance by media people.

Media day was very successful and generated much publicity for the Discovery Room. In the morning, almost every Toronto television station, including Global, OECA, CTV, and CBC French Network, was represented. The press was invited to come in the afternoon, and it, too, turned out in full force. The result was a most extensive coverage of the opening of the Room.

The press release tried to convey the impression that the Discovery Room was fun as well as educational. It stressed the novelty of the Room's appeal to the senses and linked this to the changing philosophy of museums.

The description of the Room's content was written so that the reader would see the Discovery Room not only as a springboard into the ROM but also as an extension of the Museum. Having visited the Room once, it was hoped that the reader would want to explore further.

It was important to emphasize that the Room was designed for everyone over the age of six. As far as possible, adults were present when the media visited. The poster that was designed to advertise the Discovery Room showed a senior citizen, an adult, and two children.

Of particular importance to the Museum at this time was the fact that the Discovery Room is one phase of the ROM's expansion and renovation programme. This theme was picked up repeatedly in the press and on the radio.

An additional fact sheet, called "Community Pitches In", which was distributed on media day, outlined the contributions of other institutions to the Room. Both this information sheet and the news release mentioned that the Discovery Room was accessible to the visually handicapped, and that many of the information cards were also prepared in Braille.

The Discovery Room has been publicized as a place for all members of the community, "a truly international place of exploration", where information cards, labels, and other written material are available in several languages. The fact that a number of the volunteers in the Room speak languages other than English was also mentioned.

As many vehicles of communication as possible were used to publicize the Discovery Room, both before and after its opening on July 15. The summer issue of *Rotunda*, the ROM magazine, featured an article by Bette Shepherd about the Room. *Preview*, a pamphlet that outlines upcoming Museum events, featured the Discovery Room on several occasions. Pictures, articles, and notices appeared in *Preview* in the July/August and September 1977, and January 1978 issues.

Future ROM Events, a publication distributed to media people, and *What's on at the ROM*, a brochure that is available to the public, have also regualrly featured the Discovery Room. The Awareness Boards have been used to communicate news about the Room to the staff. A poster campaign was launched following the opening of the Room, and several thousand posters were placed in the subway and in stores in the community. An orientation brochure for the Discovery Room has been published by the Programmes and Public Relations Department.

Public response has been very favourable and only a few negative letters have been received. A few people have complained about the restriction that prohibits children under six from entering the Room, but because the rule seems necessary, an attempt was made to publicize it as widely as possible. Many letters of praise, including some from museums with similar facilities, have been received.

Response by the media has been exceptionally good. Not only newspapers but also magazines have written articles. Some of the publicity has extended beyond the borders of Ontario.

Operating the Discovery Room

Staffing

The Discovery Room has a permanent, full-time manager who is responsible for the day-to-day operation of the Room (which includes the supervision of maintenance of the components and daily evaluation) and the training and supervision of volunteer and paid staff. The manager is also responsible for setting and meeting the Discovery Room budget.

Because the Discovery Room is a place where Museum objects are openly accessible to the public, it must be staffed at all times. Since the varied duties of the manager made it evident that help would be required for the daily staffing of the Room, the ROM's volunteers were approached and about sixty signed up. The applicants were screened and the successful candidates (all but a very few of the original applicants) were trained shortly before the Room opened.

During the first six months of operation, a number of Discovery Room volunteers resigned, but a larger number of new volunteers applied. All newcomers are screened and trained before they become members of the staff. The manager schedules one training session each month. All Discovery Room contact with Museum volunteers is carried out by the manager.

Volunteers provide staff every day during the hours when the Room is open to the general public. Special group visits, booked for the morning hours, are supervised by the manager and, in the case of school visits, by the accompanying teachers and members of the Education Services Department. On weekdays the volunteers work in two shifts of two or two-and-one-half hours each. On week-ends there is only one volunteer shift.

In spite of enthusiastic and generous volunteer support, it soon became evident that there were certain times of the day, and certain days of the week--late weekday afternoons and week-ends--when the Discovery Room could not depend on volunteer staffing, and so a search was made for part-time paid support staff to work at these times. For the first two months, a series of museology students supplied the need. Then, in October, two high school students were hired.

Another problem which arose was that of week-end supervisory staff. For the first ten weeks, the manager was routinely providing week-end supervision. Although a certain amount of week-end and/or evening work had been included in the job description, it was understood that this was to be on exceptional occasions only. Consequently, a search was made and a third part-time paid staff member was hired. This person provides supervision for the Room on week-ends and holidays.

STAFF DUTIES

Discovery Room staff, volunteer and paid, function as guides rather than as teachers. They welcome visitors, show them the various components, explain the concept and organization of the Room, and encourage them to make use of it. The constant presence of staff also ensures that the Room is not misused and that the risk of pilfering and damage to components is minimized.

Encouragingly, there has been a remarkably small amount of theft and destruction in the Room. With only three or four exceptions, all the damage sustained has been the result of the kind of wear-and-tear that one would expect in a room that is used by hundreds of people every week. Sceptics predicted a far higher incidence of both theft and damage. Fortunately, experience has proved them wrong.

The Discovery Room staff is also responsible for carrying out daily evaluations of the Room and its operation. An hourly attendance count is kept. At the end of each shift, the volunteers complete an evaluation sheet on which they list the components that require maintenance, the components that were the most popular, and those that created some kind of problem. They also note any suggestions, remarks, or criticisms that occur to them or that are passed

on to them by visitors. At the end of each day, the manager
and the part-time paid staff member can add their own observations. This routine is followed seven days a week. Any
necessary maintenance work noted on the evaluation forms is
carried out immediately. The comments and suggestions are
compiled once a month and presented to the Discovery Room
Working Group for consideration.

The continuing evaluations have a two-fold purpose:

(1) They have a teaching value for the ROM. As a concept,
     the Discovery Room is a novel way of involving the public
     in some of the work of a museum. As a reality, the Room
     is a new gallery in the ROM. It is experimental in nat-
     ure and, in every sense, a "discovery" room. To guide
     the future development of the Room, it is necessary to
     study it closely.

(2) The evaluations also ensure that the Room remains respon-
     sive to the visiting public. This is essential if it is
     to be a place of public involvement in the Museum. Vis-
     itors must feel assured that this is *their* room. And if
     visitors know that their suggestions and comments are be-
     ing considered, then their interest and involvement in
     the Room, indeed in the entire Museum, will increase.

Rules of Use

The Discovery Room operates under the following rules:

The Room has a maximum capacity of twenty visitors at any one
time.

Children under six are not admitted.

Children between the ages of six and nine must be accompanied
by an adult, with one adult for two children.

The Room must be staffed at all times and will be closed to
the public when staff is not available.

The Room is open to the general public only during certain
hours:

Monday through Friday   –   12:00 Noon - 5:00 p.m.
Saturday, Sunday and Holidays   –   1:00 p.m. - 5:00 p.m.

Summer hours:

Monday through Friday	–	11:00 a.m. – 5:00 p.m.
Saturday, Sunday and Holidays	–	1:00 p.m. – 5:00 p.m.

The morning hours are reserved for special groups such as school classes, the blind or otherwise handicapped, the very elderly, special interest groups, etc. These are booked into the Room during the morning hours by previous arrangement with the manager.

The Room operates successfully under these guidelines, which are posted outside the entrance. The only policy that has caused any difficulty or dissatisfaction is the one that restricts admission to children under the age of six. The Discovery Room admitted children of four and five years for a brief trial period, but the experiment was not successful.

There were a number of valid reasons for establishing the age limit. The Discovery Room was designed to appeal to, and to be used by, the widest possible range of ages. Very young children's needs are different from those of other Museum visitors. There is a great deal of written material in the Room and most of the components deal with rather complex concepts (though on a relatively simple level). Some of the objects pose a hazard for the very young child because of weight, sharp edges, etc.

In order to enable children under the age of six to use the Room successfully, far more guidance, supervision, and direction would be required, and this would not be in keeping with the intended spirit of the Room. Moreover, the existence and the continuing development of the Room depend on Museum material, and therefore on curatorial cooperation. In many cases, the support of the curators was won only by assurances that children under six would not be admitted.

The majority of volunteers who offered to staff the Discovery Room agreed to do so only if the Room did not become a "day-care centre" or a "romper room". Volunteer support is essential to the Room's operation, for the Museum cannot afford the number of full-time paid staff that would be necessary to keep the Room open.

When visitors question the age limit, they are given as an explanation the first of the three reasons described previously. The second and third reasons, although valid from the ROM's point of view, would only increase bad feelings on the

part of an already disappointed visitor. The majority of
visitors who try to bring in a child under six are willing
to observe the age limit once the reason has been explained.
Occasionally a visitor does not cooperate, however, lodges
a complaint, or creates an unpleasant situation. Such situations have to be dealt with as tactfully as possible.

Nevertheless, there is a very real need to provide facilities
for pre-schoolers. The question of making Museum activities
available to very young children seems to be focussed at the
moment on the Discovery Room. It is hoped that eventually a
Museum programme will be designed specifically for these
children. Such a programme is not only desirable; it is
necessary.

Attendance and Patterns of Use

Because the Room is a new kind of gallery, evolving and re-
sponsive to the visiting public, flexibility in its operations is essential. In the summer when the Room is constantly
busy (up to 400 visitors every day), three volunteers are
needed for each shift. During the school year when the Room
is not so crowded (up to 200 visitors every day), two volunteers are adequate for each shift.

Visitors spend a shorter time in the Discovery Room during
the summer. The average length of visit is thirty minutes.
Few people stay longer than forty-five minutes and some stay
for only fifteen minutes.

During the winter, visitors remain for a longer time and some
stay for as long as two or three hours. The average length
of stay during the school year is one hour. Visitors during
the winter also become more involved with the components.
Some work carefully through every box and identification unit;
some pick out particular components together with the relevant reference books and work with them; some make prolonged
studies of the skeletons; some sketch; some bring in their
own natural specimens either to compare them with those in
the Room or to identify them. Because the Room's summer hours
are not appropriate during the school year, it opens one hour
later between Labour Day and the end of June.

Visitor attendance (excluding advanced scheduled groups) for the first six months of operation is presented in Table I. Also listed are the number of hours per week that the Room was open and the average hourly number of visitors.

Table I _____

Discovery Room Attendance: 18 July, 1977 – 15 January, 1978

Week	Hours Open	Total Attendance	Average/Hour
July 18–24	46	1,510	33
July 25–31	43	1,948	45
August 1–7	32	1,607	50
August 8–14	39	2,014	52
August 15–21	39	1,686	43
August 22–28	38	1,800	47
August 29–Sept. 4	38	1,602	42
September 5–11	36	941	26
September 12–18	38	784	21
September 19–25	38	876	23
September 26–Oct. 2	38	995	26
October 3–9	28	782	28
October 10–16	24	649	27
October 17–23	29	731	25
October 24–30	30	818	27
October 31–Nov. 6	37	1,228	33
November 7–13	37	1,312	35
November 14–20	37	998	27
November 21–27	35	1,294	37
November 28–Dec. 4	33	981	30
December 5–11	34	813	24
December 12–18	33	1,012	31
December 19–25	25	567	23
December 26–Jan. 1	25	1,321	53
January 2–8	33	866	26
January 9–15	32	893	28
Overall Total	897	30,028	

Samples of the hourly use of the Room for one summer and one winter week are presented in Table II. The total Museum attendance in the main building, where the Discovery Room is located, is also given. These figures provide an indication of the proportion of Museum visitors who also visited the Discovery Room.

Table II

Sample hourly attendance of a summer and a winter week.

8-14 August, 1977

TIME	MON.	TUES.	WED.	THURS.	FRI.	SAT.	SUN.	TOTAL
11-12	30	38	70	35	40	–	–	213
12-1	55	49	47	41	50	2	–	244
1-2	40	45	62	37	50	28	44	306
2-3	107	40	71	60	35	24	70	407
3-4	89	49	61	43	81	47	71	441
4-5	62	40	72	71	65	38	55	403
TOTAL	383	261	383	287	321	139	240	2,014
MAIN BLDG. TOTAL	2,007	1,958	2,624	2,070	1,815	2,034	2,035	14,543

31 October - 5 November, 1977

TIME	MON.	TUES.	WED.	THURS.	FRI.	SAT.	SUN.	TOTAL
11-12	–	32	–	15	–	–	–	47
12-1	38	46	47	53	45	–	–	229
1-2	11	45	16	67	23	40	54	256
2-3	26	37	19	48	58	116	79	383
3-4	6	14	16	17	37	32	69	191
4-5	8	11	4	4	15	46	34	122
TOTAL	89	185	102	204	178	234	236	1,228
MAIN BLDG. TOTAL	932	1,611	1,540	1,322	1,863	1,967	2,574	11,809

Use of the Room by School Classes

During the planning of the Discovery Room, the committee envisaged family groups as the main users of the Room and selected components that best suited this type of group. Experience has proved that the Room functions better with small groups (three or four persons) than with large groups. In the fall of 1977, it was decided that school classes should be allowed to use the Room under certain conditions in order to determine whether the Room could provide students with worthwhile educational experiences.

Classes that represented a wide range of ages and abilities were invited to visit the Room during times when it was not open to the public. Teachers were expected to visit the Discovery Room beforehand so that they could familiarize themselves with its contents and plan programmes for their classes. Teachers were to be in charge of their groups, and Museum staff would be available only in a support role. Evaluation forms for teachers and students were prepared and were completed after the visit.

For many students "discovery learning" is not new. A large number of classrooms have "wonder tables" or "discovery corners" where learning is based on the same pedagogical principles as the Discovery Room. The individual is introduced to a new set of facts or situations which, because of their nature or manner of presentation, stimulate him to undertake further investigation of the topic. The advantage of the Discovery Room at the ROM is the large variety of human and physical resources that it can draw upon.

By December 31, 1977, sixteen school groups had used the Room under the conditions stipulated for the trial period. The classes ranged from grades one to eight and included several special education classes as well as one from the provincial school for the learning handicapped. According to the evaluation forms received from students and teachers, the boxes, the microscopes, the skeleton, and the identification units provide the most enjoyment. The junior division classes (ages nine to twelve) seem to profit the most. Some of the material is too sophisticated for primary classes and yet not sophisticated enough for the intermediate students. The ideal length of visit appears to be from thirty to forty minutes. The Room can comfortably accommodate from fifteen to twenty students. However, with a few more items such as microscopes, it could easily handle a class of thirty students.

Every teacher who came for a preliminary visit with the manager decided that it was impossible to set up a "programme" for students to follow while in the Discovery Room. Instead, teachers have described the content and philosophy of the Room to their students and then have let them follow their own interests.

From the manager's point of view, students between the ages of six and nine work best if there is a ratio of three or four children to one adult. Students over the age of nine do not need as much supervision--perhaps one adult for five students. During their individual visits, a number of teachers said that they did not think the Room was suitable for a large group, such as a class, and that they would recommend that their students visit the Room after school or on a weekend.

Other Special Groups

Groups of the visually, mentally, and physically handicapped made arrangements to visit the Discovery Room during the morning hours. These groups provided their own specially trained supervisors and came with a high ratio of supervisors to visitors.

Handicapped people use the Room extremely well. Many of them expressed a wish for a return visit. The visually handicapped work with particular success in the Room because of the tactile nature of many of the components and the provision of Braille cards.

Groups of elderly people also visit the Discovery Room. They enjoy it but tire easily and so their visits tend to be short (30 minutes on the average). The very elderly usually come with a companion.

Financial Requirements for Setting up the Room

Funds for the development of the Discovery Room and for the initial six months of its operation were provided by the ECTF and from general Museum operational accounts. Expenditures can be broken down into direct recoverable costs, direct non-recoverable costs, and indirect costs.

Direct recoverable costs included items that were considered to be transferable to any future "discovery" gallery. The $25,000 expenditure was allocated as follows:

cases	$10,000
I.D. units and containers	$ 5,000
equipment, artifacts, materials, and library	$ 5,000
graphics, labelling, tables, chairs, and other miscellaneous materials	$ 5,000

These figures are approximate.

Direct non-recoverable costs include charges incurred largely as a result of the preparation of the Room, e.g., electrical service, carpeting, etc. Developmental staff for ten months was funded as non-recoverable, one-time research and development costs. Included in staff costs were funds for a manager and assistants to carry the Discovery Room through the first six months of operation. Evaluation costs are also considered part of the research and development expense and are therefore non-recoverable.

Indirect costs include salaries of Museum staff. It is important that the ROM employ people who are skilled in such areas as design, public relations, photography, preparation, art, conservation, and carpentry.

Many departments, both curatorial and non-curatorial, spent a great deal of time on the development of this project. The committee time alone, forty meetings, was extensive. The indirect staff costs would be considerable if estimates included all the time contributed by the various departments. After the initial development and testing, the Room became the operating responsibility of the Education Services Department.

Further Budgetary Considerations

Many conclusions have emerged after six months of operating the Discovery Room. A continuing budget is essential. The need for part-time staff was not contemplated in the planning of the Room, but the first few weeks of operation made this requirement evident and part-time staff were hired. Other financial requirements arise from the need for maintenance and adjustment of existing components, both of which sometimes involve the repair of components or the purchase of replacements.

The success of the Room resulted in a decision to develop new components, which required funds for both staff and material costs. Some of these expenditures will only occur once. However, a certain amount of continuing development work is inherent in the nature of the Discovery Room which must evolve in response to public reaction. There is always room for improvement. To set a limit on the Room's future development would be to lose sight of its original concept and purpose.

Findings and Conclusions

Findings

The findings and conclusions that follow have been drawn from the Discovery Room Evaluation (Appendix B) which was carried out during the first six months of the Room's operation.

The Discovery Room Is a Success

- Visitors' overall reactions to the Discovery Room were very positive.

- Visitors clearly understood the purpose of the Room and appreciated the opportunity to touch Museum objects.

- Most visitors involved themselves with at least one component in the Room.

- Many visitors wanted to see more use made of the "discovery" concept in the Museum.

- Since many people who came to the Discovery Room had heard about it from previous visitors, it would appear that the Room provides an enjoyable experience.

- Visitors to the Discovery Room usually spent more time there than they did in most of the other ROM galleries.

- Most visitors indicated that they had learned something from their visit to the Discovery Room.

The Discovery Room Is More Successful with Children than with Adults

- There are variations in the ways in which children and adults perceive and use the Discovery Room. Children, on their own or in family groups, involved themselves more with the components of the Room than did adolescents and adults without children.

31

- Children became involved immediately with the components in the Room, whereas adults, and to a lesser degree adolescents, were more hesitant in their approach.

- Adults accompanied by children tended to become more involved with the components than did adults without children. Similarly, it appeared that adults found the Room more easy to use when some assistance from a docent was available.

- Although all age groups indicated that they found the Room to be unique and informative, children tended to be more enthusiastic in their responses.

- The answers to survey questions and the overall observations indicated that many adults perceived the Room as a facility intended for use by children.

- Many more adults than children indicated that they had not learned anything in particular from the Room.

Physical Organization of the Discovery Room

- The Skeleton appeared to be effective in attracting visitors into the Room.

- Similar types of component were often grouped together in a way that did not encourage circulation throughout the Room. Consequently, only a small proportion of the visitors saw all of the components.

- Components such as the boxes, the microscopes, the luxolamps, and the ultraviolet lamp, which involve the visitor actively, were the most popular. Because they were located in one part of the Room, that area frequently became congested.

- The adult visitors were most attracted to components such as the Skeleton, the Stumpers, and the Tree Unit which are immediately visible and easily comprehended. (Boxes, I.D. units, etc. require more participation.) Because these components are grouped around the entrance, adults often did not circulate throughout the Room.

- Adults tended to find the layout of the Room somewhat cramped and confusing.

The Discovery Room Enhances the Entire Museum

- Visitors indicated that the Discovery Room enlivened their impression of the ROM.

- Visitors regarded the Discovery Room as an exciting change within the Museum because of its novel approaches to providing information and presenting Museum objects.

- The Discovery Room was a factor in attracting people, especially repeat visitors, to the ROM.

- The most frequent comment was that the Discovery Room made the ROM more interesting for visitors by providing explanations and descriptions of relationships rather than simple identification of objects.

- The Discovery Room does not, however, appear to stimulate specific interest in related galleries.

Success of the Discovery Room Components

- Boxes were the most popular component in the Room.

- The microscopes, luxo-lamps with attached magnifying glasses, and the ultraviolet lamp were also very popular. Although they were intended to be used both for independent research and in conjunction with Discovery Room components, they were used almost exclusively with the boxes.

- The Skeleton was the component which had the most general appeal.

- Although the I.D. units and the library were designed as reference resources, neither was used by visitors for this purpose. A small proportion of the visitors found certain elements of the I.D. units (the butterflies and bugs in particular) interesting to observe. The library was not used at all.

- Although the cross-section of the tree in the Tree Unit appealed to many visitors, the component as a whole was not very successful. Many visitors indicated that they did not like it.

- The Live Exhibit, the Stamp Display, the Mirror Display, and the Bird Display were the least popular components.

- Straightforward activities were popular with all visitors but especially with children. Microscopes, luxo-lamps with attached magnifying glasses, and the ultraviolet lamp were all well liked. For example, the magnifying glasses enhanced the Stamp Display.

- Relationships between components became apparent only when the visitor had to perform some activity common to each. In the case of the boxes, this might involve using a microscope, a magnifying luxo-lamp, or the ultraviolet lamp.

- Components which visitors could relate to their own experience were popular, e.g., the Skeleton, boxes such as the one that dealt with teeth, the Insect and Butterfly I.D. units, and the tree cross-section that correlated man's history with tree growth.

- Components in the form of traditional ("hands-off") displays created an initial barrier, particularly for adults.

- Visitors were frustrated when they could not easily accomplish an activity, e.g., seeing the Buddha in the Mirror Display or seeing the colours in the Glowing Rocks Box.

Attraction of the Discovery Room

- Most visitors to the Discovery Room include it in a general visit to the ROM. Most visitors neither came specifically to see the Room nor had heard about the Room prior to their visits to the Museum.

- In the short period of time following its opening, the Room was attracting an increasing proportion of return visitors.

- The most common source of information for those visitors who had heard about the Room in advance was other visitors.

- The Room attracted higher proportions of children, of adolescents, and of family groups than the ROM as a whole.

- Discovery Room visitors were drawn from the same geographical areas as visitors to the ROM in general.

Overall Conclusions

The survey results clearly indicate that the Discovery Room is successful, and that a "discovery room" would be a positive addition to the expanded Museum. The Room has achieved the objectives set out by the Discovery Room Working Group:

The Discovery Room will provide an enjoyable learning experience.

- The Discovery Room provides an environment in which visitors are stimulated to learn in an enjoyable way by exploring and by actively involving themselves with a variety of components.

The components of the Discovery Room should be oriented to discovery learning.

- All aspects of discovery learning are successful, namely, the approaches to providing information, the techniques of presenting Museum objects, and the opportunities to become actively involved with Museum artifacts and specimens.

The Discovery Room should experiment with the discovery learning concept (using various approaches) to determine its applicability elsewhere in the ROM and outside the Museum.

- Because visitors enjoy their experiences in the Discovery Room, their impression of the ROM as a whole is often enlivened. The success of the discovery learning concept indicates the potential of this approach outside the ROM, e.g., the Extension Services programme could incorporate boxes into its mobile exhibits.

The Discovery Room should be oriented to everyone, but experience has shown that family groups tend to be the primary audience; therefore, components should be designed accordingly. Where possible, the text should be available multilingually and in Braille.

- Although family groups are the most frequent visitors to the Room, unaccompanied children and adolescents constitute a relatively high proportion of the visitors.
- Furthermore, the evaluation has shown that children and adults use the Discovery Room in very different ways. (Adolescents use the Room more like adults.) Combining activities that appeal to children with those that are designed for adults and adolescents does not appear to be successful, at least not in an area the size of the current Discovery Room. If it is decided that a Discovery Room should be intended for all age groups, the following changes are suggested:

    (1) Some form of orientation is required to accustom visitors to handling Museum exhibits. Adults in particular seem to be very cautious.

    (2) Adults could be encouraged to make greater use of the Room by a notice at the entrance that there are activities designed for them. For example, a display on the wall opposite the Touch Wall could indicate that the Room also offers a reference centre.

(3) Adults would probably feel more comfortable in a larger space.

(4) To increase adult participation, boxes could be developed which would express, in combination with other boxes and/or other components in the Room, more complex concepts.

The use of all senses interacting together should be encouraged.

● While the Discovery Room encourages visitors to use all their senses, most components involve only sight and touch. Components which appear to be traditional displays often call for the use of sight alone.

The components of the Discovery Room should relate to the galleries and departmental collections. In this way, the content of the Discovery Room would reflect that of the ROM. However, attempts to make the Room representative of all divisions and departments should be secondary to the need to develop the best examples.

● The components in the Discovery Room relate directly to the galleries and departmental collections of the ROM. However, it does not appear that an interest in a specific component stimulates interest in the related galleries.

Conclusions That Relate to Individual Components

● Visitors spend more time with the components which require active participation and appear to enjoy and learn most from then. However, it is worthwhile to offer a variety of activities that will allow for individual interests and differing time commitments.

● The success of the boxes indicates that this type of component should be expanded.

● Components which are not successful should be either removed, altered by incorporating activities that require more participation, or strongly related to already successful components such as boxes and microscopes. For instance, an activity that would involve the use of the Moon Map could be included in the Moon Box.

- Components should be organized according to their popularity and the type of activity they involve. In this way, they can be arranged so that the space in the Discovery Room is employed efficiently and so that the use of complementary components is encouraged. For example, the juxtaposition of a very attractive component such as the Tree Unit with a component that involves more participation such as one of the boxes would achieve both objectives.

- Components that are designed for children need to be within their reach and in their line of vision, unlike the Bird Displays and some of the Stumpers.

- Relationships between components in the Discovery Room and related galleries are best conveyed through participatory activities. For example, the Pattern Box could indicate the different galleries in the ROM where visitors could look for the recurrence of a specific design both in nature and in the artifacts of various cultures.

Summary and Recommendations

Summary

The Discovery Room has been an important challenge, both for
the Discovery Room Working Group and for the Museum, that
appears to have been met successfully. Bold initiatives
were taken in a number of areas of museum display with the
result that there are attractions for everyone, not just for
the hobbyist and the collector. Both children and adults,
in increasing numbers, are now able to work with Museum
specimens. For the blind, the Room is a mini-museum which,
because there is so much to handle and because many of the
components are labelled in Braille, can now be "seen". The
multilingual approach of the Room permits many who would
otherwise feel excluded to appreciate some of the material
that ROM offers.

Recommendations

The activities of the Discovery Room Working Group, comments
from Urban Design Consultants, from the Discovery Room staff,
and from the visiting public have resulted in a number of
recommendations for the future of discovery rooms in the ROM.

SHORT-TERM

(1) The Discovery Room had set a maximum attendance rate
of twenty-five people per half-hour. However, the
size of the present Room and the length of visits indicate that the gallery would better serve twenty
people for forty-five-minute time periods. The noise
level would be lower; control would be easier; there
would be ample seating and table space; and everyone
would have access to the special equipment.

(2) The DRWG has been conscious of the need for adult participation and it feels that the Room has met this need reasonably well. To ensure continuing interest, components designed especially for adults should be developed. The study-centre concept will be particularly appropriate in carrying out this recommendation.

(3) The Wood Unit should be redesigned so that the space can be condensed and herbarium information and large print labels can be added.

(4) It is important to add an active element to the Stamp Display (i.e., stamps in plastic that can be used with hand lens) and to acquire a commitment from the Post Office to renew the collection periodically.

(5) It is recommended that the Cactus Unit be removed.

(6) The Room should continue to respond to outside events, special exhibitions, or seasonal changes.

(7) An archaeological stratigraphy display, such as finds from a well, might be effective in adding a new element to the Room.

(8) Because the boxes are the most successful component, it is recommended that a second box bank be provided, to be filled by duplicates of particularly popular boxes and by the additional boxes listed below:

> Wood Smells Box
>
> Sound Box, with two head sets and a tape player
>
> Coin Box
>
> Calligraphy Box
>
> Weight Box
>
> Threads Box

(9) A bulletin board for items of interest and for special notices is suggested.

(10) A time chart on the wall with earth time to the present is requested.

(11) It is recommended that no audio-visual equipment be installed, since the Room operates effectively in its current form by providing an opportunity for personal discovery.

(12) It is recommended that the print on all labels, present and future, be enlarged and made to contrast for easy viewing.

LONG-TERM

(1) It is recommended that the Museum provide adequate space, staff, and funds for future "discovery" experiences.

(2) Any new Discovery Room should have a minimum floor space of $420m^2$ (approx. 4,500 square feet). The present Room has been too small for the range of material that could be presented and for the seasonal demand for access to the Room.

(3) The DRWG foresees a need for suitable spaces for three additional special galleries within the expanded Museum. Tests in the present Room indicate that a gallery for children who are six years and younger, a tactile gallery for the visually handicapped, and naturalist and archaeological study centres would be well received by visitors to the Museum. To accommodate these needs, a space that is between five and six times the present area would be required.

These special galleries could be clustered to enable staff to be shared, and to encourage interrelated use. Visually handicapped people could then use the gallery without feeling segregated. Alternatively, the naturalist/archaeology centre could be relocated near associated galleries. A novel museum experience adjacent to the more conventional galleries would then be possible.

(4) A special gallery work group should be established to have responsibility for the preparation of proposals and the development of additional special galleries in the existing Museum for evaluation and possible inclusion in some form in an expanded Museum. This working group should have about half its active members drawn from the curatorial departments and should prepare its proposals within the guidelines for gallery development.

The long-term relationship of the curatorial staff to "discovery" type experiences should be clearly defined. In order to develop new components as well as to maintain present components at optimum functioning capacity, the curators should be invited to attend working meetings.

(5) There is a continuing need to make the Room, as well as the rest of the Museum, more accessible for the handicapped. Within the Discovery Room, consideration should be given to wheelchair visitors, who require more space to manoeuvre if they are not to interfere with other visitors. To assist the visually handicapped, an effort should be made to make other museum exhibits more easily accessible by providing Museum guides in large type or Braille and large clear labels throughout the building.

(6) The limited activity available in the Discovery Room indicates a definite need for a multi-purpose, large-scale activity complex in the same area as the Room. The Discovery Room itself is *not* an activity room, it is an "accessibility" room.

A Curatorial Point of View

Most curators have received the discovery concept favourably
insofar as it allows visitors to become closely involved
with objects from the collections. However, they are concerned that the experience be as authentic as possible and
that the integrity of the artifacts and specimens used in
the Room be preserved. Perhaps their principal contribution to the planning of the Room has been in the development of a concept that, within obvious limitations, allows
the visitor's experience to resemble as closely as possible
actual museum practice.

Early in the deliberations it became clear that one problem
to be solved was that of balancing pure discovery (i.e., the
manipulation and examination of museum objects) and natural
science identification. It was decided that both types of
activity would be used in the Room, and that each would,
where possible, draw upon the techniques of the other. Thus,
I.D. units would allow as much manipulation of objects as
was consistent with the safety of the material, while conventional discovery components, such as the boxes, would
frequently employ identification as an activity.

Many highly creative ideas for the Discovery Room were
generated by the enthusiasm of the planning group. However,
many of these, involving display-type components, could
readily be implemented in a more traditional type of museum
gallery. It was felt that the Discovery Room should be
restricted to those components whose use required the freer
atmosphere of this unique type of gallery. Other suggested
components involved activities related either to the origin
or the original use of museum objects, with the use of models or substitute materials to create a sort of synthetic
discovery experience. Again, it was felt that other ROM
programmes such as the Saturday Morning Club were more appropriate contexts for these activities. It has not been

possible, nor is it desirable, to eliminate entirely either display or activity concepts from the experimental Discovery Room, for both are valid elements of the discovery experience. Nevertheless, as the Discovery Room grows and develops within the Museum, care must be taken to ensure that neither obliterates the original discovery concept.

Other concerns have been recognized: the need to protect artifacts and specimens from excessive wear and tear; the need to distinguish between consumable and irreplaceable objects; the obligation to see that the Room is used for its proper purpose; the relative difficulty of devising suitable components from the Art and Archaeology departments; and the problem of introducing idea-oriented as contrasted with object-oriented disciplines into the Room. In resolving these problems it has sometimes been necessary to resort to use of the less desirable display and activity techniques.

It has become apparent that the operation of the Discovery Room requires a staff with specialized skills and training. With the increasing demands on curatorial staff for educational activities of all types, curatorial departments have found it difficult to contribute as much skilled labour to the production of components as they would have liked. There is an evident need within certain departments, such as Conservation, Preparators, and Exhibit Design Services, for primary skills and training in the preparation of specimens for research collections and in the mounting and handling of specimens, so that the staffs of these departments can participate more actively in the development of new Discovery Room components.

In sum, it is fair to say that the DRWG has evolved a new and more realistic definition of "discovery" in a museum context than the one with which it began its task. Museum discovery should permit the visitor to share the kind of experience enjoyed by curatorial staff, whose work with the collections constitutes the unique and most essential aspect of museum experience. Allowing visitors to enter into this experience in some degree is the most creative and substantial contribution that any museum can make.

Appendix A

Details of Components

MICRO-MARVELS BOX

A. Description

1. What is it?   - This box contains a large assortment of ordinary material that takes on new dimensions when viewed with a microscope. The material relates to many areas of the Museum and can undergo constant change without altering the box's appeal.

- The box contains:

    - 8 slides: - shark's skin
      - aphid
      - cat flea (ctenocephalides felis)
      - hind wing of pearl crescent butterfly
      - fore wing of pearl crescent butterfly
      - bee sting
      - fish scale from a Silver Redhorse Sucker
      - porcupine quill

    - a shark tooth, requiem shark (genus - Carcharinus)

    - a piece of sponge

    - a burr

    - a feather

    - 2 dentist's tools embedded in plastic (used for root canal work)

    - 2 pictures

    - 1 colour transparency

    - 8 cloth samples

    - a penny (embedded in plastic)

    - a stamp (embedded in plastic)

    - a small pair of tweezers

    - information cards

2. Who will use it? - Age 12 and over although a younger child could use it with supervision

3. How long will it take? - 25 minutes

   Is this a repeat activity? - Yes

4. How will visitors use it? - Visitors will place materials under the microscope.

5. Why were these items chosen? - Most items are a part of daily life.

   - Many items relate to different Museum areas.

B. Statement of Objectives

   - to stimulate an interest in microscopic analysis.

   - to generate curiosity about the structure of all matter.

This box could also be used as a curator's tool for the differentiation of species (e.g., wings) and so illustrate another common Museum tool for the visitor.

SPICE OF LIFE BOX

A. Description

   1. What is it? - The box contains:

      - bottles of 12 volatile oils and
        12 plant samples from which they
        are derived

      - directions for a matching game

      - a map of historical trade routes
        and spices' origins

      - cards with detailed information
        about spices

   2. Who will use it? - Age 12 and over

   3. How long will it take? - From 15 to 20 minutes

      Is this a repeat activity? - Yes

   4. How will visitors use it? - Visitors will iden-
      tify and match 12 spices by using
      their sense of smell and sight.

      - Visitors can read the cards in
      each box to learn more about the
      origin, history, and preparation
      of spices.

      - Visitors can follow the old
      trade routes on a map.

   5. Why were these items chosen? - The items are
      designed to show that spices and
      flavourings come from different
      parts of plants and that the true
      spices in the box were historically
      important in trade-route commerce.

      - The spices in the box derive from
      tropical, temperate climates in
      many parts of the world.

      - The samples underline the every-
      day use of spices and invite the
      visitor to concentrate on his sense
      of smell and, indirectly, taste.

B. Statement of Objectives

- to show the use of volatile oils (flavouring and fragrances obtained from plant materials) and their importance in the development of world trade patterns.

- to teach the visitor, who is encouraged to smell materials of plant origin, that smell is an important sense in identifying materials of organic origin.

- to show the visitor the value invested in flavourings and fragrances.

- to indicate to the visitor how the difficulty of cultivation of certain spices influenced historical trade patterns.

- to demonstrate, that, through interconnection of taste and smell, flavourings and fragrances contribute to man's appreciation of life and food.

METEORITES BOX

A. Description

1. What is it? - The box contains:

   - amphibolite
   - iron meteorite
   - iron slag
   - dirty limestone
   - lava
   - a magnet
   - direction cards
   - a magnifying glass
   - a pamphlet on meteorites

2. Who will use it? - Age 8 and over

3. How long will it take? - From 5 to 7 minutes

   Is this a repeat activity? - Yes

4. How will visitors use it? - Visitors will read accompanying cards and will attempt to distinguish the real iron meteorite from the four others in the box by using the magnet.

   - Visitors will gain information by reading the cards.

5. Why were these items chosen? - The items show the visitor one real meteorite and four others that are often mistaken for meteorites.

   - The subject relates to the Geology gallery and to the Planetarium.

B. Statement of Objectives

        - to teach the visitor: - that meteorites are rare

                                           - that they are often incorrectly identified

                                         - that there are three types of meteorite based on composition

                                         - that large meteorites form craters when they fall

                                         - that most meteorites are four and one-half billion years old.

        - to allow the visitor to handle and to look at a piece of "outer space".

FOSSILS BOX

A. Description

1. What is it? — The box contains:

  - 10 fossil specimens accompanied by photographs of the living equivalent

  - information about the age of the fossil and other related details

2. Who will use it? — All ages

3. How long will it take? — From 10 to 20 minutes

   Is this a repeat activity? — No

4. How will visitors use it? — Visitors will examine fossil specimens and use the questions as a guide to learn about the age and the distribution of fossil remains and about pre-fossil form.

5. Why were these items chosen? — The contents of the box relate to the I.D. unit, to the Vertebrate Palaeontology gallery and, indirectly, to the Botany and Invertebrate Zoology galleries.

B. Statement of Objectives

- to make the visitor realize that at one time fossils were living organisms.

- to enable the visitor to recognize a number of general fossil groups, including cephalopods, gastropods, etc.

- to show the visitor that although the material may be millions of years old, it is from the surrounding area.

- to familiarize the visitor with the technical vocabulary used with fossils.

SKIN BOX

A. Description

      1. What is it? — The box includes:

                    — a study skin of a bird

                    — the skin of a mammal

                    — a small fish that has been preserved

                    — several large fish scales

                    — a preserved frog

                    — snake skin that has been shed

                    — a magnifying glass

                    — information cards

      2. Who will use it? — All ages

      3. How long will it take? — From 5 to 45 minutes

        Is this a repeat activity? — No

      4. How will visitors use it? — Visitors will use their sense of sight and touch to examine and compare the objects.

      5. Why were these items chosen? — The items illustrate kinds of integument on various types of vertebrate animals.

            — The subject relates to the Life Sciences departments.

B. Statement of Objectives

- to teach the visitor, through a comparison of skin types, something about their uses and growth.

- to show the visitor specifically that:

    - Cold-blooded and warm-blooded animals have different characteristics.

    - Reptiles shed their skin.

    - Scales grow with the fish.

    - Scales have growth rings.

    - There is a principle of countershading.

    - Mammals are characterized by the presence of hair.

    - Birds are characterized by the presence of feathers.

    - Amphibians may breathe through their skin.

TEETH BOX

A. Description

1. What is it? - The box contains:

    - the upper jaw of a racoon
    - the incisor of a beaver
    - the tooth of a dog
    - the molar of a horse
    - a human tooth
    - a small hand mirror
    - cards with diagrams

2. Who will use it? - Ages 9 to 12

3. How long will it take? - From 5 to 15 minutes

    Is this a repeat activity? - No

4. How will visitors use it? - Visitors will look at and compare the teeth in the box with their own teeth.

5. Why were these items chosen? - The animals from which the teeth were taken are all common and therefore familiar to the visitor.

B. Statement of Objective

- to enable the visitor to distinguish between the three types of teeth found in most mammals.

NESTS BOX

A. Description

    1. What is it?   – The box contains:

            – 5 types of nest and pictures of 4 more

            – explanation cards

            – 2 photographs of nests with eggs

    2. Who will use it?   – All ages

    3. How long will it take?   – From 5 to 10 minutes

       Is this a repeat activity?   – No

    4. How will visitors use it?   – Visitors will pick up and examine the nests and look at the accompanying photographs.

    5. Why were these items chosen?   – The items illustrate various types of nest construction.

            – The subject relates to the Ornithology Department.

B. Statement of Objectives

    – to teach the visitor about: – basic types of nest

                             – the materials used to build nests

                             – how nests are used

                             – how abandoned nests are re-used

MATCH-A-SOUND BOX

A. Description

1. What is it? - The box contains:

- 5 types of bean or seed (on display)

- 5 opaque containers of the same kind of bean, i.e., pot barley, kidney beans, rice, poppy seeds, and soup peas

2. Who will use it? - Ages 6 to 10

3. How long will it take? - 5 minutes

Is this a repeat activity? - No

4. How will visitors use it? - Visitors will pick up each container, shake it to determine which kind of bean or seed is inside, and then place it in front of the appropriate display. The container can then be opened to verify the match.

5. Why were these items chosen? - The seeds or beans, which are part of the average visitor's diet, have different shapes and sizes.

B. Statement of Objectives

- to allow the visitor to use his sense of hearing to identify an item that may be seen and felt.

- to encourage the visitor to ask why beans and seeds of different sizes make different sounds.

ARCHAEOLOGY BOX

A. Description

1. What is it? - The box contains:

   - 5 sherds from two objects (a jug and a plate)
   - silhouette pictures of all types of wares from the same site
   - information cards
   - a roll of tape

2. Who will use it? - All ages

3. How long will it take? - From 5 to 10 minutes

   Is this a repeat activity? - No

4. How will visitors use it? - Visitors will use their sense of touch and sight to fit the pottery sherds together into their original shape.

   - Visitors can read about the way in which artifacts are unearthed at an archaeological dig and they can use question-and-answer cards.

5. Why were these items chosen? - The visitor will experience the piecing together of artifacts in the same manner as an archaeologist.

   - The objects are familiar to the visitor and they make the Canadian past more tangible.

   - The objects are related to archaeological functions at the ROM.

B. Statement of Objectives

- to acquaint the visitor with Canadian archaeology and the methods used in reassembling artifacts.

- to stimulate a general interest in archaeology.

- to involve the visitor in the excitement of reconstructing part of the past.

CRYSTAL CAVE BOX

A. Description

1. What is it? - The box contains:

> - pyrite crystals
> - amethyst quartz crystal
> - rock quartz crystal
> - calcite geode
> - mica
> - a salt shaker with halite (salt)
> - a magnifying glass
> - a felt square
> - 6 photographs of mineral crystals inside box lid

2. Who will use it? - Age 10 and over

3. How long will it take? - From 10 to 15 minutes

   Is this a repeat activity? - No

4. How will visitors use it? - Visitors will handle specimens in order to examine them and will look at photographs of six minerals.

5. Why were these items chosen? - The specimens demonstrate that some minerals form crystals and others possess cleavage.

   - The subject relates to the Mineralogy gallery.

B. Statement of Objectives

- to enable the visitor to discover that some minerals form crystals of various shapes which identify them.

- to enable the visitor to discover that some minerals have cleavage properties which allow them to be broken along smooth flat planes.

PATTERNS BOX

A. Description

    1. What is it?   - The box contains the following natural materials used by ancient man to decorate pottery:

- plasticine
- a smoothing roller
- bamboo reeds
- a pig incisor
- a rope
- 2 sherds of West Asian pottery
- a cylindrical seal

The first five of these items were used by Iron-Age Britons to create patterns.

    2. Who will use it? - Age 10 and over

    3. How long will it take? - 20 minutes

Is this a repeat activity? - Yes

    4. How will visitors use it? - Visitors will use plasticine and tools to make patterns similar to those of ancient cultures.

    5. Why were these items chosen? - The items are similar to those used by archaeologists trying to duplicate ancient pottery patterns.

- The subject relates to the Art and Archaeology departments.

B. Statement of Objectives

- to teach the visitor one archaeological technique.

- to provide information about the cultures of ancient Britain and West Asia.

- to show the visitor a new perspective on ancient pottery.

FEATHERS BOX

A. Description

    1. What is it? - The box contains:

                - a variety of feathers

                - a hand lens

                - information cards

    2. Who will use it? - All ages

    3. How long will it take? - From 5 to 10 minutes

       Is this a repeat activity? - No

    4. How will visitors use it? - Visitors will use a hand lens to examine various types of feathers and to relate them to the avian activities for which the feathers are adapted.

    5. Why were these items chosen? - The items show feathers and their uses.

                - The subject relates to the Ornithology Department.

B. Statement of Objectives

    - to teach the visitor that feathers are adapted to perform various functions for the bird.

    - to teach the visitor about flight, about bird behaviour, and about the structure, purpose, and weight of feathers.

HIDDEN COLOURS BOX

A. Description

1. What is it? — The box contains:

     - 3 envelopes
     - mineral hackmanite
     - 3 shells
     - a blue glass dish
     - a glass sherd
     - a white cloth

2. Who will use it? — All ages

3. How long will it take? — From 5 to 7 minutes

   Is this a repeat activity? — Not unless visitors bring their own specimens

4. How will visitors use it? — Visitors will examine the items under an ultraviolet light (some of the items will glow a different colour and some will not).

5. Why were these items chosen? — All the items are familiar to visitors.

   — Some of the items have "hidden colours" when they are exposed to ultraviolet light.

B. Statement of Objectives

   - to encourage the visitor to find the "hidden colours" in the box.

   - to prompt the visitor to question what makes objects glow with colours.

   - to encourage the visitor to ask himself what other ordinary objects might have similar properties.

SEA SHELLS BOX

A. Description

1. What is it? — The box contains:

    - 11 kinds of sea shell
    - information cards

2. Who will use it? — All ages

3. How long will it take? — From 5 to 7 minutes

   Is this a repeat activity? — Yes

4. How will visitors use it? — Visitors will examine shell specimens in a box and will then read the accompanying cards for an explanation of each.

5. Why were these items chosen? — Each specimen represents a different kind of shelled animal.

    - The specimens are familiar to the visitor.

    - The subject relates to the Invertebrate Palaeontology Department.

B. Statement of Objectives

- to show the variety of sea shells.

- to arouse the visitor's curiosity about the different kinds of shell.

- to stimulate an interest in the Invertebrate Palaeontology gallery.

TRACKS BOX

A. Description

1. What is it? - The box contains:

    - 12 cards with pictures of animals
    - 12 cards with their footprints

2. Who will use it? - Age 10 and over

3. How long will it take? - From 10 to 15 minutes

    Is this a repeat activity? - Yes

4. How will visitors use it? - Visitors will study the footprints and match them to the appropriate animal. They will base their choices on their own knowledge and on the animal's body size, shape and behaviour.

5. Why were these items chosen? - Animals are indigenous to southern Ontario and familiar to the visitor.

B. Statement of Objectives

- to give the visitor a skill in identifying wild animals before actually seeing them.

- to increase the visitor's appreciation of the life sciences and his enjoyment of the outdoors.

GLOWING ROCKS BOX

A. Description

1. What is it? - The box contains:

- 5 rocks with the following
  fluorescent
  minerals: - calcite
            - hackmanite
            - scapolite
            - sodalite
            - willemite

- 2 rocks without fluorescent
  minerals: - granite
            - sandstone

2. Who will use it? - Age 8 and over

3. How long will it take? - From 10 to 15 minutes

   Is this a repeat activity? - Not unless visitors
        bring their own specimens

4. How will visitors use it? - Visitors will place
        a rock specimen under ultraviolet
        light to see if it contains fluores-
        cent minerals and then they will iden-
        tify the mineral by the colour of
        light that is given off.

5. Why were these items chosen? - The rock samples
        demonstrate that some minerals glow
        with brilliant colours when exposed
        to ultraviolet light.

        - The subject relates to the
        Mineralogy gallery.

B. Statement of Objectives

- to show the visitor that some minerals glow
  brightly when exposed to ultraviolet light.

- to demonstrate that fluorescent minerals can be
  identified in part by their colour.

MOONLIGHT BOX

A. Description

    1. What is it? - The box contains:

          - 19 photographs of the phases
           of the moon

          - a diagram that explains the
           phase changes

          - a list of the ways in which
           the moon affects the earth

          - a related map of the moon
           (attached to wall)

    2. Who will use it? - Age 12 and over

    3. How long will it take? - From 10 to 12 minutes

      Is this a repeat activity? - No

    4. How will visitors use it? - Visitors will
          place the photographs in sequential
          order.

          - Visitors will read the accompany-
          ing information.

    5. Why were these items chosen? - The items prov-
          ide information about the moon, the
          only extraterrestrial part of the
          solar system that man has visited.

          - The items were chosen to explain
          the visible changes in the moon and
          its effects on the earth.

          - The subject relates to the
          Planetarium.

B. Statement of Objectives

- to teach the visitor about the moon's effects on the earth.

- to provide information about gravitational pull.

- to encourage the visitor to acquire more information from the Discovery Room's moon map and from the McLaughlin Planetarium.

MINERAL MYSTERY BOX

A. Description

    1. What is it? - The box contains:

                  - 7 minerals   - barite
                                 - calcite
                                 - galena
                                 - gypsum
                                 - hematite
                                 - hornblende
                                 - magnetite

                  - a magnet

                  - 2 or 3 streak plates

                  - 8 question cards

    2. Who will use it? - Age 10 and over

    3. How long will it take? - From 10 to 15 minutes

       Is this a repeat activity? - Not unless visitors
           bring their own specimens

    4. How will visitors use it? - Visitors will use
           sight and touch to test each of
           seven minerals for certain physical
           properties (streaking, hardness,
           density, and magnetism) in order to
           identify the specimens.

    5. Why were these items chosen? - The minerals
           clearly show the properties by
           which they are to be identified.

           - The subject relates to the
           Mineralogy gallery.

B. Statement of Objective

    - to teach the visitor that different minerals
      which resemble each other can be identified by
      simple tests of their physical properties.

NATURE'S TOOLS BOX

A. Description

1. What is it? - The box contains:

- 8 artifacts: - adze
              - flesher
              - shaped antler
              - shaped columella
              - flint point
              - 2 pieces of pipe
              - curved piece of
                              shell
              - shell pendant

- 8 natural materials:
              - 2 mussel shells
              - piece of antler
              - basalt
              - beaver tooth
              - lower jaw of a
                              beaver
              - flint
              - conch
              - cow bone

- a guide booklet

2. Who will use it? - Age 12 and over

3. How long will it take? - 10 minutes

Is this a repeat activity? - No

4. How will visitors use it? - Visitors, using the
      guide booklet, will select two or
      three objects of similar-looking
      material and discover ways to dis-
      tinguish the materials.

5. Why were these items chosen? - The natural mat-
      erials were important to Native peo-
      ples of Canada.

      - The man-made materials resemble
      the natural ones.

      - The subject relates to the
      Ontario Archaeology gallery.

B. Statement of Objectives

        - to enable the visitor to distinguish between natural and man-made materials.

        - to convey Native peoples' uses of natural materials in their daily lives.

SECRETS IN STONE BOX

A. Description

1. What is it? — The box contains:

   — a sample of 18 rock specimens, some igneous, some sedimentary, some metamorphic

   — a magnifying glass

   — a set of information cards

2. Who will use it? — Age 9 and over

3. How long will it take? — 8 minutes

   Is this a repeat activity? — Yes

4. How will visitors use it? — Visitors will examine the rocks with a magnifying glass and will read through the information cards.

5. Why were these items chosen? — All the rocks are relatively common specimens and are easy to find.

   — The samples are representative of the three major classifications of rock.

   — The subject relates to the Geology gallery.

B. Statement of Objectives

   — to introduce the visitor to the three major rock classifications.

   — to teach the visitor about the formation of the three rock classifications.

   — to encourage the visitor to explore further in the Geology gallery.

STUMPERS

A. Description

1. What is it? - All the individual objects are related to various ROM galleries and may change seasonally or as more are contributed.

   - The Stumpers include:

      - the world's largest seed
      - an ostrich egg
      - a spittoon
      - a grinding stone (for use)
      - a whale bone
      - a beaver stump
      - a printer's box
      - a corn planter
      - a piece of kiln-warped pottery
      - an Egyptian weight
      - a papyrus
      - a fossiliferous limestone rock
      - a Sandhill Crane mounted in flying position
      - an owl
      - a bird skeleton
      - a bat
      - a fish in alcohol

2. Who will use it? - All ages

3. How long will it take? - The time varies according to the Stumper but the unit was designed for a short-term interest of several minutes.

   Is this a repeat activity? - No

4. How will visitors use it? – Visitors will
        arbitrarily select a Stumper,
        pick it up, look at it, perhaps
        use it, and read the attached
        label.

        – The unit involves the sense of
        sight, touch, and hearing.

5. Why were these items chosen? – The items are
        novel, some are exotic, and all
        are designed to stimulate curio-
        sity.

        – Some items relate to boxes in
        the Discovery Room as well as to
        a department in the ROM.

B. Statement of Objectives

    – to entertain the visitor.

    – to encourage the visitor to investigate a
      related box or gallery for further information
      about an item.

ONTARIO ARCHAEOLOGY I.D. UNIT

A. Description

1. What is it?   Spearpoints

- This part of the unit consists of:

    - 6 drawers of arrowheads, spear-
      points, and stone tools arranged
      with an introductory drawer and
      then chronologically, from late
      Woodland to Palaeo Indian

    Prehistoric pottery

    - This part of the unit consists of:

    - 4 drawers of ceramics arranged
      with an introductory drawer and
      then chronologically and by
      tribe

2. Who will use it? - All ages

3. How long will it take? - From 5 to 50 minutes

   Is this a repeat activity? - Yes, especially
             for collectors and students

4. How will visitors use it? - Visitors will remove
        drawers and take them to the table
        for examination through a glass lid.

        - Visitors with their own specimens
        will be asked to fill out a form
        that describes their own tentative
        identification for the department.

5. Why were these items chosen? - The items are
        representative of stone tools,
        ceramics, and pottery of Ontario.

        - The visitor should be able to
        recognize the objects and estimate
        the approximate age.

        - The unit is based on current Arch-
        aeological classification and state
        of research.

- The unit relates to both the Archaeology and Nature's Tools boxes.

B. Statement of Objectives

- to show the visitor the changes in projectile point form and pottery decoration over 10,000 to 12,000 years in Ontario and the Great Lakes region.

- to identify and date specific artifacts by placing them in a cultural context.

- to contribute to current research by reporting finds.

- to supplement the Archaeology Box experience.

- to provide a reference collection for identification purposes.

<u>FOSSILS I.D. UNIT</u>

<u>A. Description</u>

    1. What is it? - The unit consists of:

           - 9 drawers: - 1 introductory
                            - 6 with different
                              types of fossils
                            - 1 of fossils
                              and non-fossils
                            - 1 for the visitor
                              to identify
                              specimens

          - cards that illustrate the pre-
            fossil form of each specimen

    2. Who will use it? - All ages

    3. How long will it take? - From 5 to 50 minutes

       Is this a repeat activity? - Yes

    4. How will visitors use it? - Visitors will pull
               the drawers out, examine the spec-
               imens, and use the microscopes and
               the reference library if they wish.

    5. Why were these items chosen? - The specimens
               represent the quality of fossils
               often found in Ontario.

               - The cards were drawn to show
               entire fossils, with the specimens
               on display indicated.

<u>B. Statement of Objectives</u>

    - to familiarize the visitor with common fossils
      found in Ontario.

    - to teach a basic procedure and the vocabulary
      related to fossil identification.

    - to provide a reference collection for identifi-
      cation purposes.

BUTTERFLIES I.D. UNIT

A. Description

1. What is it? - The unit contains:

    - 10 double-glazed drawers with male and female specimens of 100 species of Ontario butterfly and 15 species of larger moth

    - reference books

    - identified specimens in bottom drawer

2. Who will use it? - All ages

3. How long will it take? - From 10 to 60 minutes

    Is this a repeat activity? - Yes

4. How will visitors use it? - Visitors will search through and inspect the specimens in the drawers and will use the reference books for supplementary information.

    - The drawers may be turned over to look at the undersides of the specimens.

    - The visitors may use the unidentified specimens provided or bring their own.

5. Why were these items chosen? - Butterflies generate more interest than any other insect group.

    - The specimens can be found in Ontario.

    - Butterflies are easy to identify by species.

    - There is extensive literature available.

B. Statement of Objectives

- to encourage an appreciation of Ontario Lepidopteran Fauna.

- to help the visitor understand the methodology involved in species identification for entomological research using a reference collection.

- to acquaint the visitor with basic storage methods for specimens in research collections (i.e., dried and pinned with label information).

- to teach the visitor the common and scientific Latin classifications.

- to give the visitor a clearer idea of lepidopteran anatomy, size, and weight.

- to provide a reference collection for identification purposes.

INSECTS I.D. UNIT

A. Description

1. What is it? - The unit consists of:

     - 5 drawers that contain several dozen insect specimens preserved in plastic or dried and pinned in small, plastic jewellery boxes

     - an explanation sheet about structural features that are evident

     - a list of identifications in the introductory drawer

2. Who will use it? - All ages

3. How long will it take? - From 10 to 30 minutes

   Is this a repeat activity? - Yes, especially if visitors bring their own specimens

4. How will visitors use it? - Visitors will search through the introductory and specimen drawers.

     - Visitors will select and examine specimens under a microscope.

     - They will refer to the reference library for further information if they wish.

5. Why were these items chosen? - Many people have a general interest in insects, especially during the summer.

     - There appears to be a great interest in the microscopic structures of insects.

     - The items were chosen for their identification value.

B. Statement of Objectives

- to encourage an appreciation of the diversity and beauty of insects.

- to increase the visitor's knowledge of common and Latin names.

- to promote an awareness of the structural complexity of insects.

- to acquaint the visitor with the procedure for insect identification.

- to provide a reference collection for identification purposes.

STAMPS I.D. UNIT

A. Description

1. What is it? - The unit consists of 5 drawers:

   - 3 about the evolution of the Canadian stamp (from pre-postage covers and threepenny beavers to the 1977 Christmas stamp) arranged chronologically

   - 1 of special interest stamps

   - 1 of plants and animal stamps

2. Who will use it? - All ages

3. How long will it take? - From 5 to 25 minutes

   Is this a repeat activity? - Yes, especially if visitors bring their own stamps

4. How will visitors use it? - Visitors will bring drawers to the table to examine stamp specimens.

5. Why were these items chosen? - Visitors have daily contact with stamps and mail.

   - The specimens show the evolution of all types of postage and stamp design in Canada.

   - Stamps appeal both to the layman and to the collector.

B. Statement of Objectives

- to provide a history of Canadian stamp design and changes that have occurred in postage types.

- to encourage collectors to use the display for reference and study.

SKELETON UNIT

A. Description

1. What is it? - The unit consists of:

    - a human skeleton mounted in an upright position with the limbs freely movable

    - 3 illuminated radiographs

    - 2 panels and 2 human bones that demonstrate various afflictions

    - a human skull

    - photographs of skeletons from other ROM departments

2. Who will use it? - Young children are interested only in the spectacular aspect, but those over the age of 11 may be interested in joint movements, abnormalities, and the value of radiography to archaeology and palaeopathology.

3. How long will it take? - From 10 to 30 minutes

   Is this a repeat activity? - Yes

4. How will visitors use it? - Visitors will handle the Skeleton and will move the parts to see how the joints work and how the bones are related to the joints.

    - The radiographs that show fractures and deformities will clearly refer back to the Skeleton.

5. Why were these items chosen? - The Skeleton attracts attention quickly.

    - Most visitors have had x-rays taken and therefore can relate directly to the radiographs and can study body disorders.

B. Statement of Objectives

- to teach the visitor about basic anatomy and about the framework that supports the human body.

- to illustrate simply how arm and leg motions occur.

- to convey the impact of injury or disease.

- to encourage an appreciation of the use of radiography in archaeology and bone diseases.

- to demonstrate how archaeologists use skeleton fragments to derive information about previous cultures (state of healing art, state of nutrition).

TREE UNIT

A. Description

1. What is it? - The central attraction is a large cross-section of a tree that has 150 years in time marked on it with man's achievements on one side and an explanation of the rings on the reverse. Smaller display items for handling and examination under a magnifying glass include:

   - sections of 15 native Ontario trees, woods and their labels

   - examples of wood products

   - a Queen Anne chair

   - an herbarium that includes tree and leaf samples

   - a map of the trees in Queen's Park

   - a wooden barrel that contains items such as a hockey stick, a table leg, a baseball bat

2. Who will use it? - All ages

3. How long will it take? - The unit can be scanned in less than 5 minutes but it would take 20 minutes to study it thoroughly.

   Is this a repeat activity? - No

4. How will visitors use it? - Visitors will look at and touch all parts of the display, comparing the different textures, weights, sizes, colours, patterns, and species.

5. Why were these items chosen? Although the material is readily available, it is seldom displayed elsewhere.

   - The different woods are easily handled and compared.

- Both common and more unusual types of wood allow the visitor to see the differences between species.

- The unit is attractive and therefore makes an impact upon the visitor.

- The unit is related to the ROM collection in many ways (especially to the Botany Department and to all other departments that deal with wood artifacts).

B. Statement of Objectives

- to teach the visitor:

- what the inside of a tree looks like

- about tree age and growth pattern

- about the relationships of tree rings to grain in lumber

- the differences between wood types

- about the source of knots in wood

- the uses of wood for secondary products and the way it is used for crafts

- how to recognize indigenous trees and leaves by using the herbarium.

STAMP DISPLAY

A. Description

    1. What is it? - The unit consists of an exhibit compiled by the Canadian Post Office that includes:

- envelope stamp specimens
- first-day issues
- 2 enlarged stamps
- thematic stamp displays (e.g., Indians of Canada)
- cancellation marks
- historic and rare stamps
- 3 magnifying glasses

    2. Who will use it? - All ages

    3. How long will it take? - From 5 to 10 minutes

    Is this a repeat activity? - No

    4. How will visitors use it? - Visitors will look at stamps in the exhibit and perhaps refer to the Stamp I.D. unit.

    5. Why were these items chosen? - All visitors have daily contact with stamps and mail.

- The display provides an easy introduction to philately.

- The unit relates to both the Hidden Colours and the Micro Marvels Box.

- The unit relates to the Stamp I.D. unit.

- The exhibit can be changed periodically.

B. Statement of Objectives

- to introduce the visitor to philately.

- to demonstrate the large variety and scope of Canadian stamps and cancellation marks.

MIRROR DISPLAY

A. Description

1. What is it?   - The unit, "See Yourself Through the Ages", consists of:

   - mirrors (attached to the wall at varying levels) that represent different periods in the development of mirror technology and design
   - labels/cards that describe the original owners

2. Who will use it?   - All ages

3. How long will it take?   - From 5 to 10 minutes

   Is this a repeat activity?   - Yes

4. How will visitors use it?   - Visitors will look at mirrors and read the accompanying label/card.

5. Why were these items chosen?   - Mirrors are familiar to everyone.

   - The mirrors were chosen to demonstrate design and technological advances as well as changes in size.

   - The unit relates to the Art and Archaeology departments.

B. Statement of Objectives

- to provide an aesthetic experience for the visitor.

- to demonstrate technological progress in glass silvering.

- to show evolution in one aspect of interior design.

BIRD DISPLAY

A. Description

      1. What is it? - The unit consists of:

                - a skeleton

                - 6 different sizes of bird

                - a bat

          The birds and bat are suspended from the ceiling or on display stands.

      2. Who will use it? - All ages

      3. How long will it take? - From 1 to 5 minutes

        Is this a repeat activity? - No

      4. How will visitors use it? - Visitors will look at and touch the specimens to make comparisons.

          - Some visitors may wish to use the library or go to related ROM galleries for further information.

      5. Why were these items chosen? - The items were available and show the size of the birds and the bat.

          - The unit relates to the Ornithology and Mammalogy departments.

          - The unit relates to the Feathers Box.

B. Statement of Objectives

      - to increase a visitor's understanding of the actual size of birds, the arrangement of the feathers, and the shape of the body and beak.

      - to illustrate the differences between bats and birds.

      - to teach the visitor about flight.

TOUCH WALL

A. Description

    1. What is it? - The unit consists of:

        - about 32 fragments of various materials (organic and inorganic) mounted on a display wall

    2. Who will use it? - All ages

    3. How long will it take? - From 1 to 10 minutes

      Is this a repeat activity? - Yes

    4. How will visitors use it? - Visitors will touch, scratch, stroke, and smell the various textures.

      - The unit involves sight, touch, and smell.

    5. Why were these items chosen? - The items were chosen for their interesting textures.

      - The items are familiar by name and/or sight but generally not by touch.

B. Statement of Objectives

    - to attract people, to encourage them to participate, and then to draw them into the Discovery Room.

    - to make the visitor aware of the enormous variety of textures to be found in familiar items.

LIVE EXHIBIT (Xeric Terrarium)

A. Description

1. What is it? - The unit consists of:

    - a plexiglass front built into a display wall that contains sandy soil and live desert vegetation (xeric plants)

    - labels that explain how cacti have adapted to desert conditions

    - photographs of desert scenes

2. Who will use it? - Age 8 and over

3. How long will it take? - 5 minutes

    Is this a repeat activity? - No

4. How will visitors use it? - Visitors will look at the cacti in the terrarium and will read the label information.

5. Why were these items chosen? - The display was set up to show the principles of plant adaptation to survival in extreme environments.

    - The unit relates to a proposed ROM Botany department and has expert advice available from the University of Toronto Botany Department.

    - The plants enhance the Discovery Room's appearance.

B. Statement of Objectives

- to teach the visitor that natural selection has produced plant varieties that have overcome, in a number of ways, the stresses of a desert habitat.

- to increase the visitors' appreciation of the complexities of nature in coping with a hostile environment.

- to encourage the visitor to relate what he has learned from the unit to his own experience with houseplants.

TORTOISES DISPLAY (Removed from Room)

A. Description

1. What is it? — The display consists of:

   - a terrarium with 4 box turtles (Terrapin Carolina)
   - an attached supplementary unit with several shells to handle
   - graphics of other kinds of turtles
   - fossil history and reasons for longevity

2. Who will use it? — All ages

3. How long will it take? — From 5 to 15 minutes

   Is this a repeat activity? — No

4. How will visitors use it? — Visitors will observe the turtles resting, working, or feeding.

   - The shells and live turtles may be handled to show that the soft parts of the turtle are entirely covered by bony plates.

5. Why were these items chosen? — Box turtles are hardy, odourless, and easy to sustain and their shells may be handled safely.

   - The turtles illustrate several biological principles such as a highly evolved protective shell, an omnivourous diet, and the ability to withstand draughts.

   - The turtles represent a long fossil history.

   - There are discernible differences between males and females.

- The unit relates to the Herpet-
ology and Vertebrate Palaeontology
departments.

- The unit involves the sense of
sight and touch.

B. Statement of Objectives

- to demonstrate an example of a highly specialized and successful adaptation for protection
against predators, despite a lack of speed.

- to show that turtles can be used as climatic
indicators in palaeo sites.

- to show the uses made of turtle shells by
Native peoples.

PRINTED RESOURCE MATERIALS

A. Description

    1. What is it? - The materials consist of:

        - reference books, which are related to Stumpers, I.D. units, and boxes, scattered throughout the Room near these components

    2. Who will use them? - All visitors (depending on motivation, time, and immediate accessibility)

    3. How long will it take? - From 2 to 10 minutes approximately

    Is this a repeat activity? - Yes

    4. How will visitors use them? - Visitors will have their interest aroused by the boxes, Stumpers, or I.D. units and will be motivated to find more detailed information.

    - The books will be used in the manner of any reference material.

    5. Why were these items chosen? - The books were chosen for their accuracy and ease of use.

    - The books were chosen to augment learning units and to encourage further study.

B. Statement of Objectives

    - to promote easy and frequent use of reference material.

    - to provide a facility for visitors to investigate their own interests.

A given day is considered successful when 10% of the book collection is used.

Appendix B

Evaluation

Introduction

Purpose of Evaluation

The purpose of the evaluation was to provide an assessment of the success of the Room, and to assist the DRWG both in developing new components and in redesigning or adjusting the existing ones.

Although detailed evaluation based on the objectives of individual components was not undertaken, this evaluation provides some indication of which components are working and which are not.

Methods

Two methods were used in conducting the evaluation: (1) the "tracking" of the visitors; (2) the administration of a questionnaire. A sample of visitors were observed while they were in the Discovery Room. Their circulation paths were recorded, as well as activities such as stopping, reading, touching objects, etc. After leaving the Room, these visitors were approached by the people who had observed them, and were asked to respond to the questionnaire. Samples of both the format for recording the tracking observations and of the questionnaire are included.

SAMPLING PROCEDURE

The survey was conducted during five days in August and seven days in December. Surveys were conducted both on weekdays and on week-ends.

One in every eight persons over nine years of age who entered the Discovery Room was tracked for the duration of his visit and then interviewed.[1] Interviews and tracking observations were conducted with casual visitors only, and excluded members of school groups, Saturday Morning Club groups, special groups, and ROM staff.

A total of 193 tracking observations was undertaken and 131 questionnaires were administered. Fewer completed questionnaires than tracking observations were obtained since some visitors refused to be interviewed (usually because of lack of time or language problems).

ANALYSIS OF DATA

Although the evaluation format was standard for all visitors, specific data relate to particular portions of the sample population. The population to which each table refers is clearly identified by n = sample population. Changes in the sample are due to three factors:

(1) Specific questions were directed to particular portions of the sample population (e.g., visitors with children between the ages of six and nine).

(2) Some data were obtained from tracking observations and some from the interviews.

---

[1] It was a policy of the Discovery Room that children under six years of age would not be admitted and that children between the ages of six and nine would only be admitted when accompanied by an adult. It is important to note that the age limit was determined visually by the survey team, and that although children between the ages of six and nine were not tracked or interviewed, they were included in the determination of the composition of groups.

(3) The data were analyzed in specific categories (e.g., by age, group, or month).

In addition, where analysis of the data indicated that the visitors' observed behaviour patterns and/or questionnaire responses differed according to age groupings (i.e., adult, adolescent, and child) and where the differences were significant, the data were separated into these groupings.

ALTERATIONS BETWEEN SURVEY PERIODS

This survey was designed as a formative type of evaluation that involved a continuous process: development of objectives; implementation of these objectives; evaluation; implementation of any necessary changes to respond to the evaluation; implementation; evaluation, etc. Properly carried out, formative evaluations should provide continual feedback about the degree to which objectives are being fulfilled.

While small changes have been continually taking place in the Discovery Room, the first survey formally identified some areas that needed alteration. With the limited amount of time available, only some of the alterations could be made after this initial evaluation. The second evaluation continued to test the objectives of the Room in general, and the results of these changes in particular. The effects of the alterations will be discussed in conjunction with the individual component evaluation. The alterations were as follows:

- The Micro-Marvels Box was added.
- The Herbarium I.D. Unit was combined with the Tree Unit.
- Unidentified specimens/artifacts were added to I.D. units (bottom drawer).
- New labels and photographs were provided for the I.D. units.
- The Stumpers were changed continually.
- A Moon Map was displayed on the wall.
- The Tortoise Display was removed.
- The Puzzle was removed.
- The Mirrors Display was altered aesthetically.
- A third and simpler microscope was added.
- Stepping stools were added.

The Discovery Room
as an Attraction

THE DISCOVERY ROOM AS AN ATTRACTION

Information about the nature of the Room's attraction is organized under the following headings:

A. Attraction of the Discovery Room

B. Profile of Visitors Attracted to the Discovery Room

A. Attraction of the Discovery Room

Most visitors to the Discovery Room include it in a general visit to the ROM.

Table 1:   Percentage of Visitors Who Had Planned to Visit
           the Discovery Room (by Age of Visitor)

Came Specifically for Discovery Room	Adults (n=80)	Adolescents (n=80)	Children (n=27)	Visitors (n=131)
	%	%	%	%
Yes	21.3	8.4	18.5	18.3
No	78.7	91.6	81.5	81.7
Total	100.0	100.0	100.0	100.0

● Less than one-fifth of the visitors to the Discovery Room came specifically to see it.

The Discovery Room is attracting an increasing proportion of repeat visitors.

Table 2:   Percentage of First-Time and Repeat Visitors
            (by Month)

First Visit	August (n=62)	December (n=69)	All Visitors (n=131)
	%	%	%
Yes	93.5	87.0	90.1
No	6.5	13.0	9.9
Total	100.0	100.0	100.0

● The percentage of repeat visitors increased from 6.5% in August to 13% in December. The number of repeat visitors is significant since the Room opened in July. One month later, approximately one visitor in fifteen was returning, and five months after its opening almost one-seventh of the visitors to the Room were repeat visitors.

Table   3:   Source from Which Visitors Learned of the
             Discovery Room (by Month)

Source	August (n=62)	December (n=69)	All Visitors (n=131)
	%	%	%
Had Not Heard About It	58.1	53.6	55.7
Another Person	17.8	23.2	20.6
Newspaper/Magazine	14.5	7.2	10.7
ROM Staff	3.2	5.8	4.6
Floor Plan	–	5.8	3.1
Television/Radio	1.6	3.0	2.3
"Preview" Brochure	1.6	1.4	1.5
Poster	3.2	–	1.5
Total	100.0	100.0	100.0

● Of the visitors to the Room, 20.6% had heard about it
  from other visitors, and this proportion increased considerably between August and December. The ability to
  generate enthusiasm in its visitors is a further indication of the attractiveness of the Room.

B. Profile of Visitors Attracted to the Discovery Room*

Although the majority of visitors to the Room are adults, the new gallery attracts higher proportions of children, adolescents, and family groups than the ROM as a whole.

Table 4:   Comparison of Age and Sex of Visitors to the Discovery Room and Visitors to the ROM as a Whole

Respondent	Discovery Room Visitors	Visitors to ROM
	%	%
Female Adult	35.8	44.9
Male Adult	32.1	37.2
Female Adolescent	9.3	5.7
Male Adolescent	6.7	5.6
Child	16.1 [1]	6.8 [2]
Total	100.0	100.0

[1] Only children estimated to be over nine years old were tracked and interviewed in this survey.

[2] Only children estimated to be over five years old were interviewed in the *Visitor Perception and Profile Survey*.

- Of the visitors to the Discovery Room, 32% were children or adolescents (between nine and nineteen years of age).

*All information on profile characteristics of visitors to the ROM as a whole is drawn from the *Visitor Perception and Profile Survey*, which is based on a comprehensive sample taken over an entire calendar year. This survey is published as Part I of *Mankind Discovering*, Volume I.

- The proportion of children or adolescents who were recorded as visitors to the Discovery Room was twice that of those who visited the ROM as a whole. The actual proportion, including those between six and nine years who were excluded from the sample, would be substantially higher.

- Although the proportion of adults visiting the Discovery Room was lower than those visiting the ROM as a whole, 68% of the visitors to the Room were adults.

Table 5:   Types of Groups in Which Visitors Came to the
            Discovery Room (by Age of Visitor)

Type of Group	Adults (n=80)	Adolescents (n=24)	Children (n=27)	All Visitors (n=131)	ROM Visitors (n=4861)
	%	%	%	%	%
Single	16.0	12.9	6.5	14.0	17.5
Family Group [1]	48.9	29.0	41.9	44.0	31.8
Group of Adults[1] Only	35.1	–	–	24.4	43.8
Group of Children/ Adolescents only [1]	–	58.1	51.6	17.6	6.9
Total	100.0	100.0	100.0	100.0	100.0

[1]To determine the type of a group, all children (i.e., six years and over) in the group accompanying the individual being interviewed were included.

- Almost half of the visitors to the Discovery Room came in family groups and yet family groups represent less than one-third of the general ROM population.

- Most of the children and adolescents visiting the Room came independently of adults. More than twice as many unaccompanied children and adolescents visit the Discovery Room as visit the ROM as a whole.

Discovery Room visitors are drawn from the same geographical areas as visitors to the ROM in general.

Table 6: Visitors' Places of Residence (by Month)

Place of Residence	August (n=62)	December (n=69)	All Visitors (n=131)	ROM Visitors (n=4861)
	%	%	%	%
City of Toronto	22.6	26.2	24.4	27.3
Boroughs	14.5	39.0	27.5	21.2
Surrounding Municipalities[1]	11.3	14.6	13.0	15.1
Rest of Ontario	11.2	11.6	11.4	12.6
Other Provinces	11.3	2.9	6.9	4.4
U.S.A.	21.0	4.3	12.2	15.7
Other Countries	8.1	1.4	4.6	3.7
Total	100.0	100.0	100.0	100.0

[1] For the purpose of this study, the surrounding municipalities were defined as Metropolitan Toronto's commuting area, i.e., the area bounded by Hamilton, Barrie, Peterborough, and Oshawa.

- The proportion of visitors from the Boroughs during December was particularly high.

- As with the ROM in general, a large number of tourists, particularly from the U.S.A., visited the Discovery Room during the summer.

Visitors' Overall Reactions
to the Discovery Room

The Discovery Room is very successful. Its attraction is
evident both in visitors' responses to general questions
about the Room, and in their observed behaviour, when it
is compared to typical behaviour patterns in other ROM
galleries.[1] Their responses and behaviour are organized
under the following headings:

A.   Time Spent by Visitors in the Discovery Room

B.   Visitors' Impressions of the Discovery Room

C.   How Visitors Used the Discovery Room

D.   Visitors' Recommendations for Improvements to the
     Discovery Room

E.   The Effect of the Discovery Room on Visitors' Impres-
     sions of the ROM

---

[1] As noted in the *Overall Visitor Tracking and Satisfaction Survey* published
as Part II of *Mankind Discovering*, Volume II.

A. Time Spent by Visitors in the Discovery Room

Table 7:   Total Time Spent in the Discovery Room
           (by Age of Visitor)

Amount of Time Spent In Room	Adults (n=131)	Adolescents (n=31)	Children (n=31)	All Visitors (n=193)
	%	%	%	%
Short (1 to 5 minutes)	38.1	45.2	13.0	32.5
Medium (6 to 15 minutes)	27.5	25.8	29.0	27.5
Long (16 minutes and up)	34.4	29.0	58.0	37.3
Total	100.0	100.0	100.0	100.0

- The Room is relatively small and a visitor who is not interested in participating in the activities that it offers can easily view the entire area and depart within five minutes.

- The average time spent by a visitor was ten minutes, and 37.3% of the visitors spent sixteen minutes or more in the Room.

- Children spent the most time in the Room. Over 80% spent six minutes or more, and of these, two-thirds spent sixteen minutes or more.

- Almost half of the adolescents who visited the Room left in less than five minutes.

- The proportion of adults who spent more than five minutes in the Room is probably skewed because many adults were visiting with their children, and therefore adjusted the length of their stay accordingly.

B. Visitors' Impressions of the Discovery Room

In order to discover visitors' reactions, visitors were asked to indicate their rating of the Room according to a pair of descriptive adjectives on a scale from 1 to 5. An examination of these ratings indicates that reactions are generally very positive.

Table 8:   Rating of Visitors' Impressions of the Discovery Room (by Age of Visitor)

Adjective Pairs Rated on a scale of 1-5[1]	All Visitors (Median)	Adults (Median)	Adolescents (Median)	Children (Median)
Enjoyable/Unpleasant	1.35	1.33	1.42	1.34
Inviting/Unattractive	1.42	1.48	1.50	1.25
Informative/ Unenlightening	1.44	1.41	1.50	1.46
Unique/Ordinary	1.51	1.54	1.42	1.55
Exciting/Boring	1.76	1.78	2.13	1.46
Orderly/Cluttered	1.36	1.41	1.36	1.25
Organized/Confusing	1.37	1.50	1.36	1.14
Spacious/Cramped	2.44	2.89	2.04	1.82

Adjective Pairs Rated on a scale of 1-5[2]				
Too Bright/Too Dim	2.97	2.98	3.00	2.89
Too Cold/Too Hot	3.14	3.12	3.17	3.19

[1] In this first group of adjectives the most positive rating is 1.0 and the most negative is 5.0. Visitors rated the adjective pairs on a scale of 1 to 5. The median response was calculated on a scale of 0.5 to 5.5. The first adjective in each pair is the most positive response possible and the second adjective the most negative (although it should be noted that the pairs were not organized in this manner in the questionnaire).

[2] In this group of adjectives 3.0 is the most positive rating and both 1.0 and 5.0 are negative responses. Visitors rated the adjective pairs on a scale of 1 to 5. The median response was calculated on a scale of 0.5 to 5.5. Both adjectives represent negative responses and the most positive response is the midpoint between these pairs.

- Generally, visitors found the Room to be enjoyable (1.35), orderly (1.36), and organized (1.37).

- Children usually rated the Discovery Room higher than either adults or adolescents.

- The only impressions that indicate a more negative view were the exciting/boring scale and the spacious/ cramped scale. Adults, and to some degree adolescents, tended to find the Room cramped. Adolescents found the Room less exciting than adults or children.

Visitors' responses about the purpose of the Discovery
Room make it evident that they understand its concept.

Table 9:   Visitors' Perceptions of the Purpose of the
           Discovery Room (by Age of Visitor)[1]

Purpose	Adults (n=80)	Adolescents (n=24)	Children (n=27)	All Visitors (n=131)
	%	%	%	%
To teach	27.5	37.5	55.6	35.1
For children	32.5	-	25.9	25.2
To discover/explore	23.8	25.0	22.2	23.7
To use all senses	27.5	12.5	7.4	19.8
Participation	13.8	12.5	7.4	12.2
To stimulate interest	12.5	16.7	3.7	11.5
Information	10.0	12.5	11.1	10.7
Don't know	1.3	8.3	3.7	3.8
Science	3.8	4.2	-	3.1
For fun	2.5	4.2	-	2.3

[1] This question was open-ended in that respondents were allowed to give
more than one answer; therefore the percentages do not total 100%.

- It is evident that visitors had little difficulty in
  understanding the concept of the Room. When they were
  asked the purpose of the Room, almost all their responses
  related to the overall objectives.

- It is interesting to note, that a third of the adults
  felt that the Room was primarily for children.

Visitors' enthusiasm is further indicated by the large proportion of visitors from within commuting distance who express a desire to return to the Discovery Room.

Table 10:   Proportions of Visitors from Metro Toronto and Commuting Area That Would Like to Return to the Discovery Room Soon

Plan to Return	All Visitors (n=131)
	%
Yes	82.3
No	7.3
Not Certain	10.4
Total	100.0

- A large proportion of the visitors to the Discovery Room who came from within commuting distance (82%) indicated that they would like to return soon. This finding is certainly a positive measure of the Room's success. The intention to return is corroborated by the actual pattern of return visits noted previously (Table 2).

Some components are viewed by more visitors than others. The popularity of particular components varies with different age groups.

Table 11:   Components Seen by Visitors (by Age of Visitor)[1]

Component Seen	Adults (n=131)	Adolescents (n=31)	Children (n=31)	All Visitors (n=193)
	%	%	%	%
Skeleton	48.1	61.3	64.5	52.8
Boxes	33.6	41.9	64.5	39.9
Stumpers	35.9	38.7	35.5	36.3
Tree Unit	35.1	41.9	29.0	35.2
Stamp Display	27.5	29.0	45.2	30.6
I.D. Units	26.7	16.1	25.8	24.9
Live Exhibit	18.3	16.1	12.9	17.1
Mirror Display	17.6	19.4	6.5	16.1

[1] Visitors could see any number of components; therefore percentages do not total 100%. This information was derived from tracking observations in which "seeing" was minimally defined as "focussed looking".

● The Skeleton was located in a very conspicuous position in the Room. There is evidence that this component attracted visitors into the Room.

● The Skeleton, Stumpers and, to a lesser degree, the Tree Unit and Stamp Display were all highly visible components located near the entry/exit.

● Although the boxes were less visible, they were the item that attracted the second largest proportion of visitors.

C. How Visitors Used the Discovery Room

While visitors move through the Room in a variety of ways, most visitors see a considerable proportion of the Room. The following figures illustrate the typical circulation patterns in the Discovery Room. (The findings are drawn from the analysis of the typical circulation patterns.)

- Of the visitors to the Discovery Room, 20% made a complete visit. They circulated among almost all the components (Figure 1).

- Of the visitors who entered the Discovery Room, 20% left immediately (Figure 2).

- Twenty-five per cent of the visitors followed a central path (Figure 3) and circulated around the components that were directly visible from the door.

- Nineteen per cent of the visitors followed a concentrated path around one component (Figure 4). This route most frequently consisted of a continuous pattern of movement between the boxes and a combination of the following: microscopes, ultraviolet light, tables, and luxo-lamps. The area near the boxes was frequently congested as this circulation pattern often encouraged visitors to become involved with the components (i.e., visitors, particularly children, tended to spend a considerable amount of time with the boxes).

- The remaining 17% saw about half the components in the Room, and circulated in individual patterns.

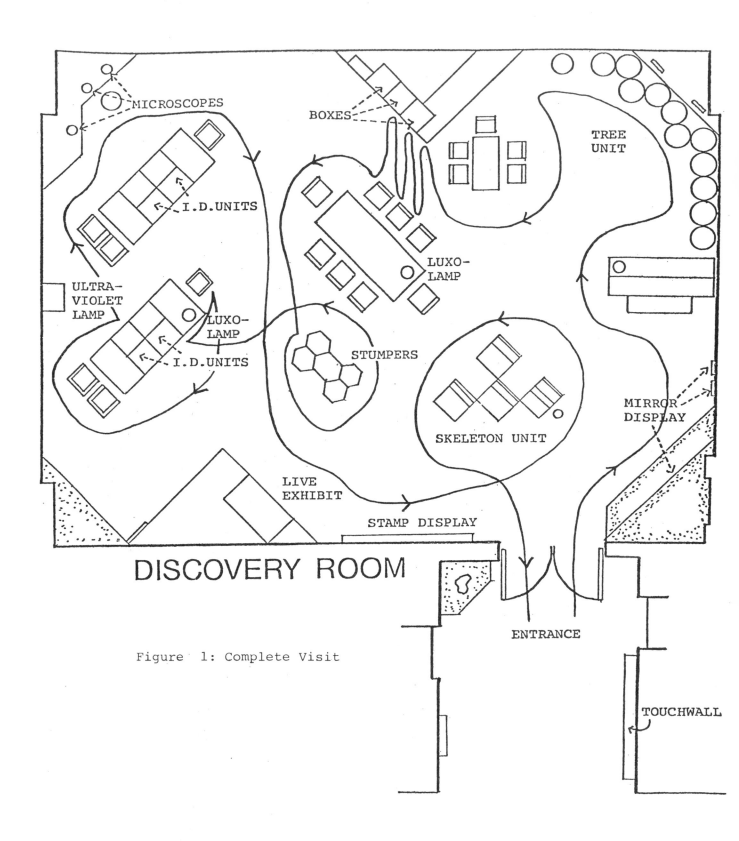

Figure 1: Complete Visit

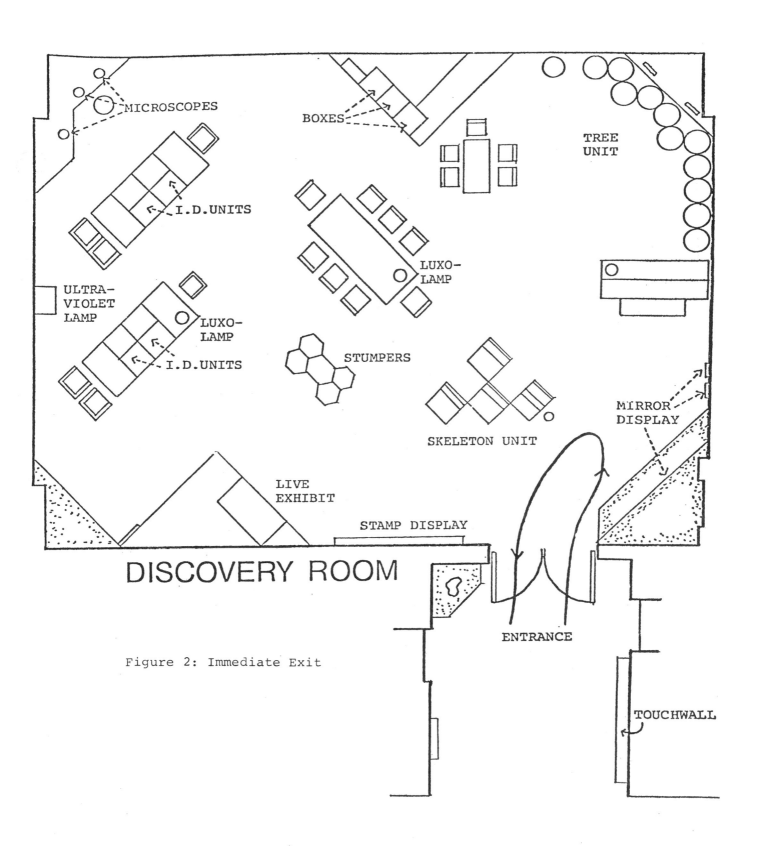

MICROSCOPES

BOXES

TREE
UNIT

I.D.UNITS

ULTRA-
VIOLET
LAMP

LUXO-
LAMP

LUXO-
LAMP

I.D.UNITS

STUMPERS

MIRROR
DISPLAY

SKELETON UNIT

LIVE
EXHIBIT

STAMP DISPLAY

DISCOVERY ROOM

ENTRANCE

TOUCHWALL

Figure 2: Immediate Exit

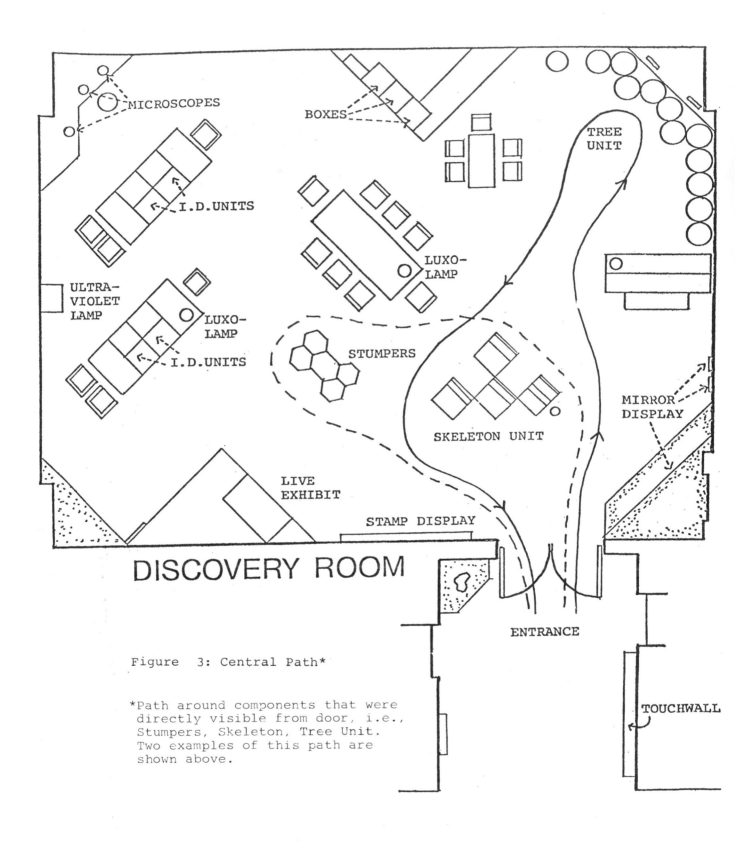

MICROSCOPES

BOXES

TREE UNIT

I.D.UNITS

ULTRA-VIOLET LAMP

LUXO-LAMP

LUXO-LAMP

I.D.UNITS

STUMPERS

SKELETON UNIT

MIRROR DISPLAY

LIVE EXHIBIT

STAMP DISPLAY

DISCOVERY ROOM

ENTRANCE

TOUCHWALL

Figure 3: Central Path*

*Path around components that were
directly visible from door, i.e.,
Stumpers, Skeleton, Tree Unit.
Two examples of this path are
shown above.

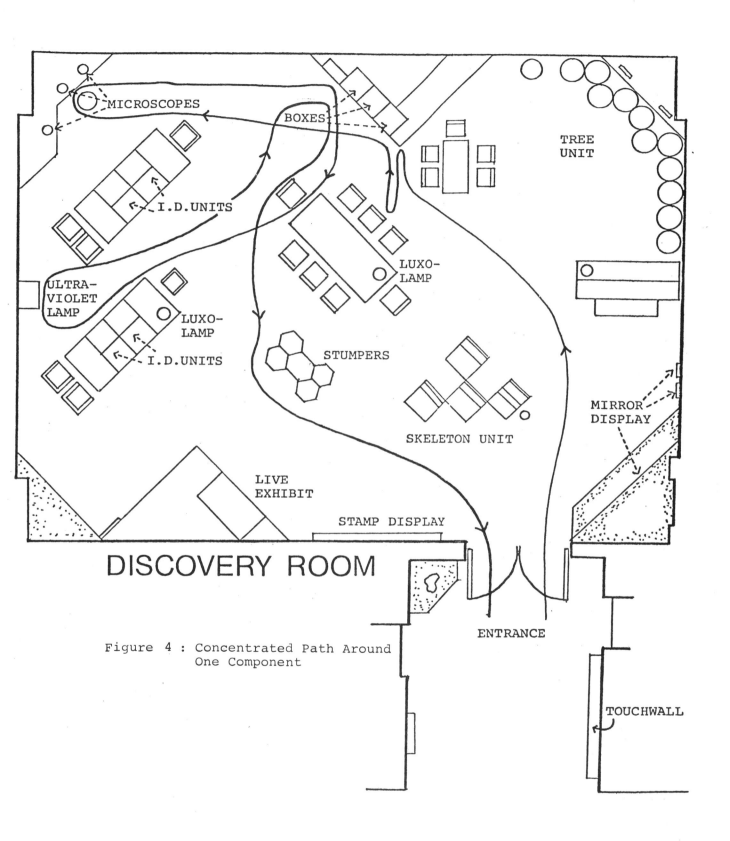

MICROSCOPES

BOXES

TREE
UNIT

I.D.UNITS

ULTRA-
VIOLET
LAMP

LUXO-
LAMP

LUXO-
LAMP

I.D.UNITS

STUMPERS

SKELETON UNIT

MIRROR
DISPLAY

LIVE
EXHIBIT

STAMP DISPLAY

DISCOVERY ROOM

ENTRANCE

TOUCHWALL

Figure 4 : Concentrated Path Around
One Component

D. Visitors' Recommendations for Improvements to the Discovery Room

Visitors' recommendations for improvements to the Discovery Room are not so much critical as indicative of a general enthusiasm for the Discovery Room experience, and they often include suggestions for expanding the Room (i.e., more components, a larger room).

Table 12: Improvements for Discovery Room Suggested by Visitors[1]

Improvements Suggested	Percentage of Visitors (n=131)
No improvements suggested	56.9
More variety	9.9
More space	8.4
More about body, bones, growth process in humans and animals	6.9
More components (more Boxes, more participation)	6.1
More assistance in using participatory exhibits	6.1
Live exhibits	3.8
Air conditioning	3.8
Other	3.8

[1] This question was open-ended in that respondents were allowed to give more than one answer; therefore the percentages do not total 100%. "Other" included such responses as: more about archaeology methods, an ant hill, more on chemistry, Tree Unit too big, more complementary resources, orient the room more to adults, more on electronics. Responses in this category were mentioned by two visitors or fewer.

- The majority of visitors (56.9%) did not suggest any improvements.

- The majority of the visitors who made specific recommendations expressed a desire for more space, more components, and a greater number of discovery-type experiences in the Discovery Room.

Table 13:   Improvements Suggested by Parents for Children
Between the Ages of Six and Nine[1]

Improvements Suggested	Percentage of Visitors (n=39)
	%
Larger room with more to do	20.5
Lower shelves, mirrors, stamp display etc. or else stools to stand on	10.3
More docents	10.3
More floor space for children's activities	7.7
Boxes too heavy and awkward	5.1
Other	17.9

[1]Visitors with children between the ages of six and nine years were asked this question. It was an open-ended question in that respondents were allowed to give more than one answer; therefore percentages do not total 100%. "Other" category includes suggestions, each made by only one visitor, for such improvements as more information, more open hours, question/answer exhibits, more stuffed animals, and dinosaur bones.

● The suggestions made by parents for their young children concerned physical adjustments, e.g., shelf heights, floor space, etc.

E. The Effect of the Discovery Room on Visitors' Impressions of the ROM

The Discovery Room has a very positive impact on visitors' impressions of the ROM. Visitors see the Room as a new approach, particularly to the provision of information. However, they do not make direct connections between the Discovery Room and other galleries in the Museum.

Table 14: Effect of Discovery Room on Visitors' Impressions of the ROM (by Age of Visitor)[1]

Effect	Adults (n=80)	Adolescents (n=24)	Children (n=27)	All Visitors (n=131)
	%	%	%	%
Makes ROM more interesting/provides explanations	38.8	41.7	55.5	42.7
Better for children	11.3	-	7.4	8.4
Progressive move	8.8	12.5	-	8.4
Enlivens Museum	5.0	4.2	-	3.8
Teaches in a new way	3.8	-	3.7	3.1
Exhibits may change	1.3	-	-	0.8
No effect mentioned	35.0	50.0	37.0	36.6

[1]This question was open-ended in that respondents were allowed to give more than one answer; therefore the percentages do not total 100%.

● Almost two-thirds of the visitors indicated that the Discovery Room affected the way they felt about the Museum and they gave specific reasons.

● Generally, the responses indicated that the Room was seen as a positive new approach.

● The most frequent comment was that the Discovery Room makes the ROM more interesting for visitors by providing explanations and descriptions of relationships rather than simple identification of objects.

Table 15:   Areas of the ROM in Which Interest Was Stimulated
            by a Visit to the Discovery Room[1]

Galleries	Percentage of Visitors (n=131)
	%
None in particular	66.7
Dinosaurs	8.4
Mammalogy	6.1
Egyptian	5.3
Mineralogy	5.3
Ontario Archaeology	3.1
Planetarium	3.1
Geology	3.1
Armour Court	1.5
Other: Fish, Greek and Roman, North American Native Cultures, Birds, Insects[2]	3.8

[1] This question was open-ended in that respondents were allowed to give more than one answer; therefore the percentages do not total 100%.

[2] "Other" responses were each mentioned by one person only.

- Two-thirds of the visitors indicated that they were not stimulated to visit any gallery in particular after visiting the Discovery Room.

- The galleries that visitors indicated they were going to visit were usually the galleries that were most popular and not necessarily those for which the Discovery Room contained a related component.

The Effectiveness of Components
in the Discovery Room

Subsections A to D provide a detailed examination of each type of component as well as a discussion of specific components. For the purposes of the evaluation analysis, the components are grouped into the following four categories:

A. Boxes - twenty-one subjects

B. I.D. units - four subjects

C. Display-Oriented Components - Skeleton, Stumpers, Tree Unit, Mirrors Display, Live Exhibits, Stamp Display, Bird Displays

D. Complementary Resources - microscopes, ultraviolet light, luxo-lamps with attached magnifying glasses

The first three categories are analyzed according to:

(i)   Time Visitors Spend with Components

(ii) Involvement of Visitors with Individual Components

(iii) Suggested Improvements and Indicated Learning

In addition, these three categories are examined according to their interrelationships.

Subsection F provides a comparative examination of the components in the Room. This is based on visitors' indications of the best liked and least liked aspects of the Room.

A. Boxes

(i) Time

Table 16: Time at Boxes (by Age of Visitor)

Time Spent At Boxes	Adults (n=131)	Adolescents (n=31)	Children (n=31)	All Visitors (n=193)
	%	%	%	%
No time at Boxes	66.0	58.2	35.6	60.1
Short (1 to 5 minutes)	8.5	9.6	6.4	8.3
Medium (6 to 15 minutes)	8.6	22.6	19.4	12.4
Long (16 minutes and up)	16.9	9.6	38.6	19.2
Total	100.0	100.0	100.0	100.0

- Of all visitors, 40% became involved with at least one box. Half of these visitors spent a long period of time (15 minutes or more) with them.

- More children than adults or adolescents were attracted to the boxes.

- Children tended to involve themselves more with the boxes; 39% of the children visiting the Room spent sixteen minutes or more with the boxes, whereas only 10% of the adolescents and 17% of the adults spent this amount of time with the boxes.

(ii) Involvement of Visitors with Individual Boxes

The following table indicates the proportion of visitors who became involved with each box.

Table 17:   Percentage and Number of Visitors That Saw Boxes (by Age of Visitor)[1]

Box	Adults (n=80) %		Adolescents (n=24) %		Children (n=27) %		All Visitors (n=131) %	
Match-A-Sound[2]	18.8	(15)	25.0	(6)	37.0	(10)	23.7	(31)
Teeth	13.8	(11)	8.3	(2)	29.6	(8)	16.0	(21)
Glowing Rocks	13.8	(11)	-	-	25.9	(7)	13.7	(18)
Skin	13.8	(11)	-	-	25.9	(7)	13.7	(18)
Spice Of Life	8.8	(7)	16.7	(4)	18.5	(5)	12.2	(16)
Moon	8.9	(7)	16.7	(4)	7.4	(2)	10.0	(13)
Patterns	11.3	(9)	-	-	14.8	(4)	9.9	(13)
Tracks	7.5	(6)	8.3	(2)	11.1	(3)	8.4	(11)
Fossils	6.3	(5)	8.3	(2)	14.8	(4)	8.4	(11)
Nests	7.5	(6)	-	-	14.8	(4)	7.6	(10)
Feathers	5.0	(4)	4.2	(1)	14.8	(4)	6.9	(9)
Hidden Colours	6.3	(5)	12.5	(3)	3.7	(1)	6.9	(9)
Crystal Cave	6.3	(5)	4.2	(1)	11.1	(3)	6.9	(9)
Meteorites	7.5	(6)	4.2	(1)	7.4	(2)	6.9	(9)
Archaeology	6.3	(5)	-	-	14.8	(4)	6.9	(9)
Mineral Mystery	5.0	(4)	4.2	(1)	14.8	(4)	6.9	(9)
Micro-Marvels	7.5	(6)	-	-	3.7	(1)	5.3	(7)
Secrets in Stone	2.5	(2)	-	-	18.5	(5)	5.3	(7)
See Shells	6.3	(5)	4.2	(1)	3.7	(1)	5.3	(7)
Bean Bag	2.5	(2)	12.5	(3)	3.7	(1)	4.6	(6)
Nature's Tools	3.8	(3)	-	-	-	-	3.2	(3)

[1]Visitors could see more than one box; therefore the percentages do not total 100%.

[2]The greatest proportion of visitors in each group involved themselves with this box.

- Almost 25% of all the visitors to the Room became involved with the Match-A-Sound Box.

- The Spice of Life, Teeth, Moon, Glowing Rocks, Skin, and Patterns boxes were also popular. However, Spice of Life was the only one of these that was popular with all age groups. Teeth, Glowing Rocks, Skin, and Patterns were particularly popular with children and adults. Moon was popular with adults and adolescents.

- The boxes that incorporated the most straightforward and interesting activities were the most popular. Almost all the visitors who became involved with the Match-A-Sound and Spice of Life boxes pursued the activities. In contrast, the activity involved in the Bean Bag Box was rarely carried out and the box was not popular.

- On the whole, visitors had few criticisms of the boxes. Adolescents and children in particular reacted very positively. About 15% of the adults indicated that they disliked certain boxes.

- It is interesting to note that although Match-A-Sound and Spice of Life were considered to be too easy by some, these visitors did not dislike the boxes. Similarly, although some visitors found Tracks too difficult, they did not indicate that they disliked the box.

(iii) Suggested Improvements and Indicated Learning

Table 18 gives an indication of what visitors learned from
the boxes they used and the improvements that were suggested.
Few conclusions can be drawn, however, as these comments are
representative rather than numerical. Some comments were
made by only one or two visitors while others were repeated
many times. Nevertheless, the information can help to assess
the need for improvements to individual boxes.

Table 18:   What Visitors Learned from Individual Boxes, and
            Suggested Improvements

Unit/Component	What Visitors Learned	Suggested Improvements
Match-A-Sound Box	- aware of sound - sound relates to texture	- more examples
Teeth Box	- different kinds of teeth - microscopes revealed details	- more examples and information/better labels
Glowing Rocks Box	- what kinds of rocks glow - why detergents make clothes whiter	- explain fluorescence - need rocks that glow brighter
Skin Box	- variety of skin types - specifically about weasel and kingfisher	- more examples - skin shouldn't be detached from animal
Spice of Life Box	- smells and names of spices - raw vs. processed spices	- better bottles
Moonlight Box	- effects of moon on the earth - about moon phases and tides	- more information and labels - additional box on moon life
Patterns Box	- interesting to create patterns	- more clay

Unit/Component	What Visitors Learned	Suggested Improvements
Tracks Box	- about variety of tracks	- more examples and information
Fossils Box	- about unusual sea creatures - how fossils occur	- more specimens
Nest Box	- how nests are built - what birds build what nests	- more examples - more information
Feather Box -	- variety of feather types - microscope revealed details - feathers identify birds	- more examples - more information
Hidden Colours Box	- effects of UV light	- more variety
Crystal Cave Box	- shape of quartz crystals - kind of crystals in cave	- explain pictures - <u>too difficult</u> to understand
Meteorite Box	- how to identify different types of iron	- more examples
Archaeology Box	- what archaeology is - that archaeology is like a puzzle	- more pieces, more detail
Mineral Mystery	- effect of UV light on minerals - variety of minerals	
Micro-Marvels Box[1]	- how things look magnified - how feathers compare	- more specimens and information

[1] Micro-Marvels: December only

Unit/Component	What Visitors Learned	Suggested Improvements
Secrets in Stone Box	- about different types of rock	- more explanation
Sea Shells Box	- sounds of sea in shells	- more examples - book on shells
Bean Bag Box	- variety of names of beans	- more examples and information
Nature's Tools Box	- shell fluorescence	- more information about raw materials and tools

B. Identification (I.D.) Units

(i) Time

While some visitors use the I.D. units, they do not use
them as the designers intended. The units were developed
as reference collections in the hope that visitors would
bring in their own specimens/artifacts to identify with the
help of the I.D. units. When it was discovered that visitors were not bringing in their own specimens/artifacts, unidentified artifacts/specimens were incorporated into the
I.D. Units after the first evaluation period.

Table 19: Time at Identification Units (by Age of Visitor)

Time Spent At Identification Units	Adults (n=131)	Adolescents (n=31)	Children (n=31)	All Visitors (n=193)
	%	%	%	%
No time at I.D. Units	72.7	83.9	74.3	75.1
Short (1 to 5 minutes)	19.1	3.2	16.1	16.1
Medium (6 to 15 minutes)	6.1	9.7	6.4	6.2
Long (16 minutes and up)	2.1	3.2	3.2	2.6
Total	100.0	100.0	100.0	100.0

● No visitors during either survey period brought their own
  specimens/artifacts to the Room for identification or
  examination.

● The unidentified artifacts/specimens that were incorporated into the I.D. units before the final evaluation period were not used and therefore did not increase visitor
  involvement with the I.D. units.

● Although the I.D. units were not employed in the way they
  were intended, visitors did use them to some extent.
  Table 20 shows that 25% of the visitors used at least one
  I.D. unit and spent approximately one to fifteen minutes
  with that unit. However, most of the visitors spent less
  than 5 minutes.

● More children and adults than adolescents were attracted
  to I.D. units. However, adolescents became more involved
  than either children or adults with the units.

(ii) Involvement of Visitors with Individual Identification Units

Table 20:   Percentage and Number of Visitors That Saw
            Individual Units (by Age of Visitor)

Identification Unit	Adults (n=80)		Adolescents (n=24)		Children (n=27)		All Visitors (n=131)	
	%		%		%		%	
Insects	17.5	(14)	12.5	(3)	18.5	(5)	16.8	(22)
Butterflies	18.8	(15)	8.3	(2)	11.1	(3)	15.3	(20)
Fossils	8.8	(7)	4.2	(1)	3.7	(1)	6.9	(9)
Herbarium[1]	2.5	(2)	8.3	(2)	–	–	3.1	(4)
Ontario Archaeology	2.5	(2)	4.2	(1)	–	–	2.3	(3)

[1]Herbarium was a separate I.D. unit in August: in December, it was combined with the Tree Unit.

● Of the visitors observed, 16.8% saw the Insects I.D. Unit and 15.3% saw the Butterfly I.D. Unit.   These units therefore appear to be the most attractive.

● The alterations made to the I.D. units between survey periods had no significant impact.   The proportion of visitors who used the units was consistent with the above figures during both survey periods.

(iii) Suggested Improvements and Indicated Learning

The table below gives an indication of what visitors learned from the I.D. units they used and the improvements that were suggested. These comments are representative rather than numerical. Some comments were made by one person, some were made by several.

Table 21: What Visitors Learned from Identification Units, and Suggested Improvements

Unit/Component	What Visitors Learned	Suggested Improvements
Ontario Archaeology I.D. Unit	- about settlement and development - about Indians through the ages	
Fossils I.D. Unit	- about fossil appearance	- change drawer presentation
Butterflies I.D. Unit	- about variety and classification - about appearance under microscopes	- more participation/ too catalogued - more labels/ information
Insects I.D. Unit	- about variety of insects - about appearance under microscope	- more participation too catalogued - improve labels and organization

● The suggested improvements indicate that visitors did not understand the reference function of these units.

C. Display-Oriented Components

(i) Time

Table 22:   Time at Skeleton (by Age of Visitor)

Time Spent At Skeleton	Adults (n=131)	Adolescents (n=31)	Children (n=31)	All Visitors (n=193)
	%	%	%	%
No time at Skeleton	51.8	38.7	35.5	47.2
Short (1 to 5 minutes)	42.0	61.3	58.1	47.6
Medium (6 to 15 minutes)	6.2	–	6.4	5.2
Long (16 minutes and up)	–	–	–	–
Total	100.0	100.0	100.0	100.0

● Of all the visitors, 52.8% spent time looking at the Skeleton. Most of these visitors spent between one and five minutes.

Table 23:   Time at Stumpers (by Age of Visitor)

Time Spent At Stumpers	Adults (n=131)	Adolescents (n=31)	Children (n=31)	All Visitors (n=193)
	%	%	%	%
No time at Stumpers	64.0	61.3	64.5	63.7
Short (1 to 5 minutes)	34.4	38.7	32.3	34.7
Medium (6 to 15 minutes)	1.6	-	3.2	1.6
Long (16 minutes and up)	-	-	-	-
Total	100.0	100.0	100.0	100.0

- Of all the visitors, 36.3% spent time looking at the Stumpers. Almost all of these visitors spent between one and five minutes.

- It was observed that few visitors picked up or handled the Stumpers. Visitors seemed to view them more as traditional "Don't Touch" displays.

- Specific Stumpers did not, as intended, stimulate visitor interest to investigate other related components in the Room.

Table 24:   Time at Tree Unit (by Age of Visitor)

Time Spent At Tree Unit	Adults (n=131)	Adolescents (n=31)	Children (n=31)	All Visitors (n=193)
	%	%	%	%
No Time At Trees	64.8	58.1	71.0	64.8
Short (1 to 5 minutes)	31.3	41.9	29.0	32.6
Medium (6 to 15 minutes)	3.9	-	-	2.6
Long (16 minutes and up)	-	-	-	-
Total	100.0	100.0	100.0	100.0

- Of all the visitors, 35.2% spent time at the Tree Unit. Most of these visitors were interested in the tree cross-section which is only one part of the unit. Almost all spent less than five minutes.

- This unit was more attractive to adults and adolescents than to children.

- Changes to the Tree Unit, made between the two surveys, had no significant impact. The proportion of visitors who spent time at the Tree Unit was consistent with the above figures during both survey periods.

Table 25: Time at Stamp Display (by Age of Visitor)

Time Spent At Stamp Display	Adults (n=131)	Adolescents (n=31)	Children (n=31)	All Visitors (n=193)
	%	%	%	%
No time at Stamps	72.4	71.0	54.8	69.4
Short (1 to 5 minutes)	26.8	29.0	45.2	30.1
Medium (6 to 15 minutes)	0.8	-	-	0.5
Long (16 minutes and up)	-	-	-	-
Total	100.0	100.0	100.0	100.0

- Of all the visitors, 30.6% spent time at the Stamp Display. Almost all of these spent less than five minutes.

- Proportionately more children were attracted to this display than to other exhibits. However, it was observed that the magnifying glasses, which were intended for use by children, were the elements that drew their attention.

Table 26:   Time at Mirror Display (by Age of Visitor)

Time Spent At Mirror Display	Adults (n=131)	Adolescents (n=31)	Children (n=31)	All Visitors (n=193)
	%	%	%	%
No time with Mirrors	82.4	80.7	93.6	83.9
Short (1 to 5 minutes)	16.8	16.1	6.4	15.1
Medium (6 to 15 minutes)	0.8	3.2	-	1.0
Long (16 minutes and up)	-	-	-	-

- Only 16.1% of all visitors spent time with the Mirror Display. Almost all of these spent less than five minutes.

- The Mirror Display was more attractive to adults and adolescents than to children.

- The alterations to the Mirror Display made between the two survey periods had no significant impact. The proportion of visitors who used the Mirrors was consistent with the above figures during both survey periods.

Table 27:   Time at Live Exhibit[1] (by Age of Visitor)

Time Spent At Live Exhibit	Adults (n=131)	Adolescents (n=31)	Children (n=31)	All Visitors (n=193)
	%	%	%	%
No time at live exhibit	81.6	83.9	87.1	82.9
Short (1 to 5 minutes)	18.4	16.1	12.9	17.1
Medium (6 to 15 minutes)	-	-	-	-
Long (16 minutes and up)	-	-	-	-
Total	100.0	100.0	100.0	100.0

[1] August: Tortoise Unit and Cactus Unit;   December: Cactus Unit only.

• Only 17% of all visitors spent time with the Live Exhibit and all spent less than five minutes.

• The changes to the Live Exhibit, made between the two surveys, did not affect its popularity. The proportion of visitors who spent time with this exhibit was consistent with the above figures during both survey periods.

Bird Displays: Visitors' involvement with the Bird Displays is difficult to measure since almost all of the mounts can only be viewed.* Only the standing owl receives attention, primarily from children, because it is the only mount in the Room which is both within a child's vision and reach.

• It appeared that many visitors did not see the mounts nor did the mounts appear to stimulate an interest in those who observed them.

*Because of the nature of this component, more precise data could not be collected.

(ii) Involvement of Visitors with Individual Display-Oriented Components

While all of the display-oriented components are highly visible, some are more attractive and appealing than others. Tables 28 to 30 present a summary comparison of the display-oriented components.

The Skeleton attracts the most attention and is the most popular. Tables 28 and 29 indicate the proportions of visitors who saw each component and their critical comments.

Table 28:   Percentage and Number of Visitors That Saw Each of the Display-Oriented Components (by Age of Visitor)[1]

Component	Adults (n=131)	Adolescents (n=31)	Children (n=31)	All Visitors (n=193)
	%	%	%	%
Skeleton	48.1 (63)	61.3 (19)	64.5 (20)	52.8 (20)
Stumpers	35.9 (47)	38.7 (12)	35.5 (11)	36.3 (70)
Tree Unit	35.1 (46)	41.9 (13)	29.0 (9)	35.2 (68)
Stamp Display	27.5 (36)	29.0 (9)	45.2 (14)	30.6 (59)
Live Exhibit	18.3 (24)	16.1 (5)	12.9 (4)	17.7 (33)
Mirror Display	17.6 (23)	19.4 (6)	6.5 (2)	16.1 (31)

[1]Visitors could see more than one component; therefore the percentages do not total 100%.

- Over half of all the visitors reacted in some way to the Skeleton. Children and adolescents in particular were attracted to this component.

- The Tree Unit, Stumpers and, to a lesser degree, the Stamp Display, also attracted attention. Of these, the Stumpers were liked the best, followed by the Tree Unit, which appealed more to adults and adolescents, followed by the Stamp Display, which children found more attractive.

Table 29:   Percentage of Visitors That Saw Each of the Display-
             Oriented Components and Visitors' Critical Comments [1]

Component Name:	Visitors Who Saw Each Component (n=131)	Those Visitors' Reactions To Components: Dislike	
	%	%	
Skeleton	52.8	2.3	(1)
Stumpers	36.3	4.0	(1)
Tree Unit	35.2	5.2	(3)
Stamp Display	30.6	8.3	(4)
Live Exhibit	17.1	11.5	(3)
Mirror Display	16.1	9.1	(2)

[1] Visitors could see more than one component; therefore the percentages do not total 100%.

- The Mirror Display and Live Exhibit and to some extent, the Stamp Display were the least attractive and received some criticism.

(iii) Suggested Improvements and Indicated Learning

The suggested improvements in Table 30 are representative rather than numerical. Some were made by one person, some were made by several.

Table 30:   What Visitors Learned from Display-Oriented Components, and Suggested Improvements

Unit/Component	What Visitors Learned	Suggested Improvements
Skeleton	- could relate it to how bones fit together - difference in male and female skeletons - about x-rays and broken bones	- more information - before and after picture - let visitor assemble bones - stool for children to stand on
Stumpers	- facts and details about items not normally encountered	- more information on labels - more stumpers - lower shelves
Tree Unit	- about age, structure, and variety of trees - about uses of wood - how minerals affect trees	- more examples and information - better labels
Herbarium[1]	- about flora in Queen's Park - about variety of tree species	- more information about leaves changing colour and seeds
Stamp Display	- variety of stamps - about design by using magnifying glass	- more variety - more old stamps
Live Exhibit[2]	- about turtles - about photosynthesis - about cacti	- more information
Mirrors	- how mirrors are made - about distortion of mirrors	- display them lower - Buddha hard to find

[1] Herbarium was a separate I.D. unit in August: in December, it was combined with the Tree Unit.

[2] August: Tortoise Unit and Cactus Unit; December: Cactus Unit only.

D. Complementary Resources

The complementary resources, which include the microscopes, the luxo-lamps, the ultra-violet lamp, and the library, are intended to be used both independently and in conjunction with other components. As both the objectives and the use of these facilities are linked closely with the other components, an individual evaluation was not undertaken. However, some general observations were made.

- While the complementary resources were used frequently in conjunction with other components, particularly the boxes, they were not used independently.

- The library was not used by any of the visitors.

E. Connections Between Components in the Room

It does not appear that visitors make connections between components in the Room. A number of individual components were developed to complement each other. For instance, one of the functions of the Stumpers was to encourage an interest in topics that could be investigated further in the Room, (e.g., the seed was intended to stimulate curiosity about the Seed Box). However, this plan was not successful.

- It was observed that the Moon Map was not frequently used in conjunction with the Moon Box. Similarly, visitors who saw the Feathers Box or the Nests Box rarely explored the Room to see the mounted Bird Displays and those who examined the Ontario Archaeology I.D. Unit rarely investigated the Archaeology Box.

F. Overall Analysis of Individual Components

(i) Best Liked Aspects of the Discovery Room

Boxes are the most popular component in the Discovery Room followed by the Skeleton. Aspects of the Room which are "best liked" tend to vary with the age of the visitor. Tables 31 and 32 indicate what visitors liked best in the Room.

Table 31:   Percentage of Best Liked Discovery Room Aspects
            (by Age of Visitor)

What Was Liked Best	Adults (n=80)	Adolescents (n=24)	Children[1] (n=27)	All visitors (n=131)
	%	%	%	%
Boxes	18.6	12.4	25.9	19.0
Micro-Marvels Box[2]	3.8	4.2	14.8	6.1
Archaeology Box	-	-	7.4	1.5
Spice of Life Box	1.3	-	3.7	1.5
Mineral Mystery Box	-	-	3.7	0.8
Skin Box	-	4.2	-	0.8
Match-A-Sound Box	-	-	3.7	0.8
Teeth Box	-	4.2	-	0.8
Skeleton	15.0	20.8	11.2	15.2
Tree Unit	10.0	16.6	3.7	9.9
Stumpers	5.0	8.2	3.7	5.3
Stamp Display	-	-	7.4	1.5
Fossils I.D. Unit	2.5	4.2	-	2.3
Butterflies I.D. Unit	2.5	4.2	-	2.3
UV Light	1.3	4.2	3.7	2.3
Live Butterfly[3]	2.5	4.2	-	2.3
Puzzle[4]	1.3	4.2	-	1.5
Touch Wall	1.3	-	-	0.8
Stuffed Animals	-	-	3.7	0.8
Live Exhibit[5]	1.3	-	-	0.8
Concept	12.4	-	3.7	8.4
Children's Room	2.5	-	-	1.5
Organization of Room	-	4.2	-	0.8
Docent	1.3	-	-	0.8
Everything	8.7	-	3.7	6.1
Nothing in Particular	8.7	4.2	-	6.1
Total	100.0	100.0	100.0	100.0

[1] This question was asked of children between the ages of nine and twelve. See Table 32 for children between six and nine years.

[2] Micro-Marvels Box: December only.

[3] Live Butterfly: August only.

[4] Puzzle: August only.

[5] August: Tortoise Unit and Cactus Unit; December: Cactus Unit only.

Table 32: Aspects of the Discovery Room Best Liked by Children Between the Ages of Six and Nine Years[1]

What Was Liked Best	Percentage Of Visitors (n=39)
	%
Microscopes	23.0
Skeleton	15.3
Boxes	5.1
Patterns Box	7.6
Spice of Life Box	5.1
Mineral Mystery Box	2.6
Crystal Cave Box	2.6
Skin Box	2.6
Nests Box	2.6
Bean Bag Box	2.6
Micro-Marvels Box[2]	2.6
Live Exhibit[3]	5.1
Tree Unit	2.6
Stumpers	2.6
Butterflies I.D. Unit	2.6
Insects I.D. Unit	2.6
Concept of Room	2.6
Everything	5.1
Nothing	5.1
Total	100.0

[1] This question was asked only of the adults who visited with children between the ages of six and nine years (n = total number of visitors who were asked this question).

[2] Micro-Marvels Box: December only.

[3] August: Tortoise Unit and Cactus Unit; December: Cactus Unit only.

- One-third of the visitors favoured boxes, either as a general category or individually. This finding was particularly evident among children (60% liked the boxes while only about 25% of the adults and adolescents favoured the boxes).

- Micro-Marvels was the most popular box with all age groups. The proportions in Table 31 are particularly significant, for this box was available only during the second survey period. (It should be noted that the box required the use of microscopes.)

- The second most popular component was the Skeleton (15%). Adolescents liked this component more than adults or children.

- Twenty-three per cent of the adults who responded for children between the ages of six and nine (Table 32) mentioned microscopes as the most popular component. General observation indicated that the microscopes were used extensively, particularly in conjunction with boxes. It is probable that most visitors did not mention microscopes as their favourite component because they did not consider them as an independent component.

- Both the Tree Unit and Stumpers were popular. Both were liked best by adolescents.

- Although the Archaeology Box and the Stamp Display are popular among children, they were not mentioned either by adults or adolescents.

- It is interesting to note that adults and, to some extent, children mentioned that they particularly liked the concept of the Room; i.e., they enjoyed the discovery approach and the opportunity to touch. Adolescents favoured the organization of the Room, and the freedom to explore on their own.

Table 33:   Visitors' Reasons for Choosing Best Liked Aspect of the Discovery Room (by Age of Visitor)[1]

Reason	Adults (n=80)	Adolescents (n=24)	Children (n=27)	All Visitors (n=131)
	%	%	%	%
No reason mentioned	46.3	29.2	33.3	38.2
Discovery Approach	25.0	41.7	33.3	29.8
Informative/Clear Explanations	8.8	12.5	18.5	11.5
Subject Matter	5.0	8.3	3.7	5.3
Interesting	3.8	4.2	7.4	4.6
Historical (Tree Cross-Section)	5.0	4.2	-	3.8
Use of microscopes to examine things	1.3	-	11.1	3.1
Compare Skeleton with self	3.8	4.2	-	3.1
Other[2]	3.8	4.2	7.4	4.6

[1] This question was open-ended in that respondents were allowed to give more than one answer; therefore the percentages do not total 100%.

[2] "Other" responses were mentioned by two persons or less and include: the room feels alive; something was difficult; the visitor was a collector.

- About half the visitors gave very general reasons for their preferences. These reasons reflected their general enthusiasm for the Room rather than for an individual component. For example, 30% of all responses related to the appeal of the discovery approach.

- The only specific comments concerned the tree cross-section, the Skeleton, and the microscopes. Adults and adolescents enjoyed the historical aspect of the tree cross-section; they also liked the opportunity to compare the Skeleton with themselves. Children enjoyed using the microscopes.

(ii) Least Liked Aspects of the Discovery Room

Less than one-third of the visitors mentioned an aspect of
the Discovery Room which they liked least. It was observed
that visitors were reluctant to criticize because of their
general enthusiasm for the Room.

Table 34:   Least Liked Aspects of Discovery Room
             (by Age of Visitor)

What Was Least Liked	Adults (n=80)	Adolescents (n=24)	Children[1] (n=27)	All Visitors (n=131)
	%	%	%	%
Nothing	64.3	70.7	63.0	65.8
Tree Unit	3.8	12.5	11.1	6.9
Boxes	-	4.2	-	0.8
Glowing Rocks Box	2.5	-	-	1.5
Skin Box	2.5	-	-	1.5
Mineral Mystery Box	-	-	3.7	0.8
Crystal Cave Box	-	4.2	-	0.8
Nests Box	-	-	3.7	0.8
Fossils Box	1.3	-	-	0.8
Patterns Box	-	-	3.7	0.8
Fossils I.D. Unit	1.3	-	-	0.8
Butterflies I.D. Unit	-	4.2	-	0.8
Insects I.D. Unit	1.3	-	-	0.8
Live Exhibit[2]	2.5	-	-	1.5
Stumpers	2.5	-	-	1.5
Mirrors	1.3	-	-	0.8
Stamps	1.3	-	-	0.8
Skeleton	1.3	-	-	0.8
Stuffed Birds and Animals	-	-	7.4	1.5
Microscopes/UV Light	1.3	-	3.7	0.8
Physical Features (shape of room, temperature, rug, space)	5.2	4.2	-	4.0
Organization/Lack of guidance	3.8	-	3.7	3.1
Rule about Children under 6 years old	2.5	-	-	1.5
Total	100.0	100.0	100.0	100.0

[1]This question was asked of children between the ages of nine and twelve.
See following table for children between six and nine.

[2]August: Tortoise Unit and Cactus Unit;   December: Cactus Unit only.

Table 35: Aspects of the Discovery Room Least Liked by
Children Between the Ages of Six and Nine[1]

What Was Least Liked	Percentage Of Visitors (n=39)
	%
Nothing	40.8
Tree Unit	15.4
Stamp Display	7.7
Boxes	2.6
Skin Box	5.1
Moon Box	2.6
Spice of Life Box	2.6
Teeth Box	2.6
Archaeology Box	2.6
Live Exhibit	5.1
Stumpers	5.1
Skeleton	2.6
Fossils I.D. Unit	2.6
Organization	2.6
Total	100.0

[1]This question was asked only of the adults who were visiting with
children between the ages of six and nine.

• The Tree Unit was the only component that received any
  significant degree of criticism, although the historical cross-section portion seemed popular. The groups
  who criticized the Tree Unit were children, adolescents,
  and parents answering for younger children.

• The only other criticism which was mentioned by more than
  two people, concerned a physical feature of the Room (size,
  temperature, organization). These concerns were expressed
  only by adults and adolescents.

- Less than 15% of all visitors gave reasons for their dislikes. A number of specific reasons were mentioned, but no pattern was evident.

Tracking Form and Questionnaire

ROM...DISCOVERY ROOM EVALUATION

OBSERVATION

CASE I.D. [1][ ][ ]

INTERVIEWER₅ [ ][ ]   DATE [ ] [ ][ ] [ ][ ]   ENTRY TIME [ ][ ]

TIME IN ROOM [ ][ ]

1. Is the person visiting with anyone? (circle I.D. of trackee,
   and enter number of persons in group in appropriate categories
   below)

   Yes/Who   No   [ ]
                                                          [ ]
   1. Female adult_____2. Male adult_____3. Female Senior_____   [ ]
   4. Male senior_____5. Infant_____6. Child_____   [ ]₁₈
   7. Female adolescent_____8. Male adolescent_____

COMMENTS:

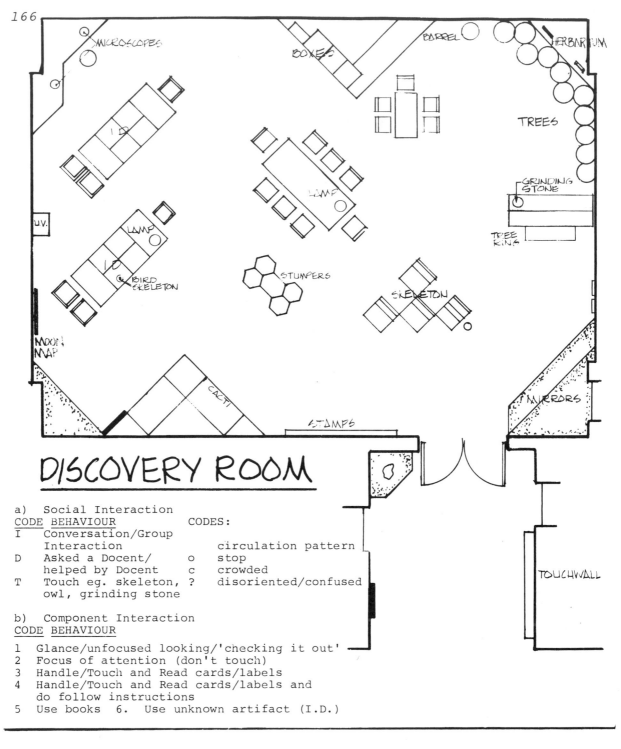

DISCOVERY ROOM

a) Social Interaction

CODE	BEHAVIOUR		CODES:
I	Conversation/Group Interaction		circulation pattern
D	Asked a Docent/ helped by Docent	o c	stop crowded
T	Touch eg. skeleton, owl, grinding stone	?	disoriented/confused

b) Component Interaction

CODE BEHAVIOUR

1 Glance/unfocused looking/'checking it out'
2 Focus of attention (don't touch)
3 Handle/Touch and Read cards/labels
4 Handle/Touch and Read cards/labels and
do follow instructions
5 Use books 6. Use unknown artifact (I.D.)

TRACKING DATA:

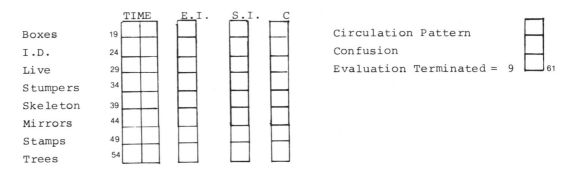

	TIME	E.I.	S.I.	C	
Boxes	19				Circulation Pattern
I.D.	24				Confusion
Live	29				Evaluation Terminated = 9
Stumpers	34				61
Skeleton	39				
Mirrors	44				
Stamps	49				
Trees	54				

ROM...Discovery Room Evaluation
Questionnaire

Since this is an experimental room the Royal Ontario Museum is especially interested in finding out your reaction to it. We would appreciate a few minutes of your time to ask you some questions about how you feel about the Discovery Room.

1. Is this your first visit to the Discovery Room?
   1. Yes   2. No   62 ☐

2. How did you hear about the Discovery Room?
   1. poster 2. radio/T.V. 3. "Previews" 4. pamphlet
   5. ROM staff 6. newspaper/magazine 7. another person
   8. didn't hear 9. other _____   ☐☐

3. Did you come to the museum today specifically because you wanted to see the Discovery Room?
            1. Yes   2. Partially   3. No   ☐

4. Generally, do you feel the Discovery Room is-

   exciting   1—2—3—4—5 boring
   unpleasant   1—2—3—4—5 enjoyable
   inviting   1—2—3—4—5 unattractive
   ordinary   1—2—3—4—5 unique
   informative   1—2—3—4—5 unenlightening
   cramped   1—2—3—4—5 spacious
   orderly   1—2—3—4—5 cluttered
   confusing   1—2—3—4—5 organized

5. Thinking about your comfort do you find this room to be-

   too bright   1—2—3—4—5 too dim
   too cold   1—2—3—4—5 too hot

6. What do you feel the purpose of the Discovery Room is?

   _____
   _____

7. Is there anything in particular that you found out by visiting the Discovery Room?

   _____ _____
   _____

8. Has your visit to the Discovery Room affected the way you feel about this museum?
            1. Yes/How   2. No

   _____
   _____

9. What did you like best? Why?

   _____
   _____

10. What did you like least? Why?

   _____

11. Do you feel that this room is for-
            1. children only   2. adults only   3. everybody

12. Now I would like to ask you a couple of questions about each of the things in the Discovery Room which you saw. I noticed that you saw the _____

   REPEAT FOR EACH COMPONENT WITH WHICH THE VISITOR INTERACTED.

Component BOXES:	Saw 1. Yes 2. No	Did you like it? 1. Yes 2. Somewhat 3. No	What did you find out from it?	Did you find it? 1. too easy 2. OK 3. too difficult	Are there any improvements you would suggest to make it better? 1. Yes/What? 2. No
Archaeology 01	33				
Mineral Mystery 02	41				
Crystal Cave 03	49				
Glowing Rocks 04	57				
Meteorites 05	65				
Moon Light 06	73				
Skin 07	1 2 / 3 4 5				
Feathers 08	13				
Match a Sound 09	21				
Nests 10	29				
See Shells 11	37				
Spice of Life 12	45				
Nature's Tools 13	53				
Teeth 14	61				
Hidden Colour 15	69				
Secrets in Stone 16	77			5	
Bean Bag 17	9				
Fossils 18	17				
Micro Marvels 19	25				
Tracks 20	33				
Patterns 21	41				

Component	Saw 1. Yes 2. No	Did you like it? 1. Yes 2. Somewhat 3. No	What did you find out from it?	Are there any improvements you would suggest to make it better? 1. Yes/What 2. No
I.D. UNITS:				
Cdn.Archaeology 30	☐ 49	☐		☐ ☐
31	☐ 56	☐		☐ ☐
Fossils 32	☐ 63	☐		☐
Butterflies 33	☐ 70	☐		☐
Bugs 34	☐ 77	☐		☐ 1 ☐ 2 ☐ 3 ☐ 4
OTHER:				
Skeleton Unit 40	☐ 8	☐		☐
Tree Unit 41	☐ 15	☐		☐
Mirrors 42	☐ 22	☐		☐
Live Exhibit 43	☐ 29	☐		☐
Stamp Exhibit 44	☐ 36	☐		☐
45	☐ 43	☐		☐
Stumpers 46	☐ 50	☐		☐

56

12. Is there anything which you would like to see in this room
    to make it better?
                    1. Yes/What?   2. No

    _____

    _____

13. Having visited the Discovery Room is there any area in the
    museum which you want to visit?
                    1. Yes/Which?   2. No

    _____

    _____

    IF TRACKEE IS ADULT WITH CHILD/CHILDREN UNDER 9 YEARS OLD.

14. What do you think your child liked the best? Why?

    _____

    _____

15. What do you think your child liked the least? Why?

    _____

    _____

16. Is there any way you would improve the Discovery Room to
    make it better for children like yours?
    1. Yes/What?   2. No

    _____

    _____

17. Do you live in Metropolitan Toronto?

    Yes - The City of which Borough?   No - Where do you live?
    _____

    01. York   04. Etobicoke   08. Western Ontario   11. Other Prov.
    02. East York   05. Scarborough 09. Eastern Ontario   12. U.S.A.
    03. North York   06. Toronto   10. N. Ontario   13. Other
            07. Central Ontario

18. Would you like to come back
    to the Discovery Room soon?

    1. Yes   2. No   3. DK